Spirituality and Psychiatry

Second Edition

Spirituality and Psychiatry

Second Edition

Edited by
Christopher C. H. Cook

Andrew Powell

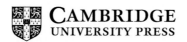

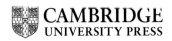

Shaftesbury Road, Cambridge CB2 8EA, United Kingdom

One Liberty Plaza, 20th Floor, New York, NY 10006, USA

477 Williamstown Road, Port Melbourne, VIC 3207, Australia

314–321, 3rd Floor, Plot 3, Splendor Forum, Jasola District Centre, New Delhi – 110025, India

103 Penang Road, #05–06/07, Visioncrest Commercial, Singapore 238467

Cambridge University Press is part of Cambridge University Press & Assessment, a department of the University of Cambridge.

We share the University's mission to contribute to society through the pursuit of education, learning and research at the highest international levels of excellence.

www.cambridge.org
Information on this title: www.cambridge.org/9781911623304

DOI: 10.1017/9781911623311

© Royal College of Psychiatrists 2022

This publication is in copyright. Subject to statutory exception and to the provisions of relevant collective licensing agreements, no reproduction of any part may take place without the written permission of Cambridge University Press & Assessment.

First edition published 2009
Second edition published 2022

A catalogue record for this publication is available from the British Library

Library of Congress Cataloging-in-Publication data
Names: Cook, Chris (Christopher C. H.), editor. | Powell, Andrew (Andrew S.), editor.
Title: Spirituality and psychiatry / [edited by] Christopher C. H. Cook, Andrew Powell.
Description: Second edition. | New York : Cambridge University Press, 2022. | Includes bibliographical references and index.
Identifiers: LCCN 2022007454 (print) | LCCN 2022007455 (ebook) | ISBN 9781911623304 (paperback) | ISBN 9781911623311 (epub)
Subjects: LCSH: Psychiatry–Religious aspects. | Spirituality. | BISAC: MEDICAL / Mental Health
Classification: LCC RC455.4.R4 S67 2022 (print) | LCC RC455.4.R4 (ebook) | DDC 616.89–dc23/eng/20220601
LC record available at https://lccn.loc.gov/2022007454
LC ebook record available at https://lccn.loc.gov/2022007455

ISBN   978-1-911-62330-4   Paperback

Cambridge University Press & Assessment has no responsibility for the persistence or accuracy of URLs for external or third-party internet websites referred to in this publication and does not guarantee that any content on such websites is, or will remain, accurate or appropriate.

....

Every effort has been made in preparing this book to provide accurate and up-to-date information which is in accord with accepted standards and practice at the time of publication. Although case histories are drawn from actual cases, every effort has been made to disguise the identities of the individuals involved. Nevertheless, the authors, editors and publishers can make no warranties that the information contained herein is totally free from error, not least because clinical standards are constantly changing through research and regulation. The authors, editors and publishers therefore disclaim all liability for direct or consequential damages resulting from the use of material contained in this book. Readers are strongly advised to pay careful attention to information provided by the manufacturer of any drugs or equipment that they plan to use.

Contents

The colour plate section can be found between page 90 and page 91

Figures

Tables

Boxes

Contributors

Gwen Adshead
Consultant Forensic Psychotherapist, Broadmoor Hospital, West London NHS Trust, UK

Joanna Barber
Honorary Researcher, Birmingham and Solihull Mental Health NHS Foundation Trust, Birmingham, UK

Cherrie Coghlan
Former Consultant in General Adult Psychiatry, Central and North West London NHS Foundation Trust; medical member of the Mental Health Tribunal, UK

Christopher C. H. Cook
Professor Emeritus, Institute for Medical Humanities, Durham University; Chair, Spirituality and Psychiatry Special Interest Group, Royal College of Psychiatrists, UK

Nicola Crowley
Retired consultant psychiatrist, UK

Rachel J. Cullinan
Specialist Trainee in Old Age Psychiatry, Gateshead Health NHS Trust, Cumbria, Northumberland, Tyne & Wear NHS Trust, and Newcastle University, UK

Simon Dein
Honorary Professor, Centre for Psychiatry, Queen Mary University of London, UK

Mary Lynn Dell
Adjunct Professor of Psychiatry and Behavioral Sciences, and Adjunct Instructor of Pediatrics, Tulane University, New Orleans, LA, USA

Glòria Durà-Vilà
Honorary Lecturer, Department of Mental Health Sciences, University College London; Consultant Child and Adolescent Psychiatrist and Medical Lead for Autism Spectrum Disorder in Surrey and Borders NHS Foundation Trust, UK

Sarah Eagger
Retired consultant psychiatrist and honorary senior clinical lecturer, previously at Imperial College, London; Executive Committee Member, Spirituality and Psychiatry Special Interest Group, Royal College of Psychiatrists and Section on Religion, Spirituality and Psychiatry, World Psychiatric Association; Chair of the Janki Foundation, UK

Robert D. Enright
Aristotelian Professor in Forgiveness Science, Department of Educational Psychology, University of Wisconsin-Madison; Founding Board Member of the International Forgiveness Institute, Madison, WI, USA

Peter Fenwick
Emeritus Consultant Neuropsychiatrist, Maudsley Hospital Epilepsy Unit, and Emeritus Senior Lecturer, Institute of Psychiatry.

Cristina Gangemi
Director, The Kairos Forum; DTh student, University of Roehampton; Disability Adviser to the Roman Catholic Bishops of England and Wales, UK

Paul Gilbert
Professor of Clinical Psychology,
University of Derby, UK; Visiting
Professor, University of Queensland,
Australia

Lucy Grimwade
Consultant Child and Adolescent
Psychiatrist, Tees Esk and Wear Valleys
NHS Foundation Trust; Executive
Committee Member, Spirituality and
Psychiatry Special Interest Group, Royal
College of Psychiatrists, UK

Paramabandhu Groves
Retired consultant psychiatrist in
addictions, Camden and Islington NHS
Foundation Trust; Founding Director of
Breathing Space, London Buddhist
Centre, UK

Julia H. Head
Therapist in private practice; Former
Specialist Chaplain and Bishop John
Robinson Fellow in Pastoral Theology and
Mental Health, South London and
Maudsley NHS Trust, UK

Gillie Jenkinson
Director, Hope Valley Counselling, UK;
UKCP accredited psychotherapist

John F. Kelly
Elizabeth R. Spallin Professor of Psychiatry
in the Field of Addiction Medicine,
Harvard Medical School; Director,
Recovery Research Institute, Massachusetts
General Hospital, Department of
Psychiatry, Boston, MA, USA

Robert M. Lawrence
Consultant and Honorary Senior Lecturer,
Psychiatry of Old Age and Neuropsychiatry
(Richmond); Associate Medical Director/
Research & Development, South West
London & St George's Mental Health Trust,
London, UK

Francis G. Lu
Luke and Grace Kim Endowed Professor in
Cultural Psychiatry, Director of Cultural
Psychiatry, and Associate Chair for Medical
Student Education at the UC Davis Health
System, Davis, CA, USA

Susan Mitchell
Former consultant psychiatrist in
rehabilitation, and Medical Director, The
Retreat, York. UK

Sarah Mullally
The Bishop of London; Formerly Chief
Nursing Officer and Director of
Patient Experience for England,
1999–2004, UK

Andrew Newberg
Professor, Department of Integrative
Medicine and Nutritional Sciences,
Professor, Department of
Radiology, and Research Director,
Marcus Institute of Integrative Health,
Thomas Jefferson University, Philadelphia,
PA, USA

Michelle Pearce
Professor, Graduate School, University of
Maryland, Baltimore, MD, USA

John R. Peteet
Associate Professor of Psychiatry,
Harvard Medical School, Boston,
MA, USA

Andrew Powell
Founding Chair, Spirituality and
Psychiatry Special Interest Group, Royal
College of Psychiatrists; formerly
Consultant Psychotherapist and Senior
Lecturer in Psychiatry, St George's
Hospital and University of London,
and Consultant Psychotherapist
and Honorary Senior Lecturer, the
Warneford Hospital and University of
Oxford, UK

Oyepeju Raji
Consultant Psychiatrist in Learning
Disabilities and Associate Clinical Director,
Neurodevelopmental Disorders Service,
South West London and St George's
Mental Health Trust, London, UK

Jason Roach
Bishop of London's Researcher and Adviser
on Policy and Strategy; formerly Clinical
Editor, *BMJ Clinical Evidence*, and Hospital
Doctor at King's College Hospital,
London, UK

Glenn Roberts
Former consultant psychiatrist in
rehabilitation, Devon Partnership NHS
Trust; Lead on Recovery for the Royal
College of Psychiatrists (2006–2011);
Academic Secretary to the Faculty of Social

and Rehabilitation Psychiatry, Royal
College of Psychiatrists; Co-Founder,
Recovery Devon, UK

Linda Ross
Professor of Nursing (Spirituality), School
of Care Sciences, Faculty of Life Sciences
and Education, University of South
Wales, UK

Jacqueline Y. Song
Program Director, International
Forgiveness Institute, Madison, WI, USA

John Swinton
Professor in Practical Theology and
Pastoral Care, School of Divinity, History
and Philosophy, King's College, University
of Aberdeen, UK

Foreword to the Second Edition

Psychiatry stands out among its medical counterparts in that to do the job well, you need to be able to go beyond the clinical aspects by being able to appreciate and understand the spiritual side in everyone. Being able to handle this sensitively and empathetically has a significant potential impact upon the relationship between psychiatrist and patient, and therefore on the eventual treatment outcome.

This second edition comes at a time when the world is emerging from a truly unprecedented period. The COVID-19 pandemic has presented all of us with a period of uncertainty and unpredictability. It has also given us opportunities to reflect on our own lives and what we value both as individuals and within our communities. We have all questioned our mortality and have been gifted time in which to think and to contemplate issues far bigger than we would have previously imagined.

As this book lays out, although spirituality is difficult to define, it is ultimately about the core beliefs, values and experiences of human beings. It is what has helped many survive the past two turbulent years. The COVID-19 pandemic has created and is leaving a legacy of economic, health and social uncertainty and insecurity. The Centre for Mental Health predicted in October 2020 that, in England, up to 10 million people (almost 20% of the population) will need either new or additional mental health support as a direct consequence of the crisis (O'Shea, 2020). With more than half of service users holding spiritual or religious beliefs that they see as important in helping them to cope with mental illness (Royal College of Psychiatrists, 2016), it continues to be an important consideration in the relationships we have with our patients.

The book provides a rich understanding of how psychiatrists are well placed to consider the spirituality of those we care for, as well as highlighting what more we could do in this area. It tackles difficult issues such as the impact of spirituality and religion on our prevailing cultural views about suicide, as well as how spirituality and religious beliefs can be handled appropriately within the lives of children and adolescents.

As President of the Royal College of Psychiatrists, I have made championing equality, diversity and inclusion one of my priorities for my three-year term. I am proud that the College has been putting in place measures to keep this issue centre stage via its Equality Action Plan (Royal College of Psychiatrists, 2021).

All people, psychiatrists and patients alike, should be treated fairly, regardless of gender, race, disability, sexual orientation, gender re-assignment, marriage and civil partnership, pregnancy and maternity, religion and belief, or age. This book is a great contribution to helping us further our understanding of each other's experience, and the inclusive nature of spirituality is entirely aligned with that non-discriminatory ambition.

I am delighted that the College remains supportive of and engaged with the Spirituality and Psychiatry Special Interest Group (SPSIG), currently expertly chaired by the lead editor of this book, Professor Chris Cook.

Adrian James

References

O'Shea, N. (2020) *COVID-19 and the Nation's Mental Health: Forcasting Needs and Risks in the UK: October 2020*. London: Centre for Mental Health; www .centreformentalhealth.org.uk/sites/default/ files/publication/download/ CentreforMentalHealth_COVID_MH_ Forecasting3_Oct20_0.pdf

Royal College of Psychiatrists (2016) *Spirituality (SPSIG)*. London: Royal College of Psychiatrists; www.rcpsych.ac.uk/members/ special-interest-groups/spirituality

Royal College of Psychiatrists (2021) *Equality Action Plan*. London: Royal College of Psychiatrists; www.rcpsych.ac.uk/about-us/ equality-diversity-and-inclusion/equality- action-plan

Foreword to the First Edition

During my presidency I became more and more convinced of the importance of promoting mental health and well-being, alongside the treatment of mental illness. But I see mental health as the responsibility of everyone, not just health and mental health professionals. The social care, criminal justice and education sectors and faith-based organisations should all be involved in asserting the centrality of mental health in society, in contributing to the prevention of mental illness and in supporting individuals with mental disorders.

The World Health Organization in 2004 estimated that 40–50% of mental illness could be prevented through primary intervention. Meanwhile, the World Bank has recognised the contribution of social capital (the extent to which people help each other) to the wealth and well-being of a country (Dasgupta and Serageldin, 2005). The contribution of mutual trust, wilful reciprocity of help and participation in civic society are described as three particular markers of social capital. When social capital is high, individual coping capacity increases, but when social capital is low, crime rates, divorce and family violence all increase.

As psychiatrists we work with people with serious mental disorders, many of whom may have lost meaning and purpose in their lives. Each person's journey of recovery will seek to find new meaning and purpose, hopefully supported by friends and family who have shared values (Care Services Improvement Partnership, Royal College of Psychiatrists and Social Care Institute for Excellence, 2007). Spirituality, defined in this book in part as being 'concerned with matters of meaning and purpose in life, truth and values', is clearly relevant. This sharing of values and belief systems with other members of one's community, and achieving a personal equilibrium, seem intuitively likely to improve one's coping capacity.

I welcome this book, which brings together so many excellent explorations of the difficult to measure construct of spirituality, which is nevertheless highly rated by service users as a fundamental marker of a good mental health service.

I believe that acquiring the understanding and skills needed to allow our patients to express and explore their own spirituality in relation to their well-being is fundamental. However, many students and practitioners will have had little or no training in how to enquire about an individual's spirituality or religious faith. The absence of spirituality in the curriculum must be addressed by educators.

You, the reader, will be the judge of whether the editors have achieved their aim to write a textbook of psychiatry that approaches the field from a new perspective – that of integrating spirituality into traditional theoretical and service models of mental health and mental illness.

Professor Sheila Hollins

References

Care Services Improvement Partnership, Royal College of Psychiatrists and Social Care Institute for Excellence (2007) *A Common Purpose: Recovery in Future Mental Health Services (Joint Position Paper 8)*. London: Social Care Institute for Excellence.

Dasgupta, P. and Serageldin, I. (2005) *Social Capital: A Multifaceted Approach*, Vol. 1. Oxford: Oxford University Press.

World Health Organization (2004) *Prevention of Mental Disorders: Effective Interventions and Policy Options: Summary Report*, Geneva: World Health Organization.

Preface to the Second Edition

Thirteen years have elapsed since the publication of the first edition of *Spirituality and Psychiatry* in 2009. Much has happened during that time. Research on spirituality, religion and psychiatry has continued to increase year on year, so that the evidence base is now huge. In 2011, the Royal College of Psychiatrists published for the first time a position statement, *Recommendations for Psychiatrists on Spirituality and Religion*, which was subsequently revised (Cook, 2013). Since 2011, following this lead, at least four other national psychiatric associations have also published guidance for psychiatrists on this important topic, and in 2016 a position statement was published by the World Psychiatric Association (Moreira-Almeida et al., 2016). (The original English version has now been translated into six other languages.) The place of spirituality within psychiatry has continued to be debated vigorously in professional journals and at conferences around the world. In 2016, Andrew Powell, Andrew Sims and I edited a volume titled *Spirituality and Narrative in Psychiatric Practice* (Cook et al., 2016). This volume was intended to be complementary to *Spirituality and Psychiatry* rather than to replace or update it, but it did draw attention to some of the gaps in the first edition. Since then, the need for a second edition of *Spirituality and Psychiatry* has become increasingly apparent, on the grounds of both the growth in the scientific evidence base and the vigorous continuing professional debate concerning the nature and boundaries of good clinical practice.

The aims of the second edition, which has been extensively revised, updated and expanded in scope, remain essentially the same as those set out in the preface to the first edition. The editors are seeking to make an argument for the importance of spirituality, in both research and clinical practice, in psychiatry. The book is intended primarily as a clinical handbook, but we have been mindful throughout of the need to ground clinical practice in the research evidence base. We have been mindful also of the needs of trainees, although (as explored in Chapter 1) we would like to see the attention to spirituality and religion in the curricula for psychiatrists in training become better established both in the UK and around the world. As before, the book is largely 'by psychiatrists for psychiatrists', but we have sought to raise the profile of contributions by non-psychiatrists. There are eight completely new chapters/subchapters in the second edition, including one by a patient and three by psychologists. Nurses, clergy/chaplains and a neuroscientist have joined as new co-authors of three other chapters. Similarly, we hope that our readers will include other mental health professionals, patients and carers, and those with broader interests in spirituality and mental health.

Completely new chapters cover a number of topics that did not appear in the first edition, namely common mental disorders, forensic psychiatry, DSM-5, spiritual interventions and the patient perspective. A glossary now provides summary information and further reading on other important topics, especially those that did not warrant an entire chapter. The chapter on assessment has been completely rewritten. New chapters, by different authors, have replaced the chapters on child and adolescent psychiatry, spiritual care in the NHS, and religion and religious experience that were included in the first edition. The list of contributors now includes colleagues from the USA as well as the UK, and we have endeavoured to address a broader international readership. We have sought to be more interdisciplinary, and this is reflected in various places in enhanced contributions from the humanities, the social sciences and neuroscience. However, there are still some gaps. For example, the book does not include chapters on eating disorders or personality disorders. The research base on spirituality and psychiatry is still, to date, heavily biased towards Western, and particularly Judeo-Christian, perspectives, and our book inevitably reflects this. Notwithstanding these lacunae, we believe that the second edition provides a broader coverage of the topic than did the first edition, and we are very grateful both to the new authors and to the original ones, all of whom have helped to make this possible.

I have taken the decision to use the word 'patient' throughout the book as the term for an individual who is being assessed or treated by mental health professionals. This is the preferred term among many (but not all) people who are suffering from mental illness (McGuire-Snieckus et al., 2003). There has been much debate about its merits and demerits by comparison with other terms, such as 'service user' or 'client' (Christmas and Sweeney, 2016), but the spiritual significance of the term seems to have been almost entirely overlooked. It is often said, either on etymological grounds or as a criticism of the medical model, that the term 'patient' implies passivity. However, I would suggest that the term might also be taken as a reminder that experiences of illness require that we be 'patient', and that we nurture the virtue of patience in the face of suffering and adversity. Patience is not passive. It requires cognitive reappraisal and emotional regulation – active coping strategies – which are facilitated by spirituality/ religion (Schnitker et al., 2017). Patience is recognised as a virtue in all of the world's major faith traditions, and is correlated with measures of religiosity and spirituality (Schnitker and Emmons, 2007).

Spirituality is every bit as important in psychiatry now as it was when the first edition of *Spirituality and Psychiatry* was published 13 years ago. It focuses our attention on the things that matter most to people – the relationships with self, others and a wider reality that provide motivation, meaning and purpose in life. The ways in which people understand these things are extraordinarily varied, and their effects upon the diagnosis and treatment of mental disorders are similarly diverse. If we are to understand our patients well, and if they are to experience us as doing our best to understand them as whole people – body, mind and soul – in their social and cultural context, we need to pay attention to spirituality in psychiatry. This book is offered with the aim of assisting the clinician in fulfilling this important responsibility. It is about finding the heart in psychiatry.

Christopher C. H. Cook
Lead Editor
February 2022

References

Christmas, D. M. and Sweeney, A. (2016) Service user, patient, survivor or client ... has the time come to return to 'patient'? *The British Journal of Psychiatry*, 209, 9–13.

Cook, C. C. H. (2013) *Recommendations for Psychiatrists on Spirituality and Religion.* London: Royal College of Psychiatrists.

Cook, C. C. H., Powell, A. and Sims, A., eds. (2016) *Spirituality and Narrative in*

Psychiatric Practice: Stories of Mind and Soul, London: RCPsych Publications.

McGuire-Snieckus, R., Mccabe, R. and Priebe, S. (2003) Patient, client or service user? A survey of patient preferences of dress and address of six mental health professions. *Psychiatric Bulletin*, 27, 305–308.

Moreira-Almeida, A., Sharma, A., Van Rensburg, B. J., Verhagen, P. J. and Cook, C. C. H. (2016) WPA position statement on spirituality and religion in psychiatry. *World Psychiatry*, 15, 87–88.

Schnitker, S. A. and Emmons, R. A. (2007) Patience as a virtue: religious and psychological perspectives. *Research in the Social Scientific Study of Religion*, 18, 177–207.

Schnitker, S. A., Houltberg, B., Dyrness, W. and Redmond, N. (2017) The virtue of patience, spirituality, and suffering: integrating lessons from positive psychology, psychology of religion, and Christian theology. *Psychology of Religion and Spirituality*, 9, 264–275.

Preface to the First Edition

What kind of book is this, and what is it about? Spirituality is not easily defined. Although many perceive it as very important, its controversial nature has led to it being defined in diverse ways. The definition that we have taken, with a view to inclusiveness, is concerned with human experience of relationship, meaning and purpose. This includes a transcendent, or transpersonal, dimension of experience that has traditionally been regarded as being more the domain of religion and theology than of psychiatry. However, it also encompasses experiences that are very familiar to psychiatry – life within family and society that has usually been viewed in a secular and non-spiritual sense. Such experiences have generally been taken as reflecting personal or interpersonal dynamics, emotions, cognitions and beliefs, which obey the 'laws' of sciences such as psychology, sociology and neurobiology. Immediately, then, this book raises the question of why anything more than science should be necessary. Cannot 'spirituality', whatever it is, be reduced to scientific discourse, a matter of objective consideration without any transcendent or transpersonal dimension?

As will become apparent, the contributors to this book have various implicit or explicit responses to this question. First, there is a growing body of research that supports the importance of spirituality as an independent and dependent variable of some significance, arguably not reducible to a purely biopsychosocial level. For some issues approached in this book, such as substance misuse, neuroscience and old age psychiatry, the body of research of this kind is already quite considerable. For others, however – such as child psychiatry, learning disability psychiatry and the transpersonal perspective – research is still in its infancy.

Second, there are the voices of service users who assert that spirituality is a dimension of their experience that they wish to be able to discuss without it being labelled in pathological terms. The book contains many examples of this kind drawn from clinical practice. In Chapter 3, for instance, we find the story of Julie, whose therapist apparently failed to understand that thoughts as well as actions can be understood as culpable. Such a notion is familiar to philosophers, theologians and priests, but is easily misunderstood phenomenologically by psychiatrists as magical thinking or delusion. Further, in Chapter 5,[1] we encounter Liam, whose physical illness led him to a profoundly spiritual reflection upon his life – a story that does not have a 'happy' ending. This could have all too easily been misunderstood by his family or by professionals seeking to help him as evidence of affective disorder, but the spiritual perspective reminds us that 'negotiating terms' with pain and suffering is a universal and primarily spiritual task for human beings, which offers evidence of spiritual health, not psychopathology.

A third answer to our question arises from the experiences of the authors and other members of the Royal College of Psychiatrists' Spirituality and Psychiatry Special Interest Group, who have found that their reflections upon clinical practice are not complete within the biopsychosocial mode of thought. In Chapter 2, Larry Culliford and

---

[1] Please note that, in the second edition, this version of Chapter 5 has been replaced by a completely new chapter by a different author.

Sarah Eagger, quoting David Hay, argue that spirituality has supraordinate and integrating significance in the proper assessment of patients. In Chapter 3, Susan Mitchell and Glenn Roberts remind us that working with patients who have psychosis can be deeply challenging for professionals, whose own spirituality offers a potentially sustaining resource – hope. Again, in Chapter 6, Andrew Powell and Christopher MacKenna remind us that spirituality – that of the therapist as well as that of the patient – is an aspect of the therapeutic alliance that is easily neglected, yet holds great power for good.

This book is, then, at least in part a response to the questions posed by researchers, service users and clinicians concerning the importance of spirituality as a 'fourth dimension' of mental healthcare. But if it is a book that argues for the importance of this fourth dimension, and warns of the pitfalls of neglecting spirituality in both research and clinical practice, what kind of book is it? Is it primarily a textbook offering guidance for evidence-based practice, an academic book pushing at the frontiers of research or a handbook for clinicians seeking to describe new territories?

As originally conceived within the Spirituality and Psychiatry Special Interest Group Executive Committee, the book was intended to be a clinical textbook. We share a concern to positively influence clinical practice. Authors have therefore been encouraged to keep in mind the needs of the trainee preparing for postgraduate examinations in psychiatry and the clinical realities of psychiatric practice. Although they were urged to pay attention to the evidence base insofar as it offers support for their beliefs, they were not asked primarily to address methodological issues or to chart current research controversies. We hope you will agree that they have endeavoured to address their remit. However, it also became clear to us when reviewing the authors' contributions that in fact this could not possibly be a textbook in the usual sense. Along with the contributors, we share the conviction of the importance of spirituality in mental healthcare, but we also have diverse perspectives about what exactly that means. Nor would it be reasonable to expect that a textbook on spirituality and psychiatry could be written in the same way as one on, say, psychopathology or substance misuse, or any other area of psychiatry.

This book offers perspectives from various subspecialties of psychiatry, as well as considering the generic task of assessment (Chapter 2), the generic perspectives of neuroscience, the transpersonal paradigm and religion (Chapters 9, 11 and 12 respectively), and issues of integrating spiritual care in service delivery (Chapter 10). It also includes an important reminder (in Chapter 13) that there is a 'dark side' to spirituality. However, the book does not attempt to cover systematically all psychiatric diagnoses in the way that a postgraduate textbook of psychiatry would be expected to do. Thus, there are important areas of omission. Notably, affective disorders, eating disorders and those disorders traditionally referred to as 'neuroses' have not received the attention that they might otherwise have had. Furthermore, within some subspecialities of psychiatry it was felt that too little work has been done to date to warrant devoting specific chapters to them; thus, forensic psychiatry and rehabilitation psychiatry are not represented here. We have felt these omissions keenly and hope that future publications will be able to remedy them.

There is, perhaps, another more important reason why this book is not a comprehensive textbook. The field of spirituality and psychiatry is currently at such a stage of development that this book must, of necessity, chart areas of research and promise for the future as much as it can say anything about what is agreed in relation to good clinical practice for the present. It will therefore pose more questions than it offers answers and, in places, it will be provocative. For example, we do not expect all readers to find that they agree with Mike Shooter in his analysis of the case of Liam in Chapter 5. Neither do we expect all readers to share the transpersonal perspective offered by Tim Read and Nicki Crowley in Chapter 11, any more than we expect all readers to identify with one of the religious traditions described in Chapter 12.[2] However, we do share a concern that psychiatrists and other mental healthcare professionals should at least be familiar with the questions that are posed and the traditions and other explanatory frameworks that are described here. It is the joint task of exploring and reflecting upon such questions with patients and colleagues, valuing those traditions and frameworks of belief, and seeking to integrate them with respect and sensitivity into a person's mental healthcare that is properly the spiritual concern of the good psychiatrist.

Christopher C. H. Cook
Andrew Powell
Andrew Sims

---

[2] Please note that, in the second edition, these versions of Chapters 5, 11 and 12 have been replaced by completely new chapters by different authors.

Acknowledgements

As lead editor, I (Christopher C. H. Cook) would particularly like to thank Andrew Powell, Founding Chair of the Spirituality and Psychiatry Special Interest Group of the Royal College of Psychiatrists, for his editorial collaboration during the process of planning, writing and editing this volume. I have greatly valued his spiritual, friendly, thoughtful and constructively critical support. His comments on my own chapters, and his wisdom in managing some of the more difficult issues that have arisen with the book as a whole, have been invaluable.

In working on the second edition, Andrew and I have greatly missed the editorial contribution of our friend and colleague Andrew Sims. However, his influence upon the book has continued in this revised and expanded edition, and we are pleased to acknowledge the debt that we owe to him in this regard.

We are grateful for conversation and debate over a period of more than two decades with colleagues in the Spirituality and Psychiatry Special Interest Group of the Royal College of Psychiatrists. This has been formative in our thinking and has provided the context within which the first edition of this book was initially conceived, and in which the second edition has now taken shape.

We are also grateful to colleagues at Cambridge University Press, and especially Jessica Papworth, Olivia Boult and Beth Pollard for their wonderful support in the planning, completion and production of this second edition. An anonymous reviewer provided constructive comments on the manuscript, which helped to improve the academic rigour of the final text. Warm thanks are due to Jo Hargreaves for her meticulous and careful copy editing. Her attention to detail, patience and genuine interest in the book have been enormously appreciated.

The Spirituality and Psychiatry Special Interest Group of the Royal College of Psychiatrists: A Personal Reflection

Andrew Powell

The commissioning of this second edition of *Spirituality and Psychiatry* by Cambridge University Press coincided with the twentieth anniversary of the Spirituality and Psychiatry Special Interest Group (SPSIG) of the Royal College of Psychiatrists. Having myself reached a certain age, it also felt to be the right time for me to retire from the SPSIG Executive Committee while taking the opportunity as Founding Chair to put on record how the SPSIG began. I would like to give a brief account of the work we have undertaken so far and what faces us in these insecure times, not least due to the pandemic that at the time of writing presents an immense challenge to humanity.

The account that follows is, at the outset, more personal than professional, for I became convinced of the need to form a Spirituality Special Interest Group as a result of developments that shaped my life over a number of years. With hindsight, as is often the case, there is a seeming inevitability about the path taken and where it led, although when I set out on this journey it would never have crossed my mind that psychiatry and spirituality could be related in any useful way.

My psychiatric training began in 1970 under the renowned Dr William Sargant. Sargant treated most of his patients with combined antidepressants and frequently with electroconvulsive therapy (ECT). The heady *furor therapeuticus* in his department at St Thomas' Hospital, London, was driven by Sargant's conviction that all mental disorder was simply a result of aberrant brain chemistry. The person's psychological history was considered largely irrelevant, and we prescribed without conversing in any real depth with our patients.

Sargant suggested that I ought to sit the membership examination of the Royal College of Physicians, otherwise no colleague of note would take me seriously. This I did, immersing myself in the surreal and compelling world of hospital medicine, where therapeutic elation comingled with the heartache of death and dying. On the one hand, there was the body to be diagnosed and treated, with its myriad and intricate parts, and on the other, one's anxious patient facing the unknown and hoping to be given good news. I was finding out that there was much more to medicine than the science.

I applied to the Maudsley Hospital, London, to undertake specialist training in psychiatry. This was a very different world, where the mind took precedence over the body except on those rare occasions when the symptoms were organic in origin. Yet the academic focus struck me as somewhat disconnected from the patient as a person, who was more often talked about than talked with. Seeking a deeper and more human encounter with the workings of the mind, I ventured into personal psychoanalysis and then headed for the psychotherapy department at the Maudsley.

The explanatory power of Sigmund Freud's theories impressed me greatly; psychoanalysis seemed to have an answer for almost everything in those days. I went on to train in group analysis, before being appointed senior lecturer and consultant psychotherapist at St George's Hospital, London.

Some years later, I became interested in the work of Carl Jung. In contrast to Freud's determinedly secular outlook, Jung dared to speak of the soul, and I found myself powerfully drawn to this more expansive vision of what it means to be human. Jung's observation that 'what was divided on a lower level will reappear, united, on a higher one' (Jung, 1941, p. 189) affirmed my intuition that psychological reality is nested within the broader compass of spiritual reality, in which wholeness of being is far more than the sum of the parts.

I should add here that I had been raised in the Anglican Church, and although I was not a churchgoer at this time, awareness of the spiritual dimension of life had been indelibly impressed on me. Yet, up to this point in my life, I had always considered this to be a private matter that had no bearing on my professional work.

Around this time, I began taking part in the Scientific and Medical Network, an international forum for exploring themes that bridge science, consciousness and spirituality. Here was a fertile exchange of ideas between leading thinkers who challenged the prevailing cultural norm of physicalism – the view that the only reality is that of the material universe. Quantum physics was opening up a new realm of possibilities that suggested primacy of mind over matter, with profound implications for the healing process. I was coming to the conclusion – to paraphrase Teilhard de Chardin – that we are not so much human beings on a spiritual journey as spiritual beings on a human journey.

In my middle years, I left London to take up a consultant post in Oxford. By now, the psychological treatment services were increasingly being run by clinical psychologists who favoured short-term cognitive–behavioural therapy. Psychiatrists were under pressure primarily to treat the severely mentally ill, time was in short supply and there was a growing climate of greater reliance on psychopharmaceuticals.

How else, in these circumstances, might a patient be helped to draw on their inner resources simply and easily? I had earlier trained in psychodrama, in which participants imaginatively embark on an inner journey to find a place of therapeusis or healing. Now, where appropriate, I began encouraging patients, by means of active imagination, to 'go within' and commune with their innermost self. Often, to their great surprise, and despite the traumas that they had endured, they would become aware of a wellspring of love and wisdom that they had not known they possessed. Such therapy was simple to initiate and was always helpful. Through inner dialogue with the soul, as it was most often felt to be, the patient would be deeply moved to find answers that they had never foreseen. A full account of soul-centred therapy can be found in *The Ways of the Soul* (Powell, 2017) and *Conversations with the Soul* (Powell, 2018).

Working in this way emboldened me to think how more generally we might try to bridge a longstanding historical divide between spirituality and psychiatry. The issue had been raised on a number of occasions previously. The patron of the Royal College of Psychiatrists, HRH The Prince of Wales, had addressed the College in 1991, when he spoke of the need to value spirituality as integral to good psychiatric practice. Two past presidents of the College, Professor Andrew Sims and Professor John Cox, had similarly highlighted the importance of the spiritual, religious and cultural dimensions of mental health care (Cox, 1994; Sims, 1994). George Carey, the then Archbishop of Canterbury, had also given an address to the College on transcending the barriers between religion and psychiatry (Carey, 1997). However, such appeals did not appear to be leading to any noticeable change.

In the USA the situation was rather different. The subject of spirituality was being both taught and researched in medical schools and universities. In 1991, David Larson, a psychiatrist at Duke University, had founded the National Institute for Healthcare Research, a think tank that aimed to bridge the gap between spirituality and health (Larson and Larson, 1994, Larson et al., 1998). I corresponded with David, who encouraged me to explore what could be done in the UK. Indeed, I personally was touched by his support, which continued until his untimely death at the age of 54 in 2002. Three of his papers are available in the Spirituality and Psychiatry Special Interest Group's publications archive, and were among the first that I uploaded.

In 1998, the *Handbook of Religion and Mental Health*, edited by Harold Koenig and David Rosmarin, was published in the USA. This academic database on the importance of spirituality and religion in mental health was to strengthen our hand for a UK initiative. Subsequent years saw the publication of two editions of the *Handbook of Religion and Health* (Koenig et al., 2001, 2012) and, most recently, the *Handbook of Spirituality, Religion, and Mental Health* (Koenig and Rosmarin, 2020).

Why was there such a bias against spiritual matters within psychiatry in the first place? The answer may lie in how spirituality and religious beliefs have traditionally only been taken into account as a feature of mental disorder – as in the case of religious delusions, to name just one example. Most likely because of this association of spirituality with pathology, it had not been considered important to explore spirituality in its own right, even though spiritual values and beliefs express a fundamental aspect of selfhood and personal identity.

In disregarding a person's spirituality, psychiatrists miss out on a valuable opportunity to engage with their patients – one that has both diagnostic and empathic implications. We know that up to half of patients draw on their religious and spiritual beliefs to help them get through a crisis, yet they have not felt comfortable talking about such matters with their psychiatrist (Faulkner, 1997). As a result, the area of spirituality is prone to communication failures. I recall one patient, who happened to be a member of the clergy, relating how she tried to talk with the admitting psychiatrist about the importance of the Holy Ghost, only to be asked in the ward round the next day if she had been seeing ghosts!

It struck me that in order to reach a well-informed diagnosis, as well as establish a positive therapeutic alliance, the psychiatrist needs to engage with this hinterland so as to earn the confidence and trust of the patient. This is made much more difficult if the psychiatrist knows nothing about the patient's faith tradition or spiritual leanings. Furthermore, if the psychiatrist is unaware of research that shows the benefit of spirituality and religion to mental health, the whole subject is likely to be glossed over. Unsurprisingly, many psychiatrists neglect to ask about their patients' spiritual and religious beliefs.

Not so long ago, it was considered intrusive to ask directly whether patients had suffered sexual abuse. We now know that this area of enquiry, when handled with respect and sensitivity, leads to a better understanding of problems that have arisen and of how best to help the person concerned. This example might seem a far cry from asking our patients about their spiritual and/or religious beliefs and practices, but when exploring how individuals see themselves and what may have contributed to their becoming ill, an understanding of their beliefs and practices can assist in determining the best way to find healing and recovery. There are, of course, occasions when enlisting the help of chaplaincy to explore spiritual concerns is the appropriate option. Frequently, however, no more is needed than a tactful enquiry on the part of the psychiatrist.

I already knew from informal exchanges with psychiatrist colleagues that although many were unhappy with the secular climate of scientific reductionism, they felt that to speak openly about spirituality would risk censure. What we needed was a professional forum, supported by the College, where we could freely explore and debate the subject – a group that would align psychiatry with its intended meaning of *psyche* (soul) and *iatros* (doctor). The College already had provision for a number of Special Interest Groups, so why not have one on spirituality? As a first step, I contacted around 200 psychiatrists whom I thought might be interested, and found that the idea met with considerable support. Since only 120 signatures would be needed when applying to the College, it seemed we had a good chance of success.

I approached several colleagues whom I knew were keen to be involved, and we formed a working group that included Professor Andrew Sims, Dr Julian Candy, Dr Larry Culliford, Dr Peter Fenwick and Dr Chris Holman. With the millennium fast approaching, a proposal was submitted to the Royal College of Psychiatrists, setting out that the new special interest group was intended to:

> facilitate the exchange of ideas on a wide range of topics, including the significance of the major religions which influence the values and beliefs of the society in which we live, also taking into account the spiritual aspirations of individuals who do not identify with any one particular faith and those who hold that spirituality is independent of religion. (Shooter, 1999, p. 310)

Happily, the College supported our application, and the inaugural meeting of the SPSIG was held on 24 September 1999, in the former home of the College at 17 Belgrave Square (Royal College of Psychiatrists, 1999). Since then, the group has steadily grown to include more than 4,600 psychiatrists – slightly less than one in four of the College membership.

Here, we must record our thanks to the members of the SPSIG Executive, past and present, who have given so generously of their time and energy over and above the demands of clinical work, and also to the College for providing ongoing administrative support, website facilities and a venue for our meetings.

From the start, the aim has been to encourage psychiatrists to explore a wide range of subjects beyond the limits of scientific materialism and, in particular, experiences that are invested with spiritual meaning. Topics have included the misunderstanding that can arise between patient and psychiatrist, the importance of an integrative (mind/body/spirit) approach, existential questions about the purpose and meaning of life, protective factors that help to sustain individuals in crisis, the problem of good and evil, the significance of the near-death experience, the nature of mystical and trance states, and the nature of anomalous experiences such as reported visitations from deceased loved ones following bereavement.

We have also been concerned throughout to centre the work of the SPSIG on the inclusive nature of spirituality, in line with the broad definition offered in Chapter 1. While a number of faith traditions are represented, the ethic has been one of respect for differences while seeking common ground as clinicians.

A landmark event for the SPSIG was the publication of *Recommendations for Psychiatrists on Spirituality and Religion* in 2011, followed by a revised version in 2013. This achievement can rightly be attributed to Professor Chris Cook, who at the time was also our Chair. The draft recommendations put forward were contested by some psychiatrists, who felt that to raise the subject of spirituality and/or religion with patients was to cross a boundary that breached professional ethical standards. The dialogue that followed was important and necessary, and meticulous re-drafting was called for. In the event, approval was granted and the position statement was published by the College (Royal College of Psychiatrists, 2013). The question of boundaries continues to be debated, and is a topic that Chris Cook explores in Chapter 1.

The SPSIG has set a number of educational goals, which include the following: learning about the difference between healthy and unhealthy spirituality; how to distinguish between mental illness and spiritual emergency; awareness of the evidence base for spirituality and religion in improving mental health outcomes; and how to make a spiritual assessment (Eagger, 2011).

With regard to spiritual assessment, the psychiatrist needs to ascertain whether the patient's spirituality or religion is experienced as supportive or stressful, how it affects the way that the patient perceives their problem, whether there are spiritual or religious issues that the patient would like to discuss in therapy, and when support from chaplaincy would be beneficial. This approach has been endorsed by the College and is now included in the College CPD online module 'Exploring Spirituality with People who use Mental Health Services'.

In 2009, the first edition of *Spirituality and Psychiatry* was published by the College, having been conceived by the SPSIG Executive and with chapters largely contributed by SPSIG members. The success of the volume has led to the publication of this expanded and revised second edition by Cambridge University Press. A further book, *Spirituality and Narrative in Psychiatric Practice: Stories of Mind and Soul*, was proposed by the SPSIG and published in 2016 by the College (Cook et al., 2016). We trust that both books will continue to attract the attention of a wide readership, including mental health professionals, service users, carers, and spiritual advisers – indeed all who seek to understand the suffering that characterises mental disorder.

As well as alerting psychiatrists to the spiritual dimension implicit in whole-person care, we have produced for service users and carers a leaflet with the title *Spirituality and Mental Health*, which can be downloaded from the College website.[3] It is written in everyday language, and it makes reference to the benefits of non-religious spiritual pursuits such as meditation, spending time with nature, music and the arts, contemplative reading and poetry.

During the early years of the SPSIG, our meetings in London, held at the former premises of the Royal College, were of necessity small in size. With the College's move to 21 Prescot Street in 2013, access to full conference facilities on site became available, enabling

---

[3] www.rcpsych.ac.uk/mental-health/treatments-and-wellbeing/spirituality-and-mental-health

many of our subsequent events to be open to the general public, with online registration for forthcoming conferences. In order to have the widest possible outreach, the SPSIG website[4] is fully in the public domain. The SPSIG publications archive holds over 200 author-indexed papers written by mental health professionals, as well as theme-based access to past programmes, all of which can be downloaded for free.[5] In addition, for the wider public, the SPSIG has produced the video *Spirituality in Psychiatry for Today's World* (Royal College of Psychiatrists, 2016), available on the SPSIG website and YouTube, and in line with current social media, we now have a College-based Twitter account.

Over time, the SPSIG has developed links with a number of other professional bodies, including the National Institute for Mental Health in England; the Scientific and Medical Network; the Dutch Foundation for Psychiatry and Religion; the Spirituality, Religion and Psychiatry Caucus of the American Psychiatric Association; and the Psychiatry and Religion Section of the World Psychiatric Association (WPA), which has now published its own position statement (Moreira-Almeida et al. 2016). Encouragingly, sections or special interest groups devoted to spirituality and religion are now being supported by psychiatric associations across many nations.

In these uncertain times, it is hard to predict what the future may bring and how mental health services can best respond. However, we already know that psychiatrists are seeing a growing number of people who are experiencing extreme levels of stress as they try to cope with the demands of modernity, heightened by ethnic, cultural, religious, educational and economic disparities. Casting a shadow over all humanity, the COVID-19 pandemic is having an unforeseen and incalculable impact on the physical and mental health of human-kind, especially for a whole generation of children. As if that were not enough, the ravages of war in one country after another are inflicting unbearable suffering on countless lives.

In a world that so often judges its winners and losers by material achievement, in which competition outpaces collaboration and where little value is placed on caring and com-passion, many people are left feeling disheartened, lacking in confidence and vulnerable to depression. Although physical treatments continue to benefit some of our patients, the era of naive faith in psychopharmaceuticals as a cure-all is long past. Regardless of diagnostic labels, human distress needs to be met with sensitivity and psychological understanding. The complex factors that determine mental health and well-being call for a holistic approach, which must also include the exploration of our patients' spiritual concerns, values and aspirations. Such person-centred care includes taking into account the spiritual significance of anxiety, doubt, guilt and shame on the one hand, and love, altruism and forgiveness on the other, as well as the potential benefits of meditation or prayer for some patients. It is no coincidence that, in recent years, mindfulness therapy, compassion-focused therapy, forgiveness therapy and religiously integrated cognitive–behavioural therapy have all contributed to mental well-being.

The many neuroscientific advances that have been made within the profession are to be applauded, but need to balanced with the nourishment of genuine dialogue, by 'getting alongside' our patients, taking time to explore what really matters to them and helping them to affirm and value what they hold most dear. In the language of spirituality, this is about meeting soul to soul, and, regardless of the specifics of the treatment, it is sure to play its part in the patient's recovery and well-being.

Looking back over the two decades since the founding of the SPSIG, I remain convinced that psychiatry, as with all of medicine, is at its best when guided by the golden rule 'Do to others as you would have them do to you.' The doctor and the patient have complementary roles, and as we meet on the path of life, there is one medicine that is constantly at our disposal and freely available. This is the power of love, lending hope, giving comfort and helping to bring peace to the troubled mind.

References

Carey, G. (1997) Towards wholeness: transcending the barriers between religion and psychiatry. *British Journal of Psychiatry*, 170, 396–397.

Cook, C., Powell, A. and Sims, A. (2016) *Spirituality and Narrative in Psychiatric Practice: Stories of Mind and Soul*. London: RCPsych Publications.

Cox, J. L. (1994) Psychiatry and religion: a general psychiatrist's perspective. *Psychiatric Bulletin*, 18, 673–676.

Eagger, S. (2011) Spirituality in psychiatry: implementing spiritual assessment. Talk given at the Royal College of Psychiatrists' Annual Meeting, 29 June 2011. Available at: www.rcpsych.ac.uk/docs/default-source/members/sigs/spirituality-spsig/spirituality-special-interest-group-publications-eagger-implementing-spiritual-assessment.pdf

Faulkner, A. (1997) *Knowing Our Own Minds*. London: Mental Health Foundation.

HRH The Prince of Wales (1991) Lecture by HRH the Prince of Wales, as Patron, to the Royal College of Psychiatrists, Brighton, Friday 5 July 1991. *British Journal of Psychiatry*, 159, 763–768.

Jung, C. (1941/1968) Paracelsus as a spiritual phenomenon. In H. Read, M. Fordham and G. Adler, eds., *C. G. Jung: The Collected Works. Volume Thirteen: Alchemical Studies*. London: Routledge, pp. 109–190.

Koenig, H. G. and Rosmarin, D., eds. (1998) *Handbook of Religion and Mental Health*. London: Academic Press.

Koenig, H. G. and Rosmarin, D., eds. (2020) *Handbook of Spirituality, Religion, and Mental Health*. London: Academic Press.

Koenig, H. G., McCullough, M. E. and Larson, D. B., eds. (2001) *Handbook of Religion and Health*, New York: Oxford University Press.

Koenig, H. G., King, D. E. and Carson, V. B., eds. (2012) *Handbook of Religion and Health*, 2nd ed. New York: Oxford University Press.

Larson, D. B. and Larson, S. S. (1994) *The Forgotten Factor in Physical and Mental Health: What Does the Research Show?* Rockville, MD: National Institute for Healthcare Research.

Larson, D. B., Sawyers, J. P. and McCullough, M. E., eds. (1998) *Scientific Research on Spirituality and Health: A Consensus Report*. Rockville, MD: National Institute for Healthcare Research.

Moreira-Almeida, A., Sharma, A., van Rensburg, B. J., Verhagen, P. J. and Cook, C. C. H. (2016) WPA position statement on spirituality and religion in psychiatry. *World Psychiatry*, 15 (1), 87–88.

Powell, A. (2017) *The Ways of the Soul. A Psychiatrist Reflects: Essays on Life, Death and Beyond*. London: Muswell Hill Press.

Powell, A. (2018) *Conversations with the Soul. A Psychiatrist Reflects: Essays on Life, Death and Beyond*. London: Muswell Hill Press.

Royal College of Psychiatrists (2013) *Recommendations for Psychiatrists on Spirituality and Religion*; www.rcpsych.ac.uk/docs/default-source/improving-care/

better-mh-policy/position-statements/
ps03_2013.pdf?sfvrsn=eb247792_4

Royal College of Psychiatrists (2016)
Spirituality in Psychiatry for Today's World;
www.youtube.com/watch?v=
72RkcfzwFpU&t=5s

Shooter, M. (1999) Proposal for a special
interest group in spirituality and
psychiatry. *Psychiatric Bulletin*, 23, 310.

Sims, A. (1994) 'Psyche' – spirit as well as
mind? *The British Journal of
Psychiatry*, 165, 441–446.

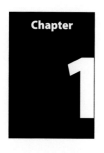

Spirituality and Religion in Psychiatry

Christopher C. H. Cook[1]

Spirituality is about the things that matter most – to all of us. For many patients it is a fundamental aspect of their experience of the human condition that they hope will not be neglected, but about which they may be hesitant to talk to their psychiatrist for fear of censure or misunderstanding. For some psychiatrists, spirituality is fundamental to their vocational calling and may influence their clinical practice (hopefully for good – but potentially also for ill) in diverse visible or invisible ways. For others it is a cause for concern, perhaps even something that they would rather avoid. Spirituality appears in religious and non-religious forms. Even for the minority of people who self-identify as neither spiritual nor religious, their world view, their sense of meaning and purpose in life (or lack of it) and their experience of deeply important relationships with self, others and a wider universe all share many of the central concerns of spirituality. Spirituality is therefore relevant to the work of all psychiatrists.

Spirituality in Psychiatry: A Brief History

Historically, much psychiatric care was provided within a religious context. The first specialist institution for the care of the mentally ill appears to have been established in Christian Byzantium in the fourth century. An Islamic facility was established in Fez in North Africa from at least as early as the seventh century (Zilboorg and Henry, 1941, p. 561). The shrine of St Dympna, at Gheel in Belgium, became a place of pilgrimage for people with mental health problems from around the seventh century, with reports of miraculous cures drawing large numbers of pilgrims and, in the thirteenth century, supported a church and a house for the treatment and confinement of the insane (Zilboorg and Henry, 1941, p. 562). In 1247 the hospital of St Mary of Bethlehem was founded in Bishopsgate in London. By the sixteenth century it had developed a special reputation for the care of the insane, and became known as 'Bedlam'. After two moves within London, it relocated to Kent in 1930 and merged with the Maudsley Hospital, in Southwark, in 1948 (Shorter, 2005, pp. 42–43).

More important than institutions, however, are the attitudes to care which they embody. The Spanish Renaissance philosopher, Juan Luis Vives (1493–1540), a contemporary of Erasmus and Thomas More, gave considerable attention to the humane treatment of the mentally ill, recognising them as suffering from *illness* and treating

---

[1] I am pleased to acknowledge the contribution made to this chapter in the first edition of *Spirituality and Psychiatry* by my friend and colleague Andrew Sims. I have missed his partnership in writing for the second edition. Remnants of his writing will still be evident here, but much of the text is completely new and what remains has been extensively revised.

them with compassion and respect (Zilboorg and Henry, 1941, pp. 180–195). Sadly, a very different approach emerged in the later Middle Ages, with mental illness attributed to demonic possession, albeit that by the end of this period such attributions appear to have been made only in respect of a minority of those suffering from mental disorder (Kemp and Williams, 1987).

The divisions between religion and what we now call psychiatry date back to the European Enlightenment in the seventeenth and eighteenth centuries, and the emergence of empirical, scientific methods for studying the mind and brain (Ansah-Asamoah et al., 2021). Christian care for the mentally ill continued well into this period, increasingly in engagement with humanism and non-religious approaches to care. The so-called 'moral approach' to the care of the insane brought about a revolution in care for the mentally ill in the late eighteenth century. Leading figures in this movement were Philippe Pinel (1745–1826) in France, Vincenzo Chiarugi (1759–1820) in Italy, and William Tuke (1732–1822), a Quaker, who established the Retreat at York in 1791 for the humane care of people suffering from mental disorders, in England. In 1856, John Conolly (1794–1866), superintendent of Hanwell Asylum, published *The Treatment of the Insane without Mechanical Restraints*. That book, and his example of good practice in a major London asylum, were influential in changing practice more widely.

Psychiatry, as a distinct discipline, traces its origins to the beginning of the nineteenth century, when there were remarkable developments in brain localisation and neurohistology, especially in Germany. For Wilhelm Griesinger (1817–1868), all mental illnesses could be understood in relation to brain disease (Shorter, 2005, pp. 119–120). The contribution of this organic, biological approach to psychiatry, neuropathology and especially classification was immense, but at the interface of religion and psychiatry these discoveries encouraged an attitude of reductionism. Mental disorders, as well as healthy mental processes and behaviour, could now be 'reduced' to material processes, the human being understandable only as the sum of its biological parts. Reductionism is clinically and philosophically problematic (Karlsson and Kamppinen, 1995), as well as theologically and spiritually objectionable, and this approach to psychiatry was to have a long-lasting and unhelpful influence.

Meanwhile, French psychiatry had reached reductionism by a different route: complex behaviour was thought to occur as a result of unconscious mechanisms, ultimately influenced by the state of the brain. Jean-Martin Charcot's pupil, Pierre Janet (1859–1947), who was a psychologist and neurologist, had established the beginnings of psychotherapy by the end of the nineteenth century. Religion and faith were not seen as necessary in the quest for explanations of human behaviour.

In Britain, following the publication of Charles Darwin's *On the Origin of the Species* in 1859, the concepts of 'natural selection' and 'survival of the fittest' had profound consequences for the care of the mentally ill. In part this was due to a trend towards discounting everything about the human being, including history and personality, which could not be shown to be clearly organic. In part it was also due to another negative influence on treatment, arising from the theory of degeneration. Popularised by Bénédict-Augustin Morel (1809–1873), notably in his *Treatise on Degeneration* published in 1857, this theory ascribed psychiatric illness to inherited causes (Shorter, 2005, pp. 181–182). Unlike Darwin, Morel believed that acquired characteristics could be inherited by offspring, and that they would then become more severe in subsequent generations. Whilst the inheritance of acquired characteristics would later be called into question, these influences presaged modern approaches to psychiatric genetics. They also ushered in several decades of therapeutic nihilism in psychiatry in Britain and elsewhere, inhibiting the search for new, effective methods of treatment.

In the late nineteenth and early twentieth centuries, the influences of psychoanalysis and behaviourism further increased the rift between psychiatry and religion. Sigmund Freud (1856–1939) asserted that monotheistic belief was an illusion, and that religion was a neurosis. For the behaviourists, human behaviour was 'nothing but' Pavlovian or Skinnerian conditioning. By the middle of the twentieth century, with science dedicated to material realism, and with the arrival of modernism in philosophy, reductionism had come to dominate medicine. Human beings were understood as little more than intelligent apes. Psychoanalysis was in conflict with traditional religious attitudes, and many churches identified Freud, psychoanalysis and, by association, the whole of psychiatry with atheism, antagonism to religion and a challenge to conventional morality.

By the 1960s, there was little recognition that the patient's religious beliefs contributed significantly to the psychiatric history, formulation or planning of treatment, and spiritual aspects of the patient's problem were usually ignored. Biological psychiatry was in the ascendent. In the standard British textbook of the 1960s and 1970s, by Mayer-Gross, Slater and Roth, there were only two references to religion in the index, and religion was assumed to be for 'the hesitant, the guilt-ridden, the excessively timid, those lacking clear convictions with which to face life' (Slater and Roth, 1979, p. 180).

In the last decades of the twentieth century, things began to change (Ansah-Asamoah et al., 2021; Cook, 2020). A seminal paper by Allport and Ross (1967), from the USA, showed not only that religiosity took different forms, but also that these different forms had differing implications for human well-being. Importantly, subsequent research has repeatedly shown that intrinsic (inwardly motivated) but not extrinsic (socially motivated) religiosity is good for mental health.

In 1986, David Larson and his colleagues published a systematic review of research on religious variables published between 1978 and 1982 in four leading psychiatric journals, including the American, British and Canadian journals of psychiatry (Larson et al., 1986). Among 2,348 articles that reported quantitative research, only 59 articles could be found in which a religious variable was quantified, and in only three of these was religion the major focus of the study. By the end of the century, research interest in spirituality and religion had increased dramatically. Publications on spirituality in the psychological and healthcare literature increased in exponential fashion during the 1990s (Cook, 2004a).

In 1991, the Patron of the Royal College of Psychiatrists in the UK, HRH The Prince of Wales, urged an approach to mental health care which encompassed body, mind and spirit. Successive presidents of the College (Professor Andrew Sims, and then Professor John Cox) took up the subject in their addresses at College meetings in 1993, and a series of conferences on religion and psychiatry was held at the Institute of Psychiatry in London. In 1997 the Archbishop of Canterbury addressed a joint annual meeting of the Royal College of Psychiatrists and the Association of European Psychiatrists. In 1999 the inaugural meeting of the Spirituality and Psychiatry Special Interest Group was held at the Royal College of Psychiatrists (as discussed later in this chapter; see also the personal reflection on this by Andrew Powell at the beginning of the present volume).

In 1994, the newly published revision of the *Diagnostic and Statistical Manual of Mental Disorders* (DSM) of the American Psychiatric Association, namely DSM-IV, included for the first time a category of 'Religious or Spiritual Problem'. Until this time, references to religion in the DSM had been almost entirely negative, associating it with pathology (Richardson, 1993). The new V code (V62.89) acknowledged that spiritual and religious problems were not necessarily pathological, and encouraged clinicians to be more discerning about the nature of spiritual and religious concerns communicated by their patients.

What Is Spirituality?

Spirituality is an abstract concept that is difficult to define. The word 'spirituality' has a long history, and its meaning has changed over the centuries. In the English language it derives from the Latin, *spiritualitas*, a word which first appears in the early fifth century, where its use draws on Christian understandings (particularly those of St Paul in the New Testament) of the human spirit as that which is led by the Spirit of God (Principe, 1983). In the twelfth century, use of the term began to change, presaging modern distinctions in which spirituality is opposed to material or bodily aspects of life. In seventeenth-century France the term grew in popularity, but it also acquired a pejorative sense when used to attack 'la nouvelle spiritualité' of such writers as Madame Guyon (1648–1717). In the late nineteenth and early twentieth century, the term began to be used by members of religious traditions other than Christianity.

During the course of the twentieth century, the term grew in popular usage, and people started to self-identify as 'spiritual but not religious' (SBNR). The SBNR are, in general, less likely to believe in God as a personal being, are more individualistic and disavow exclusivism, religious authoritarianism and religious institutions (Fuller, 2001; Mercadante, 2014; Wixwat and Saucier, 2020). However, the SBNR category may be more about morality and politics than about beliefs or empirical differences (Ammerman, 2013). It can serve to characterise 'religion', from a certain unsympathetic perspective, as morally and politically objectionable.

It has been suggested that 'spirituality' is merely a privatised, and experience orientated, form of religion (Streib and Hood, 2011) or a mystical religion (Houtman and Tromp, 2021). It shares key features with religion. For example, Linda Mercadante has drawn attention to common concerns such as belief in, and desire to connect with, a transcendent reality, and the use of various rituals and practices to aid this connection (Mercadante, 2014, pp. 5–6). The shared emphasis on transcendence is debatable, and in many ways spirituality untethered to religion is as much concerned with the immanent order as with the transcendent (Cook, 2013c; Houtman and Tromp, 2021). It is also debatable as to whether or not spirituality untethered to religious tradition is actually as individualised and fragmented as it is portrayed to be. For example, Houtman and Tromp (2021) have identified a coherent worldview within 'post-Christian' spirituality which emphasises such things as the 'immanence of the sacred' and the interconnectedness of things. Within this worldview, experience and emotions play an important part as manifestations of the spiritual/sacred within the self.

There are many possible definitions of the word *spirituality*. For the first edition of this book we provided authors with the following working definition of spirituality as a starting point:

> Spirituality is a distinctive, potentially creative and universal dimension of human experience arising both within the inner subjective awareness of individuals and within

communities, social groups and traditions. It may be experienced as relationship with that which is intimately 'inner', immanent and personal, within the self and others, and/or as relationship with that which is wholly 'other', transcendent and beyond the self. It is experienced as being of fundamental or ultimate importance and is thus concerned with matters of meaning and purpose in life, truth and values. (Cook, 2004a)

This definition was developed from a study of the way in which the concept of spirituality is used in the literature on addiction and spirituality, but it applies equally well to other areas of psychiatry. It emphasises the universality of spirituality as a subjective dimension of the experience of being human, whilst attempting to recognise that this is still, nonetheless, a socially situated phenomenon. Spirituality has come to be perceived as a more inclusive term than religion, acknowledging that a significant number of people in Western countries now see themselves as SBNR. However, a lot of people see themselves as neither spiritual nor religious. In one study in England, 19% of people identified as SBNR, but 46% identified as neither spiritual nor religious, and 35% as predominantly religious (King et al., 2013).

Koenig has argued that spirituality is distinctive by virtue of its connection with the transcendent, or sacred (Koenig et al., 2012, p. 46). As noted earlier, this is debatable. Some spiritual practices are very much about the immanent order, whether or not they also have a transcendent context (Cook, 2013c). Some, perhaps many, people who might consider themselves 'spiritual' do not relate to words such as 'transcendent' or 'sacred'. In clinical practice, conversation about spirituality often comes down to those things that matter most – intimate relationships, love, creativity, meaning and purpose in life. One may well ask whether the word is helpful if it can mean so many different things to different people, but it does appear to be helpful in practice. Many patients do want to talk about spirituality (Mental Health Foundation, 2002) and, to this extent, it is at least a word that seems to be good at opening up conversations, not least within the context of psychiatric practice.

Religion

It has been suggested by some that religion is 'giving way' to spirituality (Heelas and Woodhead, 2005), or else that the world is becoming more secular. However, the majority of people worldwide are religious. In 2010, 88.2% of the world's population identified as belonging to a religion. Whilst the comparable figure in 1910 was 99.8%, this has not been a steady decline. In 1970 almost 20% of the world's population identified as either agnostic (14.7%) or atheist (4.5%). The resurgence of religion since then may be partly attributable to the collapse of European communism (Johnson et al., 2013, pp. 11–12).

Religion, like spirituality, is susceptible to widely varying definitions. Some definitions emphasise the personal and others the social, some emphasise belief and others behaviour, some emphasise tradition and others function, and so on (Bowker, 1999, p. xv). In contrast to religion in general, any religion in particular may be defined in terms of the loyalty of its adherents (Johnson et al., 2013, p. 139). It is not necessarily so much about dogma, beliefs or practices as it is about following, belonging and identity. A religion holds a unique place in the lives of those who see themselves as belonging to it. For our present purpose, it might be helpful to emphasise that religion is also concerned with socially and traditionally shared beliefs and experience, but in placing this emphasis we must not lose sight of its personal and subjective dimension. Most religious people see their spirituality as bound up with their religion. Relatively few people see themselves as 'religious but not spiritual'.

In 2010, out of a world population of a little less than 7 billion people, almost a third (nearly 2.3 billion) identified as Christian, with Islam (nearly 1.6 billion) and Hinduism (nearly 1 billion) as the second and third most popular religions, respectively (Johnson et al., 2013). (For consideration of other religions, see Chapter 16.) For clinicians practising in any particular country, the local picture may of course look very different. Much of the research on spirituality and religion in relation to mental health has been conducted in North America and Europe, and so reflects the predominantly Judeo-Christian religious demographics and culture of these continents.

Despite the majority of believers of all creeds living peacefully together, the concept of religion has become associated in the minds of many with fanaticism and violence. For some, as discussed earlier, religion is seen as the antithesis of spirituality. In practice, talk about spirituality may therefore provide an easier way in to conversation about the things that matter. However, in research it has not proved possible to separate distinct factors of spirituality from confounding psychological variables (Koenig, 2008). In research, religiosity is easier to measure.

Religion, religions and religious experiences will be discussed further in Chapter 16. At this point it is important simply to note that most people, worldwide, understand their spirituality in a religious context.

Mysticism

Mysticism is yet another term that is difficult to define and has undergone changes of meaning over the centuries. The term has its origins in ancient Greek religions and was taken up by early Christianity. Medieval Christians distinguished between 'speculative' theology (which we might understand as an intellectual endeavour) and theology of the affect, or 'mystical theology' (which we might understand as Christian spirituality) (Tyler et al., 2018). Today, a mystical element is identifiable within almost all religious traditions, and arguably is fundamental to all religion, but is also identifiable outside of these traditions.

Psychiatry is – or ought to be – concerned with mysticism for a number of reasons. The Group for the Advancement of Psychiatry (GAP), in its 1976 report, identified mysticism as a significant social force, which gives rise to movements that challenge the social order and are attractive to young people of 'marginal mental health' (Group for the Advancement of Psychiatry, Committee on Psychiatry and Religion, 1976, p. 812). The GAP report was controversial at the time (Deikman, 1977), and did not show much appreciation of the positive value of mysticism for mental and spiritual well-being. However, some of its conclusions do apply to the aberrant forms of spirituality discussed later in this book (see Chapter 17).

More importantly, mystical experiences share phenomenology with some psychiatric disorders or, to put things the other way around, psychiatric disorders sometimes evidence mystical phenomenology. Mysticism and mystical experience are touched upon in several chapters of this book, and the problem of misdiagnosis is very real (Cook, 2004b). For some, the overlap leads to a conclusion that experiences which might otherwise be considered as evidence of psychosis or dissociation (and historically as hysteria) should be normalised. For others, it supports the opposite conclusion, that much mystical experience should be diagnosed as psychiatric disorder. To take either of these conclusions to the extreme is not helpful, but there is some truth in both of them, and it is to the credit of the committee that produced the GAP report that it acknowledged its inability to make a clear distinction between mystical and psycho-pathological states (Group for the Advancement of Psychiatry, Committee on Psychiatry and Religion, 1976, p. 815).

The GAP report identified mysticism as involving 'a relationship with the supernatural which is not mediated by another person', the goal of which is 'mystical union' (Group for the Advancement of Psychiatry, Committee on Psychiatry and Religion, 1976, p. 717). For adherents to a perennialist philosophy, mystical union is understood as a core, common experience identifiable within all religions and (we might now also add) among those who identify as SBNR. However, such views have come under strong criticism from those who would argue that all experience is socially constructed and interpreted, and that there are significant differences between various kinds of mystical experience. W. T. Stace and R. C. Zaehner offer widely cited examples of the contrasting positions.

Stace (1973), in *Mysticism and Philosophy*, suggested that mystical states may be 'introvertive' (looking inwards, into the mind) or 'extrovertive' (looking outwards), but concluded that both types of mystical states are expressions of a fundamental experience of the unity of all things. The commonality of the experiences is thus emphasised over their diversity.

Zaehner (1973), in his influential book *Mysticism, Sacred and Profane*, identified at least three types – nature mysticism, monistic mysticism and theistic mysticism. In nature mysticism, according to Zaehner, including some drug-induced experiences and those associated with mental disorder, as well as others that occur spontaneously in the absence of any diagnosable disorder, the experience is essentially an atheistic one – an experience of 'all as one and one as all' (Zaehner, 1973, p. 28). Monistic mysticism (as in some Eastern religions) takes this a step further, denying the multiplicity of reality, and asserting that there is only one reality, of which the self is a part. This is not really an experience of mystical 'union' at all, for there is only one reality. In theistic mysticism (as, for example, in Islam and Christianity), in contrast, the experience of union, the distinction between God and self, is maintained and emphasised. Although the Christian or Muslim may experience a sense of union with God, he/she will always be other than God.

Mysticism may thus be understood as being about experiences of unmediated relationship with God, but it is not necessarily about union, or about God. In his Gifford Lectures in 1901–1902, William James proposed four 'marks' of mystical experience – ineffability, noetic quality, transiency and passivity (James, 1902). For James, mystical experience was concerned with relationship with a transcendent, or 'ultimate', reality. This relationship could be understood in a very individualistic way, and James rather over-emphasised the personal and subjective nature of the experience. In fact, mysticism is concerned with experiences of the relationship of an individual with both a transcendent reality and a community (often, but not always, a community of faith).

The features of mysticism overlap with those of psychosis and can sometimes present a challenge to diagnosis (Cook, 2004b). The nature of the relationship has been much debated, with some arguing that certain forms of psychosis are associated with spiritual growth, or else that mysticism may sometimes manifest features of psychosis (Lukoff, 1985). For instance, ecstatic mood, a sense of newly gained knowledge, auditory and visual hallucinations, and concern with mythological themes provide common ground which can sometimes be difficult to interpret phenomenologically.

Psychiatrists Interested in Spirituality and Religion

Psychiatrists have, as a profession, often been seen as dismissive of religion. However, the profession has been more sympathetic than sometimes portrayed. In a presidential address to the American Psychiatric Association (APA) in 1956, R. Finley Gayle suggested that the relationship between religion and psychiatry at that time might be understood as one of 'peaceful co-existence' (Gayle, 1956). In a presidential address to the Royal College of Psychiatrists (RCPsych) in the UK in 1993, Andrew Sims spoke of the tendency of psychiatrists to ignore and avoid the spiritual (Sims, 1994). What has been needed, at least until recent decades, has been a willingness to countenance a more positive and active engagement with spirituality and religion, something that both Gayle and Sims have strongly supported.

A more positive approach to spirituality and religion within North American psychiatry eventually emerged in the early 1980s (Aist, 2012). However, an ad hoc Committee on Relations between Psychiatry and Religion was authorised at the APA as early as 1956. In 1958 this became a standing committee. The present APA Caucus on Spirituality, Religion and Psychiatry was first convened in May 2012 to facilitate communication and collaboration among members interested in spirituality and religion as a dimension of their work as psychiatrists.[2]

The Spirituality and Psychiatry Special Interest Group (SPSIG) of the Royal College of Psychiatrists in the UK was inaugurated in 1999, at the initiative of Andrew Powell, in order to facilitate an exchange of ideas among psychiatrists, and to study 'experiences invested with spiritual meaning' (Shooter, 1999). Its meetings are designed to enable colleagues to investigate and share, without fear of censure, the relevance of spirituality to clinical practice. The SPSIG aims to contribute a framework of ideas of general interest to the College, stimulating discussion and promoting an integrative approach to mental health care. The diversity of its interests has been reflected in the very wide range of topics discussed at meetings, addressing almost all sub-specialties within psychiatry, as well as such matters as professional boundaries, the nature of evil, prayer, suffering, consciousness and spiritual care within the NHS.

At the time of writing, we are aware of sections or special interest groups devoted to spirituality/religion within the national psychiatric associations of at least seven other countries in addition to the UK and USA, including Austria, Canada, Germany, Hungary, Indonesia, South Africa and Thailand.

The World Psychiatric Association Section on Religion, Spirituality and Psychiatry was established in 2003 to influence clinical practice, encourage research, disseminate findings and develop educational programmes in relation to spirituality/religion and psychiatry (Verhagen, 2019, pp. 23–46).

---

[2] I would like to extend my thanks to John Peteet for advice on the dates and developments outlined in this paragraph.

The Spirituality and Religiosity of Patients

It has long been observed that there is a mismatch between the religiosity of patients and their mental health professionals, the former being more likely to believe in God and/or identify as religious than the latter. This is usually referred to as the 'religiosity gap'. Quantitatively, the size of the gap is difficult to measure, and is very variable in different studies, according to the measures used, nationality and the nature of the comparison groups (if any) (Cook, 2011a). Qualitatively, the gap is manifested by patient reports of perceived disrespect, discomfort, misunderstanding or misinterpretation (Van Nieuw Amerongen-Meeuse et al., 2019). Even if this only happens occasionally, it is a real cause for concern.

Religion or, more correctly, religiosity is a protective factor in and from mental illness. The work that demonstrates this is drawn together in two editions of *The Handbook of Religion and Health* (Koenig et al., 2001, 2012) and also in a separate volume, *Religion and Mental Health* (Koenig, 2018). Generally speaking, this now extensive body of published research shows that greater religiosity is associated with less depression, less suicidal ideation, less substance misuse and less delinquency and crime. It is also associated in some studies with less anxiety, but here the evidence is more mixed. Many of the studies are cross-sectional, and the possibility of reverse causation is highly problematic. Individuals may be more anxious because religion makes them so, or else because people pray more and go to church when they are anxious. Where randomised controlled trials of spiritual/religious interventions have been conducted, they generally show that such interventions reduce both anxiety and depression.

During illness, or in times of stress, people use their religious beliefs and spiritual practices as a way of coping. Generally, this appears to be helpful for mental health. However, rates of spiritual/religious coping vary around the world, and evidence for the benefits of such coping is weaker for studies undertaken in relatively more secular parts of the world (e.g., East Asia, and former communist countries). This may again be due to the effects of reverse causation (Koenig, 2018, pp. 59–68). However, there clearly are some circumstances in which religious coping seems to make things worse. So called negative religious coping, in particular religious or spiritual 'struggles', fall into this category. Some believers have difficulties with their understanding of, or relationship with, God. Others struggle with their doubts, or with other religious people or forms of spirituality/religion. Cause and effect are very difficult to disentangle, and research to date leaves some doubt as to whether negative religious coping makes mental health worse, or whether poor mental health generates negative religious coping. Quite possibly, causation works in both directions (Koenig, 2018, pp. 177–204). However, in such circumstances it is questionable whether or not religion and mental health can be adequately separated for the purposes of research. For a religious person, mental health and faith are inextricable, each to a large extent being a reflection of the other.

Nevertheless, it has been shown that, in some circumstances, religion can have an unambiguously negative impact on mental health (Koenig, 2018, pp. 295–309) This may be because of:

- a form of spirituality/religion that is harmful to self or others
- a particularly rigid or inflexible (or excessive) way of interpreting and practicing spirituality/religion (e.g., non-adherence to medication due to perceived conflict with beliefs, or a particularly judgemental approach to self or others)

- the use of religion to manipulate people
- the use of religion to avoid and neglect social responsibilities (e.g., clergy who spend all their time at work, or lay people who spend all their time at church).

Pathological spirituality of various kinds is discussed further in Chapter 17.

Spiritual Practices

Where patients are religious, their spiritual practices and their religious practices will be more or less the same thing. The individualistic and subjective emphasis that has become attached to the concept of spirituality in recent years may confer a sense that some things are more religious and others are more spiritual. Thus, for example, private prayer might more widely be thought of as a spiritual practice, whereas congregational worship might more often be seen as a religious practice. However, such distinctions are dubious, and tell us more about the way in which the use of the word 'spiritual' has developed than they do about any inherent or empirical differences between spiritual/religious practices.

Traditional religious practices will be discussed further in Chapter 16. What about the spiritual practices of those who self-identify as SBNR? To some extent, those who are SBNR draw from mainstream religious traditions in a selective and personal way, according to what they find most helpful. This has led to unsympathetic allegations that such spirituality is actually 'pick-and-mix' or 'do-it-yourself' religion (Houtman and Aupers, 2007). However, a very wide range of other practices, not traditionally thought of as religious, are also understood as spiritual outside the mainstream traditions (and also by some people within them). This diversity of 'spiritual' practices stretches the conventional boundaries of what might be considered spiritual or religious. For example, in a 1996 collection of essays titled *Spirituality and the Secular Quest* (Van Ness, 1996), chapters were included on, among other things, holistic health practices, psychotherapies, Twelve-Step programmes, struggles for social justice, naturalistic recreations, ecological activism and sport. Stretching the boundaries in this way might broaden the concept of spirituality so as to be almost meaningless, but that should not distract from the important sense in which such activities are perceived by many as being practical outworkings of their spirituality.

In the influential Kendal Project (Heelas and Woodhead, 2005), more than 50 'holistic milieu activities' associated with spirituality outside of congregational religious contexts were identified, including such things as aromatherapy, circle dancing, foot massage, herbalism, nutritional therapy, play therapy, rebirthing, reflexology, tai chi and yoga groups. To those who practice them, such things may well be understood as a turn towards a spirituality centred on wholeness of being, that seeks to find a balance of body, mind and spirit. They may (or may not) also represent a turning away from material concerns and institutional structures. However, more critically, it has been pointed out that spirituality is a commodity which has been exploited in the corporate world for financial gain (Carrette and King, 2005). Those who are vulnerable by virtue of mental illness may easily find meaning and hope in offerings advertised within this marketplace. However, this does not mean that all such practices are exploitative, or that there is no spiritual value in something that also has a cash value.

One part of the clinical challenge, then, is to explore each patient's individual sense of what is spiritual and to identify the practices that bring meaning and purpose to life. Sometimes these will be familiar within traditional religious frameworks, and sometimes they will not. However, it should never be assumed that the patient who says that they do not pray or meditate is unspiritual. Spirituality can take many forms.

Spirituality in Mental Health Research

Koenig has rightly drawn attention to the tautological and meaningless way in which much research has contaminated its measures of spirituality with the vocabulary of good mental health (Koenig, 2008). Such traits and qualities as optimism, meaning and purpose, sense of peace or feeling positive about life are as much (or more) measures of mental well-being as they are features of spirituality. Koenig therefore proposes that either spirituality should be defined differently, or else it should be 'eliminated' as a research variable. Taking predominantly the latter approach, his research focus in recent years has been on religion or (more precisely) religiosity, rather than spirituality, on the basis that this is measurable without the problems of confounding with mental health variables.

As discussed in more detail in Chapter 16, religion is much more difficult to define than Koenig allows, and the variables that he and others resort to in their quest for the definable, measurable and uncontaminated construct are actually measures of religiousness, or religiosity – the personal expression of religion – rather than religion per se. The word 'spirituality' (at least in the English language) does not so easily allow itself to be adapted to distinguish between the conceptual and the personal as the word 'religion' does. However, in principle, we can imagine objective measures of 'spiritualness' or 'spiritosity' which are not confounded with mental health, in the same way that many of the measures of religiosity proposed by Koenig are not thus confounded.

Given that most people in the world are religious, these measures of spiritosity will actually be measures of religiosity. Or, to put things the other way around, religiosity is the measurable manifestation of religious spirituality. This is all well and good in countries where most people are religious (including the Bible Belt in the USA, where Koenig lives and works), just as long as the measures of religiosity work well for members of different religious traditions participating in research. This is not necessarily so easy to achieve. For example, Question 3 in the widely used Duke University Religion Index (DUREL; Koenig and Büssing, 2010) does not work well if you are a member of a non-theistic religion (see Table 1.1). However, where research participants are SBNR, different measures are required. Those who are SBNR do not attend religious meetings, do not tend to have conventional theistic beliefs, and their personal spiritual practices (as discussed earlier) are diverse, but that is not to say that they are not in principle objectively measurable. Houtman and Tromp (2021), for example, have designed a seven-item Post-Christian Spirituality Scale (PCSS) for use in healthcare research that enquires about beliefs in such things as the relationship between spirituality and religion, the nature of the spiritual 'self', the encounter of the divine within each person, and the spiritual source of the universe.

A challenge for future research is thus to address the tension between the specific and the general in the measurement of spiritosity/religiosity. On the one hand, research tools are needed to address the specific identities, experiences and practices of those who are SBNR, or otherwise non-theistically spiritual/ religious. On the other hand, instruments are needed that enable greater inclusiveness across all spiritual/religious traditions (including those who are SBNR).

Table 1.1. Proposals for a research measure of spirituality that is not confounded with mental health outcomes

Question	Duke University Religion Index (DUREL)	Proposed Durham University Spirituality Index (DUSpir)
1	How often do you attend church or other religious meetings? (Organisational Religious Activity)	How often do you attend spiritual or religious meetings? (Organisational Spiritual Activity)
2	How often do you spend time in private religious activities, such as prayer, meditation or Bible study? (Non-Organisational Religious Activity)	How often do you spend time in private spiritual activities, such as prayer, meditation or study of spiritual texts? (Non-Organisational Spiritual Activity)
3	In my life, I experience the presence of the Divine (i.e., God) (Intrinsic Religiosity)	In my life, I experience the presence of a spiritual reality (e.g., God, ultimate reality or a life force) (Intrinsic Spirituality)
4	My religious beliefs are what really lie behind my whole approach to life (Intrinsic Religiosity)	My spiritual beliefs are what really lie behind my whole approach to life (Intrinsic Spirituality)
5	I try hard to carry my religion over into all other dealings in life (Intrinsic Religiosity)	I try hard to carry my spirituality over into all other dealings in life (Intrinsic Spirituality)

By way of example, and as a basis for discussion and reflection, Table 1.1 suggests a possible rewording of the DUREL so as to be inclusive of spirituality as well as religion.

How Do Spirituality/Religion Help Mental Health?

Koenig (2018, pp. 153–176) suggests that spirituality/religion influences all of the six known determinants of mental health:

1 *Genetic associations.* Genes associated with spirituality/religiosity have also been shown to be associated with altered risk for mental disorder. For example, Anderson et al. (2017) have shown that reported importance of spirituality/religion is associated with particular alleles in the dopamine DRD2, oxytocin, serotonin and vesicular transporter genes in people at low familial risk for depression. A minor allele of the DRD2 gene also appears to increase risk for depression in this group. The associations appear to be suppressed in people at high familial risk for depression. Association does not prove causation, but what we might have here is a biological mechanism by way of which spirituality/religiosity is suppressed and risk for depression is increased. Whether or not this is true, it draws attention to the often neglected scientific evidence that there may be a neurobiological basis for spirituality, as well as for some mental disorders (Perroud, 2009). Spirituality is not a separate domain of life, disconnected from the material (in this case, genetic), but is integrally expressed within the biopsychosocial matrix.

2 *Biological processes*, such as chronic inflammation, immune/endocrine function, modification of brain structure and chromosomal telomere length. For example, Miller et al. (2014) have shown that a thicker cortex in various brain regions is associated with high reported importance of spirituality/religion, and that this may confer resilience against depression in those who are at high familial risk. Although this study in itself does not prove the causal link, we may anticipate that future research will increasingly attend to such processes with a view to establishing (or

refuting) the part that they play. Again, we cannot assume that the underlying mechanisms are not biological, or that if they were this would in any way invalidate the importance of the spiritual. So-called 'hard science' has its part to play in understanding the relationship between spirituality/religion and mental health.

3   *Psychological factors*, such as coping resources (discussed earlier), priorities in life, attachment to God or image of God. An interesting example in this regard is provided by Silton et al. (2014), who showed that belief in a punitive God is positively associated with psychiatric symptoms (social anxiety, paranoia, obsessions and compulsions), whereas belief in a benevolent God is negatively associated with the same symptoms. Based upon this study, at least, belief in God in itself was not significantly related to mental health. However, beliefs about God almost certainly are important. In another study of psychiatric patients, negative images of God were shown to be associated with borderline, avoidant, schizotypal, schizoid, dependent and paranoid personality disorders (Schaap-Jonker et al., 2002).

4   *Social factors*. Religiosity is associated with a series of social variables known to be associated with good mental health, such as social support and marital stability/satisfaction, as well as providing some resilience in relation to discrimination and stigma.

5   *Environment*. The religiosity of parents may, directly or indirectly, influence the developmental environment for children during pregnancy and early life, through such factors as reduced substance use, better social support, and better coping with trauma and deprivation when these do occur.

6   *Personal choice*. Religion provides a set of values and expectations that guide prosocial choices (e.g., volunteering), reduce crime and build social capital.

There is thus no shortage of possible mechanisms whereby religion might be understood to exert a beneficial influence in regard to mental health. Some, any or all of them may be important in respect of different disorders or populations.

Most of this research has focused on measures of religiosity. We might speculate that these mechanisms apply also to spirituality as much as to religion, although, as we have noted, research on spirituality – as opposed to religion – encounters particular methodological problems. There is also some reason to believe that being SBNR may not have the same protective effects against mental disorder as does religion (King et al., 2013).

Spirituality in Psychiatric Treatment

Spirituality is increasingly being included as a component of psychiatric treatment, at least in some countries (notably the USA, but to a lesser extent also the UK and other European countries), in the form of some specific interventions, and also as an independent and dependent variable in treatment research. Furthermore, a variety of faith-based organisations (FBOs) are providing care for people with mental health problems (Koenig, 2005).

Psychotherapy and counselling that are based upon religious frameworks of belief (Rosmarin, 2018), that integrate spiritual approaches, or that are offered within the context of a faith community potentially bring great benefit. FBOs offer a variety of advantages to the delivery of mental health care in such a way as to facilitate the addressing of spiritual/religious concerns, but they also present particular complications and challenges (Leavey and King, 2007). Clergy are often not well informed about mental illness, just as psychiatrists are not always well informed about spirituality and religion, and the explanatory models that patients bring in respect of their condition may clash with those presented by medicine and science.

A number of different spiritual and religious interventions with a growing evidence base are considered further in Chapter 14. It is also possible to explore spirituality in the secular treatment setting. Organisations such as Alcoholics Anonymous explicitly adopt a spirituality that is open to people of all faith traditions or none (see Chapter 8).

Greater integration of spirituality into psychiatric treatment raises a number of significant questions concerning good professional practice and boundaries.

Boundaries and Policy

In 1990 the Committee on Religion and Psychiatry of the APA established guidelines for good practice that were intended to address, in particular, possible conflicts between psychiatrists' religious commitments and their clinical practice (American Psychiatric Association, 1990). In 2011 the Royal College of Psychiatrists in the UK approved a position statement, *Recommendations for Psychiatrists on Spirituality and Religion* (Cook, 2011b), which makes a series of seven recommendations covering various aspects of clinical and professional practice. They address, respectively:

1 assessment of spirituality/religion
2 respect and sensitivity towards the spiritual/religious beliefs and practices of patients
3 prohibition against proselytising, and an affirmation of the importance of professional boundaries
4 development of organisational policies that promote good practice
5 collaborative working with chaplains and faith leaders
6 respect for and sensitivity towards the spiritual/religious beliefs and practices of colleagues
7 psychiatric training and continuing professional development.

Since then, various other national psychiatric associations have formulated similar policy documents, and the World Psychiatric Association, drawing upon recommendations published by the Royal College of Psychiatrists (Cook, 2013b), has since approved its own position statement (Cook, 2017).

Policy documents and guidelines are helpful to some extent, but they cannot possibly address every clinical situation, and the boundaries of good practice often remain unclear (Poole et al., 2019). The ongoing debate as to what good practice looks like in relation to spirituality/religion has often focused on the importance of good boundaries (Cook, 2013a). It is generally expected that professionals should not operate outside the limits of their training, expertise or competence. They should not impose their personal views about spirituality/religion (whether these are spiritual, religious or atheistic) upon their patients. Perhaps even more controversial is the boundary between the secular and the spiritual/religious. Secular space, it is argued, protects patients against proselytising. However, it can also be experienced as unsafe by patients who want to discuss their spiritual/religious problems with a mental health professional and yet fear that they will encounter a negative and judgemental attitude if they do so. The history of separation between religion and psychiatry, with the legacies of Freud, the behaviourists and some strands of biological psychiatry, have left a suspicion that psychiatry is anti-spiritual and anti-religious. Added to this, there is the so-called 'religiosity gap', with patients more likely to be religious than their mental health professionals. The good clinician therefore needs to be sensitive to all of these considerations in making the consulting room a safe space in which to discuss anything and everything that the patient would like to talk about, including spirituality and religion.

The Royal College of Psychiatrists' position statement (Cook, 2013b) identifies four possible attitudes that patients (or colleagues) may have towards spirituality/religion:

- identification with a particular social or historical tradition (or traditions)
- adoption of a personally defined, or personal but undefined, spirituality
- disinterest
- antagonism.

Any opening question about spirituality/religion has to be worded and delivered in such a way as to be sensitive to any or all of these possible attitudes. Mishandling of this risks alienating the patient and causing harm. Although some clinicians seem to have a more or less instinctive ability to get such things right, there is also reason to believe that it is easy to get it wrong. There is therefore a need for better training to address the relevant clinical skills and attitudes that enable the clinician to negotiate such encounters successfully and safely.

Training in Spirituality and Psychiatry

Training in spirituality/religion should begin with undergraduate medical education, and is important within all medical professions, including nursing, clinical psychology, psychotherapy and occupational therapy. The focus here will be on postgraduate education, and especially that directed towards the training of psychiatrists.

The World Psychiatric Association and the Royal College of Psychiatrists both have recommendations in their respective position statements concerning the importance of training on spirituality/religion in psychiatry. In the Royal College of Psychiatrists' position statement, the recommendation is that:

> Religion and spirituality and their relationship to the diagnosis, aetiology and treatment of psychiatric disorders should be considered as essential components of both psychiatric training and continuing professional development. (Cook, 2013b)

A recent report by a Royal College of Psychiatrists' working group has also advised that person-centred care, in which spirituality is identified as one key aspect, should occupy a central place in the practice and training of psychiatrists (Royal College of Psychiatrists, 2018; Royal College of Psychiatrists Person-Centred Training and Curriculum Scoping Group, 2019). The World Psychiatric Association includes religion and spirituality within 'general aspects' of its core training curriculum for psychiatry, but provides no detail as to exactly what this should include (López-Ibor et al., 2002). Around the world, policies and curricula have developed differently. In the USA, in 1994 the Accreditation Council for Graduate Medical Education (ACGME) made spirituality/religion a mandatory component of psychiatric residency programmes (Puchalski et al., 2001).

In the UK, the Competency Based Curriculum for Specialist Core Training in Psychiatry introduced in 2006 by the Royal College of Psychiatrists made passing reference to spirituality and religion, but largely left these factors implicit within consideration of the cultural context. In the April 2020 revision, spiritual factors were explicitly mentioned only once (in relation to clinical history taking), but again a lot more was said about cultural context, within which religion (if not also spirituality) is arguably an important consideration. The new core curriculum, adopted in 2021, makes no specific reference to spirituality or religion in its high-level learning outcomes, but spirituality/ religion have been included in the key capabilities that expand upon what is required in support of each of these outcomes. Spirituality is also included within the draft person-centred holistic model of psychiatry outlined in the 'Silver Guide' that provides guidance for psychiatric training in the UK. It remains to be seen whether or not the new curriculum will measure up in practice to the Royal College of Psychiatrists' position statement recommendation that:

> Religion and spirituality and their relationship to the diagnosis, aetiology and treatment of psychiatric disorders should be considered as *essential* components of both psychiatric training and continuing professional development. (Cook, 2013b, my emphasis)

Whether or not spirituality and religion are actually addressed in practice during psychiatric training is another matter, and research on this is limited. Since 1994, attention to this element of the curriculum appears to have increased in the USA, but even there only a minority of programs actually teach spirituality/religion to their residents. Elsewhere in the world much less information is available (Bowman, 2009). For example, some interesting work on the curriculum for psychiatric residents has emerged from Brazil (as discussed later in this chapter), but without any information (to date) about how many residents actually receive such training in practice.

What should be taught? It is clear that most psychiatrists will not become experts in the study of religion, and that an in-depth knowledge of the beliefs and practices of all of the world's major faith traditions is likely to be acquired by very few, if any, medical practitioners. In any case, a patient-centred approach does not require that the doctor should know all about his or her patient's religion, but rather that he or she should be able to show awareness of the importance of spirituality/religion, and enquire sensitively into what it means to the person seeking his or her help. Many religious people do not adopt or accept all of the orthodox beliefs and practices of their faith tradition, and so assumptions cannot be made. Many people draw on elements of a variety of traditions. For those who identify as SBNR, spirituality is likely to be highly individualistic and subjective.

Curricula for psychiatric training in the USA and UK now commonly include attention to knowledge, skills and attitudes for each of their learning outcomes. Thus, for example, in relation to a learning outcome for assessment, it is clear that the trainee/ resident should have the knowledge to recognise the ways in which patients draw on spiritual/religious resources to cope with illness and adversity, the skills to elicit information about the patient's spiritual/religious beliefs/practices, and an attitude of respect towards these beliefs/practices. Other learning outcomes for which spirituality/religion should be considered especially relevant include those for formulation/diagnosis, investigation, treatment (especially in relation to spiritually integrated psychotherapies) and risk assessment (especially for risk of self-harm). Teaching on the causes of mental disorder requires that attention be given to spirituality/religion as – potentially – both protective and risk factors (usually the former rather than the latter). Communication and collaboration with patients and professional colleagues (including clergy, chaplains and other religious leaders) are also important components of training within which attention to spirituality/religion should be given particular attention. (For an example of knowledge, skills and attitudes in relation to learning objectives for a psychiatric curriculum in the USA, see Puchalski et al., 2001.)

Kozak et al. (2010) describe a curriculum for psychiatric residents, which was introduced in Seattle in 2003. It is spread across the entire four years of training, and includes didactic teaching as well as rotational clinical experience, grand rounds, case conferences, fieldwork and involvement in a programme of feedback. The stated objectives of the programme were to:

- familiarise residents with the research literature on spirituality/religion in psychiatry
- expose residents to a variety of spiritual/religious traditions
- develop competency in engaging with spirituality/religion in assessment, formulation, differential diagnosis and treatment planning
- consider how patients' spirituality/religion may affect treatment
- address clinical ethical issues
- consider spirituality/religion in a developmental context
- provide a forum for discussion of residents' own spirituality/religion and the impact of this on their professional work.

A group of Brazilian psychiatrists (De Oliveira e Oliveira et al., 2020) have recently proposed a curriculum for a 12-hour course, covering historical context, the World Psychiatric Association position statement, assessment of spirituality/religion, spiritual/religious traditions, differential diagnosis and integration of spirituality/religion into treatment. The course employed mixed methods of teaching, including group work, clinical skills (history taking, formulation and diagnosis), discussion of clinical cases, fieldwork and individual supervision, as well as didactic teaching. A residency programme in the USA has also found community partnerships helpful (De Oliveira e Oliveira et al., 2020).

Does training actually make a difference? In a study in Texas of a three-year curriculum for psychiatry residents, McGovern et al. (2017) reported that residents ($n = 12$) who completed the programme found it to have been helpful, and that 77% of them considered the spiritual/religious needs of patients to be important. However, this study did not compare attitudes before and after training. In another study, from Stanford, California, involving an evaluation of a process-orientated approach to training of psychiatry residents, a six-session course was found to produce a statistically significant improvement in perceptions of competency, and changes in professional practice (Awaad et al., 2015). Unfortunately, this study lacked a comparison group and there was no longer-term follow-up to assess whether or not the changes were enduring.

Furthering Spirituality in Mental Health Care

Spirituality and religion have evoked strong feelings within psychiatry, both among patients and among professionals. Mutual respect for the beliefs of those from different faiths, as well as those not aligned with any faith tradition, are needed, recognising that we can make more headway collectively than individually. It is important that all those who consider religious and spiritual aspects of psychiatry to be important feel able to work together, whether in local mental health services, in national or international professional bodies or in research. It is also important that professionals and researchers are able to collaborate together with those who do not consider spirituality and religion to be important.

This book aims to make a contribution to tolerance and mutual respect within mental health care. In order to meet the aspirations of our patients, and the appropriate standards of good professional practice, psychiatrists need to be aware of the current debates and controversies, familiar (at least to a basic level) with both the scientific evidence base and the wider field of knowledge concerning spirituality/religion, and competent in the relevant clinical skills. The case for the importance of spirituality/ religion in psychiatry is easily overstated or understated, and a measured estimate is required.

In recent years, mental health statutory and voluntary organisations have both become much more aware of the spiritual aspirations of both patients and professional staff (Cook et al., 2012). Faith communities, too, have an important part to play in supporting and caring for people with mental health problems (Corrigan, 2020). By drawing on the insights of faith communities, the experiences of those who are SBNR, and working together across professional and disciplinary boundaries, we can best help our patients to feel safe and listened to. By improving training and continuing professional development, to expand the vision of clergy and mental health professionals alike, we can better ensure mutual respect and understanding. Diversity of spiritual and religious identities of patients and staff brings a greater breadth of perspective to mental health care; recognition and appreciation of this diversity is necessary if patients are to have confidence in the professionals who provide their care.

Conclusion

As Swinton puts it (2001, p. 174), psychiatrists and other mental health professionals need to be bilingual, 'fluent in two languages: the language of psychiatry and psychology ... and the language of spirituality that focuses on issues of meaning, hope, value, connectedness and transcendence'. We might add here that the many languages of religion are also important. It is probably fair to say that for too long psychiatry has neglected the languages of spirituality and religion to the detriment of the profession and – more importantly – to the detriment of patients. That the language of spirituality is now being heard more widely spoken within the consulting room is very encouraging, but like all languages this one requires practice. Psychiatrists need to be receptive to the words their patients use when talking about religion or spirituality and, at the same time, find ways to translate the language of psychiatry into a vocabulary familiar to their patients – one that includes, and values, spiritual and religious concerns.

Whilst this process of translation is vital, it should not be taken to indicate that spirituality is reducible to the vocabulary of psychiatry, neuroscience and psychology. Spirituality addresses things that are important to deeper understanding of the human condition. The language of spirituality needs to permeate our relationships with our patients and our colleagues, and our whole understanding of the field of psychiatry.

References

Aist, C. S. (2012) The recovery of religious and spiritual significance in American psychiatry. *Journal of Religion and Health*, 51, 615–629.

Allport, G. W. and Ross, J. M. (1967) Personal religious orientation and prejudice. *Journal of Personality and Social Psychology*, 5, 432–443.

American Psychiatric Association (1990) Guidelines regarding possible conflict between psychiatrists' religious commitment and psychiatric practice. *American Journal of Psychiatry*, 147, 542.

Ammerman, N. T. (2013) Spiritual but not religious? Beyond binary choices in the study of religion. *Journal for the Scientific Study of Religion*, 52, 258–278.

Anderson, M. R., Miller, L., Wickramaratne, P. et al. (2017) Genetic correlates of spirituality/religion and depression: a study in offspring and grandchildren at high and low familial risk for depression. *Spirituality in Clinical Practice (Washington, DC)*, 4, 43–63.

Ansah-Asamoah, E., Hacker-Huges, J., Hankir, A. and Cook, C. C. H. (2021) Religion, spirituality and mental health. In G. Ikkos and N. Bouras, eds., *Mind, State and Society: Social History of Psychiatry and Mental Health in Britain 1960-2010*. Cambridge: Cambridge University Press, pp. 373–383.

Awaad, R., Ali, S., Salvador, M. and Bandstra, B. (2015) A process-oriented approach to teaching religion and spirituality in psychiatry residency training. *Academic Psychiatry*, 39, 654–660.

Bowker, J., ed. (1999) *The Oxford Dictionary of World Religions*. Oxford: Oxford University Press.

Bowman, E. S. (2009) Teaching religious and spiritual issues. In P. Huguelet and H. G. Koenig, eds., *Religion and Spirituality in Psychiatry*. Cambridge: Cambridge University Press, pp. 332–353.

Carrette, J. and King, R. (2005) *Selling Spirituality: The Silent Takeover of Religion*. London: Routledge.

Cook, C. C. H. (2004a) Addiction and spirituality. *Addiction*, 99, 539–551.

Cook, C. C. H. (2004b) Psychiatry and mysticism. *Mental Health, Religion & Culture*, 7, 149–163.

Cook, C. C. H. (2011a) The faith of the psychiatrist. *Mental Health, Religion & Culture*, 14, 9–17.

Cook, C. C. H. (2011b) *Recommendations for Psychiatrists on Spirituality and Religion*. London: Royal College of Psychiatrists.

Cook, C. C. H. (2013a) Controversies on the place of spirituality and religion in psychiatric practice. In C. C. H. Cook, ed., *Spirituality, Theology and Mental Health*. London: SCM, pp. 1–19.

Cook, C. C. H. (2013b) *Recommendations for Psychiatrists on Spirituality and Religion*. London: Royal College of Psychiatrists.

Cook, C. C. H. (2013c) Transcendence, immanence and mental health. In C. C. H. Cook,, ed., *Spirituality, Theology and Mental Health*. London: SCM, pp. 141–159.

Cook, C. C. H. (2017) Spirituality and religion in psychiatry: the impact of policy. *Mental Health, Religion & Culture*, 20, 589–594.

Cook, C. C. H. (2020) Spirituality, religion & mental health: exploring the boundaries. *Mental Health, Religion & Culture*, 23, 363–374.

Cook, C. C. H., Breckon, J., Jay, C., Renwick, L. and Walker, P. (2012) Pathway to accommodate patients' spiritual needs. *Nursing Management*, 19, 33–37.

Corrigan, P. W. (2020) Challenges to welcoming people with mental illnesses into faith communities. *British Journal of Psychiatry*, 217, 595–596.

De Oliveira e Oliveira, F. H. A., Peteet, J. R. and Moreira-Almeida, A. (2020) Religiosity and spirituality in psychiatry residency programs: why, what, and how to teach? *Brazilian Journal of Psychiatry*, 43, 424–429.

Deikman, A. J. (1977) Comments on the GAP report on mysticism. *Journal of Nervous and Mental Disease*, 165, 213–217.

Fuller, R. C. (2001) *Spiritual, But Not Religious: Understanding Unchurched America*. Oxford: Oxford University Press.

Gayle, R. F. (1956) Conflict and cooperation between psychiatry and religion. *Pastoral Psychology*, 7, 29–36.

Group for the Advancement of Psychiatry, Committee on Psychiatry and Religion (1976) *Mysticism: Spiritual Quest or Psychic Disorder?* New York: Group for the Advancement of Psychiatry.

Heelas, P. and Woodhead, L. (2005) *The Spiritual Revolution: Why Religion Is Giving Way to Spirituality*. Oxford: Blackwell Publishing Ltd.

Houtman, D. and Aupers, S. (2007) The spiritual turn and the decline of tradition: the spread of post-Christian spirituality in 14 western countries, 1981–2000. *Journal for the Scientific Study of Religion*, 46, 305–320.

Houtman, D. and Tromp, P. (2021) The Post-Christian Spirituality Scale (PCSS): misconceptions, obstacles, prospects. In P. L. Ai, P. Wink, R. F. Paloutzian and K. A. Harris, eds., *Assessing Spirituality in a Diverse World*. Cham: Springer International, pp. 35–57.

James, W. (1902) *The Varieties of Religious Experience: A Study in Human Nature*. New York: Longmans, Green & Co.

Johnson, T. M., Grim, B. J. and Bellofatto, G. A. (2013) *The World's Religions in Figures: An Introduction to International Religious Demography*. Oxford: Wiley-Blackwell.

Karlsson, H. and Kamppinen, M. (1995) Biological psychiatry and reductionism: empirical findings and philosophy. *British Journal of Psychiatry*, 167, 434–438.

Kemp, S. and Williams, K. (1987) Demonic possession and mental disorder in medieval and early modern Europe. *Psychological Medicine*, 17, 21–29.

King, M., Marston, L., Mcmanus, S. et al. (2013) Religion, spirituality, and mental health: results from a national study of English households. *British Journal of Psychiatry*, 202, 68–73.

Koenig, H. G. (2005) *Faith and Mental Health*. Philadelphia, PA: Templeton Foundation Press.

Koenig, H. G. (2008) Concerns about measuring "spirituality" in research. *Journal of Nervous and Mental Disease*, 196, 349–355.

Koenig, H. G. (2018) *Religion and Mental Health: Research and Clinical Applications*. London: Academic Press.

Koenig, H. G. and Büssing, A. (2010) The Duke University Religion Index (DUREL): a five-item measure for use in epidemological studies. *Religions*, 1, 78–85.

Koenig, H. G., Mccullough, M. E. and Larson, D. B., eds. (2001) *Handbook of Religion and Health*. New York: Oxford University Press.

Koenig, H. G., King, D. E. and Carson, V. B., eds. (2012) *Handbook of Religion and Health*. New York: Oxford University Press.

Kozak, L., Boynton, L., Bentley, J. and Bezy, E. (2010) Introducing spirituality, religion and culture curricula in the psychiatry residency programme. *Medical Humanities*, 36, 48–51.

Larson, D. B., Pattison, E. M., Blazer, D. G., Omran, A. R. and Kaplan, B. H. (1986) Systematic analysis of research on religious variables in four major psychiatric journals, 1978–1982. *American Journal of Psychiatry*, 143, 329–334.

Leavey, G. and King, M. (2007) The devil is in the detail: partnerships between psychiatry and faith-based organisations. *British Journal of Psychiatry*, 191, 97–98.

López-Ibor, J. J., Okasha, A., Ruiz, P., Katona, C. and Mak, F. L. (2002) *World Psychiatric Association Institutional Program on the Core Training Curriculum for Psychiatry*. Yokohama, Japan: World Psychiatric Association.

Lukoff, D. (1985) The diagnosis of mystical experiences with psychotic features. *Journal of Transpersonal Psychology*, 17, 155–181.

McGovern, T. F., Mcmahon, T., Nelson, J. et al. (2017) A descriptive study of a spirituality curriculum for general psychiatry residents. *Academic Psychiatry*, 41, 471–476.

Mental Health Foundation (2002) *Taken Seriously: The Somerset Spirituality Project.* London: Mental Health Foundation.

Mercadante, L. (2014) *Belief Without Borders: Inside the Minds of the Spiritual but Not Religious.* Oxford: Oxford University Press.

Miller, L., Bansal, R., Wickramaratne, P. et al. (2014) Neuroanatomical correlates of religiosity and spirituality: a study in adults at high and low familial risk for depression. *JAMA Psychiatry*, 71, 128–135.

Perroud, N. (2009) Religion/spirituality and neuropsychiatry. In P. Huguelet and H. G. Koenig, eds., *Religion and Spirituality in Psychiatry.* Cambridge: Cambridge University Press, pp. 48–64.

Poole, R., Cook, C. C. H. and Higgo, R. (2019) Psychiatrists, spirituality and religion. *British Journal of Psychiatry*, 214, 181–182.

Principe, W. (1983) Toward defining spirituality. *Studies in Religion*, 12, 127–141.

Puchalski, C. M., Larson, D. B. and Lu, F. G. (2001) Spirituality in psychiatry residency training programs. *International Review of Psychiatry*, 13, 131–138.

Richardson, J. T. (1993) Religiosity as deviance: negative religious bias in and misuse of the DSM-III. *Deviant Behavior*, 14, 1–21.

Rosmarin, D. H. (2018) *Spirituality, Religion, and Cognitive-Behavioral Therapy: A Guide for Clinicians.* New York: Guilford.

Royal College of Psychiatrists (2018) *Person-Centred Care: Implications for Training in Psychiatry.* London: Royal College of Psychiatrists.

Royal College of Psychiatrists Person-Centred Training and Curriculum Scoping Group (2019) Training in psychiatry: making person-centred care a reality. *BJPsych Bulletin*, 43, 136–140.

Schaap-Jonker, H., Eurelings-Bontekoe, E., Verhagen, P. J. and Zock, H. (2002) Image of God and personality pathology: an exploratory study among psychiatric patients. *Mental Health, Religion & Culture*, 5, 55–71.

Shooter, M. (1999) Proposal for a Special Interest Group in spirituality and psychiatry. *Psychiatric Bulletin*, 23, 310.

Shorter, E. (2005) *A Historical Dictionary of Psychiatry.* Oxford: Oxford University Press.

Silton, N. R., Flannelly, K. J., Galek, K. and Ellison, C. G. (2014) Beliefs about God and mental health among American adults. *Journal of Religion and Health*, 53, 1285–1296.

Sims, A. (1994) 'Psyche' – spirit as well as mind? *British Journal of Psychiatry*, 165, 441–446.

Slater, E. and Roth, M. (1979) *Clinical Psychiatry.* London: Baillière Tindall.

Stace, W. T. (1973) *Mysticism and Philosophy.* London: Macmillan.

Streib, H. and Hood, R. W. (2011) 'Spirituality' as privatized experience-oriented religion: empirical and conceptual perspectives. *Implicit Religion*, 14, 433–453.

Swinton, J. (2001) *Spirituality and Mental Health Care.* London: Jessica Kingsley Publishers.

Tyler, P., Mclean, J. and Cook, C. C. H. (2018) Introduction: mystical theology: renewing the contemplative tradition. In C. C. H. Cook, J. Mclean and P. Tyler, eds., *Mystical Theology and Contemporary Spiritual Practice: Renewing the Contemplative Tradition.* London: Routledge, pp. 1–8.

Van Ness, P. H. (1996) *Spirituality and the Secular Quest.* London: SCM.

Van Nieuw Amerongen-Meeuse, J. C., Schaap-Jonker, H., Schuhmann, C., Anbeek, C. and Braam, A. W. (2019) The 'religiosity gap' in a clinical setting: experiences of mental health care consumers and professionals. *Mental Health, Religion & Culture*, 21, 737–752.

Verhagen, P. J. (2019) *Psychiatry and Religion: Controversies and Consensus: A Matter of Attitude*. Duren: Shaker Verlag.

Wixwat, M. and Saucier, G. (2020) Being spiritual but not religious. *Current Opinion in Psychology*, 40, 121–125.

Zaehner, R. C. (1973) *Mysticism: Sacred and Profane*. Oxford: Oxford University Press.

Zilboorg, G. and Henry, G. W. (1941) *A History of Medical Psychology*. New York: Norton.

<table>
<tr><td>

Chapter

2
</td><td>

Spiritual Assessment

Linda Ross, Lucy Grimwade and Sarah Eagger[1]
</td></tr>
</table>

Introduction

For many people the spiritual dimension is an important anchor as they seek to navigate life's often turbulent journey. In the literature the spiritual dimension has long been regarded as the unifying force that holds everything else together (Ross, 1997; Swinton, 2020). If it is important when people are well, it will be just as important, if not more so, when they are ill. This chapter focuses specifically on people with mental illnesses who may benefit from an assessment of their spiritual needs. In order to carry out any assessment it is important to know what is being assessed. We therefore begin this chapter by exploring the nature of spirituality. We ask 'why' psychiatric patients' spiritual needs should be addressed, before moving on to look at the questions of 'how', 'who' and 'when' (Koenig, 2013). We explore some of the thorny issues and considerations that arise when conducting such an assessment. Finally, we consider what happens after the assessment. If you do not have time to read the entire chapter but are looking for a quick guide on how to include a spiritual assessment, we would direct you to the Royal College of Psychiatrists (RCPsych) leaflet titled *Spirituality and Mental Health* (Cook and Grimwade, 2021).

Understanding Spirituality

How spirituality is understood has been hotly debated and contested for decades, with a rich variety of understandings. (See also Chapter 1 and, for the relationship with religion, Chapter 16.) Swinton (2010) offers three different lenses through which spirituality might be 'experienced', as opposed to defined (Swinton, 2020), namely the lens of religion, the lens of biology and the generic lens. It is the latter lens that has largely been adopted within health care (Ross and McSherry, 2021). In 2013, international experts met to seek consensus in mapping out the spiritual territory (Puchalski et al., 2014). Organisations such as the European Association of Palliative Care (EAPC) and nursing

---

[1] The authors wish to record their thanks to Dr Larry Culliford, co-author of this chapter in the first edition, for his valued suggestions during the preparation of this new chapter. We are also grateful to consultant psychiatrists Dr Russell Razzaque and Dr Rob Waller for their helpful comments on the manuscript and for their advice on current psychiatry texts and approaches to documentation in the UK. Thanks also to Information Services at the Royal College of Psychiatrists for their help with the literature review, and to James Michael Turner for assisting with the referencing.

and midwifery educators across Europe (McSherry et al., 2020) have accepted this understanding: 'Spirituality is the dynamic dimension of human life that relates to the way persons (individual and community) experience, express and/or seek meaning, purpose and transcendence, and the way they connect to the moment, to self, to others, to nature, to the significant and/or the sacred' (Nolan et al., 2011, p. 88).

The spiritual field is multidimensional, containing:

1 existential challenges (e.g., questions concerning identity, meaning, suffering and death, guilt and shame, reconciliation and forgiveness, freedom and responsibility, hope and despair, love and joy)
2 value-based considerations and attitudes (what is most important for each person, such as relations to oneself, family, friends, work, things, nature, art and culture, ethics and morals, and life itself)
3 religious considerations and foundations (faith, beliefs and practices, the relationship with God or the ultimate) (Nolan et al., 2011).

In psychiatry, spirituality has been referred to as:

a distinctive, potentially creative, and universal dimension of human experience arising both within the inner subjective awareness of individuals and within communities, social groups and traditions. It may be experienced as a relationship with that which is intimately 'inner', immanent, and personal, within the self and others, and/or as relationship with that which is wholly 'other', transcendent and beyond the self. It is experienced as being of fundamental or ultimate importance and is thus concerned with matters of meaning and purpose in life, truth, and values. (Cook, 2004, pp. 548–549)

Concept analyses (Tanyi, 2002; Weathers et al., 2015; Murgia et al., 2020) have distilled the multiple aspects of spirituality into three key elements:

- meaning
- connection (with self, others or nature/a higher power)
- transcendence.

It is well known in psychiatry that absence of meaning, and feelings of disconnection from self, or from what is important (others or a higher power), are linked with mental illness. Spirituality is therefore of particular relevance to psychiatrists, and it is at the heart of many therapies (Cook, 2015; Koenig et al., 2020a). Spirituality is now generally understood as broader than religion. However, the terms 'spirituality' and 'religion' are often used interchangeably, with 'religion' having become favoured by some leading researchers in the USA, such as Harold Koenig. Empirical research studies often choose to measure religion, religiosity or religious involvement rather than spirituality, believing that these concepts may be easier to define. (This is discussed further in Chapters 1 and 16.) We therefore refer to spirituality/religion in this chapter.

Spiritual Assessment: Why?

There are various reasons for including a spiritual/religious assessment in psychiatry. These include the following:

1 The beneficial effects that spirituality can bring to a patient's mental health by providing motivation, hope and feelings of connection, belonging and being valued.

With an increasing focus on a strengths-based approach to care (Allott et al., 2020), inclusion of an assessment of a person's spirituality would seem essential to identifying spiritual strengths that could improve resilience and longer-term wellness (e.g., identifying times, examples and aspects of spirituality that have been supportive in the past).

2   Patient/carer preference, which largely shows a desire to have spirituality/religion acknowledged and taken into account, both in mental health care (Stanley et al., 2011; Pargament and Lomax, 2013; Moreira-Almeida et al., 2014) and in other healthcare settings (Balboni et al., 2017; Selman et al., 2017; Ross and Miles, 2020), even if patients do not expect that this will actually happen (Pujol et al., 2018). Multiple patient organisations, such as the Spiritual Crisis Network,[2] make a similar plea, and a patient-led instrument that includes spirituality as one aspect of recovery has been developed to help make this happen (Barber, 2012). Despite this call from patients and carers, few mental health clinicians include a spiritual/religious assessment in their clinical practice (Moreira-Almeida et al., 2014). This means that there is potentially huge unmet patient and carer need. Studies show that taking a spiritual history in psychiatry has a number of benefits, so failure to do so is at odds with best practice. The benefits include greater satisfaction with care, feeling valued and treated as a whole person, feeling less depressed, improved quality of life (QoL), increased likelihood of using positive coping strategies, enhanced trust in clinicians (Moreira-Almeida et al., 2014) and improved treatment adherence (Huguelet et al., 2011).

Although their study was not specifically related to mental health, Selman et al. (2017) asked patients ($n = 74$) with advanced disease and their carers ($n = 71$) from nine countries to describe the most important elements of 'spiritual care' and its prerequisites. Their responses are summarised in Box 2.1.

Box 2.1   Spiritual care and its prerequisites (Selman, 2017)

Elements of spiritual care:

Help with integrating personal faith into the illness experience
Providing a safe space
Sympathetic and confidential listening and counselling
Providing existential support
Human connection at a difficult time
Care that goes beyond the physical.

Prerequisites to spiritual care:

Approaches to care that facilitate connection:

- Putting the patient first
- Making an extra effort
- Being reliable and present
- Seeing spiritual care as integral to all care
- Not stereotyping or categorising
- Providing individualised care

---

[2] https://spiritualcrisisnetwork.uk/directory (accessed 20 December 2020).

Box 2.1 *(cont.)*

Personal attributes of the clinician:

- Openness
- Respect
- Genuineness
- Non-judgement
- Hopefulness
- Honesty
- Empathy
- Kindness
- Being spiritually aware
- Not proselytising or being prescriptive

Although many studies are small and limited, emerging evidence suggests that spiritual care is linked to greater patient satisfaction with care (Balboni et al., 2017) and enhanced mental well-being/QoL in palliative care (Steinhauser et al., 2017; Ross and Miles, 2020) and in primary care (Kevern and Hill, 2015; Gibbon and Baldie, 2019). One small retrospective study found primary care chaplaincy was as effective as antidepressants (Macdonald, 2017). Another reported reduced patient time spent with GPs and improved staff resilience, with reduced sickness and absence (Snowden et al., 2018). In an era when patient-reported outcome measures (PROMs) are increasingly being used within value- based care, the Scottish PROM looks promising as a validated measure of spiritual care as delivered by chaplains (Snowden and Telfer, 2020). In addition, staff who provide spiritual care may personally benefit from greater job satisfaction and self-growth.

3   The relationship between spirituality/religion and mental health.

The last decade has seen an escalation in research pointing to a link between the spiritual/religious aspects of people's lives and their health, QoL and ability to cope with life's many challenges (Koenig et al., 2012; Steinhauser et al., 2017; see also Chapter 1). Policy stakeholders highlight the importance of including spiritual, religious and cultural aspects of people's lives within an holistic construct (European Commission, 2010; Welsh Government, 2015). The World Health Organization considers spirituality to be a dimension of quality of life (World Health Organization, 2006). Within psychiatry specifically, hundreds of studies have demonstrated the largely positive correlation of spirituality/religion with substance use disorders and reduced risk of suicide, and the moderately positive correlation of spirituality/religion with reduced risk of depression, some trauma-related disorders and antisocial personality disorders, with mixed results for other disorders such as bipolar disorder, anxiety and schizophrenia. Recent research is focusing on moral injury (Koenig, 2012; Koenig et al., 2020b). None of these studies prove cause and effect, and the mechanisms underlying the effects are unclear (Kao et al., 2020).

Based on this strong evidence, psychiatric associations across the world have highlighted the importance of including a spiritual/religious assessment. These include the Royal College of Psychiatrists in the UK (RCPsych) (Cook, 2013), the American Psychiatric Association (APA) in the USA (American Psychiatric Association, 1990) and the World

Psychiatric Association (WPA) (Moreira-Almeida et al., 2016). The National Institute for Health and Care Excellence (NICE) (2020) recommends that professionals assessing children and young people with depression should ask about, and be ready to advise on, self-help materials, including 'faith groups'. The *Diagnostic and Statistical Manual of Mental Disorders* makes a similar recommendation for all age groups in its 'Cultural Formulation Interview' (Lewis-Fernandez et al., 2016).

However, despite these evidence-based recommendations it seems that the assessment of spirituality/religion is given little attention. For example, a key psychiatry text in the UK, *The Maudsley Handbook of Practical Psychiatry*, sixth edition (Owen et al., 2014), makes no mention of spirituality/religion. The same applies to another key text, *Companion to Psychiatric Studies*, eighth edition (Johnstone et al., 2010). The tide may be turning, however, with the inclusion of a chapter on 'Psychiatry and spirituality' in the tenth edition of *Kaplan & Sadock's Comprehensive Textbook of Psychiatry* (Sadock et al., 2017). Although the World Psychiatric Association (2002) recommends that spiritual/religious assessment should be covered in the didactic curriculum, it is given scant attention in psychiatry residency programmes in the USA (de Oliveira et al., 2020) and in the new RCPsych core curriculum (Royal College of Psychiatrists, 2020) (see Chapter 1). Instead the latter focuses on person-centred treatment. We look at some of the reasons for this mismatch in the section on 'Thorny issues and other considerations', later in this chapter.

The first step in clinical treatment is the assessment. This chapter seeks to fill a vital gap by considering how psychiatrists may go about including a spiritual assessment within their clinical practice.

Spiritual Assessment: How?

Basic Principles

The psychiatric assessment takes place within a dynamic clinician–patient relationship. Therefore any suggestions on how to ask about spirituality should be used flexibly according to the level of rapport built, permission given, the patient's choice of words and their type of need.

When approaching a new patient, the clinician does not know in advance whether they are spiritual, religious, both or neither. The initial question therefore has to be sensitive to all of these potentialities – including the possibility that the patient might be offended by any assumption that they are spiritual or religious (Cook, 2013). The clinician must communicate an acceptance and respect for all patients' worldviews. Spirituality is personal, intimate and sometimes mocked by society. A patient who is already experiencing the stigma of a mental illness does not want to expose him- or herself to more. An off-the-cuff comment made by the clinician, felt as rejection of the patient's belief, may destroy the therapeutic rapport and shut down communication. Rapport can be enhanced by exploring the positive impact of spirituality on coping, resilience and self-esteem.

We are not merely seeking to describe a person's spirituality, but crucially, to understand how it relates to the illness, and whether it relates to care planning. Spirituality and mental illness are similarly intangible, and both are expressed in thoughts, feelings and behaviours. They can easily become entangled with one another, each influencing the other in ways that might be difficult for the patient to discern. The purpose of the assessment is partly to enable the patient to reflect on their spirituality and how this relates to their illness. The clinician is well placed to do this, as he or she has expertise in mental health and communication skills, whereas the patient is the expert in his or her own spirituality. Sadly, it is not always the illness that distorts the spirituality, but sometimes the spirituality that is in itself the stressor. Listening and gentle, timely questioning will be required in order to expose any difficult, stressful or even abusive or pathological aspects of the patient's spirituality. This can only be done if respect for the person's spirituality has already been established.

Tools

A mesmerising array of spiritual assessment tools has sprung up in recent years to help the clinician to include spirituality/religion within the clinical assessment, so how does one choose? The tools can largely be categorised according to their purpose – tools for research, clinical measurement and audit are mainly quantitative, whereas tools to encourage exploration of spiritual matters are mainly qualitative.

Tools for Research, Clinical Measurement and Audit

A plethora of instruments, described in several reviews (Koenig, 2011; Monod et al., 2011; Selman et al., 2011; Higginson et al., 2013) and book chapters (Büssing, 2019), purport to measure different facets of spirituality. For example, one review by Monod et al. (2011) identified 35 spiritual assessment instruments, which claimed to measure 'general spirituality' ($n = 22$), 'spiritual well-being' ($n = 5$), 'spiritual coping' ($n = 4$) and 'spiritual needs' ($n = 4$). However, few of these focused on the patient's current spiritual state, and only three were suitable for directing spiritual interventions. The Functional Assessment of Chronic Illness Therapy–Spiritual well-being (FACIT-Sp) and the Spirituality Index of Well-Being were the best validated tools (see Table 2.1). Spirituality is sometimes 'confused with mental health itself, resulting in the inclusion of mental health indicators in measures of spirituality, thus ensuring a positive relationship with mental health' (Koenig and Al Zaben, 2017, p. 427). The use of quantitative tools for spiritual assessment in the clinical setting has been criticised for pigeon-holing patients into responding in predetermined ways that may not fit with their experience.

Table 2.1. Tools for research, clinical measurement and audit

Tool	Authors
FACIT-Sp	Brady et al. (1999)
Spirituality Index of Well-Being	Daaleman et al. (2002)
Spiritual Quality of Life	World Health Organization (2002)
Spiritual Suffering | Spiritual Distress	NANDA International[a]
Spiritual struggle	Fitchett and Risk (2009)
Spiritual injury	Fitchett (2012)
Multidimensional measurement of religiousness/spirituality for use in health research	Fetzer Institute (1999)
Assessment of Spirituality and Religious Sentiments (ASPIRES) Scale	Piedmont (2012)

[a] www.nandanursingdiagnosislist.org/functional-health-patterns/spiritual-suffering/ (accessed 24 November 2020).

Tools to Aid Exploration of Spiritual Matters in Clinical Practice

In clinical practice, qualitative tools are usually preferred as they provide the flexibility that allows patients to express themselves in ways that are meaningful to them.

Although the terminology surrounding exploration of spiritual matters differs between Europe and the USA, there are essentially three approaches: (1) initial brief 'screening', which can be undertaken by any member of the healthcare team; (2) spiritual history, which can be conducted by any member of the healthcare team; and (3) more in-depth ongoing assessment, undertaken by a specialist such as the healthcare chaplain or therapist if required. A brief overview of each approach is provided here.

Screening

The literature overwhelmingly recommends that, at the very least, every patient should have a brief spiritual screening. This screen serves several purposes. It may facilitate the provision of practical necessities such as a special diet or religious artefacts. It signals permission for the subject to be talked about or returned to later if the patient prefers, and it identifies those patients who may benefit from further conversation.

There are a number of generic approaches to screening:

1   *The 2 Question Spiritual Assessment Model (2Q-SAM)*. Ross and McSherry (2018) offer two questions to guide nurses in assessing patients' spiritual needs in order to promote person-centred, co-produced, needs-led and prudent care: 'What's most important to you?' and 'How can we help?' The tool is part of a European toolkit to help nurses to incorporate spiritual care within everyday nursing practice (McSherry et al., 2020). The model is currently being field tested. It is one of the assessment tools recommended by the European Association for Palliative Care (EAPC) for multidisciplinary palliative care teams (Best et al., 2020). Application of the model in situations where the patient has difficulty in articulating their needs (e.g., the unconscious or heavily sedated patient, or the person with dementia) is covered in detail in McSherry et al. (2019).

2   *Existential enquiry*. Many authors make similar suggestions for starting the conversation about spiritual matters (e.g., Eagger and McSherry, 2011; Griffith, 2012), but the most recent examples can be found in the RCPsych leaflet titled *Spirituality and Mental Health* (Cook and Grimwade, 2021) and the RCPsych Continuing Professional Development module (Eagger and Ferdinando, 2018). These are

'What gives you hope?' or 'What keeps you going in difficult times?' or 'What is really important in your life?', followed by 'Do you have any faith or belief that is important to you?' or 'Would you say you are spiritual or religious in any way?'

3   *Other questions*. Other well-tested questions used in palliative care, such as 'Are you at peace?' (Balboni et al., 2017) and 'Do you have spiritual pain?' (Mako et al., 2006), borrowing Saunders' notion of 'total pain' (Saunders, 1996), may be particularly useful in liaison and old age psychiatry.

Spiritual History

If indicated in the introductory 'screening', Cook (2013) and Koenig et al. (2020b) recommend moving on to probe more deeply about a person's religious, spiritual or personal beliefs and practices to identify aspects that might be important to include in treatment.

Brief Literature Review –– Moreira-Almeida et al. (2014) identified clinical guidelines for spiritual assessment in mental health, drawing upon a review of 985 empirical studies and reviews (1998–2013), health guidelines and other published health and spirituality resources, and a previous systematic review of 25 spiritual history instruments rated on 16 attributes (Lucchetti et al., 2013). In this chapter, we have drawn upon this strong evidence base, supplementing it only where our own brief review[3] and knowledge of other clinical approaches has added to it since 2014. Of the other nine papers that we identified in our review, one critiqued existing tools (Raffay, 2014) and five stressed the importance of including a spiritual assessment (Harrington, 2016; Payman, 2016), three of which based this on research in patients with schizophrenia (Huguelet et al., 2011; Mohr and Huguelet, 2014) and serious or terminal illness (Koenig, 2015).

Only three papers in our review shed new light on spiritual assessment. One paper (Loynes and O'Hara, 2015) identified how spiritual assessment should be adapted for people with learning disabilities. Another paper (Starnino et al., 2014) provided guidelines for including patients' 'spiritual strengths' in a recovery plan using the 'Spiritual Strengths Assessment' tool; however, this tool did not feature in the article. The final paper (Rosmarin et al., 2011) proposed six statements (e.g., 'God loves me immensely', 'God ignores me') that may be helpful in assessing Christian and Jewish patients with a personal concept of God. The questions can be used as a qualitative tool or as a quantitative measure, both clinically and in research.

We draw upon this literature throughout the chapter. In this section we cover general mnemonic tools, tools specific to mental health that may help the clinician to probe a little deeper, and new approaches for specific patient groups.

Generic Mnemonic Tools –– The same generic mnemonic tools that were highly rated by Moreira-Almeida et al. (2014) continue to feature in the recent literature, and some of these are outlined in Box 2.2. Moreira-Almeida et al. (2014) reported studies in which spiritual assessments conducted using tools such as these were particularly well received by patients and staff, and could be completed quickly.

Assessment Tools Specific to Mental Health
Royal College of Psychiatrists (Cook and Grimwade, 2021) –– Moreira-Almeida et al. (2014) identified only two instruments specifically for assessment in the mental health setting, and only one of these was highly rated, namely the RCPsych Assessment, which has been updated multiple times. The most recent version (Cook and Grimwade, 2021) provides examples of topics that a patient may wish to talk about (see Box 2.3) and is centred around five aspects (Cook, 2015):

---

[3] The databases PsycINFO and Medline were searched from 2009 to 2020 using the following search strategy: (AB 'spiritual* assess*' or 'assess* spiritual*' or 'assess* of spiritual*' or 'assess* the spiritual*') AND (AB mental or psychi* or psychol*) in October 2020. A total of 64 sources were identified after removal of duplicates. Abstracts were scrutinised by the authors, and books, book reviews, theses and editorials were removed. The 42 remaining abstracts were screened to identify papers that might provide new insights into conducting a spiritual assessment in the clinical setting. We removed papers that obviously focused on instrument testing, exploring associations between spirituality/religion and health outcomes, and those that reinforced the importance of undertaking an assessment. Unanimous agreement was reached on 10 papers.

> **Box 2.2   Examples of mnemonic tools**
>
> **FACT** (LaRocca-Pitts, 2009) explores four areas:
>
> **F**aith or belief (including meaning and purpose)
> How **A**ctive the person is in their faith community and how **A**vailable, **A**ccessible and **A**pplicable that support is
> **C**oping strategies, **C**omfort these may provide, potential **C**onflict and **C**oncerns the person may have about their condition or treatment
> Appropriate **T**reatment.
>
> **FICA** (Puchalski and Romer, 2000) was developed for all patients, and covers:
>
> **F**aith and belief (what helps with coping, and provides meaning)
> **I**mportance (in their life and for their health)
> **C**ommunity (whether they belong to a specific group)
> **A**ddress in care or action (implications for health and the patient's spiritual journey).
>
> **HOPE** (Anandarajah and Hight, 2001) covers four areas in the general practice setting:
>
> What provides **H**ope, meaning, comfort, strength, peace, love and connection
> **O**rganised religion
> **P**ersonal spirituality and practices
> **E**ffects on health care and end-of-life issues.
>
> **SPIRIT** (Maugans, 1996) explores:
>
> **S**piritual belief system
> **P**ersonal spirituality
> **I**ntegration with a spiritual community
> **R**itualised practices and restrictions
> **I**mplications for medical care
> **T**erminal events planning.

1   *Identity.* Does the patient identify as religious? Spiritual but not religious? Neither? Is this important for self-understanding?
2   *Relationships.* Which are the most important (e.g., people, God, faith)? Are they supportive or do they cause stress?
3   *Practices.* Supportive and harmful spiritual/religious practices.
4   *Meaning and purpose.* What is really important? What is fulfilling? What causes anxiety?
5   *Implications for treatment.*

Koenig (2020b) -- Koenig, one of the co-authors of the paper by Moreira-Almeida et al. (2014), has subsequently offered a list of similar topic guides (see Box 2.4), but the language focuses more on 'religion' and 'faith' rather than on 'spirituality' (as in Box 2.3), possibly reflecting the different nuances in the USA and Europe. The guides also focus on the past as well as the present to inform treatment for the future, which was one of the key recommendations made by Starnino et al. (2014) for recovery planning.

The Spirituality Flower: A Tool for Psychiatrists (Cook, 2015) -- Developed by a working group including patients and staff at Tees, Esk and Wear Valleys NHS Foundation Trust in the UK, the Spirituality Flower has five petals that represent five aspects of spirituality, as shown in Figure 2.1 (Cook, 2015). The assessor can simply ask

Box 2.3 Topic guide for religion/spirituality assessment from the Royal College of Psychiatrists' *Spirituality and Mental Health* leaflet (Cook and Grimwade, 2021).

(After the screening questions)

Talking about your spirituality

It can be difficult to know where to start. You could think about:

1. **Beliefs and questions:**

   - What is life all about? What gives you a sense of meaning or purpose?
   - If you do believe in God - how do you understand your relationship with God?
   - What is God like? What does he think about you?
   - If you could ask God anything, what would you ask?
   - Do you find yourself asking 'Why is this happening to me?', 'Can I be forgiven?', 'Am I lovable?', 'Who can I trust?'.
   - What do you think happens after death?
   - Do your spiritual beliefs make you uneasy about any parts of your treatment plan?

2. **Spiritual practices**

   You may:

   - Spend time in meditation, mindfulness, prayer, deep reflection.
   - Spend time in reflective reading (of literature, poetry or scripture).
   - Play or sing sacred music.
   - Belong to a faith tradition.
   - Take part in services, rituals, symbolic practices or worship.
   - Go on pilgrimages or retreats.
   - Engage in fasting or other lifestyle disciplines.
   - Spend time enjoying nature.
   - Like to be creative – painting, sculpture, cookery, gardening, etc.
   - Help other people.

   How do these help you? Is there anything about them that creates problems for you?

3. **Spirituality and your community**

   What support and/or difficulties do you get from your family, friends, school/work or faith community?

4. **Spiritual experiences**

   Have you had any spiritual experiences? What did they mean to you?

5. **How your spirituality affects you**

   Does it make you feel: loved, accepted, belonging and forgiven – or rejected, guilty and ashamed; safe or afraid?

This material was published in Cook and Grimwade (2021, pp. 5–7), and is reproduced here with permission.

the patient 'Are any of these relevant to you?' and 'Would you like to discuss any of them further?'

New Approaches for Specific Patient Groups –– The need for a tailored approach to assessment for specific patient groups was evident from our brief literature review. In particular we would draw attention to the needs of children and adolescents, and those with intellectual disabilities.

Spirituality is as relevant to children and adolescents with mental health problems as it is to everyone else. Nye (2011) uses cameos to illustrate how children's spirituality can

Box 2.4 Religion/spirituality assessment guide suggested by Koenig (2018, p. 342)

1. Do you consider yourself a religious or spiritual person or neither?
2. If religious or spiritual, ask: 'Explain to me what you mean by that'.
3. If neither religious nor spiritual, ask: 'Was this always so?'

If no, ask: 'When did that change and why?' [Then end the spiritual history for now, although may return to it after therapeutic relationship established.]

4. 'Do you have any religious or spiritual beliefs that provide comfort?'
5. If yes, ask 'Explain to me how your beliefs provide comfort'.

If no, ask: 'Is there a particular reason why your beliefs do not provide comfort?'

6. 'Do you have any religious or spiritual beliefs that cause you to feel stressed?'
7. If yes, ask: 'Explain to me how your beliefs cause stress in your life'.
8. 'Do you have any spiritual or religious beliefs that might influence your willingness to take medication, receive psychotherapy, or receive other treatments that may be offered as part of your mental healthcare?'
9. 'Are you an active member of a faith community, such as a church, synagogue or mosque?'
10. If yes, ask: 'How supportive has your faith community been in helping you?' If no, ask: 'Why has your faith community not been particularly supportive?'
11. 'Tell me a bit about the spiritual or religious environment in which you were raised. Were either of your parents religious?'
12. 'During this time as a child, were your experiences positive or negative ones in this environment?'
13. 'Have you ever had a significant change in your spiritual or religious life, either an increase or a decrease?' If yes, ask: 'Tell me about that change and why you think the change occurred'.
14. 'Do you wish to incorporate your spiritual or religious beliefs in your treatment?' If yes, ask: 'How would you like this to be done?'
15. 'Do you have any other spiritual needs or concerns that you would like addressed in your mental healthcare?'

This material was published in Koenig (2018, p. 342) and is reproduced here with permission. © Elsevier 2018.

be a source of recovery or adjustment, and how it can be a stressor that contributes to the aetiology of an illness. The taboo on speaking about spirituality may be strong with children, when clinicians fear imposing their own viewpoint on a vulnerable child. However, avoiding the subject altogether risks communicating that spirituality is a banned topic, thus promoting a specifically secular viewpoint. The first step is to give the child permission to speak about this subject, simply by asking a screening question.

Young children may lack the language to express their spiritual experiences and needs. Nye (2011) suggests the use of stories, creative arts and ritual to help children to express themselves. Sexson (2004) suggests observation, and talking to both parents and the child. Older children can express themselves verbally, but still need developmentally appropriate language.

Exploration of the spirituality of adolescents will include questions about beliefs, practices, experiences, feelings and social aspects. Adolescents in the developmental stage of individuation are questioning and developing their beliefs. Their spirituality may take

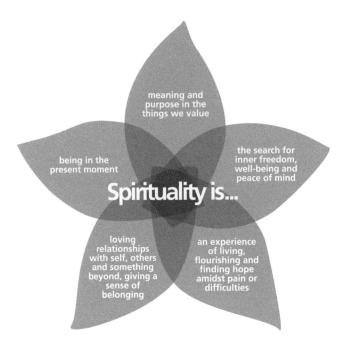

Figure 2.1 The spirituality flower. The petals of the flower represent five aspects of spirituality that may be of importance.
Are any of these relevant to you?
Would you like to discuss any of them further?
Copyright © 2011 Tees, Esk and Wear Valleys NHS Foundation Trust. Reproduced with permission.

the form of existential questions rather than fully formed beliefs. Sexon (2004) quotes work by Fosarelli, who found that the question 'If you could get God to answer one question, what one question would you ask God?' was powerful in identifying the issues that young people were grappling with. As adolescents separate from their parents, the opinions of peers become more important. We can enquire about how the adolescent's spirituality is supported by or causes conflict with family, faith community, teachers and peers (Cotton et al., 2010).

A review of spiritual care for patients with intellectual disabilities argues that people with intellectual impairment have just the same need for spiritual fulfilment, but face more barriers to achieving this. For example, the rigid thinking style of autism may make the interpretation of religious metaphor quite difficult. However, symbolism and personal relationships may be key to facilitating spiritual development. In addition to language-adjusted forms of the questions described earlier, photos or other visual images, which rely less on verbal skill, can be used to explore spiritual well-being. Spiritual assessment is more than a discreet set of questions, as it requires an ongoing willingness to explore spiritual meanings in the patient's experiences as they arise (Loynes and O'Hara, 2015).

In-Depth Spiritual Assessment

Occasionally an in-depth assessment by a specialist such as a chaplain will be indicated (as discussed in more detail in the next section). An array of in-depth tools has been developed (see Table 2.2), mainly by chaplains for the palliative care setting, and these are adequately described and evaluated elsewhere (Fitchett, 2012; Balboni et al., 2017; Best et al., 2020). We have selected two which seem particularly relevant to mental health,

Table 2.2. Tools for in-depth spiritual assessment

Tool, and aspects covered	Author
Pruyser's Spiritual Assessment Model Faith, providence, holiness, grace, gratefulness, repentance, communion, vocation	Pruyser (1976)
Discipline for pastoral care giving Meaning, hope, community, holiness	Lucas (2001)
Spiritual lifemaps	Hodge (2005)
MD Anderson's Spiritual Assessment Model Spiritual distress	Hui et al. (2011)
7 × 7 model Belief and meaning, vocation and obligations, experience and emotions, doubt (courage) and growth, ritual and practice, community, authority and guidance	Fitchett (2012)
Spiritual Distress Assessment Tool Spiritual distress	Monod et al. (2012)
Spiritual AIM Spiritual distress	Shields et al. (2015)

namely the spiritual 'lifemaps' of Hodge (2005) and the 7 × 7 model of Fitchett (2012). Spiritual lifemaps are 'client-constructed pictorial narratives of a spiritual journey' (Hodge, 2005, p. 77) which acknowledge patients as the experts, thus empowering them to work in partnership with clinicians to facilitate therapeutic interventions. In addition, the process of constructing such a map can promote self-esteem and enhance self-image, because the patient is the key player. Spiritual lifemaps link with Fowler's six developmental 'stages of faith' across the lifespan Fowler (1981), and also with Piaget's, Erikson's and Kohlberg's developmental stages (Culliford, 2007).

Fitchett's 7 × 7 model is designed to provide an in-depth ongoing means of assessing a patient's spiritual needs and resources. It is designed as an 'interpretative framework based on listening to the patient's story as it unfolds in the clinical relationship' (Fitchett, 2012, p. 299). The model assesses seven aspects of spirituality (outlined in Table 2.2) across seven dimensions: medical, psychological, psychosocial, family systems, ethnic/racial/cultural, social and spiritual.

Post Assessment

Formulation

Formulation makes sense of the information gathered and observations made by identifying first the patient's presentation, and then predisposing, precipitating, perpetuating and protective factors. Further prompts are given by considering the biological, psychological and social aspects of the patient's life. Including a spiritual history allows this process to be completed through what may be referred to as a bio-psycho-socio-spiritual formulation.

Within the spiritual part of the formulation, the information gathered in the assessment will be reflected upon by the clinician and patient together. Spirituality and illness

Table 2.3. A spiritual formulation[a]

	Impact of spirituality on illness	Impact of illness on spirituality
Healthy	What are the positive aspects of the patient's spirituality which could be harnessed for recovery and resilience?	Are there existential questions or a desire to explore their spirituality as a result of their circumstances?
Unhealthy	Are there any unhelpful aspects of the patient's spirituality that contribute to the aetiology of the illness?	Has the illness distorted or become confused with the patient's spirituality?

[a] Adapted from Grimwade and Cook, 2019, p. 36; used with permission.

can each affect the other in healthy and unhealthy ways, thus giving four potential areas for intervention (see Table 2.3).

Focusing on positive areas of spirituality first demonstrates respect for the person's spirituality. Beliefs and practices that are identified as positive can build recovery and resilience, and these can be incorporated into a care plan.

The experience of becoming ill may have prompted existential questions, such as 'Am I lovable?', 'Why is this happening to me?' or 'Who can I trust?', or may simply have inspired the person to develop their personal spirituality. Seeking answers to these questions or starting a spiritual journey would be directed by the patient, not the clinician, and a chaplain or other appropriate person may be called on to provide guidance.

Sadly, people who are struggling with their mental health may often have experienced an unhealthy or pathological spirituality. This can take many forms, such as abuse or control by a faith community, beliefs that generate feelings of condemnation or hatred, or practices that exacerbate an illness. Great care must be taken to give the patient the freedom to come to this conclusion, while working with them to cherish and strengthen the positive aspects of their spirituality.

Finally, the illness itself can distort the person's spirituality. Hallucinations may be interpreted as a spiritual reality, or depression may distort beliefs in such a way as to generate guilt or feelings of disconnection with a God previously experienced as loving. The clinician's role is to help the person to reflect on this rather than to impose their own assessment. Ideally a chaplain or trusted faith leader knowledgeable about and experienced in dealing with people with mental health problems would be needed to discern which elements arise from the illness and which arise from an unhealthy spirituality. Sadly, people with this skillset are in short supply, which highlights the need for greater collaboration and more cross-professional teaching and learning (in both directions) than is currently the case.

Spiritual Assessment: When?

The spiritual assessment is more than a tick-box exercise. It requires a clinician with the skills already outlined under 'basic principles', together with an environment in which the patient is comfortable; this will usually be a quiet safe space. A trusting meaningful relationship will take time to develop, as the patient learns to trust that what they have divulged initially is not ridiculed or ignored but is respected and considered important enough to be included in their treatment plan. Therefore a spiritual assessment is likely to be continuous throughout the patient's treatment (McSherry et al., 2019).

Spiritual Assessment: Who?

Everyone

No single profession or lay group has sole responsibility for the provision of spiritual care – all have a part to play (UK Board of Healthcare Chaplaincy, 2015). This includes the entire multidisciplinary team (MDT), such as nurses, midwives, doctors, occupational therapists, social workers, physiotherapists, paramedics and support workers. For example, recognising the importance of spirituality for health, undergraduate students from most of these professions in Wales will need to demonstrate that they meet four core spiritual care competencies developed from a European project (van Leeuwen et al., 2021), as part of new curricula that came into effect between 2020 and 2022 (McSherry et al., 2020). Although healthcare chaplains are the specialist spiritual caregivers, they are too few and far between to see every patient, and are likely to rely on other professionals to refer patients.

Nurses and Doctors

Internationally, patients tell us that the people they most want to engage with about their spiritual concerns are nurses, healthcare assistants and doctors (Selman et al., 2017). In other words, they want to engage with those with whom they have established relationships and who have an ongoing role in treating their illness, provided that they display the attributes, such as openness and kindness, highlighted earlier in Box 2.1. Mental health nurses and psychiatrists are key individuals who also have a professional requirement to include a spiritual assessment within holistic person-centred care.

The International Council of Nurses states that nurses, including those specialising in mental health, are to respect the 'spiritual beliefs of the individual, family and community' (International Council of Nurses, 2012, p. 2). In the UK this means assessing people's spiritual needs and using 'that information to develop person centred evidence-based interventions and support' (Nursing and Midwifery Council, 2018, p. 13). For example, in Wales it is a legal requirement for mental health service users in secondary care to have their 'social, cultural or spiritual' needs assessed and included in their Care and Treatment Plan (Domain 7).[4] Part of the assessment will involve establishing which people and networks are supportive rather than harmful to the patient's mental health, and this is discussed in more detail later in this chapter.

For doctors in the UK, the General Medical Council (GMC) states that the assessment should take account of the patient's 'history (including the symptoms and psychological, spiritual, social and cultural factors)' (General Medical Council, 2013a, p. 7). The Royal College of Psychiatrists' position statement on religion and spirituality recommends that 'exploration of patients' religious beliefs and spirituality should routinely be considered and will sometimes be an essential component of clinical assessment' (Cook, 2013, p. 10). The WPA makes similar recommendations (Moreira-Almeida et al., 2016).

---

[4] www.mentalhealthwales.net/mental-health-measure/

In addition, Cook and Grimwade (2021) point out that mental health professionals need to be able to distinguish between a spiritual crisis and a mental illness, particularly when these overlap.

Spiritual assessment is therefore a concern for all clinical disciplines, but especially for nurses and psychiatrists. In more complex cases it may be necessary to refer the patient to a specialist, namely the healthcare chaplain. However, distinguishing between a 'spiritual crisis' and a 'mental illness' is particularly challenging, and we shall return to this later in the chapter, in the section on 'Thorny issues and other considerations'.

The Specialist: Healthcare Chaplain

The healthcare chaplain is the only member of the healthcare team with sole responsibility for and specialist training in addressing the spiritual and religious needs of service users and staff of all faiths and none (Snowden et al., 2020). This specialist remit is reflected in the competencies and standards for healthcare chaplaincy practice, which are at a higher level than that expected of non-specialists such as nurses in many countries, such as the UK (UK Board of Healthcare Chaplaincy, 2020) and North America (Jobin, 2020; Peery, 2020). In Europe, chaplaincy organisations have been established to enhance evidence-based spiritual care practice, namely the European Research Institute for Chaplains in Healthcare (ERICH)[5] and the European Network of Healthcare Chaplaincy (ENHCC).[6] Many chaplains work within multifaith teams, and some specialise in mental health (Peng-Keller and Neubold, 2020), although exactly how many there are and what 'mental health' training they have received is unclear. Referral to a chaplain should be considered in more complex cases where the chaplain's contribution can be invaluable (see their benefits to patients and staff outlined earlier in point 2 in the section on 'Spiritual Assessment: Why?'), not only for their specialist expertise, but also for their links to supportive services within health services and other communities.

Thorny Issues and Other Considerations

Documentation

In mental health care a key individual will normally be responsible for the patient's assessment and for ensuring that the patient collaborates as fully as possible in the planning of appropriate, helpful interventions towards recovery, including the meeting of his or her spiritual needs. This individual is also likely to be responsible for documenting the assessment, agreed plans, reassessments and outcomes. This information will usually be documented in a patient record, often in electronic form. However, there is great variation in documentation by clinicians. Most records have a box for 'religion' in the demographic section, but this immediately excludes people who identify as 'spiritual not religious' or 'neither'. Some countries are more inclusive in their wording – for example, the term 'religious/spiritual affiliation', which

---

[5] www.pastoralezorg.be/page/erich/ (accessed 16 December 2020).
[6] www.enhcc.eu/ (accessed 16 December 2020).

includes 'secular spirituality, atheist, other', is used in a hospital in Quebec, Canada (Bélanger et al., 2020), and the term 'faith community' is used in a hospital in Belgium (Vandenhoeck, 2020). Usually there is a section for recording more detailed information about spirituality/religion – in England a 'spiritual needs' section (Care Programme Approach document), in Wales a 'social, cultural or spiritual' section (CTP domain 7 in Wales) and in Scotland a free-text box for 'patient preferences' – but it is unclear exactly what should be documented. As England moves towards a more holistic, person-centred care model, with clinicians controlling the agenda less (see, for example, the Strengths Model), as advocated by Starnino et al. (2014), it will be interesting to see if and how the documentation of spirituality changes. Of course, the questions contained in the document are only part of the story. As we have already seen, what – if anything – is documented will depend on the clinician and the importance they attribute to spirituality within a patient's care. Chaplains have separate processes for documenting what they do, with great variation internationally, adding further complexity to the information that is gathered and shared (Peng-Keller and Neubold, 2020).

Sharing Information

It is common for the patient record to be shared with other members of the MDT to inform and enable joined-up, person-centred care. However, unlike many other countries where chaplains are able to access and contribute to these records (Peng-Keller and Neubold, 2020), in the UK chaplains are frequently prevented from doing so, in effect being excluded from the MDT (Ross and McSherry, 2020). This means that both they and the healthcare team may miss out on vital information that would help a patient's recovery, and this increases the likelihood that care will be disjointed, conflicting and less effective. The reasons for chaplains not being considered part of the MDT in the UK are complex, but include the following: the fact that registration with a professional body, and by default abiding by a code of professional practice, is voluntary (Snowden et al., 2020); lack of a common approach to documentation and sharing of information within chaplaincy teams; concerns and complexities around boundaries, disclosure, confidentiality, data protection and data privacy; and fear of litigation (Ross and McSherry, 2020). In Germany, Frick (2020) has sought to address some of the concerns around teamworking within a mental health setting by (1) 'insist(ing) on the capacity to navigate between disclosure and non-disclosure and to respect both the physician's and the patient's boundaries' (Frick, 2020, p. 177), and (2) by keeping the focus of treatment on 'understand(ing) a sick person and . . . shar(ing) this understanding in the caring team' (Frick, 2020, p. 178). However, cultivation of an environment like this can be difficult to achieve, especially if a culture of fear has set in, and if institutional norms are unsupportive.

Time

Concern that including spirituality/religion within the psychiatric assessment may take more time is understandable in current resource-challenged health services. Ultimately, however, it may actually save time. For example, some nursing students who tested the 2Q-SAM (mentioned earlier in the section on screening) reported that patients' most pressing problems were identified and resolved, resulting in earlier discharge.

Moreira-Almeida et al. (2014) point out that the history need not necessarily take long, and in some cases need only take six minutes to be of benefit.

Spiritual and Religious Issues Are Part of the Problem

In the earlier section on 'The relationship between spirituality/religion and mental health', we highlighted the largely inverse correlation between spirituality/religion and some, but not all, mental illnesses. There are situations in which spirituality/religion exerts no effects or has deleterious effects, particularly in some personality disorders, bipolar disorder, anxiety and chronic psychotic disorders (e.g., schizophrenia). Religious delusions, hallucinations, and feelings of rejection (by God or a faith group) and excessive guilt or shame may be part of the presenting problem. Concern that spirituality/religion may be a root cause of the mental health problem may make some clinicians decide it is best left well alone. However, these 'symptoms' may also relate to 'spiritual struggle' as a precursor to 'spiritual growth', and may be beneficial (Cook, 2020). Determining which spiritual/religious beliefs and practices are positive and should be supported, and which are harmful and should not, will require a careful spiritual assessment by a sensitive clinician with a significant degree of spiritual maturity. Making this distinction is challenging. Koenig et al. (2020a, 2020b) offer some guidance to help the clinician making this assessment. This includes checking with family and friends whether the behaviour is within the normal range, checking for other accompanying symptoms (e.g., thought disorders or behaviours associated with psychosis), and comparing behaviour across multiple visits as part of the clinician's continuous assessment. They advise against challenging the patient about his or her beliefs and behaviours. Instead they advocate a 'gentle' approach in which the clinician is the 'student' and remains 'harmlessly inquisitive', with the patient as the 'teacher'. They advise that such an approach will foster trust and advocacy, an important point reinforced by Starnino et al. (2014) in relation to recovery planning. Of course, it may not be possible to distinguish between a spiritual crisis and an episode of mental illness until after the person concerned has recovered and so can better describe what they went through (Slade and Culliford, 2004). In cases of spiritual crisis or 'emergence' the outcome is almost always positive – for example, in terms of sustained reductions in levels of anxiety, depression and addiction behaviour, greater self-esteem and improved interpersonal relationships.

Negative View of Spirituality/Religion and Differing Clinician and Patient Worldviews

Historically, mental illness was viewed as a spiritual/religious problem to be remedied by spiritual/religious interventions, such as prayer, exorcism or other rituals. With the subsequent shift away from a spiritual/religious view of mental illness in favour of a more scientific one, the spiritual/religious view came to be regarded as old-fashioned and unscientific. Freud's claim that religion was pathological fostered this negative view of spirituality/religion, which persists among many mental health professionals today (Kao et al., 2020; Koenig et al., 2020b). For example, mental health professionals tend to be less religious than the general population (Kao et al., 2020), a disparity referred to as the 'religiosity gap' (Kao et al., 2020), which combined with a predominantly negative view of spirituality/religion among mental health professionals means that these aspects are often disregarded in psychiatric assessment and treatment. Yet choosing not to enquire about a patient's spirituality/religion is to deny them the opportunity to say whether it is important for their recovery. If the patient says it is not important, then the assessment need go no further at that point, but may need revisiting later if the situation changes. If the patient indicates that their spirituality is important, then the assessment should continue. This will ensure that treatment is patient led.

Faith-based therapies, which actively draw upon the patient's faith to achieve treatment goals, are increasing in popularity and there is growing evidence of their efficacy (Koenig and Al Zaben, 2017). This presents a number of challenges. How do psychiatrists who share the patient's worldview provide treatment that adheres to GMC guidelines which state that they must not express their own beliefs 'to patients in ways that may exploit their vulnerability or are likely to cause distress' (General Medical Council, 2013b)? Koenig and Al Zaben (2017) acknowledge that 'suspending one's own beliefs and values in order to enter the world of the patient is indeed difficult'. They suggest training and reflection to minimise therapist bias, thereby keeping the focus on the patient's beliefs and values and not those of the therapist. On the other hand, it may be equally challenging for the psychiatrist whose worldview is very different from that of the patient to provide the desired treatment. If a mutual way forward cannot be agreed upon, it may be necessary to refer the patient or opt for a secular therapy that both parties are comfortable with (Koenig and Al Zaben, 2017).

Feelings of Discomfort and of Being Unprepared

Given the deeply subjective and personal nature of spirituality/religion and the ambiguity, misconceptions and complexities surrounding spirituality/religion and mental health, it is not surprising that there is controversy and scepticism amongs some psychiatrists about including it within the psychiatric assessment. This is not easy territory to navigate. Clinicians have a lot to consider: assessing whether spirituality/religion is supportive or harmful; deciding how to maintain boundaries and confidentiality; and determining how to manage potential conflict between their own worldview and that of the patient, and at what point to refer him or her. In addition, fear of not getting it right, of doing harm, of proselytising (consciously or unconsciously) or of ever achieving sufficient competence might be enough to prevent many clinicians from even trying to include spirituality/religion within the psychiatric assessment. They may feel unsure about what data are required or how to handle the information, especially if they have not received adequate training and do not have appropriate encouragement and support within the workplace. All of these concerns could be remedied, however, if the subject was included in core training and CPD, as recommended by the RCPsych and WPA, especially as studies show that physicians who have undergone training are more likely to discuss spiritual/religious issues with patients (Moreira-Almeida et al., 2014). Encouragingly, a core curriculum has been proposed and is awaiting testing by the Brazilian Psychiatric Association (de Oliveira et al., 2020). In the meantime, free training materials and resources are provided by a number of organisations (listed under 'Educational resources' at the end of this chapter; see also Chapter 1).

Conclusion

At the very heart of the person-centred approach is our ability to discover what is meaningful and important for patients, and how it affects their care. Without knowing something about the spiritual and religious aspects of patients' lives, we will always have only an incomplete picture. In 2014, Moreira-Almeida et al. called for research on the feasibility and impact of including a spiritual history, especially across different spiritual/religious groups, but there has been little evidence of follow-up. Some advances have been made internationally in proposing the inclusion of spirituality in curricula and in standard textbooks, but sadly this has not yet materialised in the UK, where there appears to be resistance to such initiatives. That gap must be filled in order to respond to the patient voice. We end by quoting the views of one patient who has grappled with bipolar disorder:

'I, personally, would like to see the issue of spirituality addressed as part of people's care plans and programmes if that is what they desire. Spiritual beliefs play an integrated role in the whole person identity, and to create a balanced, whole person it is important to start treating them in a holistic way, not just as an illness. Mind, Body and Spirit, [these are] the magic ingredients!'.[7]

Educational Resources

- Duke University, USA: https://spiritualityandhealth.duke.edu/index.php/cme-videos
- The Royal College of Psychiatrists' Spirituality and Psychiatry Special Interest Group, UK: www.rcpsych.ac.uk/members/special-interest-groups/spirituality/resources
- The EPICC Project Toolkit, which contains teaching and learning materials to promote development of spiritual care competency in student nurses and midwives across Europe: http://blogs.staffs.ac.uk/epicc/resources/epicc-adoption-toolkit/

References

Allott, K., Steele, P., Boyer, F. et al. (2020) Cognitive strengths-based assessment and intervention in first-episode psychosis: a complementary approach to addressing functional recovery? *Clinical Psychology Review*, 79, 101871.

American Psychiatric Association (1990) Guidelines regarding possible conflict between psychiatrists' religious commitments and psychiatric practice. *American Journal of Psychiatry*, 147, 542.

Anandarajah, G. and Hight, E. (2001) Spirituality and medical practice: using the HOPE questions as a practical tool for spiritual assessment. *American Family Physician*, 63, 81–89.

Balboni, T. A., Fitchett, G., Handzo, G. F. et al. (2017) State of the Science of Spirituality and Palliative Care Research Part II: screening, assessment, and interventions. *Journal of Pain and Symptom Management*, 54, 441–453.

Barber, J. M., Parkes, M., Parsons, H. and Cook, C. C. H. (2012) Importance of spiritual well-being in assessment of recovery: the Service-user Recovery Evaluation (SeRvE) scale. *The Psychiatrist*, 36, 444–450.

---

[7] Mind, body, & spirit. Sarah's blogs about the role spirituality can play in mental health treatments, 14 February 2013. Available at www.mind.org.uk/information-support/your-stories/mind-body-spirit/ (accessed 16 December 2020).

Bélanger, B., Beauregard, L., Bélanger, M. and Bergeron, C. (2020) The Quebec model of recording spiritual care: concepts and guidelines. In S. Peng-Keller and D. Neubold, eds., *Charting Spiritual Care: The Emerging Role of Chaplaincy Records in Global Health Care*. Cham: Springer, pp. 53–75.

Best, M., Leget, C., Goodhead, A. and Paal, P. (2020) An EAPC white paper on multidisciplinary education for spiritual care in palliative care. *BMC Palliative Care*, 19, 9.

Brady, M. J., Peterman, A. H., Fitchett, G., Mo, M. and Cella, D. (1999) A case for including spirituality in quality of life measurement in oncology. *Psycho-Oncology*, 8, 417–428.

Büssing, A., ed. (2019) *Measures of Spirituality/Religiosity*. Basel: MDPI.

Cook, C. C. H. (2004) Addiction and spirituality. *Addiction*, 99, 539–551.

Cook, C. C. H. (2013) *Recommendations for Psychiatrists on Spirituality and Religion. Position Statement PS03/2013*. London: Royal College of Psychiatrists.

Cook, C. C. H. (2015) Religion and spirituality in clinical practice. *BJPsych Advances*, 21, 42–50.

Cook, C. C. H. (2020) Religion and psychiatry: research, prayer and clinical practice. *BJPsych Advances*, 26, 282–284.

Cook, C. and Grimwade, L. (2021) *Spirituality and Mental Health*. London: Royal College of Psychiatrists.

Cotton, S., McGrady, M. E. and Rosenthal, S. L. (2010) Measurement of religiosity/spirituality in adolescent health outcomes research: trends and recommendations. *Journal of Religion and Health*, 49, 414–444.

Culliford, L. (2007) Taking a spiritual history. *Advances in Psychiatric Treatment*, 13, 212–219.

Daaleman, T. P., Frey, B. B., Wallace, D. and Studenski, S. A. (2002) Spirituality Index of Well-Being Scale: development and testing of a new measure. *Journal of Family Practice*, 51, 952.

de Oliveira e Oliveira, F. H. A., Peteet, J. R. and Moreira-Almeida, A. (2020) Religiosity and spirituality in psychiatry residency programs: why, what, and how to teach? *Brazilian Journal of Psychiatry*, 43, 424–429.

Eagger, S. and Ferdenando, S. (2018) *Exploring Spirituality with People Who Use Mental Health Services*. Royal College of Psychiatrists Online CPD module. https:// elearning.rcpsych.ac.uk/learningmodules/ exploringspiritualitywithpe.aspx (accessed 15 December 2020).

Eagger, S. and McSherry, W. (2011) Assessing a person's spiritual needs in a healthcare setting. In P. Gilbert, ed., *Spirituality and Mental Health*. Brighton: Pavilion Publishing, pp. 193–215.

European Commission (2010) *EUROPE 2020: A Strategy for Smart, Sustainable and Inclusive Growth*. Brussels: European Commission.

Fetzer Institute (1999) *Multidimensional Measurement of Religiousness/Spirituality for Use in Health Research*. Kalamazoo, MI: Fetzer Institute and National Institute on Aging Working Group.

Fitchett, G. (2012) Next steps for spiritual assessment in healthcare. In M. Cobb, C. Puchalski and B. Rumbold, eds., *Oxford Textbook of Spirituality in Healthcare*. Oxford: Oxford University Press, pp. 299–305.

Fitchett, G. and Risk, J. (2009) Screening for spiritual struggle. *Journal of Pastoral Care & Counseling*, 63, 1–12.

Fowler, J. (1981) *Stages of Faith*. San Francisco, CA: Harper and Row.

Frick, E. (2020) Charting spiritual care: psychiatric and psychotherapeutic aspects. In S. Peng-Keller and D. Neuhold, eds., *Charting Spiritual Care: The Emerging Role of Chaplaincy Records in Global Health Care*. Cham: Springer, pp. 171–180.

General Medical Council (2013a) *Good Medical Practice*. London: General Medical Council.

General Medical Council (2013b) *Personal Beliefs and Medical Practice*; www.gmc-uk .org/ethical-guidance/ethical-guidance-for-doctors/personal-beliefs-and-medical-practice/personal-beliefs-and-medical-practice (accessed 15 December 2020).

Gibbon, A. and Baldie, D. (2019) Community Chaplaincy Listening in a community mental health group. *Health and Social Care Chaplaincy*, 7, 57–74.

Griffith, J. L. (2012) Psychiatry and mental health treatment. In M. Cobb, C, Puchalski and B. Rumbold, eds., *Oxford Textbook of Spirituality in Healthcare*. Oxford: Oxford University Press, pp. 227–233.

Grimwade, L. and Cook, C. (2019) The clinician's view of spirituality in mental health care. In J. Fletcher, ed., *Chaplaincy and Spiritual Care in Mental Health Settings*. London: Jessica Kingsley Publishers, pp 31–43.

Harrington, A. (2016) The importance of spiritual assessment when caring for older adults. *Ageing & Society*, 36, 1–16.

Higginson, I., Evans, C., Grande, G. et al. (2013) Evaluating complex interventions in end of life care: the MORECare statement on good practice generated by a synthesis of transparent expert consultations and systematic reviews. *BMC Medicine*, 11, 111.

Hodge, D. R. (2005) Spiritual lifemaps: a client-centered pictorial instrument for spiritual assessment, planning, and intervention. *Social Work*, 50, 77–87.

Huguelet, P., Mohr, S., Betrisey, C. et al. (2011) A randomized trial of spiritual assessment of outpatients with schizophrenia: patients' and clinicians' experience. *Psychiatric Services*, 62, 79–86.

Hui, D., de la Cruz, M., Thorney, S. et al. (2011) The frequency and correlates of spiritual distress among patients with advanced cancer admitted to an acute palliative care unit. *American Journal of Hospice and Palliative Medicine®*, 28, 264–270.

International Council of Nurses (2012) *The ICN Code of Ethics for Nurses*. Geneva: International Council of Nurses.

Jobin, G. (2020) Charting spiritual care: ethical perspectives. In S. Peng-Keller and D. Neubold, eds., *Charting Spiritual Care: The Emerging Role of Chaplaincy Records in Global Health Care*. Cham: Springer, pp. 199–212.

Johnstone, E. C., Owens, D. C. and Lawrie, S. M. (2010) *Companion to Psychiatric Studies*. Edinburgh: Churchill Livingstone.

Kao, L. E., Peteet, J. R. and Cook, C. C. H. (2020) Spirituality and mental health. *Journal for the Study of Spirituality*, 10, 42–54.

Kevern, P. and Hill, L. (2015) 'Chaplains for well-being' in primary care: analysis of the results of a retrospective study. *Primary Health Care Research & Development*, 16, 87–99.

Koenig, H. G. (2011) *Spirituality and Health Research: Methods, Measurement, Statistics, and Resources*. West Conshohocken, PA: Templeton Press.

Koenig, H. G. (2012) Religion, spirituality, and health: the research and clinical implications. *ISRN Psychiatry*. DOI: https://doi.org/10.5402/2012/278730

Koenig, H. G. (2013) *Spirituality in Patient Care: Why, How, When, and What*. West Conshohocken, PA: Templeton Foundation Press.

Koenig, H. G. (2015) Religion, spirituality, and health: a review and update. *Advances in Mind-Body Medicine*, 29, 19–26.

Koenig, H. (2018) *Religion and Mental Health: Research and Clinical Applications*. San Diego, CA: Academic Press.

Koenig, H. G. and Al Zaben, F. (2017) Integrating religious faith into patient care: Commentary On... The Role of Faith in Mental Health Care. *BJPsych Advances*, 23, 426–427.

Koenig, H. G., King, D. E. and Carson, V. B., eds. (2012) *Handbook of Religion and Health*. New York: Oxford University Press.

Koenig, H. G., Peteet, J. R. and VanderWeele, T. J. (2020a) Religion and psychiatry: clinical applications. *BJPsych Advances*, 26, 273–281.

Koenig, H. G., Al-Zaben, F. and VanderWeele, T. J. (2020b) Religion and psychiatry: recent developments in research. *BJPsych Advances*, 26, 262–272.

LaRocca-Pitts, M. A. (2009) FACT: taking a spiritual history in a clinical setting. *Journal of Health Care Chaplaincy*, 15, 1–12.

Lewis-Fernandez, R., Krishan Aggarwal, N., Hinton, L. et al. (2016) *DSM-5 Handbook on the Cultural Formulation Interview.* Washington, DC: American Psychiatric Publishing.

Loynes, B. and O'Hara, J. (2015) How can mental health clinicians, working in intellectual disability services, meet the spiritual needs of their service users? *Advances in Mental Health and Intellectual Disabilities.* 9, 9–18.

Lucas, A. M. (2001) Introduction to the discipline for pastoral care giving. *Journal of Health Care Chaplaincy*, 10, 1–33.

Lucchetti, G., Lucchetti, A. L. G. and Vallada, H. (2013) Measuring spirituality and religiosity in clinical research: a systematic review of instruments available in the Portuguese language. *São Paulo Medical Journal*, 131, 112–122.

Macdonald, G. (2017) The efficacy of primary care chaplaincy compared with antidepressants: a retrospective study comparing chaplaincy with antidepressants. *Primary Health Care Research & Development*, 18, 354–365.

McSherry, W., Ross, L., Balthip, K., Ross, N. and Young, S. (2019) Spiritual assessment in healthcare: an overview of comprehensive, sensitive approaches to spiritual assessment for use within the interdisciplinary healthcare team. In F. Timmins and S. Caldeira, eds., *Spirituality in Healthcare: Perspectives for Innovative Practice.* Cham: Springer, pp. 39–54.

McSherry, W., Ross, L., Attard, J. et al. (2020) Preparing undergraduate nurses and midwives for spiritual care: some developments in European education over the last decade. *Journal for the Study of Spirituality*, 10, 55–71.

Mako, C., Galek, K. and Poppito, S. R. (2006) Spiritual pain among patients with advanced cancer in palliative care. *Journal of Palliative Medicine*, 9, 1106–1113.

Maugans, T. A. (1996) The spiritual history. *Archives of Family Medicine*, 5, 11–16.

Mohr, S. and Huguelet, P. (2014) The wishes of outpatients with severe mental disorders to discuss spiritual and religious issues in their psychiatric care. *International Journal of Psychiatry in Clinical Practice*, 18, 304–307.

Monod, S., Brennan, M., Rochat, E. et al. (2011) Instruments measuring spirituality in clinical research: a systematic review. *Journal of General Internal Medicine*, 26, 1345–1357.

Monod, S., Lécureux, M. E., Spencer, B. and Büla, C. (2012) Validation of the Spiritual Distress Assessment Tool in older hospitalized patients. *BMC Geriatrics*, 12, 13.

Moreira-Almeida, A., Koenig, H. G. and Lucchetti, G. (2014) Clinical implications of spirituality to mental health: review of evidence and practical guidelines. *Brazilian Journal of Psychiatry*, 36, 176–182.

Moreira-Almeida, A., Sharma, A., Janse van Rensburg, B., Verhagen, P. and Cook, C. C. H. (2016) WPA Position Statement on Spirituality and Religion in Psychiatry. *World Psychiatry*, 15, 77–78.

Murgia, C., Notarnicola, I., Rocco, G. and Stievano, A. (2020) Spirituality in nursing: a concept analysis. *Nursing Ethics*, 27, 1171–1173.

National Institute for Health and Care Excellence (NICE) (2020) *Depression in Children and Young People: Identification and Management.* NG134. www.nice.org.uk/guidance/ng134/resources/depression-in-children-and-young-people-identification-and-management-pdf-66141719350981 (accessed 24 November 2020).

Nolan, S., Saltmarsh, P. and Leget, C. (2011) Spiritual care in palliative care: working towards an EAPC task force. *European Journal of Palliative Care.* 18, 86–89.

Nursing and Midwifery Council (2018) *Future Nurse: Standards of Proficiency for Registered Nurses.* London: Nursing and Midwifery Council.

Nye, R. (2011) Children and young people's well-being. In P. Gilbert, ed., *Spirituality and Mental Health.* Hove: Pavilion, pp. 217–230.

Owen, G., Wessely, S. and Murray, R., eds. (2014) *The Maudsley Handbook of Practical Psychiatry.* Oxford: Oxford University Press.

Pargament, K. I. and Lomax, J. W. (2013) Understanding and addressing religion among people with mental illness. *World Psychiatry,* 12, 26–32.

Payman, V. (2016) The importance of taking a religious and spiritual history. *Australasian Psychiatry,* 24, 434–436.

Peery, B. (2020) Chaplaincy documentation in a large US health system. In S. Peng-Keller and D. Neubold, eds., *Charting Spiritual Care: The Emerging Role of Chaplaincy Records in Global Health Care.* Cham: Springer, pp. 21–52

Peng-Keller, S. and Neubold, D., eds. (2020) *Charting Spiritual Care: The Emerging Role of Chaplaincy Records in Global Health Care.* Cham: Springer.

Piedmont, R. L. (2012) Overview and development of a trait-based measure of numinous constructs: the Assessment of Spirituality and Religious Sentiments (ASPIRES) Scale. In L. J. Miller, ed., *The Oxford Handbook of Psychology and Spirituality.* Oxford: Oxford University Press, pp. 104–122.

Pruyser, P. W. (1976) *The Minister as Diagnostician.* Philadelphia, PA: The Westminster Press.

Puchalski, C. and Romer, A. L. (2000) Taking a spiritual history allows clinicians to understand patients more fully. *Journal of Palliative Medicine,* 3, 129–137.

Puchalski, C. M., Vitillo, R., Hull, S. K. and Reller, N. (2014) Improving the spiritual dimension of whole person care: reaching national and international consensus. *Journal of Palliative Medicine,* 17, 642–656.

Pujol, N., Leboul, D., Prodhomme, C. and Guirimand, F. (2018) Is spiritual care the hospital's business? A qualitative study on patients' preferences about the integration of spirituality in palliative care units (PCU).

Journal of Pain and Symptom Management, 56, E47–E48.

Raffay, J. (2014) How staff and patient experience shapes our perception of spiritual care in a psychiatric setting. *Journal of Nursing Management,* 22, 940–950.

Rosmarin, D. H., Pirutinsky, S. and Pargament, K. I. (2011) A brief measure of core religious beliefs for use in psychiatric settings. *International Journal of Psychiatry in Medicine,* 41, 253–261.

Ross, L. A. (1997) *Nurses' Perceptions of Spiritual Care.* Aldershot: Avebury.

Ross, L. and McSherry, W. (2018) The power of two simple questions. *Nursing Standard.* 33, 78–80.

Ross, L. and McSherry, W. (2020) Spiritual care charting/documenting/recording/assessment: a perspective from the United Kingdom. In S. Peng-Keller and D. Neubold, eds., *Charting Spiritual Care: The Emerging Role of Chaplaincy Records in Global Health Care.* Cham: Springer, pp. 97–116.

Ross, L. and McSherry, W. (2021) Relevance of addressing spiritual needs for clinical support: nursing perspective. In A. Bussing, ed., *Spiritual Needs in Research and Practice: The Spiritual Needs Questionnaire as a Global Resource for Health and Social Care.* Cham: Springer Nature, pp. 419–436.

Ross, L. and Miles, J. (2020) Spirituality in heart failure: a review of the literature from 2014 to 2019 to identify spiritual care needs and spiritual interventions. *Current Opinion in Supportive and Palliative Care,* 14, 9–18.

Royal College of Psychiatrists (2020) *Core Psychiatry Curriculum 2021.* London: Royal College of Psychiatrists.

Sadock, B., Sadock, V. and Ruiz P., eds. (2017) *Kaplan & Sadock's Comprehensive Textbook of Psychiatry,* 10th edition. Philadelphia, PA: Wolters Kluwer.

Saunders, C. (1996) A personal therapeutic journey. *British Medical Journal,* 313, 1599–1601.

Selman, L., Siegert, R., Harding, R. et al. (2011) A psychometric evaluation of measures of spirituality validated in culturally diverse palliative care populations. *Journal of Pain and Symptom Management*, 42, 604–622.

Selman, L.E., Brighton, L. J., Sinclair, S. et al. (2017) Patients' and caregivers' needs, experiences, preferences and research priorities in spiritual care: a focus group study across nine countries. *Palliative Medicine*, 32, 216–230.

Sexson, S. B. (2004) Religious and spiritual assessment of the child and adolescent. *Child and Adolescent Psychiatric Clinics of North America*, 13, 35–47.

Shields, M., Kestenbaum, A. and Dunn, L. B. (2015) Spiritual AIM and the work of the chaplain: a model for assessing spiritual needs and outcomes in relationship. *Palliative & Supportive Care*, 13, 75–89.

Slade, N. and Culliford, L. (2004) Heavenbound. In P. J. Barker and P. Buchanan-Barker, eds., *Spirituality and Mental Health: Breakthrough*. London: Whurr Publishers, pp. 167–190.

Snowden, A. and Telfer, I. (2020) The story of the Scottish PROM. In E. Kelly and J. Swinton, eds., *Chaplaincy and the Soul of Health and Social Care: Fostering Wellbeing in Emerging Paradigms of Care*. London: Jessica Kingsley Publishers, pp. 67–89.

Snowden, A., Gibbon, A. and Grant, R. (2018) What is the impact of chaplaincy in primary care? The GP perspective. *Health and Social Care Chaplaincy*, 6, 200–214.

Snowden, A., Enang, I., Kernohan, W. G. et al. (2020) Why are some healthcare chaplains registered professionals and some are not? A survey of healthcare chaplains in Scotland. *Health and Social Care Chaplaincy*. 8, 45–69.

Stanley, M. A., Bush, A. L., Camp, M. E. et al. (2011) Older adults' preferences for religion/spirituality in treatment for anxiety and depression. *Aging & Mental Health*, 15, 334–343.

Starnino, V. R., Gomi, S. and Canda, E. R. (2014) Spiritual strengths assessment in

mental health practice. *British Journal of Social Work*, 44, 849–867.

Steinhauser, K. E., Fitchett, G., Handzo, G. F. et al. (2017) State of the Science of Spirituality and Palliative Care Research Part I: definitions, measurement, and outcomes. *Journal of Pain and Symptom Management*, 54, 428–440.

Swinton, J. (2010) The meanings of spirituality: a multi-perspective approach to the spiritual. In W. McSherry and L. Ross, eds., *Spiritual Assessment in Healthcare Practice*. Keswick: M&K Publishing, pp. 17–35.

Swinton, J. (2020) BASS ten years on: a personal reflection. *Journal for the Study of Spirituality*, 10, 6–14.

Tanyi, R. A. (2002) Towards clarification of the meaning of spirituality. *Journal of Advanced Nursing*, 39, 500–509.

UK Board of Healthcare Chaplaincy (2015) *Spiritual and Religious Care Capabilities and Competences for Chaplaincy Support 2015*. Cambridge: UK Board of Healthcare Chaplaincy.

UK Board of Healthcare Chaplaincy (2020) *Spiritual Care Competences for Healthcare Chaplains (2020)*. Cambridge: UK Board of Healthcare Chaplaincy and NHS Education Scotland. Available at www.ukbhc.org.uk/wp-content/uploads/2020/10/UKBHC-CCs-180220.pdf (accessed 20 December 2020)

Vandenhoeck, A. (2020) The spiritual care giver as a bearer of stories: a Belgian exploration of the best possible spiritual care. In S. Peng-Keller and D. Neubold, eds., *Charting Spiritual Care: The Emerging Role of Chaplaincy Records in Global Health Care*. Cham: Springer, pp. 129–142.

van Leeuwen, R., Attard, J., Ross, L. et al. (2021) The development of a consensus-based spiritual care education standard for undergraduate nursing and midwifery students: an educational mixed methods study. *Journal of Advanced Nursing*, 77, 973–986.

Weathers, E., McCarthy, G. and Coffey, A. (2015) Concept analysis of spirituality: an evolutionary approach. *Nursing Forum.* 51, 79–96.

Welsh Government (2015) *Health and Care Standards.* Cardiff: Welsh Government. Available at https://gov.wales/health-and-care-standards. (accessed 20 December 2020).

World Health Organization (2002) *WHOQOL Spirituality, Religiousness and Personal Beliefs (SRPB) Field-Test Instrument.* Geneva: World Health Organization.

World Health Organization (2006) *The World Health Report 2006: Working Together for Health.* Geneva: World Health Organization. Available at www.who.int/whr/2006/whr06_en.pdf (accessed 15 December 2020).

World Psychiatric Association (2002) *World Psychiatric Association Institutional Program on the Core Training Curriculum for Psychiatry.* Yokohama: World Psychiatric Association.

Psychosis

Susan Mitchell and Glenn Roberts

Much Madness is divinest Sense
To a discerning Eye.
(Emily Dickinson, 1862)

Introduction

Spirituality and psychosis stretch reason to its limits; they share a sense of mystery and each is notoriously difficult to define. Although psychosis, commonly called 'madness', is at the heart of psychiatry, psychiatrists have often had difficulties with spirituality – dismissing or distrusting the spirituality that is valued by many of their patients, and also struggling to find a place for their own spirituality. We are aware of an ever present risk of engaging with psychosis in ways that lose contact with the people involved or too easily see them as 'cases', and so we start our exploration by meeting Desmond:[1]

Desmond

Desmond is fearful and wide-eyed, he appears dishevelled and is resisting the police officers who have brought him to the ward. He seems confused, and he appears to be responding to voices commanding him to kneel and pray. He's been here before and his Jamaican mother thinks that he may have been using cannabis again. He has stopped his medication as he believes it is poisoning him, and he has little trust that the staff can help him.

Every psychiatrist practising in general adult, forensic or rehabilitation specialties will be familiar with the struggle to make sense of and make progress with people who are experiencing psychosis, and to effectively support their personal journeys towards recovery. The staff and the person who has now become a patient find themselves meeting at the crossroads between personal experience and professional assessment, and it is often difficult to achieve a fully satisfactory outcome.

---

[1] All examples of lived experience described in this chapter are anonymised and have been published previously.

Psychiatric care has seldom escaped criticism, much of which relates to the failure or neglect of sensitive engagement with the person, particularly for those patients who present with psychosis. Clinicians are well aware that the bio-psycho-social model we are taught can all too easily become reduced to a 'bio-bio-bio model' in practice (Sharfstein, 2005). If we are open to listening carefully to the experience of those using our services, we find 'some [examples] of excellent care. . . . But equally [we] find that some people's experiences were poor – or worse than poor. The details make harrowing reading' (Mind, 2011). Schizophrenia, despite being the focus of the first national clinical treatment guidelines by the National Institute for Health and Care and Excellence (NICE) in 2002, has been described as 'an abandoned illness,' accompanied by stigma, discrimination, neglect, fear, poverty, rejection, alienation, premature death, workless- ness, homelessness and a lack of close or committed relationships (Murray, 2012).

These disturbing associations are expressions of wider concerns that historically the discipline of psychiatry has suffered from a regrettable lack of humanity and humility in its response to the needs of its patients, and in recognising the limits of its understanding and knowledge. In 1792, at the beginning of the modern psychiatric era, it was the inhumane care and abuse of power at the local asylum that led to the founding of The York Retreat by William Tuke, a Quaker. There he developed a personal approach in which 'The patient on all occasions should be spoken to and treated as much in the manner of a rational being as the state of his mind will possibly allow' (Tuke, 1813). The origins of the recovery movement in psychiatry date back to this spiritually inspired practice and to subsequent reform movements, which in the past 30 years have been substantially led by the advocacy and testimony of those with personal experience of psychosis (Davidson et al., 2010; Roberts and Boardman, 2013).

The Royal College of Psychiatrists in the UK has recently brought together many of the College's values-led groups, including the Spirituality and Psychiatry Special Interest Group, to formulate 'person-centred care' and the shared objective that our training and practice could and should become 'values-based, person-centred and recovery-focused' (Person-Centred Training and Curriculum [PCTC] Scoping Group, 2019). Psychiatric rehabilitation, which is primarily about enabling recovery for people experiencing psychosis (Holloway et al., 2015), is fully supported by person-centred guidelines (National Institute for Health and Care Excellence, 2020), and engagement with spiritual perspectives is now explicitly acknowledged as an important factor (Milner et al., 2020). Yet we continue to live and practice with an uncomfortable gap between these agreed, even mandated aims and approaches and the lived experience often reported by both patients and staff.

It is in this context, and against this background, that we will consider as clinicians how spirituality can be relevant to understanding the experience of people like Desmond, the relief of suffering and the provision of care.

Making Sense of Spirituality and Psychosis

Psychosis and spirituality often seem to be entwined. Early heroic fables and religious myths speak of gods, spirits and madness as both fate and punishment. Humankind, powerless before incomprehensible forces, saw madness in spiritual terms (i.e., as a mystery explained by a mystery). Equally old are the fears and suspicions that surround madness – both a fear of the mad and a fear of becoming so oneself. What is this experience that we call 'psychosis'? When a young person experiences a frightening break from reality, Western experts may regard it as a 'first-episode psychosis', whereas other cultures may conceptualise it as a 'spiritual awakening,' as illustrated by Phil Borges in his film *Crazywise* (2016).

Personal narratives (Chadwick, 2007; Cordle et al., 2011; Baker and Attwater, 2015), alongside accounts by clinicians (Cullberg, 2014; Filer, 2019), provide complementary perspectives that offer access to and understanding of the inner world of the person with psychosis. For example, David Harewood gives a rich description of his psychotic experience as 'extraordinary, vivid, exciting ... and full of fear'.[2] The phenomenon of 'hearing voices' has been richly and insightfully presented in autobiographical accounts. For example, in the words of Debra Lampshire (2018), 'I am the possessor of a mutinous mind ... but I'm not mad', and according to Eleanor Longden (2013), 'my voices were a ... source of insight into solvable problems'.

What Do We Mean by Spirituality?

The Tao that can be told is not the eternal Tao;
The name that can be named is not the eternal name.

(Lao-Tzu [c. 604–531 BCE], undated)

In a talk on 'Spirit and Life', Jung (1926) asked, 'Do we know then, for all our familiarity with the verbal concept, what spirit really is? Are we sure that when we use this word we all mean the same thing? Is not the word "spirit" a most perplexingly ambiguous term?' A hundred years later there continues to be so little agreement on the definition of spirituality that researchers prefer to engage with the more measurable concepts of 'religion' and 'religiosity' (Koenig et al., 2020). It may be that in 'spirituality' we are engaging with something of fundamental importance which, as Lao-Tzu suggests, is by definition inherently elusive.

As rehabilitation psychiatrists seeking to consider what may be the contribution of spirituality to the care and treatment of people who experience psychosis, we are aware that we personally come to this substantially informed by our practice and studies in Quaker (Mitchell, 2009) and secular Buddhist (Batchelor, 2015) perspectives. These have led us to consider that there is within all beings an integral and indefinable quality – an 'inner light' – that enables connectivity and belonging with the totality of life.

We take these concepts of 'spirit' and 'spirituality' as signposts pointing towards essential qualities of what it is to be fully human, and we have found it helpful to understand spirituality primarily from religious (cultural), ethical (moral) and existential (philosophical) perspectives. Some find support for their spirituality through developing their religious practice, path or way of life. Others may access a sense of meaning, purpose and connection through something else, such as creativity, music, poetry, nature or art. For many people, organised religion can be a relatively safe container or channel

---

[2] www.rcpsych.ac.uk/events/free-webinars/free-webinars-for-members/2020/interview-with-david-harewood-23-july-2020

for their spirituality, but this is clearly not true for all. For some, religion can have a negative connotation, being experienced as oppressive or linked with abusive experiences. Accounts of recovery by service users confirm the importance of a safe and satisfactory spiritual home, wherever that may be found.

The guiding purpose of all religions may be to connect us to the spiritual, but spirituality need not be the preserve of religion (Remen, 1993). Wittgenstein, a devastating critic of conventional religious language, nevertheless recognised that the concerns that religions engage with could have universal relevance: 'I am not a religious man but I cannot help seeing every problem from a religious point of view' (Drury, 1981). We see spirituality as part of life, inherent and innate to the natural order, rather than anything separate or optional that can come and go and which some have and others do not. However, such is the intrinsic and interwoven nature of spirituality that we may not recognise this quality within ourselves or in others unless we are first open to the possibility of its existence. It is not acquired so much as realised, and cannot be proven to someone uninterested in it or unwilling to notice it. We see this universal spiritual quality as a core characteristic of our humanity which is as valid, present and relevant for those who seek our help as it is for us.

Understanding Psychosis

> The physician knows madness in one way; he collects the symptoms of it, the causes and cure; but the madman in his way knows it far better. The terror and the glory of the illusion, which after all, are the madness itself, are open only to the madman or to some sympathetic spirit as prone to madness as he is. (Santayana, 1925, pp. 14–15)

Although the cause or causes of most forms of psychosis remain uncertain, it often arises in the context of disruptive personal challenges and disempowering psychosocial stresses. The provocations, explorations and uncertainties of adolescence and the confusions and insecurities of migration, trauma, racism, environmental isolation and social isolation have all been implicated, although none of these are specific to psychosis. Understanding the complex interaction and accumulation of such causal factors has relevance when responding to a recurring request from experience-based experts that we focus not just upon *what is wrong with someone*, but also upon *what has happened to them* (Longden, 2013; Read et al., 2014; Baker and Roberts, 2015).

The early stage of psychosis is often characterised by a turmoil of disintegrative experiences. This so-called 'pre-psychotic panic' is extremely unpleasant and may be followed by an uncanny sense of strangeness and significance, accompanied by the unravelling of previously accepted patterns of meaning. This state of distressing perplexity begins to resolve with the emergence of delusions as the new meanings attributed to the changed view of the world, and a person's perception of his or her world can be turned 'inside out', 'from a neglected, peripheral person without any power to make an impression on the world, that person suddenly becomes its centre' (Cullberg, 2014, p. 52) (see also Chadwick, 2007).

Sometimes these transitions are accompanied by an ecstatic sense of 'mystery and awe' or revelation of the interconnectedness of all things, and it is unsurprising that people may then be reluctant to lose such insights, and ambivalent about treatments that may remove them.

Jimmy

Jimmy was a well-known local eccentric who would waylay shoppers in the high street offering to 'heal' them, but only came into contact with services after he'd tried, and failed, to walk across the local river. He believed he was an incarnation of Jesus, and having confidently set off upon the water was then surprised to find himself waist deep and sinking. On the ward he expressed a basic dilemma: as Jesus he was 'someone' whereas as Jimmy he was no one. His acceptance of effective care and treatment pivoted around his estranged children coming to visit and being able to relate to him when not eclipsed by his messianic identifications. He subsequently valued supportive day care and became known by how he signed himself in – Jimmy (JC). His bracketing of his alternative identity was a key part of his recovery.

Delusions and hallucinations that were experienced as frightening and destructive in the early phases of a developing psychosis may be accommodated and then become of central significance within a changed 'perspectival world' (Cox and Theilgaard, 1994). The person can have a tenuous but committed sense of 'I know what is going on', a conviction that is not easily rescinded. For some these are brief or temporary states, and for others these initial delusional constructions are elaborated and developed into whole systems of belief, which can provide a basis for progressively reconstructing the individual's identity, meaning and purpose (Roberts, 1991). The importance of understanding this confusing and paradoxical process is relevant not only in approaches to early intervention in psychosis, but also in the later stages of recovery, as a patient caught in this confusion explains:

> There are days when I wonder if it might not be more humane to leave the schizophrenic patient to his world of unreality, not to make him go through the pain it takes to become part of humanity. These are the days when the pain is so great. I think I might prefer the craziness until I remember the immobilising terror and the distance and isolation that keeps the world so far away and out of focus. It is not an easily resolved dilemma. (Anon, 1986)

The idea that paranoid delusions may be defensive or protective for the individual against the turmoil of their inner chaos is not new (Cullberg, 2014). It was first discussed in the early psychoanalytic literature (Tausk, 1933), and more recently by behavioural psychologists. Bentall (2004) has described how, in the face of adversity, externalising personal attributions can lead to a paranoid worldview but simultaneously preserve self-esteem.

Michael

Michael, a musician, struggling to get a tune out of the ward piano, states that 'they' must have broken his fingers when he was 'in captivity'. He complains that as a consequence he can no longer reach the keys, rather than recognising that he is hopelessly out of practice, anxious and distracted, and continuing to feel traumatised by his sojourn in the police station prior to admission.

Similarly, the desperate efforts of Desmond to maintain his delusional beliefs, resisting all attempts by parents and doctors to help him believe otherwise, now become more understandable. Losing his belief system would expose him to renewed internal chaos, a painful realisation of his predicament and reconnection with whatever were the pre-psychotic provocations and traumas.

When, as part of a research study, 17 people with long-standing complex systems of delusional belief were asked to imagine what it would be like to 'discover that what they believed was not true, that their mind had been playing tricks on them' (in effect, 'What would it be like to recover?'), 14 individuals gave a range of strongly felt negative answers and considered the prospect of losing their beliefs to be very threatening (Roberts, 1991). Eight said that they would have 'nothing to live for' or that they would be 'destroyed', eight viewed the prospect as 'terrible', 'depressing' or 'frightening', five anticipated 'entering futility', 'emptiness', 'bleakness' or 'becoming inert' or 'destitute', three felt that they would be cut off from others and two believed they would 'go mad.'

Meaning and Purpose in the Experience of Psychosis

This paradoxical finding of meaning and purpose in delusional belief (illness) and anticipation of emptiness and futility on recovery (health) is consistent with Jaspers' warning about the predicament of the very mad, whose knowledge of reality has changed and whose existential fulfilment is in their beliefs, such that 'any correction would mean a collapse of Being itself, in as far as it is for him his actual awareness of existence' (Jaspers, 1963, p. 105). Sims expressed a compassionate concern for people struggling with this process of awakening to reality: 'As the delusions fade, the patient may gain insight and regard them as false beliefs "due to the illness". Such a person needs help in accepting himself as a fit repository for his own self-confidence once more. He may feel himself to be damaged, vulnerable and untrustworthy and suffer a massive loss of self-esteem' (Sims, 2003, p. 142).

Such 'awakening' on the threshold of 'going sane' may be a necessary preliminary to true recovery. It is an important spiritual principle in therapeutic care to uphold a sense of value and significance through believing in the person, even if not assenting to their beliefs, during what may be for them a crisis of losing faith with their psychosis. This respect for the person, conveyed through holding hope in the context of confusion, can become a foundation for personal recovery.

How Are We to Understand the Ununderstandable?

> Understanding or Thought is not natural to Man; it is acquir'd by means of Suffering & Distress i.e. Experience. (William Blake, 1789)

The fact that I cannot understand someone does not mean that what they are saying is without meaning or value. Meaning and value are sometimes conflated, which has profound implications for people with psychosis; as Jaspers observed, 'everything understandable has a constituent potentiality of worth. In contrast we do not value the ununderstandable as such' (Jaspers, 1963, p. 310). Jaspers recognised the importance of empathy: 'We can have no psychological understanding without empathy into the *content* (symbols, forms, images, ideas) and without seeing the *expression* and sharing the *experienced phenomena*. All these spheres of meaningful objective facts and subjective experience form the matter for understanding' (Jaspers, 1963, p. 311). Thus understanding, even if partial and hard won, can be a valued bridge to relationship and reconnection, and potently antipsychotic. Too often in the busyness of the acute ward or in the community the doctor may fail to stop and think, to put him- or herself into the shoes of the patient, and try to reach a shared understanding of that person's experience. In order to be 'person-centred', care must attend to the nature of the experiences in the context of that person's life as a whole (Davidson, 2011).

Henry

Henry, a late middle-aged man, had spent 20 years in the back wards of a hospital and continued to be troubled by a voice that said 'he buggered a pig'. It made other derogatory and critical remarks, but mostly repeated this offensive accusation. It did not seem to have occurred to anyone to wonder if it was true. On being asked for more details (for an account of making sense of voices, see Romme and Escher, 2000), he clearly recognised the voice as that of his old headmaster. With his permission we were able to track down this elderly man, who remembered our patient and that there had indeed been an embarrassing incident with a pig on the school farm. This had resulted not only in punishment, but ever after being taunted by the other children and regarded with suspicion by the staff. It was possible to gently introduce this into conversation and although the experiences persisted, there was a greater sense of compassionate understanding for his life experience, which opened a greater sense of connection and relationship.

Religious Delusions and the Need for Cultural Context

The existence of a god or gods has been denied by many writers, including Dawkins (2006), who has described religious beliefs as delusions (on the basis that religion is inherently fabricated and therefore beliefs associated with it are also false). However, psychiatric convention is that beliefs shared by people with a similar religious or cultural background are not considered to be clinical delusions. The beliefs of the mad and the religious may share some properties in form, content and quality of belief holding, but that does not make them the same. The great majority of religious believers with their creeds and congregations are recognisably different from people with psychotic illness, alone with their idiosyncratic and isolating beliefs. Delusions of clinical significance are those with morbid consequences. The clinician is fundamentally concerned with relieving suffering, not correcting what some may regard as erroneous or unshared beliefs.

People who are experiencing psychosis may present with delusions or hallucinations of a religious nature (even if they themselves do not practise a religion), and religious patients who develop psychosis are very likely to express themselves through the language and imagery of their beliefs. We need to beware of making assumptions and, like good detectives, be interested in investigating associations and making sense of each person in the context of their own background. The complex delusional system built up by a patient born on 6 June 1966 may make some sense if the doctor has a knowledge of the New Testament Book of Revelation and the significance of the number of the beast (Revelation 13:18). Similarly, some knowledge about punishment for those who wage war against Allah (Qur'ān 5:33) makes the act of cutting off his own left foot and attempting to cut off his right hand by a Muslim who believed he had sinned a little more understandable.

Sustained curiosity, patience and trust are often needed before understanding emerges:

Simon

Simon was just 18 when he was brought into hospital via the air-sea rescue service; he had attracted unwanted attention by jumping off the end of a pier into the sea tied to the wheel of a car. He had intended to kill himself, and was surprised to find he'd attached himself to a float. He eventually explained his confusing behaviour as having arisen from acting on the voices he was hearing saying he had 'harmed the little ones' and had acted out the text saying 'it would be better for a man to tie a millstone around his neck and throw himself in the sea than harm any of these little ones' (Mark 9:42). Lacking access to a millstone he thought, wrongly, a car wheel would serve the purpose. Recovery involved both relief from psychotic symptoms and a sympathetic reconnection with his faith and belief.

The Spirit of Therapy and Therapeutic Spirituality

Do justice, love kindness and walk humbly. (Hebrew Scripture, Micah 6:8)

There is a significant overlap between the ethical dimensions of spirituality, psychotherapy, recovery-based practice and person-centred care, such that an emphasis on compassion, humility, patience and kindness is common to each. Given this, do we need to cultivate spiritual awareness specifically as 'spirituality'? We think the short answer could be 'no'. Davidson is clear that working towards 'recognising and restoring a person's "personhood" is fundamentally a *loving* act' (Davidson, 2011, p. 105), and he distinguishes four different kinds of non-romantic love, all of which are important in helping the person to rebuild a sense of self and a 'self-determined and meaningful life in a community of his or her peers' (Davidson, 2011, p. 106). If we provide truly humane care there will be a spiritual aspect to all that we do. It is not something extra that we do, but 'the thoughtful integration of the spiritual dimension of the patient's life into treatment' (Lomax and Pargament, 2016, p. 62). It is as much a way of being as a way of doing (Swinton, 2001). Approaches that enhance creativity, connection, communication, meaning and purpose for the individual have been shown to be therapeutically effective, improving self-esteem and well-being. 'Spirituality' is not a special form of treatment; there are no technical routines that are inherently spiritual. It is the way in which the work is carried out that imparts the spiritual quality, whether named as such or not.

Tensions: The Value of Creative Collaboration

It can be a difficult but helpful struggle to develop constructive connections between clinical and spiritual perspectives in therapeutic settings. When it is possible these connections may be very supportive of the recovery journeys of people of faith:

Anna

Anna, a taxi driver, was admitted to a psychiatric unit having driven her car through a hedge and down a steep bank, fortunately without injury. Her explanation was that she had swerved to avoid 'an evil nun' walking across the road in the twilight. She had become increasingly depressed in response to various life difficulties, and distressed and puzzled by the experience of fleeting robed 'presences'. She had no explanation of what they were or why they had come to her, but was convinced they were evil. She sought support from the hospital chaplain, who was also the Bishop's advisor on health and healing. He suggested prayers for deliverance. The patient was keen to pursue this, and after careful thought the clinical team were willing to work alongside this wish. They sat with Anna through a quiet and respectful service of spiritual deliverance. To the patient's relief and the staff's surprise 'it worked'; she felt better and reported that the 'evil nuns' had left. She remained well and was able to leave hospital. A few weeks later, however, these experiences had returned, as had other symptoms of psychotic depression, all of which this time responded to conventional psychiatric treatments.

Sometimes the overlap between clinical and religious views creates conflict for both the patient and the team who are seeking to help:

James

James, a middle-aged man, had a strong sense of religious vocation and liked to attend Mass each day, often acting as acolyte. He believed that divine healing was more important than medication and psychological therapy, which he felt were only half the story. Yet he regularly relapsed severely into a catatonic state either when medication was reduced or if he became an informal patient and stopped taking medication on his own initiative. During relapse his religious beliefs took on an intense delusional quality.

This situation led to tension within the clinical team. Some team members saw his religious beliefs as part of his illness and concluded that he should be medicated and prevented from attending Mass (or that it should at least be limited to Sundays). Others wished to facilitate his attendance at Mass because they acknowledged his spiritual needs and respected his view that spiritual healing could play a part in his recovery. The tension was resolved by the team agreeing that he needed help in developing and maintaining a balance in his life in order to remain well. The team, having contacted his minister, now helped to validate the patient's religious experience and his need for communication with his congregation, while also encouraging other interests that have a more practical, grounding spiritual element, such as gardening, which he found helpful.

Finding out about the patient's religious and spiritual background may help us to avoid making premature assumptions, as this story illustrates:

Julie

During her first pregnancy, Julie, a young lawyer, suffered a recurrence of an earlier depression; she was anxious and fearful and gave up work. As her pregnancy continued so her mood worsened and she began psychotherapy. Before her child was born, an interpretation was made in therapy that she was having murderous thoughts towards her unborn child. Her condition deteriorated with the emergence of paranoid delusions that she was being poisoned, which progressed to a serious puerperal psychosis. She had been brought up as a Roman Catholic and, as she later explained, had been taught that thoughts could have the moral culpability of actions. She believed that she had killed her unborn child. Once she had recovered, she was very apprehensive about further psychotherapy and believed that the therapist had not taken enough time to find out about her religious beliefs.

What is important here is not so much 'taking a history' as reaching a shared understanding – being aware of the difference between 'my story of you' and 'your story of you', with all the complex overtones of 'author-ity' (i.e., whose meanings count?) (Hunter, 1991). For the therapist it is important to keep in mind three questions – 'What is your inner world like?', 'What sustains you?' and 'What has your life been like?' – and then, together with the patient, to explore how each can be understood in the context of the others (Roberts, 2006).

It is essential to recognise the need to understand the cultural values and experienced inequalities of people from different ethnic and religious backgrounds as a foundation for trust (Bhui et al., 2007, 2018). Furthermore, Loewenthal (2017, p. 66) reminds us that 'it is important to bear in mind that specific spiritual beliefs and practices are not uniform within any culture'.

Interactions With Meaning and Purpose

Laing memorably echoed the spiritual philosophy of William James in conceptualising schizophrenia as the outworking of a 'divided self' (Laing, 1960). He also wrote that 'the mad things said and done by people with schizophrenia will remain a closed book until we can see them in their existential context' (Laing, 1960, p. 17). Access to an existential appreciation of being part of and connected to that which is greater than ourselves – transcendence – is a key dimension of spirituality, often reached through the arts or contact with nature. Vincent van Gogh wrote to his brother Theo, 'In life and in painting too, I can easily do without the dear Lord, but I can't, suffering as I do, do without something greater than myself, which is my life, the power to create' (van Gogh, 1888, letter 673). However, there is a risk of art or nature being transformed in psychiatric settings into 'interventions' or 'therapies' when their value may in fact be more beneficial as everyman activities and resources, accessible to all.

Murray Cox's initiative in bringing Shakespeare, 'this great and amazing libertarian ... shaking his spear at ignorance and talking about spiritual things but in such an open way that you can take it as you like it' (Cox, 1992, p. 32), to offender patients in Broadmoor is an excellent example. Ferris, a forensic psychiatrist at Broadmoor, writes that the process of diagnosing and deciding about treatment 'actively avoids the spiritual aspects or dimensions which something like the play [*Hamlet*] taps' (Cox, 1992, p. 33).

Storytelling, being listened to, and gaining new understanding in the process of telling and listening are important in the journey of recovery and to us as practitioners (Cook, 2016). Julie Leibrich, as both service user and Mental Health Commissioner in New Zealand, created an inspirational anthology of personal recovery stories (Leibrich, 1999) as part of a national anti-stigma campaign. She also described personally how important it was to have one's own meanings and frame of reference respected if narrative inquiry was to be therapeutic:

> Yes, of *course* I sometimes ask myself am I having a mystical experience or going nuts? Am I walking towards the light or into the dark? But it is *my* question. Not someone else's. And it's *my* answer. Does that matter? Of course it does, because if someone else is defining your personal experience, your status can change overnight from valid to invalid (in-valid). That is very dangerous because then the very *ways* in which you heal might be interpreted as sick too. And no longer available to you. (Leibrich, 2002, p. 154)

If we imagine a clinician in discussion with Julie Leibrich, we can hear her raise or imply important questions: 'Are you willing to work with or within *my frame of reference*?', 'Are you willing to understand me *in my terms*?' and 'Will you believe *in me* even if you do not agree with me?' When confronted with apparent meaninglessness it is neither kind nor helpful to attempt to prove it wrong. Contradiction is often met with loss of trust and withdrawal, leading to further defensive elaboration of belief. In contrast, seeking to see through the expressed beliefs to the struggling person within offers an opportunity for cautious, tentative, respectful connection.

How does this work in practice? Here's a small example:

> You step on to the ward and are met by an agitated young woman saying 'I don't want to take the medication'. There is a nurse behind her holding an opaque plastic pot with the rejected pill . . . a familiar situation . . . but what do you do next? In an unhurried world you may be aware that you don't really know why she refuses this pill . . . and ask. She offers an apparently nonsensical answer, 'because I don't want to kill anyone' . . . you now know even less . . . what do you do? Maybe you ask again 'What makes you think that?' . . . 'I looked it up' . . . 'Where?' . . . 'In the dictionary' . . . 'Can you show me?' . . . and she goes in the office and brings out an elderly and battered copy of Webster's Dictionary and shows you that 'Quell' (as in Seroquel) means to 'kill, murder or subdue'. You look at the text together and you point out that this is linked to the ancient and now disused root 'cwellan', and that in modern times it means 'to calm'. This interaction has taken 10 minutes; she feels heard and there is now a sense of mutual understanding sufficient for her to choose to try the medication and see if it helps.

This kindly, curious and conversational approach to seeking meaning in madness fosters trust and helps to enable recovery (Roberts, 2006), and it has been further and more formally developed as various forms of narrative therapy (Rhodes and Jakes, 2009).

Implications for Practice and Practitioners

I note the obvious differences between each sort and type,
but we are more alike, my friends, than we are unalike.
(Maya Angelou, The Human Family, *1994)*

No one is ever completely mad, and looking for connection with the non-psychotic 'sane' aspect of people when their way of presenting themselves is unfathomable or unacceptable is a key issue in rehabilitation psychiatry and in recovery. If we really are 'more alike than unalike', the practitioner needs to respect and relate to the patient as someone who is and always has been a person, a person separate from his or her illness, struggling and doing his or her best to deal with confusing and sometimes horrifying experiences (Strauss, 1994; Davidson 2011). Someone like me.

The Culture of Care and the Construction of Services

As we have seen, social isolation is toxic and traumatic whereas acceptance, including recognition of the legitimacy of psychotic experience as part of being fully human, can be antipsychotic. The possibility of being restored to a community of peers may be powerfully supported by incorporation of peer perspectives in the culture of care.

The psychotic experience, which may include some compensatory 'comforts', is mostly exquisitely uncomfortable, being characterised by disruption and disturbance, immobilising terror, distance and isolation (Sayer, 1989). It is a sobering realisation that these profound personal struggles can be compounded by the ways in which our services are delivered – what Deegan (2000) called *'spirit breaking'*. The stigma, discrimination and social exclusion commonly associated with psychosis may be just as important or even more important determinants of the life experience of people with mental disorder than the disorder itself. This can apply to family members, too, who frequently become 'carers', as if they had no other role in life (Boardman et al., 2010).

Despair as well as hope is contagious. Psychiatrists need to be able to develop the capacity to witness and endure the distress of those with psychosis, to travel the long and often complex road to recovery with them and remain hopeful. This includes sustaining morale and a sense of possibility even for those for whom lengthy hospitalisations may have led to loss of agency or vision for their own lives.

Practitioners have their own needs for supportive relationships and spiritual renewal, and get into particular difficulties when they over-identify with their professional roles, neglect the importance of living a balanced life and forget that they are 'also human' (Elton, 2018). Kennard (2007, p. 207) observed that 'Mental health professionals . . . need to maintain and sometimes recover the sense of meaning and fulfilment in their work, the humanity and compassion that first brought them into the field. The day-to-day work in settings that are pressured from many directions can lead to self-protective defences such as emotional detachment, reductive labelling, them-and-us blaming, and retreat to the paperwork'.

It is a sad commentary on the realities of current practice that 'burnout' is such a common experience among psychiatrists (Summers et al., 2020). It is also uncanny and possibly meaningful that the state of demoralisation, exhaustion, detachment and loss of meaning and purpose which typifies 'burnout' (Roberts, 1997) appears to mirror the criticisms commonly applied to poorer services. This disorder of morale and vision clearly has spiritual implications. Is it primarily the vitality of the spirit that has been exhausted?

It is very important to seriously consider how we may be able to uphold and cultivate our creativity, hope and enthusiasm. How are we to sustain our own spirit to be effective holders of hope, for we cannot give what we do not have?

Although we could be trained and better prepared to care for ourselves, and there could and should be organisational responses (Roberts, 1997), the Buddhist concept of 'Sangha' may be helpful, too. It describes a way of being in relationships based on mutual support, goodwill and trust, focused on enabling spiritual growth and maturity. Sometimes called 'spiritual friendship', it may characterise a group, or be a way of relating. Looking for like-minded colleagues, companions and allies in our teams and clinical communities, joining or creating local values-based supports for recovery and progressive practice (e.g., Recovery Devon, www.recoverydevon.co.uk) and taking an interest in research that seeks to put values-led principles into practice, such as peer-supported open dialogue (Razzaque and Stockmann, 2016), can all help.

In 2011, the aspiration to understand what may be the key factors in enabling mental health systems, services and cultures to better support recovery outcomes led to the Department of Health sponsoring a programme of 'Implementing Recovery through Organisational Change' (ImROC). This has since become a leading not-for-profit service development consultancy and source of authoritative co-produced guidance on many aspects of innovative person-centred practice (https://imroc.org/about-us/).

There is also benefit in developing an international perspective through cultivating connections with groups and organisations that explicitly seek to support person-centred values. To that end, we have both found the International Society for Psychological and Social Approaches to Psychosis (ISPS) (www.isps.org) a hospitable and companionable 'broad church' that is deeply committed to compassionate care and improved lives for people with psychosis.

Diagnosis and Discernment

Psychiatric diagnosis is fundamental to practice, and in practice is fundamentally problematic. The process of reaching a diagnosis is one of discernment – of eliciting patterns of signs and symptoms that conform to diagnostic concepts described and given names in international frameworks of classification. In psychiatry, diagnoses are mostly conceptualisations to be used, not things to 'have', still less to 'be', but diagnosis and identity are easily and inappropriately conflated. When helpful they serve to orientate both clinician and patient, and guide treatment and expectations. David Harewood reminds us how important it is to discuss the diagnosis with the patient (James, 2020). However, a diagnosis can also lead to stigma and discrimination, be experienced negatively as labelling or even unwarranted accusation and create obstacles to recovery. Diagnostic practice, when framed as 'truth telling', can be deeply divisive and generate disturbing tensions between practitioners and patients and between different professionals in multidisciplinary teams.

This comes to a head with 'schizophrenia' – on the one hand considered by the World Health Organization to be the third most disabling of all medical conditions, and on the other the focus of disputes over whether it even exists. An international debate on renaming or de-naming schizophrenia has been led by Japan and other Asian countries which, since 2002, accepted family-led advocacy to change what was felt to be the socially discriminating and personally humiliating diagnosis of 'mind-splitting disease' (schizophrenia) to that of 'disintegration disorder' (Japan) or 'attunement disorder' (Korea). Crucially, the name change was accompanied by reconceptualization of the disorder with positive implications for informed consent, education, optimism for recovery and hopefulness (Maruta and Matsumoto, 2019). The debate continues in the West, where there have been other developments such as co-produced guides to diagnostic practice that seek to be more sensitive to a person-centred approach (Devon Partnership NHS Trust, 2012), and advocacy for more evidence-based diagnostic formulations (Timimi, 2014).

Madness as a Spiritual Journey?

The mystic dances in the sun,
hearing music others don't.
'Insanity', they say, those others.
If so, it's a very gentle,
nourishing sort.

(Jelaluddin Rumi, thirteenth-century Persian Sufi)

Mysticism and the characteristics of mystical experiences have been defined in Chapter 1; many mystics of different religious faiths have long been known to have experiences which, from a clinical point of view, are recognisably psychotic. This neither confirms nor invalidates their spiritual standing. William James observed that 'a religious life exclusively pursued, does tend to make the person exceptional and eccentric . . . religious geniuses have often shown symptoms of nervous instability ... subject to abnormal psychical visitations' (James, 1902, p. 29). Mystical experiences are not uncommon in the population and may be reported more frequently by people with certain personality profiles, notably schizotypy (Clarke et al., 2016).

We should consider the possibility that a person might be having both a spiritual and a psychotic experience, or the possibility that in psychosis, at the limits of reason, there may be a crack that lets in the light.[3] Jaspers (1963, p. 108) comments that 'religious experience remains what it is whether it occurs in saint or psychotic or whether the person in whom it occurs is both at once' (for further consideration of this issue, see Chapter 16).

The important issue is the way in which the psychotic phenomena are embedded in the values and beliefs of the person: 'it is not what you believe but how you believe it' (Peters, 2001, p. 207). Jackson and Fulford (2002) acknowledge the limitations of traditional descriptive diagnostic criteria in distinguishing pathological from non-pathological psychotic experiences, and they suggest the need for an additional evaluative criterion. A key arbiter of clinical concern is a guiding focus on relief of suffering; distress and unwanted preoccupations characterise psychosis, whereas spiritual experiences may be sought after and are more often associated with transformative life changes (Clarke et al., 2016). Unlike delusional belief systems, the beliefs of those with religious convictions may be accompanied by doubt, valued as the growing edge of faith (Roberts, 1991). However, Jackson observes that the distinction based on whether the experience is life enhancing or overwhelming and isolating becomes blurred in the longer term; many people see their psychosis 'as part of a process through which they reached, from their perspective, a constructive spiritual reorientation' (Jackson, 2001 p. 183; see also Chapter 16).

Seeking a Balance Between Power, Compulsion and Coercion

> The respect for patients, the emphasis on human rights and the value placed on relationships are as relevant now as they were in 1813. (Kathleen Jones, 1996)

Desmond, with part of whose story we began this chapter, was detained in hospital. Severe psychosis often results in the person feeling overwhelmed, governed by forces beyond their control or understanding which may be compounded if compulsory measures are needed in care and treatment. Power is a key dynamic in therapeutic settings; how we use it, share it and give it away may be shaped by our spiritual beliefs and ethical practices. A person cannot progress far in recovery while others are in control of their lives, and there is no such thing as 'forced recovery' (Roberts and Hollins, 2007). Practice developments to reduce the use of physical intervention and restraint (e.g., 'No force first', championed by ImROC) can be of value here. It has long been recognised that optimising choice and reshaping power relationships in therapeutic settings may be a key variable in determining whether our well-intended interventions are experienced as therapeutic or additionally traumatic (Roberts et al., 2008). However, there is a difference between being subject to involuntary interventions and being subject to coercion – for

---

[3] The Baptist Minister, John Martin, proclaimed that if Blake is cracked, 'his is a crack that lets in the Light' (Bentley, 2001, p. 176).

some this may seem to be splitting hairs, but it may be the difference between being supported to accept an unwanted necessity or being fearfully forced into submission. However, any possibility of involuntary intervention should be carefully considered in the light of potential longer-term consequences related to trauma and trust.

Spiritual Support, and Supporters, for Journeys in Recovery

> You need hope to cope. (Rachel Perkins, 2006)

Personal accounts of recovery from severe mental health challenges and mental illness are themselves a potent source of hope that supports resilience on the journey to recovery. They commonly emphasise the value of 'spiritual factors' such as the learning and healing arising from the experience of psychosis itself, relationships and connections with people, animals and nature, creativity and storytelling (Leibrich, 1999; Davidson and Lynn, 2009). These may be supported through involvement in a community and participation in its practices, whether explicitly spiritual or not, and having a therapist who is alive to spiritual values. As Peter Chadwick emphasised, 'recognition of the spiritual side of my illness and the taking of it seriously by clinicians and social workers were extremely important in my recovery' (Chadwick, 2001, p. 87).

A service needs to work with the person to support their own story and values so that their resilience is strengthened, and so that *they*, rather than the professionals, retain or regain control. Whitwell (2005, p. 158) observed that 'Personal recovery involves much more than losing symptoms. It involves becoming a person again, regaining a personal life that has some value and meaning'. The impact of a psychotic illness on the life of the individual and of their family can be devastating, redefining both. The qualities that keep a sense of humanity alive are challenged and often overwhelmed; there is a loss of meaning and purpose, and of relationships and place in the family, work and society. Unfamiliar and frightening emotions can lead to discomfort and withdrawal, and mental health institutions can be desolate and friendless places. In this situation, 'hope is not just a nice sounding euphemism. It is a matter of life or death' (Deegan, 1996, p. 3). Deegan talks of the importance of relationships in keeping hope alive. Perkins (2006, p. 119), too, acknowledges the importance of relationships – 'hope does not exist in a vacuum' – and emphasises the value of 'hope-inspiring relationships'; there is a particular challenge and opportunity for practitioners to cultivate their capacity to be 'carriers of hope'.

In Praise of Ordinary

> As van Gogh (1879, letter 154) said, 'Like everyone else, I have need of relationships of friendship or affection or trusting companionship, and am not like a street pump or lamp-post, whether of stone or iron, so that I can't do without them without perceiving an emptiness and feeling their lack'.

When confronted with the psychotic mind manifested in 'full blown madness' we can easily forget or fail to value just how important are the simple supports of ordinary living. Yet, for the most part, this is what so many people in recovery long for. In response to the question 'What makes life valuable for those of us with mental illness?', Esso Leete (1993, p. 127) stated, 'exactly what is necessary for other people. We need to feel wanted, accepted ... we need support from family and friends ... we need to feel part of the human race, to have friends. We need to give and receive love'. Davidson (2011, p. 111), too, recognises the importance of loving mutual relationships with family and friends which involve a sense of loyalty and belonging, and also states that in the process of regaining a sense of personhood it is important to be able 'to do something, to participate, to contribute and to recognise oneself as a worthwhile person based on these contributions'.

Patte Randal, a rehabilitation psychiatrist who has herself had psychotic episodes, felt stigmatised and rejected by her profession. She puts it like this:

> I have really questioned, *am I credible, am I worth listening to?* And I think you need to recover that in a relationship, you need someone to enable you to experience again that you have validity and value. You're not an invalid. You're not invalid. You have worth, value, validity, credibility. You *mean* something to someone else. I don't think you can discover that except in a relationship. (Randal, 1999, p. 142)

Cullberg also acknowledges the importance of relationships at the 'turning-point' in recovery:

> In a positive sense to tire of dependence on inner destructive forces and to decide to depend on one's own potential is a process that sometimes bears a resemblance to Christian parables of conversion. Often the event is conveyed through a personal relationship with a carer, a partner or someone who believes in the person's potential and who does it at the right time. (Cullberg, 2014, pp. 166–1677)

Professional carers can practise with these values in mind and seek to form therapeutic relationships based on partnership (Tondora et al., 2014), but these values are also what makes peer support so important.

Valuing Peer Support

> As much as possible, all servants are chosen from the category of mental patients. They are at any rate better suited to this demanding work because they are usually more gentle, honest, and humane. Jean Baptiste Pussin, in a letter written to Philippe Pinel in 1793 (Davidson et al., 2012, p. 123)

In ordinary life, maturity and wisdom are often closely associated with living through suffering, and mediated by the transformation of experience into expertise. The possibility of benefiting from the support and guidance of experience-based experts, who are now coming into the workforce as peer support workers or recovery guides, is growing (Davidson et al., 2012). Michael Cornwall's peer perspective on spiritual aspects of extreme states leads him to observe that a reductive *'medical model'* approach 'never seemed to effectively account for the mysteries of human emotional suffering and madness that I know about personally and that I witness in others. The requisite clinical gaze of a detached medical, diagnostic based approach diffuses the human warmth that I believe we all need when we are in emotional pain and distress' (Cornwall, 2014).

This 'requisite clinical gaze' has recently been described as 'psychiatry's myopia' (Braslow et al., 2021). It is striking that as an experience-based expert, Cornwall argues for the value, need and effectiveness of 'loving receptivity' as a healing force in madness – just as Pussin, in the language of his time, did in 1793. This compassionate peer perspective is also a foundation for developing the collaborative educational opportunities which have characterised the growth of Recovery Colleges, largely in NHS trusts

(Perkins and Repper, 2017). Engagement with and support for these co-produced innovations are recommended as significant contributions towards *person-centred care* (Person-Centred Training and Curriculum [PCTC] Scoping Group, 2018), which in turn is now influencing the training and qualification of psychiatrists.

What We Need to Do: Listening, Learning and Teaching, Together

The lyf so short, the craft so long to lerne. (Geoffrey Chaucer, 1380/1957, p. 310)

We began by observing that psychosis was of central significance in psychiatry. In many ways the history of psychiatry is the history of the care and treatment of people with psychosis, and for much of that time it has not been a happy or hopeful one. Yet many positive developments and values-led innovations have been advocated *by people with psychosis*, arising from how they themselves had been treated. Latterly this has led to the recovery movement, with its emphasis on experience-based expertise, peer support and recovery learning which all find a place in the hope for person-centred care. Similarly, the drive for contemporary rehabilitation approaches is to enable recovery through working with people in partnership in ways that are sensitive to meaning, purpose, choice and self-determination. Much of this pivots around how we see and value one another when in profoundly compromised and confused states of mind. A spiritual element, though not often named, is interwoven throughout.

The value of spirituality both to practitioners and to people experiencing psychosis is in its support for health, healing and wholeness, as an inspiration for acceptance, respect and understanding, and as a source of kindness and compassion, even love.

If our commitment to developing a spiritual approach to psychosis is to be practical and result in tangible benefits to those who need it, we will need to look beyond our confidential conversations and professional meetings and consider how we can influence the world in which people live, and how we can do this in the context of their lives. We will need to cultivate an approach to practice that is fully engaged with the realities of life and living in society.

The Royal College of Psychiatrists is supportive of psychiatrists working to improve services and to fulfil important leadership roles in their teams and organisations. The civil rights roots of the recovery movement suggest still wider roles and relationships, and that recovery-oriented professionals of the future should also lend their skill, authority and influence to social activism and support for social justice. This is about working not only in the community but also with the community, seeking to influence key issues in people's lives, such as income, housing, employment, social inclusion (Roberts and Boardman, 2014), equality and race (Royal College of Psychiatrists, 2018), and asking how hospitable our faith communities are to those with significant mental health challenges (Corrigan, 2020).

In this chapter, we have indicated only some of the complexities encountered in the often problematic but potentially restorative and healing relationship between spirituality and psychosis. We hope that we have encouraged our readers to enquire further and to seek for themselves answers to the questions we have raised. We hope also that we have demonstrated that to work well with people suffering from psychosis there is a need for a practical, grounded, person-centred and recovery-oriented spirituality – one that incorporates humanity and compassion while accepting the integrity of personal experience. Could the recognition, cultivation and use of our own spiritual strengths and vulnerabilities help to enable us to put this into practice? We believe so, for all good medical practice is founded on values that include compassion, honesty and humility, but in psychosis, where the loss of a sense of personhood is potentially greatest, these attributes are paramount.

References

Angelou, M. (1994) *The Complete Collected Poems of Maya Angelou.* New York: Random House.

Anonymous (1986) 'Can we talk?' The schizophrenic patient in psychotherapy. *American Journal of Psychiatry*, 143, 68–70.

Baker, E. and Attwater, M (2015) *Living with Psychosis: Recovery and Wellbeing.* London: Chipmunkapublishing.

Baker, E. and Roberts, G. (2015) Understanding madness: a psychosocial perspective. In F. Holloway, S. Kalindindi, H. Killaspy and G. Roberts, eds., *Enabling Recovery: The Principles and Practice of Rehabilitation Psychiatry*, 2nd ed. London: RCPsych Publications, pp. 79–98.

Batchelor, S. (2015) *After Buddhism: Rethinking the Dharma for a Secular Age.* New Haven, CT: Yale University Press.

Bentall, R. P. (2004) Abandoning the concept of schizophrenia: the cognitive psychology of delusions and hallucinations. In J. Read, L. Mosher and R. Bentall, eds., *Models of Madness: Psychological, Social and Biological Approaches to Schizophrenia.* New York: Brunner-Routledge, pp. 195–208.

Bentley, G. E. Jr. (2001) *The Stranger from Paradise: A Biography of William Blake.* New Haven, CT: Yale University Press.

Bhui, K., Warfa, N., Edonya, P. et al. (2007) Cultural competence in mental health care: a review of model evaluations. *BMC Health Services Research*, 7, 15.

Bhui, K. Halvorsru, K. and Nazroo, J. (2018) Making a difference: ethnic inequality and severe mental illness. *The British Journal of Psychiatry*, 213, 574–578.

Blake, W. (1789/1969) Annotations to Swedenborg's *Wisdom of Angels, Concerning Divine Love and Divine Wisdom.* In G. Keynes, ed., *Blake: Complete Writings.* Oxford: Oxford University Press, p. 89.

Boardman, J., Currie, A., Killaspy, H., et al. (2010) *Social Inclusion and Mental Health.* London: RCPsych Publications.

Braslow, J. T., Brekke, J. S. and Levenson, J. (2021) Psychiatry's myopia – reclaiming the social, cultural, and psychological in the psychiatric gaze. *JAMA Psychiatry*, 78, 349–350.

Chadwick, P. K. (2001) Sanity to supersanity to insanity: a personal journey. In I. Clarke, ed., *Psychosis and Spirituality: Exploring the New Frontier.* London: Whurr, pp. 75–89.

Chadwick, P. K. (2007) Peer-professional first-person account: schizophrenia from the inside: phenomenology and the integration of causes and meanings. *Schizophrenia Bulletin*, 33, 166–173.

Chaucer, G. (1380/1957) The Parliament of Fowls. In F. N. Robinson, ed., *The Works of Geoffrey Chaucer.* London: Oxford University Press, p. 310.

Clarke, I., Mottram, K., Taylor, S. et al. (2016) Narratives of transformation in psychosis. In C. Cook, A. Powell and A. Sims, eds., *Spirituality and Narrative in Psychiatric Practice: Stories of Mind and Soul.* London: Royal College of Psychiatrists, pp. 108–120.

Cook, C. C. H. (2016) Narrative in psychiatry, theology and spirituality. In C. Cook, A. Powell and A. Sims, eds., *Spirituality and Narrative in Psychiatric Practice: Stories of Mind and Soul.* London: Royal College of Psychiatrists, pp. 1–13.

Cordle, H., Carson, J. and Richards, P., eds. (2011) *Psychosis: Stories of Recovery and Hope*. London: Quay Books.

Corrigan, P. (2020) Challenges to welcoming people with mental illness into faith communities. *British Journal of Psychiatry*, 217, 595–596.

Cox, M. (1992) *Shakespeare Comes to Broadmoor*. London: Jessica Kingsley Publishers.

Cox, M. and Theilgaard, A. (1994) *Mutative Metaphors in Psychotherapy: The Aeolian Mode*. London: Jessica Kingsley Publishers.

Cullberg, J. (2014) *Psychoses: An Integrative Perspective*. London: Routledge.

Davidson, L. (2011) Recovery from psychosis: what's love got to do with it? *Psychosis*, 3, 105–114.

Davidson, L. and Lynn, L. (2009) *Beyond the Storms: Reflections on Personal Recovery in Devon*. Available at https://library .recoverydevon.co.uk/document/beyond-the-storms/ (accessed 1 April 2022).

Davidson, L., Rakfeldt, J. and Strauss, J. (2010) *The Roots of the Recovery Movement in Psychiatry: Lessons Learned*. Oxford: Wiley-Blackwell.

Davidson, L., Bellamy, C., Guy, K., et al. (2012) Peer support among persons with severe mental illness: a review of evidence and experience. *World Psychiatry*, 11, 123–128.

Dawkins, R. (2006) *The God Delusion*. Boston, MA: Houghton Mifflin.

Deegan, P. (1996) *Recovery and the Conspiracy of Hope*. Available at www.nyaprs.org/e-news-bulletins/2018/9/18/recovery-the-conspiracy-of-hope-pat-deegans-1996-call-to-arms-come-hear-pat-this-wednesday-at-the-nyaprs-conference?rq=deegan (accessed 25 November 2020).

Deegan, P. (2000) Spirit breaking: when the helping professions hurt. *The Humanistic Psychologist*, 28, 194–209.

Devon Partnership NHS Trust (2012) *How Can We Use Diagnosis to Support People in Their Recovery?* Recovery Devon Resource Library. Available at https://library .recoverydevon.co.uk/document/how-can-we-use-diagnosis-to-support-recovery/ (accessed 1 April 2022).

Dickinson, E. (1862/1976) Much Madness is divinest Sense. In T. H. Johnson, ed., *The Complete Poems of Emily Dickinson*. Boston, MA: Little, Brown & Co., p. 209.

Drury, M. O'C. (1981) Some notes on conversations with Wittgenstein. In R. Rhees, ed., *Ludwig Wittgenstein: Personal Recollections*. Oxford: Blackwell, p. 94.

Elton, C. (2018) *Also Human: The Inner Lives of Doctors*. London: William Heinemann.

Filer, N. (2019) *This Book Will Change Your Mind About Mental Health: A Journey into the Heartland of Psychiatry*. London: Faber and Faber.

Holloway, F., Kalindindi, S., Killaspy, H. and Roberts, G., eds. (2015) *Enabling Recovery: The Principles and Practice of Rehabilitation Psychiatry*, 2nd ed. London: RCPsych Publications.

Hunter, K. M. (1991) *Doctors' Stories: The Narrative Structure of Medical Knowledge*. Princeton, NJ: Princeton University Press.

Jackson, M. (2001) Psychotic and spiritual experience: a case study comparison. In I. Clarke, ed. *Psychosis and Spirituality*. London: Whurr Publishers, pp. 165–190.

Jackson, M. and Fulford, K. W. M. (2002) Psychosis good and bad: values-based practice and the distinction between pathological and non-pathological forms of psychotic experience. *Philosophy, Psychiatry, & Psychology*, 9, 387–394.

James, W. (1902/1960) *The Varieties of Religious Experience*. London: Collins Fontana Library.

Jaspers, K. (1963) *General Psychopathology* (J. Hoenigand J. W. Hamilton, trans.). Manchester: Manchester University Press.

Jones, K. (1996) *Foreword to Description of the Retreat, by Samuel Tuke (1813)*. London: Process Press.

Jung, C. G. (1926/1972) Spirit and life. In *Collected Works of C. J. Jung, Vol. 8: The Structure and Dynamics of the Psyche*, 2nd ed. Princeton, NJ: Princeton University Press, pp. 319–337.

Kennard, D. (2007) Things you can do to make in-patient care a better experience. In M. Hardcastle, D. Kennard, S. Grandison and L. Fagin, eds., *Experiences of Mental Health In-Patient Care: Narratives from Service Users, Carers and Professionals.* London: Routledge, pp. 205–207.

Koenig, H. G., Al-Zaben, F. and VanderWeele, T. (2020) Religion and psychiatry: recent developments in research. *BJPsych Advances*, 26, 262–272.

Laing, R. D. (1960) *The Divided Self: An Existential Study in Sanity and Madness.* London: Tavistock Publications.

Lao-Tzu. (undated) *Tao Te Ching: The Book of the Way* (S. Mitchell, trans. 1988). London: Kyle Cathie.

Leete, E. (1993) The interpersonal environment: a consumer's personal recollection. In A. Hatfield and H. Lefley, eds., *Surviving Mental Illness: Stress, Coping, and Adaptation.* New York, NY: Guilford Press, pp. 114–128.

Leibrich, J. (1999) *A Gift of Stories: Discovering How to Deal with Mental Illness.* Dunedin: Otago University Press.

Leibrich, J. (2002) Making space: spirituality and mental health. *Mental Health, Religion & Culture*, 5, 143–162.

Loewenthal, K. M. (2017) Spirituality and cultural psychiatry. In D. Bhugra and K. Bhui, eds., *Textbook of Cultural Psychiatry.* Cambridge: Cambridge University Press, pp. 59–71.

Lomax, J. and Pargament, K. (2016) Gods lost and found: spiritual coping in clinical practice. In C. H. Cook, A. Powell and A. Sims, eds., *Spirituality and Narrative in Psychiatric Practice: Stories of Mind and Soul.* London: Royal College of Psychiatrists, pp. 53–66.

Maruta, T. and Matsumoto, C. (2019) Renaming schizophrenia. *Epidemiology and Psychiatric Sciences*, 28, 262–264.

Milner, K., Crawford. P., Edgley, A. et al. (2020) The experiences of spirituality among adults with mental health difficulties: a qualitative systematic review.

Epidemiology and Psychiatric Sciences, 29, e34.

Mind (2011) *Listening to Experience: An independent Inquiry into Acute and Crisis Mental Health Care.* Available at www.mind.org.uk/media-a/4377/listening_to_experience_web.pdf

Mitchell, S. (2009) *In every one: a psychiatrist's reflections on spirituality.* The Retreat Lecture: Britain Yearly Meeting. Available at www.retreatyorkbfund.com/Retreat-Lecture

Murray, R. (2012) *The Abandoned Illness.* London: Schizophrenia Commission.

National Institute for Health and Care Excellence (NICE) (2002) *Schizophrenia: Clinical Guideline, CG1.* London: NICE.

National Institute for Health and Care Excellence (NICE) (2020) *Rehabilitation for Adults with Complex Psychosis.* Available at www.nice.org.uk/guidance/ng181

Perkins, R. (2006) First person: 'you need hope to cope'. In G. Roberts, S. Davenport, F. Holloway and T. Tattan, eds., *Enabling Recovery: The Principles and Practice of Rehabilitation Psychiatry.* London: Gaskell, pp. 112–124.

Perkins, R. and Repper, J. (2017) Editorial: When is a 'recovery college' not a 'recovery college'? *Mental Health and Social Inclusion*, 21, 65–72.

Person-Centred Training and Curriculum (PCTC) Scoping Group (2018) *Person-Centred Care: Implications for Training in Psychiatry. CR215.* London: Royal College of Psychiatrists.

Person-Centred Training and Curriculum (PCTC) Scoping Group (2019) Training in psychiatry: making person-centred care a reality. *BJPsych Bulletin*, 43, 136–140.

Peters, E. (2001) Are delusions on a continuum? The case of religious and delusional beliefs. In I. Clarke, ed., *Psychosis and Spirituality: Exploring the New Frontier.* London: Whurr, pp. 191–207.

Randal, P. (1999) Loving relationship is at the root of recovery. In J. Leibrich, ed., *A Gift of Stories: Discovering How to Deal with*

Mental Illness. Dunedin: University of Otago Press, pp. 137–143.

Razzaque, R. and Stockmann, T. (2016) An introduction to peer-supported open dialogue in mental healthcare. *BJPsych Advances*, 22, 348–356.

Read, J. Fosse, R. Moskowitz, A. et al. (2014) The traumagenic neurodevelopmental model of psychosis revisited. *Neuropsychiatry*, 4, 65–79.

Remen, N. (1993) On defining Spirit. *Noetic Sciences Review*, 27, 41.

Rhodes, J. and Jakes, S. (2009) *Narrative CBT for Psychosis*. London: Routledge.

Roberts, G. (1991) Delusional belief systems and meaning in life: a preferred reality? *British Journal of Psychiatry*, 19 (Suppl. 14), 19–28.

Roberts, G. (1997) Prevention of burnout. *Advances in Psychiatric Treatment*, 3, 282–289.

Roberts, G. (2006) Understanding madness. In G. Roberts, S. Davenport, F. Holloway and T. Tattan, eds., *Enabling Recovery: The Principles and Practice of Rehabilitation Psychiatry*. London: Gaskell, pp. 93–111.

Roberts, G. and Hollins, S. (2007) Recovery: our common purpose? *Advances in Psychiatric Treatment*, 13, 397–399.

Roberts, G. and Boardman, J. (2013) Understanding recovery. *Advances in Psychiatric Treatment*, 19, 400–409.

Roberts, G. and Boardman, J. (2014) Becoming a recovery-oriented practitioner. *Advances in Psychiatric Treatment*, 20, 37–47.

Roberts, G., Dorkins, E., Wooldridge, J, et al. (2008) Detained: what's my choice? Part 1: Discussion. *Advances in Psychiatric Treatment*, 14, 172–180.

Romme, M. and Escher, S. (2000) *Making Sense of Voices*. London: Mind Publications.

Royal College of Psychiatrists (2018) *Racism and Mental Health. Position Statement PS01/18*. London: Royal College of Psychiatrists.

Rumi, J. (1993) *Birdsong: 53 Short Poems* (C. Barks, trans.). Athens, GA: Maypop Books, p. 24.

Santayana, G. (1925) *Dialogues in Limbo*. London: Constable and Co. Ltd. Available at https://archive.org/details/dialoguesinlimbo014715mbp (accessed 25 November 2020).

Sayer, P. (1989) *The Comforts of Madness*. London: Hodder & Stoughton.

Sharfstein, S. (2005) Big Pharma and American psychiatry: the good, the bad, and the ugly. *Psychiatric News*, 40, 3.

Sims, A. (2003) *Symptoms in the Mind: An Introduction to Descriptive Psychopathology*, 3rd ed. London: Elsevier Science Limited.

Strauss, J. (1994) The person with schizophrenia as a person. *British Journal of Psychiatry*, 164 (Suppl. 23), 103–107.

Summers, R. F., Gorrindo, T., Hwang, S. et al. (2020) Well-being, burnout, and depression among North American psychiatrists: the state of our profession. *American Journal of Psychiatry*, 177, 955–964.

Swinton, J. (2001) *Spirituality and Mental Health Care*. London: Jessica Kingsley Publishers.

Tausk, V. (1933) On the origin of the "influencing machine" in schizophrenia. *The Psychoanalytic Quarterly*, 2, 519–556.

Timimi, S. (2014) No more psychiatric labels: why formal psychiatric diagnostic systems should be abolished. *International Journal of Clinical and Health Psychology*, 14, 208–215.

Tondora, J., Miller, R., Slade, M. et al. (2014) *Partnering for Recovery in Mental Health: A Practical Guide to Person-Centred Planning*. Chichester: John Wiley & Sons.

Tuke, S. (1813/1996) *Description of the Retreat, An Institution Near York, for Insane Persons of the Society of Friends*. London: Process Press.

Van Gogh, V. (1879) *The Letters of Vincent Van Gogh*. Letter 154: To Theo van Gogh. Cuesmes, between about Monday, 11 and Thursday, 14 August 1879. Available at https://vangoghletters.org/vg/letters/

let154/letter.html (accessed 23 November 2020).

Van Gogh, V. (1888) *The Letters of Vincent Van Gogh*. Letter 673: To Theo van Gogh. Arles, Monday, 3 September 1888. Available at https://vangoghletters.org/vg/letters/let673/letter.html (accessed 23 November 2020).

Whitwell, D. (2005) *Recovery Beyond Psychiatry*. London: Free Association Books.

Audiovisual references and resources

Borges, P. (2016) A Traditional Approach to Mental Illness: Crazywise. Available at www.ted.com

Cornwall, M. (2014) Providing Loving Receptivity Can Help People in Extreme States. Available at www.madinamerica.com/2014/10/providing-loving-receptivity-can-help-people-extreme-states/

Devon (2011) The Autumn Festival of Recovery and Wellbeing. Available at https://vimeo.com/35739103

James, A. (2020) Interview with David Harewood. Available at www.rcpsych.ac.uk/events/free-webinars/free-webinars-for-members/2020/interview-with-david-harewood-23-july-2020

Lampshire, D. (2018) Hearing Voices: An Insider's Guide to Auditory Hallucinations. Available at www.ted.com

Longden, E. (2013) Voices in My Head. Available at www.ted.com

Suicide

Cherrie Coghlan[1]

Suicide is a central concern in clinical psychiatry. Spirituality/religion, being concerned with life, death and meaning, is relevant to suicide for a variety of reasons which will be explored in this chapter. The chapter will consider the following: attitudes to suicide in faith traditions; membership of faith communities and spiritual practices; psychological interventions with spiritual features; spiritual issues in the clinical management of suicidal people; physician-assisted suicide; the impact of suicide on survivors; and the response of mental health professionals to suicide.

Attitudes to Suicide in Religious Traditions

Religious attitudes to suicide have traditionally been condemnatory, but have become more humane over time; the emphasis has shifted to one of compassion for the deceased and support of the bereaved. Despite generally condemnatory views in religious teachings, there is heterogeneity within and between traditions, and allowance is usually made for mental disorder as a mitigating factor.

Suicide in the Ancient World

In ancient Greece there was a taboo against suicide, resulting in the corpse being buried outside the city with the hands cut off and buried separately. Alvarez (2002) sees this as a logical extension of a taboo against killing members of one's own family. Pythagoras regarded humans as the chattels of gods who would be angered by the self-destruction of their creation, whereas Aristotle took the more pragmatic view that suicide robs the state of economic contributions.

Plato's account of the death of Socrates suggests that Socrates was opposed to suicide on both these grounds (Holland, 1969; Alvarez, 2002). Although he died by his own hand, it is arguable that Socrates' death was not suicide but a courageous acceptance of the death penalty. He did not choose to die, but neither did he choose to run away. He considered it appropriate to desire death, but not to bring it about deliberately. He did not see death as a way of escape from anything. Bille-Brahe (2000) suggests that his ideas about the blessedness of death have inspired others to commit suicide.

In ancient Rome, suicide was considered honourable for private citizens and military leaders facing defeat. It was forbidden for ordinary soldiers and for slaves who were the property of their masters.

---

[1] The author acknowledges the contribution of Dr Imran Ali to the version of this chapter that appeared in the first edition, elements of which are incorporated in this updated version.

Suicide in the Jewish and Christian Traditions

servant to kill him. One account (1 Samuel 31:1–4)[2] suggests that the servant refused and
Saul killed himself; another (2 Samuel 1:1–10) suggests that he was killed by a soldier on
request. Samson, who was held captive, blinded and humiliated, pushed against the
pillars of the temple, causing the building to collapse, killing himself and his Philistine
captors.

There are two accounts of Judas's death. In the first (Matthew 27:3–5) he hangs
himself; in another (Acts 1:18) he falls to the ground with his abdomen bursting open. In
the former account Judas returns the money given for betraying Jesus to the authorities,
before hanging himself in anguish and remorse.

There is no specific biblical condemnation of suicide (Alvarez, 2002; Koch, 2005).
However, suicide is implicitly condemned in the sixth commandment, 'You shall not
murder' (Exodus 20:13), and in Genesis 9:5, which states that 'For your lifeblood I will
surely require a reckoning'. Actual and possible suicides are recorded in Hebrew and
Christian scriptures in a factual way that neither praises nor condemns the act. The
context is generally one of personal crisis; only in the case of Saul is there evidence of
prior mood swings (Barraclough, 1992). Koch (2005) notes that those who express
suicidal ideas are treated with compassion; for example, Sarah is comforted by thoughts
of her family and prayer (Tobit 3:10–16).

A former UK Chief Rabbi, Lord Jakobovits, has written of Judaism's uncompromising attribution of value to human life: 'In Jewish thought and law, human life enjoys an
absolute, intrinsic and infinite value. Man is not the owner of his body but merely its
custodian, charged to preserve it from any physical harm and to promote its health
where this has been impaired' (Jakobovits, 1988, p. 5).

The post-Talmudic tractate of Semachot advocates denying formal funeral rites to
those who 'destroy themselves' *lada-at*, meaning wittingly (Kaplan and Schoeneberg,
1988). In Judaism, the right to take life belongs to God alone; to kill oneself is to usurp
the divine priority. Suicide also deprives the community. Kaplan and Schoeneberg (1988)
emphasise that Jewish law (*Halacha*) defines suicide rigorously, requiring clear indication that the person acted wittingly. Not only mental illness but also behavioural
abnormalities and the influence of substances reduce responsibility; suicides in secular
law may therefore not be regarded as such in Jewish law.

In Jewish history, mass suicide at the fort of Masada in 70 CE was seen as a heroic act
whereby the entire population under siege by the Romans killed themselves, rather than
submit to the destruction of their way of life. During the Holocaust, 'suicide was the
conscious decision to end the unendurable: to refuse to remain at the whim of tormentors whose cruelties were sadistically drawn out: to die at one's chosen moment' (Gilbert,
1987, p. 322).

In the Christian tradition, St Augustine (354–438 CE) first pronounced on the issue
of suicide, considering it to be a violation of the sixth commandment. He clashed with

---

[2] Quotations are from the Bible, New Revised Standard Version.

the Donatists, who sought death for the glory of martyrdom. In the Christian Church, it has been important to distinguish between martyrdom and suicide (Wood, 1986).

Augustine's views influenced future scholars, most notably Thomas Aquinas (1225–1274) (Alvarez, 2002). Aquinas believed that the act of suicide was a mortal sin, as the final repentance had not been undertaken. He argued that suicide was unnatural and damaged the community, and that life was a gift of God not to be squandered. This became the widely accepted Christian stance on suicide, prevailing for seven centuries.

Harsh condemnation of suicide as a sin was prevalent throughout the Middle Ages. This view influenced the legal status of suicide as a crime. From the Enlightenment onwards, Christian attitudes began to change, questioning why people die by suicide. The Christian teaching to care for one's neighbour led to an emphasis on prevention, as well as feelings of guilt about failing to prevent suicide (Bille-Brahe, 2000).

The Church of England had a leading role in reform of the law on suicide in the UK, following a committee set up by the Archbishop of Canterbury in 1959. It recommended that suicide should no longer be considered a crime, and that the clergy should take a pastoral interest in suicidal people (Stengel, 1965). Another example of the positive influence of the Christian Church was the founding in 1953 of Samaritans by an Anglican priest. The Roman Catholic Church has also changed its position, acknowledging that anguish can diminish responsibility for suicide (Auer and Ang, 2007).

Suicide in Islam

Islam is more overt in its condemnation of suicide than the other Abrahamic faiths; suicide rates are relatively low in countries with Muslim majorities (Cook, 2014) and among Muslim communities in countries with diverse faith traditions (Lester, 2006). However, there may be under-reporting, both where suicide is illegal and because of religious attitudes (Lester, 2006).

The Qur'an and Hadith (sayings and actions of the Prophet Muhammad) explicitly condemn suicide: 'Do not kill yourselves. Surely Allah is ever Compassionate to you' (Qur'an 4:29).[3] Muslims believe that, among the many bounties Allah has bestowed upon humankind, the most precious is life. One of the five principles of Shar'iah is protection and preservation of life. In Islam it is believed that people who die by suicide will be deprived of Allah's blessings and mercy in the afterlife.

It is recorded in Hadith that the Prophet Muhammad said 'A man was inflicted with wounds and he committed suicide, and so Allah said: "My slave has caused death on himself hurriedly, so I forbid Paradise for him"' (Al-Bukhari, 1971a, verse 445), and 'None of you should long for death, for if he is a good man, he may increase his good deeds, and if he is an evil-doer, he may stop the evil deeds and repent' (Al-Bukhari, 1971b, verse 341).

Muslims are encouraged to pray rather than to despair or wish for death, and to be aware that Allah does not test individuals beyond their capacity: 'None of you should make a request for death because of the trouble in which he is involved, but if there is no other help to it, then say: "O Allah, keep me alive as long as there is goodness in life for me and bring death to me when there is goodness in death for me"' (Muslim, 1990). There is an implicit prohibition here of physician-assisted dying as well as suicide. In an

---

[3] All quotations from the Qur'an are from the 2007 translation by Zafar Ishaq Ansari.

Indian study of Hindu and Muslim attitudes to suicide (Thimmaiah et al., 2016), Muslim subjects disagreed that "Suicide is an acceptable means to terminate an incurable disease.'

As with the other Abrahamic faiths, despite the condemnation of suicide there is understanding that abnormal states of mind commonly underlie the act. In practice, compassion is shown towards the deceased person and their family: 'Many of our religious traditions condemn suicide. The condemnation is for suicides committed with a sound mind. But I have yet to have a case in which a suicide victim seemed to be making a rational choice' (Mozaffar, 2018).

In the context of suicide and Islam, it is important to note that 'suicide bombing' is a misnomer, more appropriately considered to be a form of politically motivated violence (Acevedo and Chaudhary, 2015). 'Suicide bombing' is culturally sanctioned only within unrepresentative extremist groups. Within these groups 'the prohibition in Islamic law against suicide is, in such instances being overridden or reinterpreted as another factor, namely that of martyrdom' (Gordon, 2002, p. 285).

Suicide in Eastern Faith Traditions

Buddhism and Hinduism have a more ambiguous attitude to suicide than the Western faiths, with less condemnation of it. The idea of eternal damnation is not found. This relates to a central doctrinal difference between Eastern and Western traditions: 'In contrast with the Judeo-Christian religions, one theme dominates the world view of both Hinduism and Buddhism: the doctrine of rebirth. According to this doctrine, an individual is subject to repeated cycles of birth and death before he arrives at the ultimate salvation of Nirvana' (Bhugra, 2004, p. 13).

Buddhism and Suicide

In Buddhism, suicide is usually considered regrettable, since the potential for spiritual development that a human life represents is squandered (Harvey, 2000). The act may cause harm to others as well as depriving them of the good that one could do. Life entails suffering, but it is a distorted state of mind that leads one to take this personally (Harvey, 2000; Bhugra, 2004). Reflection on impermanence and karma is recommended to enable more patient living, as is the practice of loving-kindness towards the self. Longing for something better may not bring it about, and dying in an agitated state of mind may damage the transition into the next life. 'Suicide from despair has been seen in Buddhism as a prudential error since, given their unresolved karma, suicides will just be reborn in situations similar to those they were seeking to escape from' (Perret, 1996, p. 312).

Heroic and altruistic suicides can be revered, as in the case of certain Bodhisattvas, or monks who burned themselves in protest at the Vietnam War. The person's state of mind and intentions at the time of death influence the view of suicide adopted by Buddhism and cultures influenced by Buddhism (Becker, 1990; Keown, 1996).

Suicide in Hinduism

Bhugra (2004) reviews suicide in several different religious traditions. In Hinduism, he notes that Ayurveda (a subsection of one of the four Vedas that are traditional sources of wisdom in Hinduism) is literally translated as 'knowledge of long life', and within the

Ayurvedic system 'the cognitive triad for well-being includes desire for self-preservation, wealth and a happy future' (Bhugra, 2004, p. 10). There is some condemnation of suicide in Hinduism, such that individuals who hanged themselves could be denied funeral rites. Yet there are accounts of deaths by suicide in the Hindu scriptures, including the deaths of Rama and Sita, which are not condemned (Bhugra, 2004, pp. 26–27).

The Hindu practice of *sati*, in which the widow offers herself to be burned to death in her husband's funeral pyre, was once widely practiced in India. When a widow elected to join her husband in death, *sati* conferred blessing on the couple, their families and the congregation in the next life (Cheng and Lee, 2000; Bhugra, 2004). Political and cultural change, including women's rights, is likely to have contributed to the abolition and cessation of *sati*, which was legally abolished by the British in 1829, and has since been generally discarded by Indian society, although sporadic cases were later reported (Chadda et al., 1991).

The Effect of Spiritual Practices and Membership of Faith Communities

Émile Durkheim (1858–1917) viewed suicide from a social rather than an individual perspective, seeing it as dependent upon factors external to the individual, such as the level of social integration. This was defined along two dimensions – the individual's sense of community and the community's control over the individual – with disturbance to the balance of these two factors increasing the chance of suicide. Durkheim described four states that can threaten the equilibrium between the individual and the community: where the bond between the two is too strong, leading to either altruism or fatalism, and where the bond is too weak, resulting in egoism or anomie (Bille-Brahe, 2000).

Durkheim (1897) also observed that suicide rates were lower for Catholics than for Protestants, and ascribed this to a difference in religious emphasis between integration and individualism. He found that Judaism, although valuing freedom of thought, was not associated with a high suicide rate. He attributed this to the solidarity within Jewish communities, which were under threat from the wider society. Stack (1980) notes that suicide rates among Catholics and Protestants have converged more recently, which he attributes to changes in social attitudes and beliefs.

The question of whether spirituality/religion has an effect – either positive or negative – on suicide rates and tendencies remains a live issue which has been comprehensively reviewed (Koenig et al., 2012; Gearing and Alonzo, 2018). The focus has been mainly on religion, because definitions of spirituality overlap with general measures of health and well-being, leading to confounding of variables, thus making it difficult to study. (For further discussion of this issue, see Chapter 1.)

The nature of suicide poses challenges for research. Attempts to quantify spirituality/religion can be crude. Studies of completed suicide are usually retrospective, involving psychological autopsies which are necessarily inferential, and confounded by under-reporting resulting from stigma. There is a paucity of well-designed prospective studies (Cook, 2014).

Koenig et al. (2012) note that religious involvement is associated with various benefits, including decreased depression, loneliness and substance misuse, improved physical health, recovery from depression and ability to cope with stress, and finding meaning in life. They conducted a meta-analysis of 141 peer-reviewed quantitative studies of suicidal ideation, suicide attempts,[4] completed suicide and spiritual/religious involvement. In total, 106 studies (75%) showed an inverse correlation between spiritual/religious involvement and suicidal ideation, suicide attempts and completed suicide, 27 studies showed no relationship, and only four, which had methodological flaws, showed a positive relationship.

More recent studies that have shown a negative relationship include that by Lawrence et al. (2016). The authors asked 371 people with a diagnosis of major depressive or bipolar disorder about their religious affiliation, the importance of religion in their lives and their attendance at services. They found that suicide attempts were more common among those with a religious affiliation, and suicidal ideation was more severe in those to whom religion was important and who attended services frequently. Lawrence and colleagues acknowledge that this study was retrospective and therefore causal conclusions cannot be drawn.

Spiritual/Religious Factors

Most studies show that spirituality/religion has some protective effect. It is unclear whether the factors responsible are *extrinsic* ones, such as having a religious affiliation and attending services, or *intrinsic* ones, such as beliefs and practices including prayer, or a combination of both. For example, if service attendance is protective, does this result from social support, religious teaching on the non-acceptability of suicide and substance misuse, or a transcendent focus on the meaning of life and belief in a loving God? The extrinsic act of service attendance could lead to the adoption of intrinsic practices, and vice versa. These interactions complicate the interpretation of findings, and are not always considered during research design. A number of studies highlight this (Rasic et al., 2009; Kleiman and Liu, 2014; Lester, 2017).

Rasic et al. (2009) and Kleiman and Liu (2014) found the strongest protective effects for attendance at religious services (extrinsic religiosity), whereas Lester (2017) found a weak protective effect for intrinsic factors. However, these studies collectively have significant limitations, including factors not controlled for (e.g., severity of mental illness), diagnostic groups overlooked and limited religious affiliations studied. More recently, a large study (Chen et al., 2020) found that attendance at religious services was protective against 'deaths from despair'. These deaths were not confined to suicide, but included those related to alcohol and drug misuse.

Gender and Age

The protective effect of religion varies according to gender, being stronger for women than for men. Neeleman and Lewis (1999) found that for men the protective effect disappeared when factors such as education, divorce and unemployment were controlled for. Several studies reviewed by Gearing and Alonzo (2018) found that the protective effect of religion was stronger for women, and was related to both church attendance and intrinsic factors.

---

[4] It has become customary in practice to use the term 'deliberate self-harm', rather than 'suicidal behaviour', 'suicidal tendencies' or 'attempted suicide', as this is neutral with respect to motivation. However, many studies have not adopted this convention, and this chapter follows the terminology of the research.

Studies have also found a stronger effect in old age (Wu et al., 2015; Gearing and Alonzo, 2018). It is not surprising that communal support, beliefs and rituals can be comforting in the face of loss, declining health and approaching death. In a national study of completed suicides in Switzerland, where assisted suicide accounts for the majority of deaths by self-poisoning in those over 65, the Catholic faith was particularly strongly associated with lower suicide rates, possibly because of its religious teaching (Spoerri et al., 2010).

Some protection has also been noted in younger age groups, which is either a direct effect or mediated through lifestyle factors such as reduced substance misuse and risk-taking behaviour (Rasic et al., 2011; O'Reilly and Rosato, 2015). In a small qualitative study of 20 religiously diverse female college students in India with suicidal thoughts in the absence of illness, it was found that religious ritual, belief and prayer were a source of strength in managing stress (Francis and Bance, 2017). An Israeli study of high-school students (Wilchek-Aviad and Malka, 2016) found that a sense of the meaning of life offered similar protection against suicidal tendencies among religious and secular adolescents.

Overall, across the age groups and for the majority of people, spirituality/religion is protective to some degree. However, it is not always protective: 'religion has the potential to help people through their hardest times and it also has the potential to make bad matters worse' (Pargament, 1997, p. 10). Some people have a negative experience of religion; its message may be distorted either in the transmission or in the context of psychosis. An image of a harsh punitive God may reflect an internal world wherein early experience has resulted in the formation of a punitive superego. Particular groups may experience alienation from religion on account of its teachings. Lesbian, gay, bisexual and transgender (LGBT) people represent one such important group.

LGB people are known to be at increased risk of depression and attempted suicide, and probably also completed suicide, and are subject to adverse experiences of prejudice, violence and abuse (King et al., 2008). Homosexuality is condemned as a sin in some conservative religious traditions. This can result in LGB people experiencing estrangement from family and community, internalised homophobia, and abandonment of religion because of conflict between their spiritual and sexual identities. Transgender people likewise are a vulnerable group. A study of transgender young people (Reisner et al., 2015) found that they are at increased risk of depression, anxiety disorder, suicidal ideation, suicide attempts and self-harm without lethal intent compared with matched cisgender controls. One useful psychological model of suicide (Joiner, 2005) considers adverse, often physically injurious experience and failure to belong to be two of three key risk factors. This makes LGBT people especially vulnerable.

Leaving a religion due to conflict carries an increased risk of suicide for LGBT people beyond that of internalised homophobia, and young people are vulnerable even when they are no longer living with their parents (Gibbs, 2015). Some religious communities are inclusive and welcoming of LGBT people, and an Austrian study of mainly Catholic young people showed that religious affiliation could be both a risk factor and a protective factor against suicide attempts (Kralovec et al., 2014). These issues are highlighted by the case of Jamie.[5]

---

[5] All case studies are based on real cases, but names and details have been changed to protect anonymity.

Case study: Jamie

Jamie is 20, grew up in a strict evangelical Christian sect, and lived with his parents and older brother. He became ill in adolescence; his behaviour deteriorated and he began to strip in front of his parents and their friends. Following a brief admission, he ran away to central London where, in the company of strangers, he took drugs and was raped. He then took a life-threatening overdose.

He presented as a young gay man in conflict about his identity, who wished he could be straight like his brother. He said that he had taken the overdose to see if God loved him. Initially he was relieved to have survived, but very soon he became guilty for having 'put God to the test'.

Psychological Interventions with Spiritual Features

Some psychological interventions with spiritual features are effective approaches to treatment of people with suicidal ideation or self-harm who are at risk of suicide. These include *mindfulness-based cognitive therapy (MBCT)* (Segal et al., 2002), *dialectical behaviour therapy (DBT)* (Linehan, 2020) and existential psychotherapeutic approaches, such as logotherapy (Frankl, 1959).

The value of mindfulness meditation is now well recognised. MBCT combines key elements of cognitive therapy with mindfulness training. The latter derives from the work of Kabat-Zinn (2013), which in turn has roots in Buddhism, Taoism and yoga (see Chapter 14.1). DBT also contains modules based on Buddhist meditative practice, and is recommended in the National Institute for Health and Care Excellence (NICE) (2009) guidelines for borderline personality disorder (BPD).

MBCT

Depressed people and those experiencing suicidal ideation have been noted to have a generalised autobiographical memory with less access to specific useful memories that would demonstrate to them how they have coped with adversity in the past (Williams and Pollock, 2001). The mindfulness component of MCBT involves a focus on moment-to-moment experience, appreciating the thought as simply a mental event and observing it with a non-judgemental attitude, while maintaining an awareness of bodily sensation and breathing to which the mind can return. The aim is to create distance between the person suffering from depression or suicidal ideation and his or her destructive thoughts, and to equip him or her with the skill to observe such thoughts with acceptance but without identification ('I am not my thoughts') and thereby to escape from a downward spiral.

MBCT that addresses suicidal behaviour is described in detail by Williams et al. (2017). They found MBCT to be superior to treatment as usual and cognitive psychoeducation in reducing suicidal ideation. They studied people who were well at the time of entering treatment, but identified as having had suicidal thoughts or behaviour during depressive relapse. They note that even small downward changes of mood can activate problematic modes of thinking involving ruminations, hopelessness, self-criticism, and a futile and exhausting effort to 'fix' the gap between the real self and the ideal self, which the authors call the *driven-doing mode*. This mode focuses on the past and the future, increases despair and does not lead to any useful action. In MBCT such mental states and their triggers are noted, and the *being* mode is facilitated, which focuses on the present and compassion towards the self. There is an emphasis on returning to the body as the basis of experience in the present. The Buddha is said to have experienced awakening 'within [his] six-foot body' (Williams et al., 2017, p. 55). In the MBCT group the person is encouraged not to suppress or avoid the painful thought or experience that may arise, but to notice it, so that the ruminative driven-doing mode can be avoided.

Research on MBCT and suicidal behaviour is not confined to people with a history of depression. Existential avoidance is a factor associated with suicide, whereby death represents the ultimate escape from unbearable pain. Mindfulness techniques '[tend] to generate contact with a transcendent sense of self ... that is larger than their story' (Luoma and Vilatte, 2012, p. 267). This is reminiscent of the Jungian concept of the archetypal Self, described by Edinger (1992), and the attitude of compassion inherent in mindfulness-based treatment resembles the Jungian idea of *befriending the shadow* – that is, the dark or unwanted part of the individual. The ability to do this makes it possible to bear what might otherwise be unbearable.

DBT

In her autobiography, Linehan (2020) gives an account of DBT and its development within the context of her own life and spiritual journey. A devout Catholic, she explored Buddhist teaching to enhance her clinical work, trained as a Zen master and incorporated this into DBT. She describes how she herself suffered from serious mental health problems which manifested in adolescence with features of BPD. An inpatient for over 2 years in her late teens, she struggled with depression, intense suicidal preoccupation and self-harm. She experienced this as hell, and made a promise to God that when she got out, she would 'go back into hell and get others out' (Linehan, 2020, p. 29). This motivated both her training in psychology and her work.

While working with people with BPD she found that they experienced a traditional behavioural emphasis on change as attacking, and a purely validating one as useless; both approaches increased their distress. From this discovery her aim changed to finding a balance between support and challenge, which was worked out in a to-and-fro dialogue. Finding a degree of irreverence therapeutically useful, and having built up sufficient supportive groundwork, she could directly confront people about what they sought to gain by suicide. The finding that her clients were sensitised by tragic life histories, so that interventions could feel disproportionately painful, led to a focus on distress tolerance and radical self-acceptance.

Mindfulness training is a central feature of DBT. Seeking to address emotional dysregulation, it involves learning to access one's 'wise mind' when problem solving. This is more than a balance between logical and emotional thinking. It represents a *third way*, incorporating intuitive knowing, and has a transcendent element: 'The idea of going into wise mind is the same as recognizing and going within our connections to the universe as a whole' (Linehan, 2020, p. 284).

DBT comprises the above-mentioned features, and the teaching of a broader set of skills for living, delivered by a therapeutic team in a structured programme. Although its immediate aim is to reduce the risk of suicide, its originator's aim is for it also to help people to develop a life worth living.

Logotherapy

Victor Frankl's logotherapy takes its name from the Greek word *logos,* here translated as 'meaning'. Its focus is on the meaning of life as being a primary motivational force for each individual (Frankl, 1959).

The 'will to meaning' that Frankl describes can be subject to existential frustration. The aim of logotherapy is to make a person aware of what is vital for him or her at that point in time. What an individual may need to fulfil emerges in therapeutic dialogue. Tension is tolerated as healthy in this quest, and Frankl warns against the tendency of doctors to medicate this away, and against the deliberate pursuit of happiness. Happiness in his view is a by-product of fulfilment, and will elude those who seek it directly.

Frankl was a survivor of Auschwitz. He had written about his work before his incarceration, and his experience became a testing ground for his theories. He had concealed his notes on his person, and when they were removed on arrival his own reason for living was to recover his work. He discovered that even in the most terrible conditions, personal meaning (e.g., a past or future relationship, a project or an explicitly spiritual outlook) could maintain hope, or allow people to die with dignity, whereas the alternative was to give in to despair and give up, which was invariably fatal. Maslow's hierarchy of needs suggests that self-actualisation is an aim only when more basic needs are satisfied. However, Frankl found the reverse to be true. He quoted from Nietzsche: 'He who has a *why* to live for can bear almost any *how*' (Frankl, 1959, p. 109). Remarkably, while at Auschwitz, he set up emergency therapeutic teams, along with another medical inmate, to prevent recently arrived fellow prisoners from committing suicide through shock and despair (Frankl, 1967).

Echoing Durkheim, Frankl writes of the existential vacuum whereby the decline in the values and structure provided by religion in Western society had resulted in an increase in neurosis as a crisis of meaning. He notes that people who would previously have consulted clergy to aid them in the search for personal significance now ask help of psychiatrists.

Logotherapy brings the past and future to bear on the present situation. The past can be seen as a depository of experience – some of it good – which cannot be removed, and the future as an opportunity for choice and change. Meaning can be achieved in three realms – in achievement, in experience and in dealing with unavoidable suffering. Society tends to overvalue the first of these in terms of worldly success, which is not always attainable. The second realm refers to love, either for something abstract or within a relationship. With regard to the third realm, Frankl emphasises that although bearing inevitable suffering with courage may be inspirational, it would be masochistic not to avoid suffering where possible. His approach is not confined to a specific treatment – it is applicable in any therapeutic encounter. A suicidal person may not be asking for death, but for a personally meaningful life rather than an existence. Once immediate safety is assured and any underlying illness treated, this can be usefully explored.

Spiritual Issues in the Clinical Management of Suicidal People

Reviews of suicide and spirituality have consistently suggested that a spiritual history should be taken (Colucci and Martin, 2008; Gearing and Lizardi, 2009; Koenig et al., 2012; Gearing and Alonzo, 2018). This aids understanding of the person's illness and its context in that individual's personal world. A position statement from the Royal College of Psychiatrists (Cook, 2013) addresses the issue regarding appropriate enquiry and intervention, including the need to maintain professional boundaries. It would be inappropriate to raise the issue of religion in a proselytising way, or to suggest a spiritual intervention where a person's spiritual history is unknown, especially at the time of a suicidal crisis when the priority is to keep the person safe.

In a timely assessment (see Chapter 2) it is respectful to consider not only the person's spiritual background, but also the wishes of those who do not have a spiritual or religious inclination. Religion can be a loaded issue for better or worse, and discretion is mandatory. Assessment should include ascertaining the person's religious background or lack of it, and what this means to him or her. If religious observance has been helpful in the past, could this be something to turn to in a time of crisis? If a spiritual practice has been abandoned, why might this be? If a person's religious outlook is harmful (e.g., a belief in a punitive God), a consultation with a chaplain, to augment medical treatment, may help to develop a more life-affirming worldview from within that person's generic religious background. Reconnecting with a congregation may provide emotional support.

The idea of suicide may raise questions about faith, hope and the meaning of life, as is illustrated by the following three case studies.

Case study: Gail

Gail is a music teacher in her thirties with a history of abuse and neglect. She made a serious suicide attempt when her partner, with whom she had a turbulent relationship, left her. In the past she had found it helpful to pray. This time she was unable to do so. She spoke about this with the agency nurse doing her one-to-one observation, who suggested a poem called 'Prayer', by Carol Ann Duffy, about spiritual rhythms in daily life. Gail loved it, and it prompted her to explore poetry online. She discovered a group called 'Survivors' Poetry' which publishes the work of people with mental health problems. A year after her suicide attempt, Gail had had two poems published in the group's anthologies.

Case study: Geraldine

Geraldine, a young woman with a history of sexual abuse and borderline personality disorder, was habitually preoccupied with suicide and took frequent serious overdoses. She became aware that suicide attracted her partly as revenge on her abuser, who had never been brought to justice, and on her parents, who had not believed her. She happened to read a book about the afterlife which cast doubt on the value of suicide as punishment for the living, who would eventually meet their own karma. The book also suggested that the deceased person would still have problems to contend with in the afterlife. Reading this did not altogether stop Geraldine from self-harming, but provided a focus for therapeutic dialogue.

Case study: Margaret

Margaret, a devout Christian who had a history of abandonments, took a serious overdose when her son moved to Canada. Her daughter had previously moved to a war-torn part of Africa as a missionary, taking her children with her. Margaret was depressed with psychotic features, believing that God was condemning her for her anger with her children. In addition to her medical treatment, the team worked together with the chaplain to encourage a healthier spiritual attitude of self-acceptance and freedom to be angry.

The experience of loss of faith may emerge from a life crisis or may be a symptom of illness, bearing in mind that Beck's cognitive triad model of depression includes a negative view of the self, the future and the outside world (Beck et al., 1987). Self-criticism and self-loathing may be either depressive symptoms or a preoccupation with an unrealistic idea of how one should be.

Some themes associated with the act of suicide include the following:

- anger, violence, rage, conflict, envy, rejection, abandonment
- despair, isolation, meaninglessness, void, annihilation, nihilism
- contrast between inner and outer worlds, perfectionism
- option, autonomy, choice, control, 'last way out', regression
- destiny, sacrifice, gamble/ordeal
- afterlife, heaven/paradise, hell, escape, oblivion, rest
- reunion with deceased loved one(s), union with God/nature
- courage, altruism, political or religious ideals.

Spiritual understanding can aid psychiatric management, as death can be viewed symbolically as 'dying' to self-destructive ways of living, and the subsequent 'birth' of a more life-affirming direction. The professional challenge is to free the person from the concrete intention to find release through destruction of the body, and instead begin a journey of transformation, helped by emphasis on the unity of body, mind and spirit.

The need for revenge can be a motivating factor (as in the case of Geraldine, described earlier), with a fantasy of watching one's funeral, and the expressions of anguish, regret and love never acknowledged in life. This can be explored in a dialogue that includes the person's ideas about life after death. If appropriate, in-person meetings with relatives may be arranged, enabling the psychological work to be more grounded in life in the here and now.

Experiencing the call of a dead person to join them may result from unresolved grief, illness or personal anguish about unmet needs. In grief, it is important not to inhibit the process with inappropriate medication, but to respect the need to experience painful emotions before being able to 'let go'. Counselling, therapy and spiritual support may help the person to develop an inner dialogue with the deceased, find peace and move on. Where there are long-term unmet needs, a sense of belonging and attachment to a faith community may offer befriending outside the mental health service setting.

People may respond to questions about suicide by saying that they would do it if they had sufficient courage. In the author's experience this, and concern for family members, are the commonest reasons for desisting; both deserve respect. Concern about family implies a capacity for empathy and love which, in time, may be applied to the self. It can be useful to comment on the courage required to remain alive and struggle with adversity. The person may not have considered this before. Paul Tillich, a theologian, has written of 'the courage to accept acceptance' (Tillich, 2000, pp. 163–171). Low self-esteem and past deprivations can make it very hard for people to 'accept acceptance'. They may feel sufficiently threatened by the goodness of the therapist or mental health team to need (unconsciously) to try to subvert their treatment by acting out destructively, and so reassert the familiar experience of rejection and neglect.

Assisted Dying/Physician-Assisted Suicide (PAS)

The deliberate ending of life in cases of unbearable suffering has long divided medical and public opinion. This is reflected in the terminology – *physician-assisted suicide (PAS)* and *assisted dying* – the latter being the preferred legal term in parliamentary debates. Some countries have legislation allowing PAS in defined circumstances. These include parts of Australia, Belgium, Canada, Columbia, Luxembourg, the Netherlands, Switzerland and several US states. In New Zealand the law has recently changed to allow it. Terminal illness is a requirement for PAS in most countries outside Europe. In the UK, PAS remains illegal, although attitudes are changing and the issue is regularly debated in parliament.

Most doctors oppose a change in the law, but medical attitudes have shifted over time. The Royal College of Physicians has changed its stance of opposition to one of neutrality (Smyth, 2019). The Royal College of Psychiatrists has not taken a specific position on PAS.

A draft bill presented by Lord Falconer (Falconer, 2014), debated in the UK parliament in 2015, was defeated by 330 votes to 118. Had the bill been passed it would have required the person requesting PAS to be an adult, expected to die within 6 months, with a consistent intention to end his or her life, and to have the agreement of a judge. Two doctors would be required to confirm the intention, prognosis, capacity and lack of coercion or duress, and to ensure that the person had been made aware of the palliative care alternatives. Doctors with a conscientious objection would be exempted. It is unlikely that psychiatrists would be routinely involved except to give expert opinion in complicated questions of capacity, or where the patient's mental state might be influencing his or her decision making.

If laws more liberal than Lord Falconer's proposal were to be enacted, capacity issues would represent a greater ethical dilemma for psychiatrists. An editorial in the *British Journal of Psychiatry* (Shaw et al., 2018) which asserted, from a Swiss perspective, that it is paternalistic to suggest that people suffering from mental health conditions, including depression, cannot consent to PAS, unsurprisingly provoked concerned correspondence (Breen, 2019; Firestone, 2019; Kioko and Meana, 2019; Olie and Courtet, 2019). One opinion expressed was that 'Ultimately a request for suicide is a request for help to relieve existential suffering. It is not a request to annihilate existence' (Kioko and Meana, 2019, p. 172). All of this reflects a professional and societal fear of the 'slippery slope' that might potentially result from the passing of a UK law that allows PAS.

In practice, there are rarely prosecutions of those who help terminally ill relatives to die or to access PAS services abroad. Following a test case, the UK Law Lords decided that a distinction must be made between compassionate assistance and malicious encouragement (Hirsch, 2009). In 2010 the Director of Public Prosecutions issued guidelines to the Crown Prosecution Service (CPS) out of concern that it was not in the public interest to prosecute those who had acted out of love rather than having applied coercion or duress. Where the person assisting has acted with reluctance, out of compassion, without ulterior motives and without cover-up, the CPS may use discretion provided by public interest considerations not to prosecute (Crown Prosecution Service, 2010).

Compassion – a spiritual value – can be seen on both sides of the debate, which centres on the relative importance of personal autonomy and the sanctity of life. From the perspective of the suffering individual – that is, self-compassion – the person's inner spiritual life, including their beliefs, attitude to death and relationship with others and the transcendent (however conceived), merit consideration. Personal autonomy is highly valued in Western countries, reflecting the increasing empowerment of the individual in all areas of healthcare. In a study on attitudes to physician-provided euthanasia (a wider category than PAS), Danyliv and O'Neil (2015) found that support for legislation for PAS in the UK had risen significantly over a period of 29 years, reflecting increasing secularisation in society. Religious affiliation, particularly when accompanied by frequent church attendance, was associated with opposition to a change in the law.

The Impact of Suicide on Survivors

Suicide occurs in a social context and has a considerable impact on those left behind. Families bereaved by suicide are a vulnerable group. The support they receive is vital, as they themselves are at risk of depression and suicide. They may be reluctant to access support because of stigma, and they may mistrust the mental health services, whom they may see as having failed to help the deceased. Among their difficulties are shock, anger, guilt, blame, stigma, unfinished business, rejection, questions of 'how' and 'why', and confusion about their own beliefs and values. There may be concern about God, the afterlife and the spiritual state of the deceased, regardless of religious belief (Clark and Goldney, 2000).

In a Swiss study based on interviews with 50 mainly Christian female participants, Castelli Dransart (2018) examined spiritual and religious issues in the aftermath of suicide, and found spirituality to be an issue for all of those interviewed, including non-believers. Beliefs and practices helped survivors to say farewell. Feeling supported by their minister and community helped, as did assurance that neither they nor the deceased had been condemned. The customary respect and kindness towards the deceased and mourners that are a part of every funeral service seemed to balance the extraordinary death. Responses to the funeral included a sense of being 'carried', and of personal and transcendent support. The ceremony could also be the subject of tensions in the family – for example, conflict about who might attend, and about the burial site.

Most of the participants believed in some sort of afterlife for the deceased – as part of a spiritual journey, a presence, finding a place, or a hope of reunion. Some experienced a crisis of faith, which was not always resolved. God's will and agency in relation to humanity came into question. In the short term, belief in God's agency could divert survivors from their own responsibility or guilt. For some the crisis enabled a journey from disillusionment, anger and loss of belief to mature faith – a sense of God as 'a presence among mankind [who] does not intervene directly . . . a sympathetic witness and source of strength to help survive what happens' (Castelli Dransart, 2018, p. 14). Others found it helpful to ask for divine forgiveness for failing the deceased, in a confessional rite. People tended not to mention spiritual issues to mental health professionals. Closer working and collaboration between religious and health professionals was recommended for the benefit of both disciplines, and to facilitate positive religious coping.

Hawton (2003) suggests that specialised training for undertakers and ministers of religion may help the bereaved. They have an important role and contact with survivors, and can convey acceptance, information and a non-judgemental atmosphere. Such training could facilitate awareness of the heightened family discord that can develop as an unconscious response to the violence of suicide. The vulnerability of some mourners, such as siblings and teenage friends, may be less obvious than that of a parent or partner, and ordinarily helpful rites may be differently perceived. The experience of Harry in the following case study illustrates this.

Case study: Harry

Harry was a trainee psychiatrist and a secular Jew. His sister Susan still lived at home. Their parents were occasionally religiously observant. Susan took a fatal overdose after a long struggle with anorexia. Her illness had been a focus of family discord, with their parents hoping that Harry could save her. When she died their anger was turned on him.

Before the funeral one of the officiants made a cut in Harry and his parents' clothing in accordance with the rite of *kriah*, symbolising the physical separation between the living and the dead. He was distressed by this; it heightened his feeling that his family had been torn apart. His parents found the mourning rituals helpful, whereas these exacerbated his sense of alienation.

A year later, all found the tombstone consecration ceremony that marked the end of formal mourning helpful. The family wounds had begun to heal, and Harry was having psychotherapy.

The funeral can be a healing opportunity, allowing for truthfulness about the death and celebration of the positive attributes of the person's life so that these are not eclipsed by the manner of death. When sensitively conducted, it can allow safe expression of difficult emotions, bring the family together and enable 'letting go'. One hospital chaplain (R. Christian, 2007, personal communication) suggests that each mourner will have views about the circumstances behind the act, leading to blame and self-criticism. It is never possible to know the whole story, and he suggests that this is a reason not to persist with guilt and blame. In better moments the deceased would have wanted them to get on with their lives. The minister can remind the bereaved about this before, during and after the funeral.

Recovery may take years, and the sense of loss may be enduring. Psychiatrists should not expect 'closure', but rather they should support adaptation to the circumstances. Most bereaved individuals eventually make an adjustment, although some may continue to experience depression and relationship difficulties. Others are relieved that the deceased is no longer suffering. Many find a new, inner relationship with the deceased, and a new purpose or direction (Clark and Goldney, 2000).

The Response of Mental Health Professionals to Suicide

Suicide has variously been viewed as honourable, a sin and a human right. In clinical experience it is hard to escape the underlying mixture of anger and despair, which may be experienced as a personal or professional attack, and an attack on life itself. The severity with which suicide has sometimes been condemned reflects the threat that it poses and the abhorrence that it can evoke. Such attitudes may be culturally denied, but persist at some level and can be encountered by people who attempt or die by suicide and by their families. In the general hospital setting, for example, some nurses and doctors show negative attitudes to people who self-harm (Hawton, 2000, p. 526). That both mental health professionals and non-clinical carers may experience self-harm as an attack upon themselves and their efforts to help the person may need to be addressed in the therapeutic relationship.

Some psychiatrists may hold strong moral views about suicide. It is important to put these aside while relating to the individual, in order to appreciate the uniqueness of his or her situation. In addition, the medical imperative to 'do no harm' and medical concern about prevention (Hillman, 1997) can get in the way of understanding the personal meaning of suicide; the idea that 'where there's life there's hope' can induce an excess of medical zeal. A different kind of hope may be called for – the hope for something different. In acute mental illness and where there is substantial immediate risk, the imperative to prevent suicide may seem obvious; for chronically ill people who long for an end to their suffering, it may be less so.

It is possible to see suicide as a choice against life. The psychoanalyst Neville Symington observed that his patients who are diagnosed with narcissism are repeatedly presented with crises and opportunities for change, only to repeatedly make choices that amount to a refusal of 'the Life Giver' (Symington, 1994). Change is very difficult, perhaps because it means loss of the known inner world to which the person is deeply, if painfully, attached. The challenge echoes a passage from Hebrew scripture: 'I have set before you life and death, blessings and curses. Choose life so that you and your descendants may live' (Deuteronomy 20:19). In general psychiatry, it is worth remembering that a life-denying course of action may not feel like a choice to the person involved.

During their career most psychiatrists will experience the death by suicide of at least one patient in their care. The treating psychiatrist is bereaved, and as mentioned earlier commonly experiences the loss of a patient by suicide as both personally and professionally injurious. The experience is so painful that this may account for the relative lack of literature on the subject (Campbell and Hale, 2017). Gitlin (1999) describes his experience largely in the third person, using a pseudonym, which gives a sense of the defensive distance needed to approach it. A recent study (Gibbons et al., 2019) shows that the feelings evoked include guilt, shame, anger, isolation and fear of litigation. This can have an adverse effect on practice which is usually transient. It can lead to early retirement or a change of career. Their study has given rise to a detailed leaflet that provides advice and support for psychiatrists (Hawton et al., 2020).

Although meeting the relatives can help all parties, and some doctors attend the funeral, feelings are often too raw for the family to meet the doctor in the short term; support can be provided by a suitable professional within the NHS trust. Recovery from a patient's suicide is aided by supportive colleagues and family, and sometimes psychotherapy. Spiritual practices including mindfulness may help. The place of spirituality is to know when to move on from the facts of the case and to begin enabling acceptance and forgiveness of self and others, and recognising the inevitability of human imperfection. This in turn may free the professional to learn from the experience.

Conclusion

Spirituality and religion have contributed to prevailing cultural views about suicide. Religious traditions have in the past variously condemned the act to a greater or lesser degree, yet have also shown compassion towards those involved. The act of suicide has moral and existential implications for the individual and society. Spiritual beliefs and practices can have a positive impact on mental health and suicide prevention. Recognition of the spiritual dimension of mental health care is likely to improve the understanding and support available to patients, carers and professionals.

References

Acevedo, G. A. and Chaudhary, A. R. (2015) Religion, cultural clash, and Muslim American attitudes about politically motivated violence. *Journal for the Scientific Study of Religion*. 54, 242–260.

Al-Bukhari, M. I. I. (1971a) *The Translation of the Meanings of Sahih al-Bukhari by Muhammad Mushin Khan*, Vol. 2, Book 23, No. 455. Manama: Al Hilal Publishing House.

Al-Bukhari, M. I. I. (1971b) *The Translation of the Meanings of Sahih al-Bukhari by Muhammad Mushin Khan*, Vol 9, Book 90, No. 341. Manama: Al Hilal Publishing House.

Alvarez, A. (2002) *The Savage God*. London: Bloomsbury.

Auer, B. and Ang, J. (2007) *Torment of the Soul: Suicidal Depression and Spirituality*. Bloomington, IN: AuthorHouse™.

Barraclough, B. M. (1992) The Bible suicides. *Acta Psychiatrica Scandinavica*, 86, 64–69.

Beck, A. T., Rush, A. J., Shaw, B. F. and Emery, G. (1987) *Cognitive Therapy of Depression*. New York: Guilford.

Becker, C. (1990) Buddhist views of suicide and euthanasia. *Philosophy East and West*, 40. 543–555.

Bhugra, D. (2004) *Culture and Self-Harm: Attempted Suicide in South Asians in London*. Maudsley Monograph 46. London: Psychology Press.

Bille-Brahe, U. (2000) Sociology and suicidal behaviour. In K. Hawton and K. van Heeringen, eds., *The International Handbook of Suicide and Attempted Suicide*. Chichester: John Wiley & Sons, pp. 193–207.

Breen, E. (2019) Capacity is only one aspect of decision-making at life's end (correspondence). *British Journal of Psychiatry*, 214, 171–172.

Campbell, D and Hale, R. (2017) *Working in the Dark: Understanding the Pre-Suicide State of Mind*. Oxford: Routledge.

Castelli Dransart, D. A. (2018). Spiritual and religious issues in the aftermath of suicide. *Religions*, 9, 1–19.

Chadda, R. K., Shome, S. and Bhatia, M. S. (1991) Suicide in Indian women (correspondence). *British Journal of Psychiatry*, 158, 434.

Chen, Y., Koh, H. K., Kawachi, I., Botticelli, M. and VanderWeele, T. J. (2020) Religious service atttendance and death related to drugs, alcohol, and suicide among US health care professionals. *JAMA Psychiatry*, 77, 737–744.

Cheng, A. and Lee, C. (2000) Suicide in Asia and the Far East. In K. Hawton and K. van Heeringen, eds., *The International Handbook of Suicide and Attempted Suicide*. Chichester: John Wiley & Sons, pp. 29–48.

Clark, S. and Goldney, R. (2000) The impact of suicide on relatives and friends. In K. Hawton and K. van Heeringen, eds., *The International Handbook of Suicide and Attempted Suicide*. Chichester: John Wiley & Sons, pp. 476–484.

Colucci, E. and Martin, G. (2008) Religion and spirituality along the suicidal path. *Suicide and Life-Threatening Behaviour*, 38, 229–244.

Cook, C. C. H. (2013) *Recommendations for Psychiatrists on Spirituality and Religion. Position Statement PS03/2013*. London: Royal College of Psychiatrists.

Cook, C. C. H. (2014) Suicide and religion. *British Journal of Psychiatry*, 204, 254–255.

Crown Prosecution Service (2010) *Suicide: Policy for Prosecutors in Respect of Cases of Encouraging or Assisting Suicide*. Available at www.cps.gov.uk/legal-guidance/suicide-policy-prosecutors-respect-cases-encouraging-or-assisting-suicide (accessed 11 December 2020).

Danyliv, A. and O'Neil, C. (2015) Attitudes towards legalising physician provided euthanasia in Britain: the role of religion over time. *Social Science and Medicine*, 128, 52–56.

Durkheim, E. (1897/2006) *On Suicide* (R. Buss, trans.). London: Penguin.

Edinger, E. (1992) *Ego and Archetype*. Boston, MA: Shambhala.

Falconer, Lord. (2014) *Assisted Dying Bill [HL]*. London: The Stationery Office Limited.

Firestone, A. (2019) An odd choice for an editorial! (correspondence). *British Journal of Psychiatry*, 214, 172.

Francis, W. and Bance, L. O. (2017) Protective role of spirituality from the perspective of Indian college students with suicidal ideation: 'I am here because God exists'. *Journal of Religion and Health*, 56, 962–970.

Frankl, V. E. (1959/1992) *Man's Search for Meaning*. London: Rider Books.

Frankl, V. E. (1967) Group psychotherapeutic experiences in a concentration camp. In *Psychotherapy and Existentialism*. Harmondsworth: Penguin, pp. 95–104.

Gearing, R. E. and Alonzo, D. (2018) Religion and suicide: new findings. *Journal of Religion and Health*, 57, 2478–2499.

Gearing, R. E. and Lizardi, D. (2009) Religion and suicide. *Journal of Religion and Health*, 48, 332–341.

Gibbons, R., Brand, F., Carbonnier, A. et al. (2019) Effects of patient suicide on psychiatrists: survey of experiences and support required. *BJPsych Bulletin*, 43, 236–241.

Gibbs, J. (2015) Religious conflict, sexual identity, and suicidal behaviour among LGBT young adults. *Archives of Suicide Research*, 19, 472–488.

Gilbert, M. (1987) *The Holocaust*. London: Fontana Press.

Gitlin, M. (1999) A psychiatrist's reaction to a patient's suicide. *American Journal of Psychiatry*, 156, 1630–1634.

Gordon, H. (2002) The 'suicide' bomber: is it a psychiatric phenomenon? *Psychiatric Bulletin*, 26, 285–287.

Harvey, P. (2000) *An Introduction to Buddhist Ethics*. Cambridge: Cambridge University Press.

Hawton, K. (2000) General hospital management of suicide attempters. In K. Hawton and K. van Heeringen, eds., *The International Handbook of Suicide and Attempted Suicide*. Chichester: John Wiley & Sons, pp. 519–537.

Hawton, K. (2003) Helping people bereaved by suicide. *British Medical Journal*, 327, 177–178.

Hawton, K., Brand, F., Carbonnier, A. et al. (2020) *If a Patient Dies by Suicide: A Resource for Psychiatrists*. Oxford: University of Oxford Centre for Suicide Research.

Hillman, J. (1997) *Suicide and the Soul*. Carpinteria, CA: Spring Publications.

Hirsch, A. (2009) Debbie Purdy wins 'significant legal victory' on assisted suicide. *The Guardian*, 31 July.

Holland, R. F. (1969) Suicide. In G. Vesey, ed., *Talk of God: Royal Institute of Philosophy Lectures, Volume 2, 1967/8*. London: Macmillan, pp. 72–85.

Jakobovits, I. (1988) Some modern responses on medico-moral problems. *ASSIA – Jewish Medical Ethics*, 1, 5–10.

Joiner, T. (2005) *Why People Die by Suicide*. Cambridge, MA: Harvard University Press.

Kabat-Zinn, J. (2013) *Full Catastrophe Living*. London: Piatkus.

Kaplan, S. and Schoeneberg, L. (1988) Defining suicide: importance and implications for Judaism. *Journal of Religion and Health*, 27, 154–156.

Keown, D. (1996) Buddhism and suicide – the case of Channa. *Journal of Buddhist Ethics*, 3, 8–31.

King, M., Semlyen, J., Tai, S. S. et al. (2008) A systematic review of mental disorder, suicide and deliberate self harm in lesbian, gay and bisexual people. *BMC Psychiatry*, 8, Article 70.

Kioko, P. M. and Meana, P. R. (2019) Physician beneficence: the last stop for patients requesting assisted suicide. *British Journal of Psychiatry*, 214, 172–173.

Kleiman, E. M. and Liu, R. T. (2014) Prospective prediction of suicide in a nationally representative sample: religious service attendance as a protective factor. *British Journal of Psychiatry*, 204, 262–266.

Koch, H. J. (2005) Suicides and suicide ideation in the Bible: an empirical study. *Acta Psychiatrica Scandinavica*, 112, 167–172.

Koenig, H. G., King, D. E. and Carson, V. B. (2012) *Handbook of Religion and Health*, 2nd ed. Oxford: Oxford University Press.

Kralovec, K., Fartacek, C., Fartacek, R. et al. (2014) Religion and suicide risk in lesbian, gay and bisexual Austrians. *Journal of Religion and Health*, 53, 413–423.

Lawrence, R. E., Brent, D., Mann, J. J. et al. (2016) Religion as a risk factor for suicide attempt and suicidal ideation among depressed patients. *Journal of Nervous and Mental Disease*, 204, 845–850.

Lester, D. (2006) Suicide and Islam. *Archives of Suicide Research*, 10, 77–97.

Lester, D. (2017) Does religiosity predict suicidal behavior? *Religions*, 8, 238.

Linehan, M. M. (2020) *Building a Life Worth Living*. New York: Random House.

Luoma, J. and Vilatte, J. (2012) Mindfulness in the treatment of suicidal individuals. *Cognitive and Behavioural Practice*, 19, 265–276.

Mozaffar, O. M. (2018) This Ramadan, mental illness and suicide are on Loyola Muslim chaplain's mind. *Chicago Sun-Times*, 15 June. Available at https://chicago.suntimes.com/2018/6/14/18327965/this-ramadan-mental-illness-and-suicide-are-on-loyola-muslim-chaplain-s-mind (accessed 3 April 2022).

Muslim, A. H. (1990) *Sahih Muslim* (A. H. Siddiqi, trans.). Book 35, Chapter 4. Lahore: Sh. Muhammad Ashraf Publishers. Available at https://sunnah.com/muslim:2680a (accessed 3 April 2022).

National Institute for Health and Care Excellence (2009) *Borderline Personality Disorder: Recognition and Management*. Clinical guideline [CG78]. Available at https://www.nice.org.uk/guidance/cg78 (accessed 3 April 2022).

Neeleman, J. and Lewis, G. (1999) Suicide, religion and socioeconomic conditions: an ecological study in 26 countries, 1990. *Journal of Epidemiology and Community Health*, 53, 204–210.

Olie, E. and Courtet, P. (2019) The advocates of euthanasia in patients with mental illness are going in the wrong direction. *British Journal of Psychiatry*, 214, 171.

O'Reilly, D. and Rosato, M. (2015) Religion and the risk of suicide: longitudinal study of over 1 million people. *British Journal of Psychiatry*, 206, 466–470.

Pargament, K. I. (1997) *The Psychology of Religion and Coping*. New York: Guilford Press.

Perret, R. W. (1996) Buddhism, euthanasia and the sanctity of life. *Journal of Medical Ethics*, 22, 309–314.

Rasic, D. T., Belik, S. L., Elias, B. et al. (2009) Spirituality, religion and suicidal behaviour in a nationally representative sample. *Journal of Affective Disorders*, 114, 32–40.

Rasic, D., Robinson, J. A., Bolton, J. et al. (2011) Longitudinal relationships of religious worship attendance with depression risk, suicidal behaviours and substance use in adolescents in Nova Scotia, Canada. *Journal of Affective Disorders*, 132, 389–395.

Reisner, S. L., Vetters, R., Leclerc, M. et al. (2015) Mental health of transgender youth in care at an adolescent urban community health center: a matched retrospective cohort study. *Journal of Adolescent Health*. 56, 274–279.

Segal, Z. V., Williams, J. M. G. and Teasdale, J. D. (2002) *Mindfulness-Based Cognitive Therapy for Depression: A New Approach to Preventing Relapse*. New York: Guilford Press.

Shaw, D., Trachsel, M. and Elger, B. (2018) Assessment of decision-making capacity in patients requesting assisted suicide. *British Journal of Psychiatry*, 213, 393–395.

Smyth, C. (2019) Doctors' group drops opposition to assisted suicide after divisive poll. *The Times*, 22 March.

Spoerri, A., Zwahlen, M., Bopp, M. et al. (2010) Religion and assisted and non-assisted suicide in Switzerland: national cohort study. *International Journal of Epidemiology*, 39, 1486–1494.

Stack, S. (1980) Religion and suicide: a re-analysis. *Social Psychiatry*, 15, 65–70.

Stengel, E. (1965) *Suicide and Attempted Suicide*. Harmondsworth: Penguin Books.

Symington, N. (1994) *Emotion and Spirit*. London: Karnac.

Thimmaiah, R., Poreddi, V., Ramu, R. et al. (2016) Influence of religion on attitude towards suicide: an Indian perspective. *Journal of Religion and Health*, 55, 2039–2052.

Tillich, P. (2000) *The Courage To Be*, 2nd ed. New Haven, CT: Yale University Press.

Wilchek-Aviad, Y. and Malka, M. (2016) Religiosity, meaning in life and suicidal tendency among Jews. *Journal of Religion and Health*, 55, 480–494.

Williams, J. M. and Pollock, L. R. (2001) Psychological aspects of the suicidal process. In K. van Heeringen, ed., *Understanding Suicidal Behaviour: The Suicidal Process Approach to Research, Treatment and Prevention*. Chichester: John Wiley & Sons, pp. 76–93.

Williams, M., Fennell, F., Barnhofer, T. et al. (2017) *Mindfulness-Based Cognitive Therapy with People at Risk of Suicide*. New York: Guilford Press.

Wood, T. (1986) Suicide. In J. Macquarrie and J. Childress, eds., *A New Dictionary of Christian Ethics*. London: SCM Press, pp. 609–610.

Wu, A., Wang, J-Y. and Jia, C.-X. (2015) Religion and completed suicide: a meta-analysis. *PLoS One*, 10, e0131715.

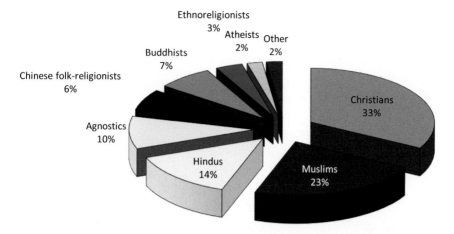

Fig. 16.1 Adherents of world religions in 2010.
Data from Johnson et al. (2013, p. 10).

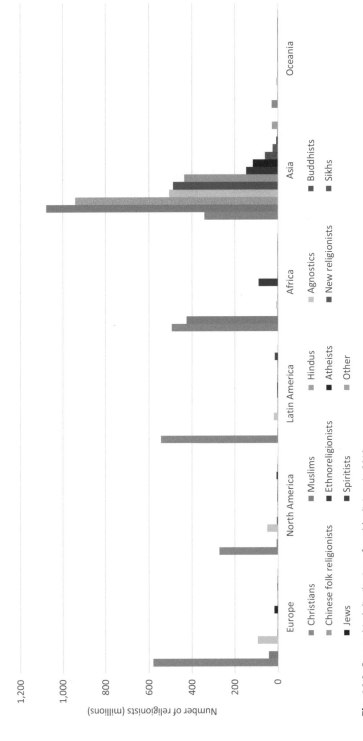

Fig. 16.2 Geographical distribution of world religions in 2010.
Data from Johnson et al. (2013, pp. 344–345).

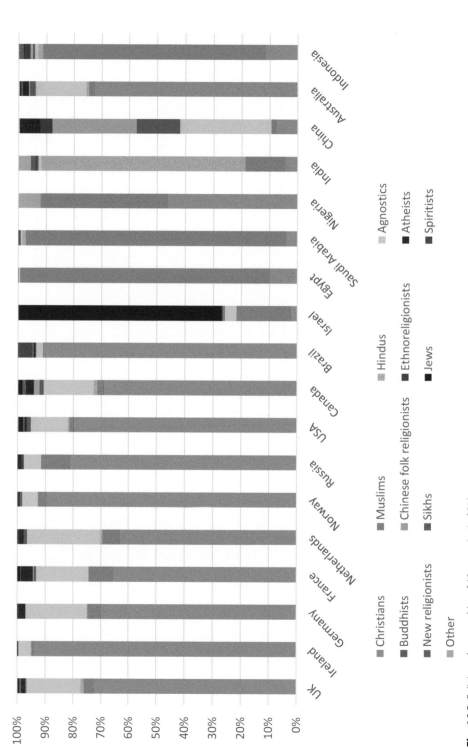

Fig. 16.3 Religious demographics of 18 countries in 2010.
Data from Johnson et al. (2013, pp. 337–345).

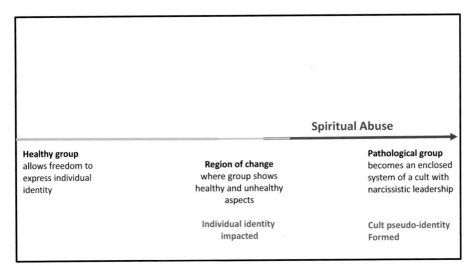

Spiritual Abuse

Healthy group	Region of change	Pathological group
allows freedom to express individual identity	where group shows healthy and unhealthy aspects	becomes an enclosed system of a cult with narcissistic leadership
	Individual identity impacted	Cult pseudo-identity Formed

Figure 17.1 Continuum of group dynamics from healthy to pathological.

Child and Adolescent Psychiatry

Mary Lynn Dell

Attention to spirituality/religion in child and adolescent psychiatry has lagged behind not only adult psychiatry, but also psychology, social work, nursing and education. Authoritative and scholarly statements, such as the World Psychiatric Association's 'Position Statement on Spirituality and Religion in Psychiatry', have summarised the past 30 years of work in this field in adult psychiatry and set the course for continued progress by highlighting the importance of patient-centred care, the roles of spirituality/religion in diagnosis and treatment, medical education and professionalism, sensitivity to differences in beliefs and practices in therapy, the awareness of both possible harms and benefits of spiritual/religious perspectives and worldviews, and the necessity of collaboration with faith leaders and communities (World Psychiatric Association, 2017). The importance of spirituality/religion in child and adolescent mental health has become appreciated more over the past two decades, as evidenced by the creation in 1999 of the Religion and Spirituality Committee at the American Academy of Child and Adolescent Psychiatry, the publication in 2004 of an issue of *Child and Adolescent Psychiatric Clinics of North America* dedicated to the topic (Josephson and Dell, 2004), and various reviews and book chapters published in the UK and mainland Europe (Shooter, 2009; Grimwade and Cook, 2019). In recent years, clinicians and researchers working in the fields of paediatric palliative medicine, child abuse, gender, trauma, diversity and cultural psychiatry have recognised the centrality of spirituality/religion to their areas of study. Now, more than ever before, the special interest area of spirituality/religion in child and adolescent psychiatry can appreciate its historical roots in psychoanalysis, the many areas of relevance in clinical work today, and the prospect that spiritual/religious beliefs and practices will continue to shape worldviews vital to the future health and welfare of children and families.

Spirituality/Religion and the Importance of Parenting

The influence of spirituality/religion – or in some cases the relative lack of influence – begins with the family unit of origin and parenting, whatever form the family takes and whoever functions in the parent or caregiver role(s). As defined by the United States Census Bureau, a family is a group of two or more individuals residing together and related by birth, marriage or adoption. In 2020, the average US family consisted of 3.15 individuals, and 41% of these households included children under the age of 18 years (Statista, 2021). According to a 2017 Gallup poll, 87% of US adults believed in God,

The author is grateful to Dr. Lucy Grimwade for her expert and thoughtful input and review of this chapter.

indicating that a certain degree of religious or spiritual belief was present in close to nine out of ten households, including those with members under the age of 18 years (Hrynowski, 2019). Even in the European Union, where one third (75 million out of 223 million) of households had children living in them and where one in five households claim not to identify with any religion, more families and parents than not acknowledge at least some degree of spiritual/religious beliefs (Pew Research Center, 2016, 2018; European Large Families Confederation (ELFAC), 2019). The influence of spirituality/ religion in the lives of children undeniably begins in the households in which they are raised, and is related to how their parenting figures choose to address this subject matter.

Of the theoretical models that have been developed to explain how parents influence their offspring's religious and spiritual lives, two have achieved prominence. *Spiritual modeling theory,* a form of observational learning, contends that children learn important spiritual/religious behaviours and beliefs by observing the actions of others. These role models, also called spiritual exemplars, exhibit spiritual/religious behaviours that are imitated and then integrated by junior observers. This paradigm leads to the conclusion that religious parents who talk about and participate in religious activities are more likely to have children who value and engage in these same activities (Bandura, 2003; Oman and Thoresen, 2003). The second theory that has been developed to describe the influence of parents upon their offspring's religious and spiritual lives is the *spiritual capital theory.* This schema hypothesises that parental relationships – along with other interpersonal relation-ships, social networks and other societal institutions – promote resources and establish environments that foster spiritual development and interactions with religious meanings. Family prayer, conversations that arise spontaneously during daily life, religious holiday rituals, the observation of spiritual or religious rites of passage, participation in organised worship and other activities in faith communities provide settings and occasions for religious socialisation. Whereas religious example is key to the child's spiritual/religious development in spiritual modeling theory, religious interaction is the core aspect of the spiritual capital model. Studies have found that young people raised in close families with parents supportive of spirituality/religion generally demonstrate greater religiosity, and youth participation in family religious practices predicts involvement of young people in future religious activity. In reality, both the spiritual modeling and spiritual capital theories are helpful explanations of parental influence upon young people's spirituality/religion. Parents often serve as spiritual/religious models or exemplars, and conversations and interactions between parents and children set the stage for the value and priority that young people give to spirituality/religion as they mature, and in their adult lives (Tamminen, 1994; King and Mueller, 2004). Further research is necessary to determine the influences, if any, of recent societal shifts in the roles and degree of family and societal participation in organised faith traditions, rituals, worship and community groups.

Most studies of parenting, religion and spirituality have demonstrated mixed effects – positive and negative – on the offspring's religious and spiritual beliefs, behaviours, interpersonal relationships, and healthy, prosocial attitudes and interactions (Goeke-Morey and Cummings, 2017; Malinakova et al., 2019). Mahoney et al. (2001) reviewed 90 studies published between 1980 and 2000, and found some, but not overwhelming, support for three general observations. First, greater parental religiousness was associated with small positive effects on marital functioning, and appeared to decrease the risk of divorce. Second, conservative Christianity was associated with a modest increase in the use and support of corporal punishment in preadolescents. Finally, increased parental reli-giousness may be associated with positive parenting and better childhood adjustment.

A review by Petro et al. (2017) of 10 articles on religion and parenting published between 2004 and 2014 and selected for methodological rigor found positive associations between religious conservatism, strict parenting and nurture, but the influence on children's spirituality was not measured specifically. Having parents who attend religious services was associated with less problematic externalising behaviours in children, and immersed the younger generation in moral, prosocial communities. However, children of parents with strict religious beliefs and practices may be more subject to issues of internalisation of emotions and behaviours. In a three-year longitudinal study of 1,198 families from nine countries and four world faith traditions (Buddhism, Catholicism, Islam and Protestantism), Bornstein et al. (2017) found that parental religiosity had positive and negative associations with parenting and adjustment of offspring. Adults and children in the study agreed that increased parental religiousness was associated with more controlling parenting, with parents viewing this as an indication of parental effectiveness and warmth, whereas children perceived the same style to be associated with parental rejection. Needless to say, additional study is warranted, especially with regard to the influence of parenting on the next generation's spirituality, the relationship to the transcendent, and religious beliefs and practices. In the meantime, general agreement exists that parental and family-of-origin spirituality/religion commonly influences beliefs and practices in relation to family size and composition, contraception, pregnancy, childbirth, paediatric and mental health care, secular and religious education, discipline, leisure, finances, politics and interpersonal relationships (Josephson and Dell, 2004).

Spirituality/Religion in Development: Rites of Passage, Faith Development Theory, God Images and God Concepts

Many developmental milestones and rites of passage throughout history and across the globe have evolved hand in hand with religious and spiritual beliefs and practices (see Table 5.1). Many of these rituals, their importance to individuals and the investment of communities are strikingly similar, although participants may be from diverse faith traditions and cultures.

Although complex theological precepts may inform these important times and ceremonies, they are frequently important to the child or adolescent because of the specific, often concrete meaning of an event (e.g., a new dress and extended family visit for a child's first communion, or a nearly 13-year-old boy attending Hebrew classes in preparation for his bar mitzvah). Many faith groups place importance on a young person's presence or participation in rites of passage that are more specific to adults, such as covering their heads and dressing as adults, or engaging in required service projects or missionary endeavours. These customs provide ways to learn about their tradition, serve others, honour elders and be included more fully in their families and religious communities.

Faith development theory has become associated chiefly with James W. Fowler (1940–2015), a United Methodist clergyman who gained his doctorate at Harvard University and spent the majority of his career as a theology professor and ethicist at Emory University in Atlanta, Georgia. Fowler sought to wed core elements of growth in understanding and religious belief with developmental psychology across the lifespan. He was influenced significantly by two theologians – H. Richard Niebuhr at Yale University, and Wilfred Cantwell Smith, founder of the Institute of Islamic Studies at

Table 5.1. Life cycle events with religious/spiritual significance[a]

Birth and infancy
- Blessings
- Religious services
- Naming of the infant
- Male circumcision (brit milah in Judaism)
- Baptisms

Childhood
- Religious education
- Consecrations at the beginning of religious and secular education
- Religious service attendance
- Roles assumed in family life based on gender and birth order
- Participation in extracurricular and group activities
- Baptisms, confirmations and first communions

Adolescence
- Coming-of-age observances (e.g., bar and bat mitzvahs)
- Confirmations and first communions
- Assuming adult responsibilities and leadership roles in houses of worship and local faith communities
- Dating and sexuality

Young adulthood
- Decisions about vocation
- Missionary service (e.g., Church of Latter-Day Saints)
- Dating and sexuality
- Marriage
- Contraception
- Gender roles
- Dress, hairstyles, head coverings
- Childbirth
- Decisions about the religious and spiritual lives of children

Middle adulthood
- Roles as religious leaders and spiritual advisors in the home and in the larger community
- Continuation of parenting responsibilities

Late adulthood
- Roles as spiritual and religious sages
- Prayers and religious/spiritual observances during illness
- Religious/spiritual beliefs and practices at the end of life
- Funerals and burial practices
- Mourning rituals
- Celebrations of life

[a] This table is reproduced from Dell and Shepherd (2021) with permission.

McGill University in Quebec and later the director of Harvard University's Center for the Study of World Religions. Fowler became expert in the life-stage developmental theory of Erik Erikson, the cognitive development theory of Jean Piaget and the moral development theory of Lawrence Kohlberg. He integrated these theological and psychological constructs with his own empirical research to form a seven-stage schema that characterises an individual's thinking, behaviours and relationships with the divine and with other human beings (see Table 5.2).

Although it was groundbreaking in the 1970s and 1980s, Fowler's faith development theory has since been subject to critiques by feminist psychologists and

Table 5.2. Stages of faith and selfhood, based on the work of James W. Fowler[a]

Primal faith (infancy)
Occurs before formal language develops
Infant develops awareness of others
Development of trust in caregivers eases anxiety when apart

Intuitive–projective faith (early childhood)
Imagination, perceptions and feelings are of great importance
Stories, gestures and symbols are not yet fully logical
Child uses imagination, stories and feelings to deal with protective and threatening powers and influences
Images, symbols and feelings created may be long-lasting

Mythic–literal faith (childhood and beyond)
Logical thinking helps to explain the world
Child has better understanding of cause and effect
Child is beginning to understand the perspective of others
Child can explain events and meaning through the use of stories

Synthetic–conventional faith (adolescence and beyond)
Enhanced ability to engage in mutual perspective taking
Can integrate different perspectives of oneself and others into a single identity
Because self-identity is more mature, can unite in solidarity of beliefs and feelings with others

Individuative–reflective faith (young adulthood and beyond)
Can reflect critically on beliefs and values through third-person perspective taking
Understands individuals and self as part of greater social order
Internal locus of control regarding responsibility, orderliness, authority and lifestyle
Self-awareness facilitates mature commitments in relationships and vocation

Conjunctive faith (early mid-life and beyond)
Appreciates paradox
Appreciates myths, symbols and metaphors as expressions of truth
Understands that there are multiple interpretations of reality

Universalising faith (mid-life and beyond)
Oneness of the individual's being with an ultimate power or higher power
Free from worldly cares and constraints, passionate yet detached
Can devote their entire being to love, justice, human rights and overcoming oppression and violence
This stage is rarely achieved – examples may include Mother Theresa, Mahatma Gandhi and Archbishop Desmond Tutu

[a] This table is reproduced from Dell and Shepherd (2021) with permission. It was originally adapted from Fowler (1981), Fowler and Dell (2004) and Fowler (1991–2008, personal communications).

theologians, in addition to liberation, black, Hispanic and other theologians, for a lack of religious, cultural, geographic and socioeconomic diversity in the initial research. Fowler acknowledged these limitations in his work, especially against a background of increasing cultural and theological diversity in the early twenty-first century. Fritz Oser, Sharon Daloz Parks, K. H. Reich and Heinz Streib have now enriched faith development theory considerably, giving attention to nuances of spirituality, multicultural populations and the rapidly changing contexts of contemporary society. Even so, faith development theory is likely to remain synonymous with James Fowler for years to come (Fowler, 1981; Streib, 2001, 2005; Fowler and Dell, 2004; Hay et al., 2006).

Although contemporary clinicians often pay little heed to Freud, the topic of God images is one that can be traced to several of his works. The term *God images* may be used to refer either to one's personal view of God generally, or more specifically to the relationship of the self to the specific divine attachment figure (God, Jesus, Allah and others). God images encompass the emotional, relational and experiential elements of the relationship, and are context specific, context sensitive and often full of affect. The image may be conceptualised as one's intellectual, explicit knowledge about God and/or one's personal and internalised experience of God. God images exist on a continuum from positive to negative, and are formed by and interact with the religious and spiritual experiences of the individual and his or her family and religious community (Hall and Fujikawa, 2013).

Freud's God images consisted of projections of parents, especially the father, exercising all-powerful protection and care over believers in the roles of innocent, dependent children. This was, by definition, pathological because the God image and belief in God were a defense mechanism against anxiety (Hall and Fujikawa, 2013). Ana-Maria Rizzuto, a psychoanalyst and object relations theorist, posited that the God image is based on characteristics of the parents and others close to the child, in addition to images created by the child to meet his or her own developing personal needs. In a sense, the God image serves as a transitional object as the individual develops a mature sense of self (Rizzuto, 1979). Attachment theorists have noted that God images often parallel mental representations of human attachment figures (Kirkpatrick, 1992; Proctor et al., 2009). Hand in hand with feminist psychologists, feminist and womanist theologians have critiqued male God representations as problematic – even traumatising – for individuals who have suffered abuse by men (Moder, 2019). The experience of human caring and nurturant behaviours, or the lack thereof, cannot help but affect the internalised God images of children and adolescents, and their spiritual and religious lives in adulthood.

Spirituality/Religion and Child Maltreatment

A review of spirituality/religion in childhood and adolescence would not be complete without consideration of how it has been misunderstood and at times misappropriated in harmful, even destructive ways. The scholarship of two particular twentieth-century scholars from different disciplines – the American historian Philip Greven and the Polish-Swiss psychologist, psychoanalyst and philosopher Alice Miller – provide insight into abuse that is either initiated or perpetuated by religion and religious institutions. Greven's research focused on the child-rearing practices of conservative religious families from the seventeenth century onwards in North America, especially the eastern seaboard in the early years of the USA. He traced the experiences and writings of individuals raised with biblical verses and understandings, such as the literal application of verses from Proverbs, that justified harsh verbal structuring, and the use of the rod and other forms of severe punishment. According to the religious convictions of those times, children are born with evil wills which dutiful parents must shape, or break, so that their offspring can live godly, faithful lives. Even if parents did not wish to discipline their children harshly, they were taught by their parents, clergy and churches that the greater tragedy would be for their children to lose their souls to sinful attitudes and behaviours that were not extinguished. Through historical methodology, Greven determined that religiously sanctioned emotional and physical abuse led to depression, apathy, or rage and paranoia (Greven 1977, 1992). Alice Miller, herself the victim of physical and emotional abuse, came to similar conclusions but from a different starting point. She described all forms of child abuse – even socially sanctioned forms such as spanking – as *poisonous pedagogy*. Abusive parents are responsible for mental illness and criminality that result from the suppressed anger and pain of the abused child. In fact, Miller believed that societal violence arises from physical beatings administered to very young children with vulnerable, developing brains that are damaged permanently by abuse (Miller 1981, 1983, 1988, 1997, 2009). In essence, Miller changed previous psychoanalytic thought about what constitutes child emotional abuse and its consequences just enough to complement and support Greven's historical work. Together, Miller, Greven and similar experts have provided alternative ways of thinking about parenting practices in all major world faith traditions, and the subsequent effects on children and their faith and mental health (Capps, 1992).

Recent research into adolescent religious development has focused on internalised and psychological perspectives of God or an ultimate being as loving or punitive. For instance, Shepperd et al. (2019) surveyed 760 adolescents at three data-collection points over a period of 18 months. The young people were asked to report the extent to which they viewed God as loving or punitive, and the extent to which they engaged in benevolent or aggressive behaviours. As one might surmise, adolescents who viewed God as loving and not punitive were more likely to engage in more benevolent and less aggressive behaviours. The importance of these studies lies in their contribution to a scientifically informed evidence base that documents findings supportive of or consistent with the historicity of scholars such as Greven, and the theories of well-trained psychologists such as Miller.

Certainly the misuse of spirituality/religion to harm children generally has been well documented, including the effects of abuse by clergy and other religious professionals (Blakemore et al., 2017). However, religion and spirituality may be as protective as other positive social determinants of health, or even more so, for young people in abusive situations (Walker and Aten, 2012; Feinson and Meir, 2015). Clinicians are encouraged not only to listen to accounts of religion that harms, but also to be alert for clues to spirituality that can be tapped in order to undergird strength, motivation, resilience and hope.

Spirituality/Religion and Psychiatric Conditions

Psychiatric conditions represent significant public health concerns worldwide, leading to incalculable suffering, diminished quality of life, economic burden, morbidity and mortality. This is true across the lifespan, with increasing prevalence in the paediatric age range, especially since the beginning of the SARS-COVID-19 pandemic. According to data collected in July 2020 in England by the Mental Health of Children and Young People Survey (MHCYP), one in six (17.6%) young people aged 11–16 years and one in five (20.0%) of those aged 17–22 years had a probable mental health disorder. Data from the administration of the same English survey in 2017 showed that 15.3% of young people aged 11–19 years had at least one mental health disorder, with 6.3% meeting the diagnostic criteria for two or more psychiatric conditions. Of the young people in that age range, 11% suffered from mood and anxiety disorders, whereas 4.3%

manifested repetitive persistent disruptive behaviours. Of significant concern, the 2017 data revealed that 32.8% of English adolescents with a mental disorder between the ages of 11 and 19 years reported harming themselves or attempting suicide, including 46.8% of those aged 17–19 years (Clarke et al., 2020). Similarly, the data available from the Centers for Disease Control and Prevention document that, in the USA, one in six children aged 2–8 years have a mental, behavioural or developmental disorder, three in four children aged 3–17 years with depression also suffer from anxiety, and these diagnoses increase in number and severity in older age groups (Centers for Disease Control and Prevention, 2021). Given the centrality of spirituality/religion to child rearing, family life and broader culture, the relationships of psychopathology, religion and spirituality should be of interest to all clinicians working in child and adolescent mental health services.

In one of the most comprehensive reviews of child and adolescent psychopathology, religion and spirituality, Mabe et al. (2010) identify key confounding variables that account for the challenges of defining cause and effect between spirituality/religion and psychopathology, whether positive or negative. First, religion and spirituality are complex and diverse constructs in and of themselves, incorporating cognitions, emotions, behaviours and community relationships. Secondly, a great diversity of religious beliefs and practices exists across the world, with many countries becoming more pluralistic than at any other time in their histories. Thirdly, there is the intertwining of psychology, culture and spirituality/religion. To illustrate this complex set of relationships, Mabe cites the 'Golden Rule' – treating others as one wishes to be treated – as an illustration of the overlap of biblical, religious, ethical and societal principles that the majority of individuals may subscribe to, albeit for a combination of different underlying reasons. Finally, psychopathology in children and adolescents is a multifactorial process even before spiritual/religious and moral elements are added into any theoretical or clinical formulations. The scientific literature in this area remains primarily descriptive, as the topic does not lend itself easily to controlled study opportunities. The corpus of work is inconsistent, in theory as well as in practice. All of these factors, in addition to the relatively limited number of methodologically sound studies and publications, should invite growing work and participation by clinicians and researchers alike to add to the fund of knowledge with an eye towards developing spiritually/religiously informed treatment strategies.

Depression

Numerous studies have documented the relationships of spirituality/religiosity to lower rates and severity of depressive disorders in adults (Koenig et al., 1998; Braam et al., 2004). However, several studies of child and adolescent religiosity and depression have revealed a plethora of relationships, including spirituality/religion as a protective factor, risk factor and neutral factor for mood disorders (Patock-Peckham et al., 1998; Miller and Gur, 2002; Horowitz and Garber, 2003; Cotton et al., 2005).

Rachel Dew and her colleagues advanced the study of adolescent depression, religion and spirituality with the publication of two papers (Dew et al., 2008, 2010). A total of 145 adolescents aged 12–18 years and recruited from two outpatient psychiatry clinics were administered the Beck Depression Inventory-II, the Fetzer Institute's Brief Multidimensional Measure of Religiousness/Spirituality, and substance abuse and perceived social support measures. The researchers found that forgiveness, negative religious support, loss of faith and negative religious coping were correlated with depression scores, and that loss of faith predicted less improvement in depression scores at 6 months. They concluded from the study that although perceived social support and substance abuse may be related to symptoms of depression, other correlations with depression exist for negative religious coping, loss of faith and forgiveness. Dew and her team suggested that religious beliefs and support from the religious community are important to adolescents' experience of depression, and clinicians are well advised to be sensitive to the spiritual/religious beliefs and values of adolescents and their families.

Jane Fruehwirth and her colleagues have studied data from the National Longitudinal Study of Adolescent to Adult Health in the USA, a longitudinal study of adolescents in grades 7–12 that was initiated in the 1994–1995 academic year. Participants were administered measures to study depression, religiosity, and information about home and school settings and related stressors (Fruehwirth et al., 2019). First, the researchers found that increased religiosity decreased the risk of severe symptoms of depression, the effects being most prominent for those adolescents with the most severe symptoms. Secondly, the benefits of religiosity in mitigating depression were explained by individual student behaviours in addition to the positive benefits of associating with religious peers or participating in religiously oriented groups. Finally, the benefits of spirituality/religion appeared to be independent of the other therapeutic effects of group involvement and socialisation without spiritual/religious meaning or content.

Finally, substantive longitudinal research highlights the relationships of spirituality/religion with the well-being of offspring of depressed mothers. Gur et al. (2005) reported that transmission of religion from mother to adult children, especially when the personal importance of religion or spirituality is considered, is muted by maternal depression. Although concordance of the religious denomination of mother and offspring mitigated the risk of depression in offspring, that protective benefit was attenuated when offspring were concordant with their depressed mothers regarding the personal importance of religion. A 10-year follow-up study of this same cohort of depressed mothers and their offspring found that when offspring and mothers shared denominational preferences, the likelihood of childhood depression and anxiety was decreased by 91% independent of maternal mood disorder (Jacobs et al., 2012). These and other studies continue to demonstrate the multidimensional nature of spirituality/religiosity, and of biological and psychosocial family risks for depression, anxiety and other psychiatric conditions (McClintock et al., 2019).

Suicide

According to statistics for 2019 released by the World Health Organization, one in every 100 deaths, or the death of 700,000 people per year, is by suicide. This exceeds the number of individuals who die from HIV, malaria or breast cancer, or as a result of war and homicide. Suicide was the fourth leading cause of death in the 15–29 years age group, after road traffic accidents, tuberculosis and interpersonal violence (World Health Organization, 2021). In the UK, according to data for 2018, there were 6,507 suicides, with a suicide rate of 11.2 deaths per 100,000 population. There was an increase in suicides among people under the age of 25 years, especially in females aged 10–24 years. All of these statistics represent a significant increase over the previous year (Office for National Statistics, 2019). In the USA, in 2020 there was a 31% increase in emergency-room visits for adolescents aged 12–17 years compared with the previous year, and for a 1-month period in early 2021, emergency-room visits for suspected suicide attempts in female adolescents aged 12–17 years were 50% higher compared with the same 1-month period in 2019 (Yard et al., 2021). This global pandemic of mental health crises and suicidality warrants a fresh look at the relationships between spirituality/religion and suicide.

Mabe et al. (2010) reviewed the literature on the relationships between spirituality/religion and suicide in children and adolescents. Religious involvement was found to be inversely related to childhood depression and suicide. Religious involvement has also been reported to be a protective factor against suicide within the African American community, largely due to higher levels of traditional religious beliefs exclusive of church attendance (Neeleman et al., 1998; Choi, 2002). One explanation for the lower rates of suicidality associated with spirituality/religion is the fact that religious beliefs increase hope, as hopelessness is a significant risk factor for suicide (Murphy et al., 2000). The past decade has seen an explosion of interest in the relationships between suicidality and spirituality/religion among sexual-minority young people and ethnic/racial minority populations. These will be discussed later in this chapter.

Psychosis

Religious content in adult psychopathology has been recognised for centuries, whether in the guise of hallucinations, delusions, bizarre beliefs and behaviours, demons and spirit possession, or in assuming the person of a divine figure. However, despite the frequency and familiarity of religiosity in adult psychosis, rigorous reviews have documented a surprising lack of consistency and methodology in studies of the biological and psychodynamic aetiologies and meanings of this particular category of psychotic expression (Cook, 2015).

Attachment theory offers an interesting hypothesis that fits with the neuropsychiatric elements of child and adolescent development. According to some attachment theorists, the *correspondence hypothesis* states that attachment of a religious/spiritual person to his or her divine being parallels the process of attachment of a child to parent. The *compensation hypothesis* posits that, if the primary attachment is insecure or inadequate, a particularly strong sense of religiosity/spirituality will arise to compensate for the deficient early human attachments. Huguelet et al. (2015) studied these hypotheses in 30 patients with psychosis and 18 controls, including qualitative and quantitative analyses of beliefs and practices pertaining to spiritual figures. The results of the study demonstrated a high prevalence of insecure attachments in patients with psychosis, with close to one in four of those individuals subsequently developing strong significant attachments to a spiritual or divine figure. This attachment paradigm may also be relevant for patients whose primary relationships with caregivers are interrupted by physical and/or psychological trauma.

Many clinicians have noted an increase in the numbers of psychotic child and adolescent patients over the last two or three decades (Stevens et al., 2014). As the numbers of psychotic young people have increased, so has interest in the religious/spiritual elements of paediatric psychotic disorders. Three studies have specifically addressed religious/spiritual phenomena and psychotic episodes. In a study that grouped religious/spiritual issues with other cultural considerations, Adriaanse et al. (2015) found that ethnic-minority young people in the Netherlands had two to three times as many significant psychotic symptoms as did non-minority Dutch peers experiencing psychotic episodes. Also in the Netherlands, Steenhuis et al. (2016) studied 337 children with and without auditory hallucinations in a population-based case–control study. They were assessed 5 years later, at the age of 12–13 years, with regard to religiosity and the presence or absence of delusions and auditory and visual hallucinations. The researchers found that moderately religious adolescents were more likely to report auditory and visual hallucinations than were non-religious or very religious young adolescents. The study subjects described the religious elements that they experienced as being supportive, useful or, at worst, neutral. Overall severity of auditory and visual hallucinations and comorbidity of the hallucinations with delusions were unrelated to religiosity (Steenhuis et al., 2016). In a more recent study, 71 adolescents with prodromal symptoms that did not yet meet the criteria for diagnosis of an Axis I psychotic disorder and 72 healthy control subjects were assessed with the Duke University Religion Index, the Structured Interview for Prodromal Symptoms, the Structured Clinical Interview for DSM-IV Disorders, the Beck Depression Inventory and the Social and Role Global Functioning Scales. Data analysis revealed that the adolescents with prodromal symptoms attended religious services less frequently than healthy control subjects, but endorsed feeling the presence of the divine more often than healthy controls. Among the adolescents with prodromal symptoms, there was no association between positive or negative psychotic symptoms and religiosity. However, greater religiosity in this higher-risk group was associated with more severe depressive symptoms (Severaid et al., 2019). Taken together, the findings of all the available studies indicate that additional research is needed to better understand the relationships between spirituality/religion and the presence, severity and prognosis of psychotic symptoms and disorders in childhood, adolescence and beyond.

Conduct Disorder and Externalising Behaviours

Historically, religion and its associated ethics, morality and behavioural guidelines have been viewed as either preventive or protective against antisocial or illegal behaviours that are potentially harmful to others and to society at large. Several studies have supported the hypothesis that spirituality/religion mitigates problem behaviours, even to the point of there being an inverse relationship between family/community religious practices and observance and adolescent delinquent behaviour. Religious attendance has been associated with less stealing, less violence, less contact with law enforcement, fewer school suspensions and expulsions, less aggression against other people, and a lower incidence of using weapons while committing theft (Ketterlinus et al., 1992; Blyth and Leffert, 1995; Donahue and Benson, 1995; Evans et al., 1996).

Some psychologists and developmental theorists have identified *risk taking* as a key factor mediating the relationship between spirituality/religion and externalising behaviours deemed undesirable to society (Hirschi and Stark, 1969; Holmes and Kim-Spoon, 2016). Religious/spiritual checks and balances on risk taking may be associated with an internal or external locus of control, or both. Adolescents may look within and to their personal relationship with the sacred to define themselves, and for meaning, comfort and guidance. Practices associated with this type of religious/spiritual orientation, such as prayer, meditation and personal devotions, may through self-discipline reinforce self-regulation and minimise risk taking (McCullough and Willoughby, 2009). External controls or limits to risk-taking behaviours are provided by active parenting practices based on faith principles, and the role models and safe controlled environments and activities provided by religious organisations and groups that foster not only faith concerns, but also healthy social relationships and constructive prosocial behaviours (Ellison, 1991; Holmes et al., 2019).

The changes in the religious landscapes of Western Europe and North America, especially since 2000, should reshape the way mental health clinicians view religious/ spiritual externalising behaviours and deviance, especially in children and adolescents. The decline in formal religious affiliations and attendance at religious services, the diminished observance and importance of many religious rituals associated with developmental milestones, and the increased polarisation of political, social and religious beliefs are all factors that call for a reconsideration of the age-old supposition that religion/spirituality is protective against conduct concerns and antisocial behaviours. Certainly there is a need for new methodologically sound studies by thoughtful researchers capable of understanding adolescent development, diversity, the changing social climate and twenty-first-century expressions of adolescent spirituality/religion.

Substance Use

Many research studies have documented that a higher degree of religiosity in adolescence is associated with lower levels of substance use, including tobacco smoking, alcohol consumption and illicit drug use (Mabe et al., 2010; Ford and Hill, 2012). However, there are few reviews of the 'next generation' of studies of religion/spirituality and substance use that go beyond simple associations. Drawing from data obtained through the 2008 National Survey on Drug Use and Health, Ford and Hill (2012) reported that religiosity decreased tobacco use, heavy alcohol consumption, prescription drug abuse, and the use of cannabis and other illicit drugs. Religiosity particularly influenced respondents' attitudes about substance use. Again using the National Survey on Drug Use and Health, Salas-Wright et al. (2012 classified 17,205 respondents into five categories: religiously disengaged (10.76%); religiously infrequent (23.59%); privately religious (6.55%); religious regulars (40.85%); and religiously devoted (18.25%). The religiously devoted group was associated with less likelihood of substance behaviours, fighting and theft, the religious regulars group was associated with decreased substance use and fighting, and the religiously infrequent and privately religious groups only evidenced a decreased likelihood of marijuana use. As the religiously devoted group had the highest rates of participation in organised religious activities and the religiously disengaged group had the lowest rates, the researchers interpreted the results as meaning that the combination of intrinsic and extrinsic religiosity, or personal and corporate expressions of religiosity, is associated with few problems with substance use, violence and delinquency.

Other researchers have studied whether adolescent religiosity affects crime and drug use among juvenile offenders. The young people's religiosity was quantified objectively by participation in religious activities, and subjectively by reports of the importance of religion/spirituality and their experiences of these. The relationship between religiosity and crime was found to be bidirectional, such that if one item increased or decreased, the other did likewise. However, the relationship between religiosity and drug use, binge drinking, cannabis and other substance abuse was unidirectional. Religiosity decreased crime and drug use (Jang, 2018).

The relationships between externalising behaviours, substance use and religion/spirituality can be expected to increase in complexity as more becomes known about the genetic and biological components, and as the societal considerations become more fluid. For instance, how might the relaxing of societal attitudes and legal prohibitions regarding cannabis interact with religious/spiritual behaviours and beliefs that are less tied to scheduled, structured religious observances and organisations than in the past? What are the relationships between substance use, religion and spirituality in a generation of teenagers whose parents grew up as places of worship and religious groups were relaxing their organisational conformity? Indeed, these relationships will keep evolving over time, promising to teach clinicians and researchers much along the way.

Obsessive-Compulsive Disorder

Religious and spiritual themes have long been recognised as a prominent feature of obsessive-compulsive disorder (OCD). *Scrupulosity,* or obsessive concerns about thinking or acting against one's religious/spiritual or moral compass, is a common expression of OCD that has fascinated psychiatrists, theologians and historians alike. Religious obsessions include fears that one has committed the 'unpardonable sin', that one has been condemned to eternal damnation despite having a pristine lifestyle, or that one has not carried out one's religious responsibilities or oblations perfectly. Examples of common compulsions include repetition of religious activities or rituals, such as praying to the point of exclusion of other activities, perpetually crossing oneself, and seeking comfort or reassurance from religious authorities so frequently as to be a hindrance to all involved (Foa and Kozak, 1995; Greenberg and Huppert, 2010). Scrupulosity as a clinical subset of OCD is associated with greater depression, anxiety and guilt, and often with poorer treatment outcomes (Huppert and Siev, 2010; Siev et al., 2011). Although scrupulosity and OCD in adults has been well described (Buchholz et al., 2019), rigorous description, study and treatment outcomes lag behind in paediatric populations, despite the longtime recognition of the existence of these conditions in children and adolescents. A recent study of 215 young people aged 7–17 years by Wu et al. (2018) found that those with religious OCD symptoms had greater illness severity overall, poorer insight and higher levels of family expressiveness, but no differences in treatment response compared with young people with OCD but no religious symptoms. Clearly, additional research is needed in this area.

Eating Disorders

Eating disorders often present with comorbid symptoms of depression, anxiety, OCD, personality disorders and suicidality (Steinhausen et al., 2021). In addition to these comorbidities, scrupulosity and other religious/spiritual considerations permeate historical writings about eating disorders, as well as the personal and family psychodynamics in contemporary societies across the world. Prominent examples of 'holy anorexics' in history include St Wilefortis in the eighth century CE, and Catherine of Siena, a fourteenth-century ascetic. Both women displayed classic symptoms of anorexia nervosa – perhaps with occasional binging and purging – that became intertwined with expressions of piety and religious devotion (Bell, 1985; Bemporad, 1996; Brumberg, 2000). Even today, food, eating and fasting practices are integral to religious observance, celebrations and other acts of commitment and obedience to the sacred in many major faith traditions. In some instances, religious and spiritual beliefs and practices may be risk factors for distorted body image and eating disorders, although up-to-date research will be helpful as patterns of religious affiliation, worship and spiritual practices are experiencing flux and transformation across the larger world religious landscape (Goulet et al., 2017).

Spirituality/Religion in Autism and Developmental Disabilities

Autism spectrum disorders and intellectual disabilities (ID) are two groups of often related conditions that entail many challenges for those affected, their families and communities, and the mental health professionals who care for them. According to the *Diagnostic and Statistical Manual of Mental Disorders, Fifth Edition (DSM-5)*, autism spectrum disorder includes 'persistent deficits in social communication and social interaction across multiple contexts', and 'restricted, repetitive patterns of behaviour, interests, or activities' that are present beginning in childhood and 'cause clinically significant impairment in social, occupational, or other important areas of current functioning' (American Psychiatric Association, 2013, p. 50.) Autism may or may not be associated with intellectual or language impairments, genetic or metabolic conditions, or other psychiatric disorders. Recent data published by the Autism and Developmental Disabilities Monitoring (ADDM) Network estimated the prevalence of autism to be 18.5 per 1,000 children aged 8 years, or one in 54 children in the USA in 2016. The prevalence was 4.3 times higher in boys than in girls (Maenner et al., 2020). Autism, with its variety of symptom expression and levels of severity, affects an estimated 52 million people worldwide (Baxter et al., 2015).

Intellectual disabilities are 'deficits in intellectual functions, such as reasoning, problem solving, planning, abstract thinking, judgment, academic learning, and learning from experience' that limit adaptive functioning and are first evident in early development (American Psychiatric Association, 2013, p. 33). As with autism, intellectual disabilities may be associated with genetic or metabolic causes, or may be acquired as a result of head injuries or disease processes affecting the brain. Analysis of 2014 data from the ADDM found that 11.8 per 1,000 eight-year-old children (1.2%) had an IQ less than or equal to 70, meeting the criteria for an intellectual disability diagnosis (Patrick et al., 2021). One meta-analysis of 52 studies that estimated intellectual disability globally in all age groups calculated a prevalence rate of 10.37 per 1,000 members of the population (Maulik et al., 2011).

Autism and intellectual disabilities are conditions that exist across the lifespan and involve parents, siblings and other caregivers in long-lasting, intimate and complex ways not experienced by individuals with typical development. In addition to their personal relationship with the sacred within their religious tradition, spirituality/religion is especially relevant to the identity, sense of community and sense of purpose in life of children and adolescents with autism and/or intellectual disabilities (Gaventa and Dell, 2018).

Historically, people with physical and intellectual disabilities have been greatly maligned, treated as sinners themselves, as the outcome of the sins of their parents, or as evil, diseased or outcasts at one extreme, and as saints and objects of worship at the other extreme (Giangreco, 2004; Bogdan et al., 2012). How such people view themselves is influenced by how they are viewed and treated by others, and that internalised identity also influences how they relate to their God. The messages of inferiority, imperfection or not belonging may make it more difficult to interact with individuals associated with religion/spirituality, or God and faith communities may undergird acceptance and feelings of self-worth. Some evidence exists that young adults with autism and intellectual disabilities who are supported in the development and nurturance of their spiritual lives are more accepting of their disability, even to the point of affirming it and seeing it as a blessing or something very positive (Liu et al., 2014). In addition to fostering loving healthy spiritual relationships between individuals with intellectual disabilities and the God they worship, faith communities can provide emotional and spiritual support through the medical, psychological, financial and other challenges faced by people with disabilities and by their families. Whether this involves providing lifts to appointments, offering special activities and social programming, or volunteering to help with companionship, supervision or respite care, faith communities may assist and support these members in both tangible and intangible ways. Finally, acceptance of individuals with disabilities fosters acceptance, learning and inclusion, which then provide purpose and meaning. Many groups do this by adapting worship services, religious education and even rites of passage (e.g., bar or bat mitzvahs, first communions and confirmations) to appropriate cognitive levels and physical abilities and shorter lengths of time, to facilitate greater participation and inclusion. Many individuals with disabilities delight in participating in small acts of service in their church, mosque or synagogue, such as setting up chairs or helping to prepare for serving refreshments after services. In turn, knowing that their family members are accepted and valued by their local religious community can be comforting to exhausted or ageing parents, especially if they have experienced rejection or felt unwelcome or judged in other settings (Ault et al., 2013; Gaventa and Dell, 2018; Ekas et al., 2019; Bertelli et al., 2020).

Certainly the religious and spiritual lives of individuals with autism and intellectual disabilities are significant and worthy of attention by psychiatrists and other mental health clinicians. We must appreciate the very personal and private nature of the spirituality of individuals, and be aware of the very real harms of religious stigma that still exist today, while encouraging and reinforcing the benefits and blessings of healthy spirituality and supportive faith communities. People with disabilities can be treasured members of families and religious communities, with gifts that enrich the spiritual and religious lives of others in unique and often surprising ways.

Spirituality/Religion and Sexual and Racial Minorities

Spirituality/religion, whether conceptualised as a subset of culture or as an area of inquiry and clinical importance that stands alone, is an essential consideration when assessing mental health and providing treatment for individuals from non-majority backgrounds. Many countries are becoming increasingly diverse and heterogenous in terms of culture and racial composition, and therefore also in terms of religious/spiritual affiliations, beliefs and practices (Pew Research Center, 2017; see also Chapter 16). Between the first and second United States Religious Landscape Surveys the proportion of Christians in the population decreased from 78.4% to 70.6%. Significant trends included a decline in the number of people self-identifying as mainstream Protestant or Catholic, and an increase in unaffiliated individuals (including some who think of themselves as spiritual people) and those claiming non-Christian faith identities (Pew Research Center, 2015).

Globally, many societies are dealing with ethnic and religious prejudices, hate and other crimes against those who differ in their beliefs and appearance, and structural disparities and implicit biases in healthcare institutions, mental health services and medical and mental health care research (Moore et al., 2020). Religious beliefs and practices play prominent roles in how minority populations understand and express physical and psychiatric symptoms and illness, relationships with healthcare professionals and organisations and, especially in mental health, the use of medications and non-biological treatment modalities.

According to a 2021 Gallup poll, 5.6% of Americans identify as lesbian, gay, bisexual or transgender (LGBT), an increase from 4.5% in the previous poll, completed in 2017. One in six of those in Generation Z (18–30 years of age) identified as LGBT in 2021 (Jones, 2021). The Williams Institute at the UCLA School of Law estimates that 9.5% of adolescents in the USA aged 13–17 years self-identified as LGBT on the 2019 Youth Risk Behavior Surveillance Survey (Conron, 2020). Although LGBT adolescents are found in all ethnic, cultural and religious groups, they are at increased risk for medical illnesses and mental health concerns compared with their heterosexual peers. LGBT young people experience significantly more mood and anxiety symptoms, bullying, rejection, isolation and suicidality than their non-LGBT peers (Hafeez et al., 2017).

The relationship between spirituality/religion and suicidality among LGBT individuals has received much attention in the last decade. Green et al. (2020) reported an online survey of 34,808 LGBT young people aged 13–24 years. Those who had participated in sexual orientation or gender identity conversion efforts were twice as likely to have reported one or more suicide attempts than their LGBT peers who had not undergone such interventions. Religious communities and leaders have historically been proponents of conversion therapies, which are now opposed by most clinical professional groups in Western countries (e.g., American Academy of Child and Adolescent Psychiatry, 2018; American Psychiatric Association, 2018). Research consistently finds that high levels of religiosity may be associated with higher rates of suicidality in LGBT young people, whereas they offer varying degrees of protection or are neutral factors with regard to suicidality in heterosexual adolescents and young adults (Gibbs, 2015; Blosnich et al., 2020; McCann et al., 2020; Price-Feeney et al., 2021; Shearer et al., 2018).

A helpful resource for understanding and addressing religious/spiritual matters in LGBTQ+ young people and their families and communities is the Family Acceptance Project, 'a research, intervention, education and policy initiative to prevent health and mental health risks and to promote well-being for lesbian, gay, bisexual, transgender and queer-identified (LGBTQ) children and youth, including suicide, homelessness, drug use and HIV – in the context of their families, cultures and faith communities' (Family Acceptance Project, 2021). Led by its director, Caitlyn Ryan, the organisation has been a leader in asserting the importance of religion/spirituality in the lives of sexual-minority young people, including the struggles and challenges involved and resources available. The Group for the Advancement of Psychiatry has also issued a booklet titled *Faith Communities and the Well-Being of LGBT Youth*. Written as a resource for faith leaders and groups from all the major world faith traditions, it reviews the evidence base for the importance of religion/spirituality in the lives of LGBTQ+ young people and their families, and describes how faith leaders and communities can collaborate in addressing the mental health needs of these children, adolescents and families (Group for the Advancement of Psychiatry, 2020).

Assessment of Children and Their Families

Assessment of spirituality/religion in psychiatry is addressed in Chapter 2 (see in particular the section on 'New Approaches for Specific Patient Groups'). Some questions appropriate to the assessment process in child and adolescent psychiatry are provided in Table 5.3.

Incorporating Spirituality/Religion in Treatment

The literature on incorporating spirituality/religion into psychiatric treatment of adults is substantial (see Chapter 14). In addition to general treatment concerns, significant evidence exists that various schools of psychotherapy lend themselves well to spiritual and religious content in therapy, or to treatment of religious and spiritual clients (Peteet, 2018). These include psychoanalytic and psychodynamic psychotherapies (Shafranske, 2009), cognitive–behavioural therapy (Hook et al., 2010; Worthington et al., 2011), dignity therapy (Chochinov et al., 2005), spiritually informed psychotherapy (Goncalves et al., 2015), forgiveness therapy (Akhtar and Barlow, 2016) and gratitude therapy (Emmons and Stern, 2013).

As one might expect, evidence-based studies of specific methods for integrating spirituality/religion into child and adolescent treatment are less robust than those for adult patients. Gathering basic historical information about the religious affiliation, beliefs, practices and observed rituals of the child and their family is often the first step in determining the centrality of spirituality/religion to the presenting problem (see Table 5.3). As important as that information may be for ongoing psychotherapy and/or medication management, clinicians must remember that a strategic inquiry consisting of only one or two questions may be advisable in emergency situations such as possible suicidality or psychosis. Knowing the relevance of a religious or spiritual variable in an emergency setting may inform the clinician about the young person's circumstances and factors that may assist or complicate stabilisation and preliminary treatment steps. In ongoing psychotherapeutic encounters, many child and adolescent therapists are able to

Table 5.3. Questions regarding religion and spirituality for children and families[a]

Questions for young children

1. Do you go to a church, synagogue or mosque? What is it like? What do you learn there?

2. What is God like?

3. What do you pray for?

4. If you could ask God to change just one thing, what would it be?

5. What is your favorite sacred text/Bible story? Why do you like it?

6. What happens when a person (you) dies?

Questions for older youth and parents or adult caregivers

1. Is religion or personal faith an important part of your life? Would you describe yourself as religious or spiritual?

2. What is your value system? How do you live out your faith or beliefs in daily life?

3. What kinds of things do you pray about?

4. Are you a part of a faith community, such as a church, synagogue or mosque?

5. With what beliefs and practices of your faith community do you agree or disagree? Why?

6. Who or what do you turn to when in trouble, scared, sick or alone?

7. What has your religious education been?

8. What does your faith community teach and what do you believe about health, illness, pain and suffering?

9. What religious practices, rituals and holidays are important to you and why?

10. What do you believe happens after death?

[a] This table is reproduced from Dell (2021) with permission.

navigate the perceived or real awkwardness that may surround religious and spiritual topics by conceptualising and handling such material in the same way as they do for other common themes in therapy, such as fears about and relationships with parents, siblings and peers. In essence, the therapeutic modalities used are those that the clinician has been trained in and is comfortable with, and the content is religious or spiritual in nature.

In recent years, spiritually sensitive therapy has come into its own, largely due to its capacity to individualise assessment and treatment according to the priorities, moral foundations, ethics, beliefs and practices of children, adolescents and families within their faith communities and cultures. This school of therapy appeals to religious/spiritual resources – intrinsic to the individual and their family, as well as external in their communities and environments – to address psychological concerns and challenges in relationships. The goals of treatment include, but are not limited to, improved psychological well-being, increased personal fulfilment, reduction in anxiety and distress, and perhaps – although not necessarily – increased spiritual well-being and inner peace (Sperry 2001, 2010). Heather Boynton and her colleagues have adapted spiritually sensitive therapy for use in clinical work with children, especially those dealing with trauma, grief and loss (Boynton and Vis, 2011). As experience with this treatment modality in children has accumulated, four characteristics or tasks of therapists have been identified:

1   an appreciation that spirituality is diverse, complex and multidimensional, and that religion and religiosity are both related to and distinct from each other

2   an appreciation that children are spiritual beings, facilitated by the therapist's holistic approach to them

3   the ability to empathise and connect deeply with children

4   an appreciation of the role of spirituality in meaning making, identity formation and supporting children who are experiencing trauma, grief and loss.

Therapists then incorporate spirituality into therapeutic work with the child by:

1   providing a safe place for the child's spiritual life through 'openness, exploration, inquiry, discussion, and validation'

2   permitting and respecting emerging spiritual expression

3   fostering spiritual growth and coping

4   'expecting the unexpected' (Boynton and Mellan, 2021, p. 3).

At its best, spiritually sensitive therapy underscores the need for a physically and emotionally safe place for children's vulnerability as they deal with the trauma, grief, loss and other events that brought them to therapy in the first place. Spiritually sensitive therapy also lends itself well to hope and healing, reinforcing its appeal both to the child and to the adult therapists who are invested in his or her treatment.

The combination of the innate physicality of children and the spirituality imbued in the practice of yoga has led to recommendations for yoga for children and adolescents for a number of psychological conditions. Although many conservative, non-Buddhist/ Hindu faith traditions in some Western countries view yoga with some suspicion, the general public views yoga as a way to integrate body, mind and spirit, and as a cornerstone of complementary and alternative medicine. It is attractive to many parents and child advocates given its emphasis on health lifestyle habits. Benefits of yoga have been documented for young people with eating disorders, anxiety and difficulties with mood and self-regulation (Sheveland, 2011; Hagen and Nayar, 2014; Ostermann et al., 2019; Borden and Cook-Cottone, 2020).

As would be expected, the issue of spirituality/religion arises regularly in family assessments and provides significant 'grist for the mill' for family therapy. Spiritual issues may contribute to conflict and misunderstandings between family members. Spirituality and religious beliefs, practices and rituals may also provide vessels for renewed, improved interpersonal relationships and healthier family functioning (Walsh, 2013). With good training, technique and patience, most schools of family therapy may be conducive to handling religious or spiritual issues that can arise in the course of treatment. Family therapy is also becoming a preferred treatment modality for addressing religious and spiritual concerns in multifaith families, very conservative or fundamentalist families of diverse major faith traditions, religious minorities, and LGBT+ young people and their families (Walsh, 2010; Harvey and Fish, 2015; Weatherhead and Daiches, 2015; Sherbersky, 2016).

Religious/Spiritual Leaders and Institutions as Helpful Resources for Children, Adolescents and Families

Spiritual leaders and religious institutions are often overlooked or underutilised sources of care and support for children, adolescents and families who are dealing with psychosocial stresses and psychiatric disorders. Recognising that every person[1] whom clinicians encounter in the course of their work has a spiritual life is essential to appreciating the roles of clergy, youth leaders, religious educators and others with regard to the faith development and relationship with God in the faith tradition to which the young person belongs. When children and adolescents are hospitalised, or when they are severely depressed, struggling with psychotic symptoms, or have experienced abuse or trauma, accepting and nurturing pastors, rabbis and spiritual mentors are additional adults who can address their youthful existential angst as well as monitor for concerning verbalisations or behaviours. They may also model prosocial attitudes and behaviours such as acceptance, forgiveness, love, hope, gentleness, empathy and helpfulness – positive qualities that are common to all of the major world faith traditions. Inpatient psychiatric hospital programmes may have access to hospital chaplains or community clergy who are available to support patients and their families, or to serve treatment teams as consultants when spirituality/religion is a prominent issue in assessment and care. Similarly, some families may be more likely to see well-trained pastoral counselors in outpatient settings than those working for secular organisations. If this is the case, it is essential that child and adolescent psychiatrists work closely with religiously based therapists to coordinate all aspects of care (Dell, 2004).

Mental health professionals must also remember that our patients have the same spiritual and religious needs as all individuals who are not receiving formal psychiatric care or mental health treatment. These needs may include individual worship, corporate worship or participation in services in group settings, religious instruction, participation in sacraments or aspects of worship or devotions espoused by their own tradition, and observance of rituals or rites of passage celebrated by their families and faith traditions. Maintaining strong religious/spiritual beliefs and practices is often cited by patients as a protective factor that is helpful both for their mental health and for adhering to their psychiatrist's treatment recommendations (Dell, 2004).

Religious communities and institutions may provide other resources of benefit to patients and families. Examples include after-school programmes for school-age children, extracurricular activities and youth groups for teenagers, sports activities and 'food banks'. Some larger churches, or even smaller congregations in close physical proximity, may sponsor or host health clinics, clothing banks, and low-cost supplies such as nappies and school equipment. Retired members of faith communities may help with childcare, tutoring or providing lifts to medical appointments. Churches and synagogues may host language classes, first-aid training and meetings of support groups such as Alateen. By addressing physical and practical needs, religious institutions often contribute in very concrete yet life-giving ways to the spiritual and mental health of young people and families who are being cared for by child psychiatrists and other clinicians (Dell, 2004).

References

Adriaanse, M., van Domburgh, L., Hoek, H. W. et al. (2015) Prevalence, impact and cultural context of psychotic experiences among ethnic minority youth. *Psychological Medicine*, 45, 637–646.

Akhtar, S. and Barlow, J. (2016) Forgiveness therapy for the promotion of mental

---

[1] However, at the same time it is important to recognise that not all people are happy to self-identify as having a spiritual life (see Chapter 1).

well-being: a systematic review and meta-analysis. *Trauma, Violence, & Abuse*, 19, 107–122.

American Academy of Child and Adolescent Psychiatry (2018) *Conversion therapy.* Available at www.aacap.org/aacap/Policy_ Statements/2018/Conversion_Therapy.aspx (accessed 1 October 2021).

American Psychiatric Association (2013) *Diagnostic and Statistical Manual of Mental Disorders*, 5th ed. Arlington, VA: American Psychiatric Association.

American Psychiatric Association (2018) *Position Statement on Conversion Therapy and LGBTQ Patients.* Available at www .psychiatry.org/File%20Library/About-APA/Organization-Documents-Policies/ Policies/Position-Conversion-Therapy.pdf (accessed 8 April 2022).

Ault, M. J., Collins, B. C. and Carter, E. W. (2013) Congregational participation and supports for children and adults with disabilities: parent perceptions. *Intellectual and Developmental Disabilities*, 51, 48-61.

Bandura, A. (2003) On the psychosocial impact and mechanisms of spiritual modeling: comment. *International Journal for the Psychology of Religion*, 13, 167–173.

Baxter, A. J., Brugha, T. S., Erskine, H. E. et al. (2015) The epidemiology and global burden of autism spectrum disorders. *Psychological Medicine*, 45, 601–613.

Bell, R. M. (1985) *Holy Anorexia.* Chicago, IL: University of Chicago Press.

Bemporad, J. R. (1996) Self-starvation through the ages: reflections on the pre-history of anorexia nervosa. *International Journal of Eating Disorders*, 19, 217–237.

Bertelli, M. O., Del Furia, C., Bonadiman, M. et al. (2020) The relationship between spiritual life and quality of life in people with intellectual disability and/or low-functioning autism spectrum disorders. *Journal of Religion and Health*, 59, 1996–2018.

Blosnich, J. R., De Luca, S., Lytle, M. C. et al. (2020) Questions of faith: religious affiliations and suicidal ideation among sexual minority young adults. *Suicide & Life-Threatening Behavior*, 50, 1158–1166.

Blythe, D. A. and Leffert, N. (1995) Communities as contexts for adolescent development: an empirical analysis. *Journal of Adolescent Research*, 10, 64–87.

Bogdan, R., Elks, M. and Knoll, J. (2012) *Picturing Disability: Beggar, Freak, Citizen and Other Photographic Rhetoric.* Syracuse, NY: Syracuse University Press.

Borden, A. and Cook-Cottone, C. (2020) Yoga and eating disorder prevention and treatment: a comprehensive review and meta-analysis. *Eating Disorders*, 28, 400–437.

Bornstein, M. H., Putnick, D. L., Lansford, J. E. et al. (2017) 'Mixed blessings': parental religiousness, parenting, and child adjustment in global perspective. *Journal of Child Psychology and Psychiatry*, 58, 880–892.

Boynton, H. M. and Mellan, C. (2021) Co-creating authentic sacred therapeutic space: a spiritually sensitive framework for counselling children. *Religions*, 12, 1–14.

Boynton, H. M. and Vis, J.-A. (2011) Meaning making, spirituality, and creative expressive therapies: pathways to posttraumatic growth in grief and loss for children. *Counselling and Spirituality*, 30, 137–159.

Braam, A. W., Hein, E., Dorly, J. H. D. et al. (2004) Religious involvement and 6-year course of depressive symptoms in older Dutch citizens: results from the Longitudinal Aging Study Amsterdam. *Journal of Aging and Health*, 16, 467–489.

Brumberg, J. J. (2000) *Fasting Girls: The History of Anorexia Nervosa.* New York: Vintage Press.

Buchholz, J. L., Abramowitz, J. S., Riemann, B. C. et al. (2019) Scrupulosity, religious affiliation and symptom presentation in obsessive compulsive disorder. *Behavioural and Cognitive Psychotherapy*, 47, 478–492.

Capps, D. (1992) Religion and child abuse: perfect together. *Journal for the Scientific Study of Religion*, 31, 1–14.

Centers for Disease Control and Prevention (2021) *Data and Statistics on Children's*

Mental Health. Available at www.cdc.gov/childrensmentalhealth/data.html (accessed 1 August 2021).

Chochinov, H. M., Hack, T., Hassard, T. et al. (2005) Dignity therapy: a novel psychotherapeutic intervention for patients near the end of life. *Journal of Clinical Oncology*, 23, 5520–5525.

Choi, H. (2002) Understanding adolescent depression in ethnocultural context. *Advances in Nursing Science*, 25, 71–85.

Clarke, A., Pote, I., and Sorgenfrei, M. (2020) *Adolescent Mental Health Evidence Brief 1: Prevalence of Disorders.* London: Early Intervention Foundation. Available at www.eif.org.uk/report/adolescent-mental-health-evidence-brief-1-prevalence-of-disorders (accessed 2 October 2021).

Conron, K. J. (2020) *LGBT Youth Population in the United States.* Available at https://williamsinstitute.law.ucla.edu/wp-content/uploads/LGBT-Youth-US-Pop-Sep-2020.pdf (accessed 17 September 2021).

Cook, C. C. H. (2015) Religious psychopathology: the prevalence of religious content of delusions and hallucinations in mental disorder. *International Journal of Social Psychiatry*, 61, 404–425.

Cotton, S., Larkin, E., Hoopes, A. et al. (2005) The impact of adolescent spirituality on depressive symptoms and health risk behaviors. *Journal of Adolescent Health*, 36, 529.

Dell, M. L. (2004) Religious professionals and institutions: untapped resources for clinical care. *Child and Adolescent Psychiatric Clinics of North America*, 13, 85–110.

Dell, M. L. (2021) Cultural and religious issues. In M. K. Dulcan, ed., *Dulcan's Textbook of Child and Adolescent Psychiatry*, 3rd ed. Washington, DC: American Psychiatric Association Publishing, pp. 539–550.

Dell, M. L. and Shepherd, J. J. (2021) Religion and spirituality in child and adolescent cultural psychiatry. In R. Parekh, C. S. Al-Mateen, M. J. Lisotto and R. D. Carter, eds., *Cultural Psychiatry with Children,*

Adolescents, and Families. Washington, DC: American Psychiatric Association Publishing, pp. 129–150.

Dew, R. E., Daniel, S. S., Goldston, D. B. et al. (2008) Religion, spirituality, and depression in adolescent psychiatric outpatients. *Journal of Nervous and Mental Disease*, 196, 247–251.

Dew, R. E., Daniel, S. S., Goldston, D. B. et al. (2010) A prospective study of religion/spirituality and depressive symptoms among adolescent psychiatric patients. *Journal of Affective Disorders*, 120, 149–157.

Donahue, M. J. and Benson, P. L. (1995) Religion and the well-being of adolescents. *Journal of Social Issues*, 51, 145–160.

Dunning, D. L., Griffiths, K., Kuyken, W. et al. (2019) Research review: the effects of mindfulness-based interventions on cognition and mental health in children and adolescents – a meta-analysis of randomized controlled trials. *Journal of Child Psychology and Psychiatry*, 60, 244–258.

Ekas, N. V., Tidman, L. and Timmons, L. (2019) Religiosity/spirituality and mental health outcomes in mothers of children with autism spectrum disorder: the mediating role of positive thinking. *Journal of Autism and Developmental Disorders*, 49, 4547–4558.

Ellison, C. G. (1991) Religious involvement and subjective well-being. *Journal of Health and Social Behavior*, 32, 80–99.

Emmons, R. A. and Stern, R, (2013) Gratitude as a psychotherapeutic intervention. *Journal of Clinical Psychology*, 69, 846–855.

European Large Families Confederation (ELFAC) (2019) Only 13% (8.5 million) of the households with children in Europe had three children or more. Available at www.elfac.org/only-13-8-5-million-of-the-households-with-children-in-europe-had-three-children-or-more/ (accessed 8 April 2022).

Evans, T. D., Cullen, F. T., Burton, V. S. et al. (1996) Religion, social bonds, and delinquency. *Deviant Behavior*, 17, 43–70.

Family Acceptance Project (2021) *Welcome to the Family Acceptance Project.* San

Francisco, CA: Family Acceptance Project, San Francisco State University. Available at https://familyproject.sfsu.edu/ (accessed 4 October 2021).

Feinson, M. C. and Meir, A. (2015) Exploring mental health consequences of childhood abuse and the relevance of religiosity. *Journal of Interpersonal Violence*, 30, 499–521.

Fitchett, G., Emanuel, L., Handzo, G. et al. (2015) Care of the human spirit and the role of dignity therapy: a systematic review of dignity therapy research. *BMC Palliative Care*, 14. Doi 10.1186/s12904-015-0007-1.

Foa, E. B. and Kozak, M. J. (1995) DSM-IV field trial: obsessive-compulsive disorder. *American Journal of Psychiatry*, 152, 90–96.

Ford, J. A. and Hill, T. D. (2012) Religiosity and adolescent substance use: evidence from the national survey on drug use and health. *Substance Use & Misuse*, 47, 787–798.

Fowler, J. W. (1981) *Stages of Faith*. New York: HarperCollins.

Fowler, J. W. and Dell, M. L. (2004) Stages of faith and identity: birth to teens. *Child and Adolescent Psychiatric Clinics of North America*, 13, 17–33.

Fruehwirth, J. C., Iyer, S. and Zhang, A. (2019) Religion and depression in adolescence. *Journal of Political Economy*, 127, 1178–1209.

Gaventa, W. and Dell, M. L. (2018) Spirituality, ethics, and people with intellectual disabilities. In J. R. Peteet, M. L. Dell and W. L. A. Fung, eds., *Ethical Considerations at the Intersection of Psychiatry and Religion*. New York: Oxford University Press, pp. 179–198.

Giangreco, M. F. (2004) "The stairs didn't go anywhere!": a self-advocate's reflections on specialized services and their impact on people with disabilities. In M. Nind, J. Rix, K. Sheehy and K. Simmons, eds., *Inclusive Education: Diverse Perspectives*. London: David Fulton Publishers in association with the Open University, pp. 32–42.

Gibbs, J. J. (2015) Religious conflict, sexual identity, and suicidal behaviors among LGBT young adults. *Archives of Suicide Research*, 19, 472–488.

Goeke-Morey, M. C. and Cummings, E. M. (2017) Religiosity and parenting: recent directions in process-oriented research. *Current Opinion in Psychology*, 15, 7–12.

Goncalves, J. P. B., Luccheti, G., Menezea, P. R. et al. (2015) Religious and spiritual interventions in mental health care: a systematic review and meta-analysis of randomized controlled clinical trials. *Psychological Medicine*, 45, 2937–2949.

Goulet, C., Henrie, J. and Szymanski, L. (2017) An exploration of the associations among multiple aspects of religiousness, body image, eating pathology, and appearance investment. *Journal of Religion and Health*, 56, 493–506.

Green, A. E., Price-Feeney, M., Dorison, S. H. and Pick, C. J. (2020) Self-reported conversion efforts and suicidality among US LGBTQ youths and young adults, 2018. *American Journal of Public Health*, 110, 1221–1227.

Greenberg, D. and Huppert, J. D. (2010) Scrupulosity: a unique subtype of obsessive-compulsive disorder. *Current Psychiatry Reports*, 12, 282–289.

Greven, P. J. (1977) *The Protestant Temperament: Patterns of Child-Rearing, Religious Experiences, and the Self in Early America*. Chicago, IL: University of Chicago Press.

Greven, P. J. (1992) *Spare the Child: The Religious Roots of Punishment and the Psychological Impact of Physical Abuse*. New York: Vintage Books.

Grimwade, L. and Cook, C. (2019) The clinician's view of spirituality in health care. In J. Fletcher, ed., *Chaplaincy and Spiritual Care in Mental Health Settings*. London: Jessica Kingsley Publishers, pp. 31–43.

Group for the Advancement of Psychiatry: Psychiatry and Religion Committee and LGBT Committee (2020) *Faith Communities and the Well-Being of LGBT Youth*. Available at https://ourgap.org/resources/Documents/GAP%20LGBT-Religion%20Project.pdf (accessed 1 September 2021).

Gur, M., Miller, L., Warner, V. et al. (2005) Maternal depression and the intergenerational transmission of religion. *Journal of Nervous and Mental Disease*, 193, 338–345.

Hafeez, H., Zeshan, M., Tahir, M. A. et al. (2017) Health care disparities among lesbian, gay, bisexual, and transgender youth: a literature review. *Cureus*, 9, e1184.

Hagen, I., and Nayar, U. S. (2014) Yoga for children and young people's mental health and well-being: research review and reflections on the mental health potentials of yoga. *Frontiers in Psychiatry*, 5, 35.

Hall, T. W. and Fujikawa, A. M. (2013) God image and the sacred. In: K. I. Pargament, ed., *APA Handbook of Psychology, Religion, and Spirituality: Vol. 1. Context, Theory, and Research*. Washington, DC: American Psychological Association, pp. 277–292.

Harvey, R. G. and Fish, L. S. (2015) Queer youth in family therapy. *Family Process*, 54, 396–417.

Hay, D., Reich, K. H. and Utsch, M. (2006) Spiritual development: intersections and divergence with religious development. In E. C. Roehlkepartain, P. E. King and L. Wagener, eds., *Handbook of Spiritual Development in Childhood and Adolescence*. Thousand Oaks, CA: Sage, pp. 46–59.

Hirschi, T. and Stark, R. (1969) Hellfire and delinquency. *Social Problems*, 17, 202–213.

Holmes, C. and Kim-Spoon, J. (2016) Why are religiousness and spirituality associated with externalizing psychopathology? A literature review. *Clinical Child and Family Psychology Review*, 19, 1–20.

Holmes, C., Brieant, A., King-Casas, B. et al. (2019) How is religiousness associated with adolescent risk-taking? The roles of emotion regulation and executive function. *Journal of Research on Adolescence*, 29, 334–344.

Hook, J. N., Worthington, E. L. Jr., Davis, D. E. et al. (2010) Empirically supported religious and spiritual therapies. *Journal of Clinical Psychology*, 66, 46–72.

Horowitz, J. L. and Garber, J. (2003) Relation of intelligence and religiosity to depressive disorders in offspring of depressed and nondepressed mothers. *Journal of the American Academy of Child and Adolescent Psychiatry*, 42, 578–586.

Hrynowski, Z. (2019) How many Americans believe in God? Available at https://news.gallup.com/poll/268205/americans-believe-god.aspx (accessed 30 May 2021).

Huguelet, P., Mohr, S., Rieben, I. et al. (2015) Attachment and coping in psychosis in relation to spiritual figures. *BMC Psychiatry*, 15, 237.

Huppert, J. D. and Siev, J. (2010) Treating scrupulosity in religious individuals using cognitive-behavioral therapy. *Cognitive and Behavioral Practice*, 17, 382–392.

Jacobs, M., Miller, L., Wickramaratne, P. et al. (2012) Family religion and psychopathology in children of depressed mothers: ten-year follow-up. *Journal of Affective Disorders*, 136, 320–327.

Jang, S. J. (2018) Religiosity, crime, and drug use among juvenile offenders: a test of reciprocal relationships over time. *International Journal of Offender Therapy and Comparative Criminology*, 62, 4445–4464.

Jones, J. M. (2021) LGBT identification rises to 5.6% in latest U.S. estimate. Available at https://news.gallup.com/poll/329708/lgbt-identification-rises-latest-estimate.aspx (accessed 3 October 2021).

Josephson, A. M. and Dell, M. L. (2004) Religion and spirituality in child and adolescent psychiatry: a new frontier. *Child and Adolescent Psychiatric Clinics of North America*, 13, 1–15.

Ketterlinus, R. D., Lamb, M. E., Nitz, K. et al. (1992) Adolescent nonsexual and sex-related problem behaviors. *Journal of Adolescent Research*, 7, 431–456.

King, P. E. and Mueller, R. A. (2004) Parental influence on adolescent religiousness: exploring the roles of spiritual modeling and spiritual capital. *Marriage and Family: A Christian Journal*, 6, 413–425.

Kirkpatrick, L. A. (1992) An attachment-theory approach to the psychology of religion. *International Journal for the Psychology of Religion*, 2, 3–28.

Koenig, H. G., George, L. K. and Peterson, B. L. (1998) Religiosity and remission from depression in medically ill older patients. *American Journal of Psychiatry*, 155, 536–542.

Liu, E. X, Carter, E. W., Boehm, T. L. et al. (2014) In their own words: the place of faith in the lives of young people with autism and intellectual disability. *Intellectual and Developmental Disabilities*, 52, 388–404.

Mabe, P. A., Dell, M. L. and Josephson, A. M. (2010) Spiritual and religious perspectives on child and adolescent psychopathology. In J. R. Peteet, F. G. Lu and W. E. Narrow, eds., *Religious and Spiritual Issues in Psychiatric Diagnosis: A Research Agenda for DSM-V*. Washington, DC: American Psychiatric Association, pp. 123–142.

McCann, E., Donohue, G. and Timmins, F. (2020) An exploration of the relationship between spirituality, religion and mental health among youth who identify as LGBT+: a systematic literature review. *Journal of Religion and Health*, 59, 828–844.

McClintock, C. H., Anderson, M., Svob, C. et al. (2019) Multidimensional understanding of religiosity/spirituality: relationship to major depression and familial risk. *Psychological Medicine*, 49, 2379–2388.

McCullough, M. E. and Willoughby, B. L. (2009) Religion, self-regulation, and self-control: associations, explanations, and implications. *Psychological Bulletin*, 135, 69–93.

Maenner, M. J., Shaw, K. A., Baio, J. et al. (2020) Prevalence of autism spectrum disorder among children aged 8 years – Autism and Developmental Disabilities Monitoring Network, 11 sites, United States, 2016. *Morbidity and Mortality Weekly Report: Surveillance Summaries*, 69, 1-12.

Mahoney, A., Pargament, K. I., Tarakeshwar, N. et al. (2001) Religion in the home in the 1980s and 1990s: a meta-analytic review and conceptual analysis of links between religion, marriage, and parenting. *Journal of Family Psychology*, 15, 559–596.

Malinakova, K., Trnka, R., Bartuskova, L. et al. (2019) Are adolescent religious attendance/spirituality associated with family characteristics? *International Journal of Environmental Research and Public Health*, 16, 2947.

Maulik, P. K., Mascarenhas, M. N., Mathers, C. D. et al. (2011) Prevalence of intellectual disability: a meta-analysis of population-based studies. *Research in Developmental Disabilities*, 32, 419–436.

Miller, A. (1981) *Thou Shalt Not Be Aware*. New York: Farrar, Straus, and Giroux.

Miller, A. (1983) *For Your Own Good*. New York: Farrar, Straus, and Giroux.

Miller, A. (1988) *Banished Knowledge*. New York: Anchor Books.

Miller, A. (1997) *The Drama of the Gifted Child*. New York: Basic Books.

Miller, A. (2009) *Breaking Down the Wall of Silence*. New York: Basic Books.

Miller, L. and Gur, M. (2002) Religiosity, depression, and physical maturation in adolescent girls. *Journal of the American Academy of Child and Adolescent Psychiatry*, 41, 206–214.

Moder, A. (2019) Women, personhood, and the male God: a feminist critique of patriarchal concepts of God in view of domestic abuse. *Feminist Theology*, 28, 85–103.

Moore, Q., Tennant, P. S. and Fortuna, L. R. (2020) Improving research quality to achieve mental health equity. *Psychiatric Clinics of North America*, 43, 569–582.

Murphy, P. E., Ciarrocchi, J. W., Piedmont, R. L. et al. (2000) The relation of religious belief and practices, depression, and hopelessness in persons with clinical depression. *Journal of Consulting and Clinical Psychology*, 68, 1102–1106.

Neeleman, J., Wessely, S. and Lewis, G. (1998) Suicide acceptability in African- and white Americans: the role of religion. *Journal of Nervous and Mental Disease*, 186, 12–16.

Office for National Statistics (2019) *Suicides in the UK: 2018 Registrations*. Available at www.ons.gov.uk/peoplepopulationandcommunity/birthsdeathsandmarriages/deaths/bulletins/

suicidesintheunitedkingdom/2018registrations (accessed 1 October 2021).

Oman, D. and Thoresen, C. E. (2003) Spiritual modeling: a key to spiritual and religious growth? *International Journal for the Psychology of Religion*, 13, 149–165.

Ostermann, T., Vogel, H., Boehm, K. et al. (2019) Effects of yoga on eating disorders – a systematic review. *Complementary Therapies in Medicine*, 46, 73–80.

Patock-Peckham, J. A., Hutchinson, G. T., Cheong, J. et al. (1998) Effect of religion and religiosity on alcohol use in a college student sample. *Drug and Alcohol Dependence*, 49, 81–88.

Patrick, M. E., Shaw, K. A., Dietz, P. M. et al. (2021) Prevalence of intellectual disability among eight-year-old children from selected communities in the United States, 2014. *Disability and Health Journal*, 14, 101023.

Peteet, J. R. (2018) A fourth wave of psychotherapies: moving beyond recovery toward well-being. *Harvard Review of Psychiatry*, 26, 90–95.

Petro, M. R., Rich, E. G., Erasmus, C. et al. (2017) The effect of religion on parenting in order to guide parents in the way they parent: a systematic review. *Journal of Spirituality in Mental Health*, 20, 114–139.

Pew Research Center (2015) *America's Changing Religious Landscape*. Available at www.pewforum.org/2015/05/12/americas-changing-religious-landscape/ (accessed 1 September 2021).

Pew Research Center (2016) *Pew-Templeton Global Religious Futures Project: Europe*. Available at www.globalreligiousfutures .org/regions/europe.pdf (accessed 20 May 2021).

Pew Research Center (2017) *The Changing Global Religious Landscape*. Available at www.pewforum.org/2017/04/05/the-changing-global-religious-landscape/ (accessed 1 September 2021).

Pew Research Center (2018) *10 Key Findings About Religion in Western Europe*. Available at www.pewresearch.org/fact-tank/2018/05/29/10-key-findings-about-religion-in-western-europe/ (accessed 23 May 2021).

Price-Feeney, M., Green, A. E. and Dorison, S. H. (2021) Suicidality among youth who are questioning, unsure of, or exploring their sexual identity. *Journal of Sex Research*, 58, 581–588.

Proctor, M., Miner, M., McLean, L. et al. (2009) Exploring Christians' explicit attachment to God representations: the development of a template for assessing attachment to God experiences. *Journal of Psychology and Theology*, 37, 245–264.

Rizzuto, A.-M. (1979) *The Birth of the Living God*. Chicago, IL: The University of Chicago Press.

Salas-Wright, C. P., Vaughn, M. G., Hodge, D. R. et al. (2012) Religiosity profiles of American youth in relation to substance use, violence, and delinquency. *Journal of Youth and Adolescence*, 41, 1560–1575.

Severaid, K. B., Osborne, K. J. and Mittal, V. A. (2019) Implications of religious and spiritual practices for youth at clinical high risk for psychosis. *Schizophrenia Research*, 208, 481–482.

Shafranske, E. P. (2009) Spiritually oriented psychodynamic psychotherapy. *Journal of Clinical Psychology*, 65, 98–109.

Shearer, A., Russon J., Herres, J. et al. (2018) Religion, sexual orientation, and suicide attempts among a sample of suicidal adolescents. *Suicide and Life-Threatening Behavior*, 48, 431–437.

Shepperd, J. A., Pogge, G., Lipsey, N. P. et al. (2019) Belief in a loving versus punitive God and behavior. *Journal of Research on Adolescence*, 29, 390–401.

Sherbersky, H. (2016) Family therapy and fundamentalism: one family therapist's exploration of ethics and collaboration with religious fundamentalist families. *Clinical Child Psychology and Psychiatry*, 21, 381–396.

Sheveland, J. N. (2011) Is yoga religious? Spiritual roots of a physical practice. *Christian Century*. Available at www .christiancentury.org/article/2011-05/yoga-religious (accessed 1 August 2021.)

Shooter, M. (2009) Child and adolescent psychiatry. In: C. Cook, A. Powell and A. Sims, eds., *Spirituality and Psychiatry*. London: RCPsych Publications, pp. 81–100.

Siev, J., Baer, L. and Minichiello, W. E. (2011) Obsessive-compulsive disorder with predominantly scrupulous symptoms: clinical and religious characteristics. *Journal of Clinical Psychology*, 67, 1188–1196.

Sperry, L. (2001) *Spirituality in Clinical Practice: Incorporating the Spiritual Dimension in Psychotherapy and Counseling*. New York: Brunner-Routledge.

Sperry, L. (2010) Psychotherapy sensitive to spiritual issues: a postmaterialist psychology perspective and developmental approach. *Psychology of Religion and Spirituality*, 2, 46–56.

Statista (2021) Average number of people per family in the United States from 1960 to 2021. Available at www.statista.com/statistics/183657/average-size-of-a-family-in-the-us/ (accessed 28 May 2021).

Steenhuis, L. D., Bartels-Velthuis, A. A., Jenner, J. A. et al. (2016) Religiosity in young adolescents with auditory vocal hallucinations. *Psychiatry Research*, 236, 158–164.

Steinhausen, H.-C., Villumsen, M. D., Horder, K. et al. (2021) Comorbid mental disorders during long-term course in a nationwide cohort of patients with anorexia nervosa. *International Journal of Eating Disorders*, 2021, 1608–1618.

Stevens, J. R., Prince, J. B., Prager, L. M. et al. (2014) Psychotic disorders in children and adolescents: a primer on contemporary evaluation and management. *Primary Care Companion for CNS Disorders*, 16, PCC.13f01514.

Streib, H. (2001) Faith development theory revisited: the religious styles perspective. *International Journal for the Psychology of Religion*, 11, 143–158.

Streib, H. (2005) Faith development research revisited: accounting for diversity in structure, content, and narrativity of faith. *International Journal for the Psychology of Religion*, 15, 99–121.

Tamminen, K. (1994) Religious experiences in childhood and adolescence: a viewpoint of religious development between the ages of 7 and 20. *International Journal for the Psychology of Religion*, 4, 61–85.

Walker, D. F. and Aten, J. D. (2012) Future directions for the study and application of religion, spirituality, and trauma research. *Journal of Psychology and Theology*, 40, 349–353.

Walsh, F. (2010) Spiritual diversity: multifaith perspectives in family therapy. *Family Process*, 49, 330–348.

Walsh, F. (2013) Religion and spirituality: a family systems perspective in clinical practice. In K. I. Pargament, ed., *APA Handbook of Psychology, Religion, and Spirituality: Vol. 2. An Applied Psychology of Religion and Spirituality*. Washington, DC: American Psychological Association, pp. 189–205.

Weatherhead, S. and Daiches, A. (2015) Key issues to consider in therapy with Muslim families. *Journal of Religion and Health*, 54, 2398–2411.

World Health Organization (2021) One in 100 deaths is by suicide: WHO guidance to help the world reach the target of reducing suicide rate by 1/3 by 2030. Available at www.who.int/news/item/17-06-2021-one-in-100-deaths-is-by-suicide (accessed 29 September 2021).

World Psychiatric Association (2017) *WPA Position Statement on Spirituality and Religion in Psychiatry*. Available at https://3ba346de-fde6-473f-b1da-536498661f9c.filesusr.com/ugd/e172f3_d1e17ded175d4f0898fad1c4ae5b1135.pdf (accessed 21 May 2021).

Worthington, E. L., Jr., Hook, J. N., Davis, D. E. et al. (2011) Religion and spirituality. In J. D. Norcross, ed., *Psychotherapy Relationships That Work*. New York: Oxford University Press, pp. 402–420.

Wu, M. S., Rozenman, M., Peris, T. S. et al. (2018) Comparing OCD-affected youth with and without religious symptoms: clinical profiles and treatment response. *Comprehensive Psychiatry*, 86, 47–53.

Yard, E., Radhakrishnan, L., Ballesteros, M. F. et al. (2021) Emergency department visits for suspected suicide attempts among persons aged 12–25 years before and during the COVID-19 pandemic – United States, January 2019–May 2021. *Morbidity and Mortality Weekly Report*, 70, 888–894.

Psychotherapy
The Spiritual Dimension
Andrew Powell[1]

We live in succession, in division, in parts, in particles. Meantime within man is the soul of the whole; the wise silence; the universal beauty, to which every part and particle is equally related, the eternal ONE. And this deep power in which we exist and whose beatitude is all accessible to us, is not only self-sufficing and perfect in every hour, but the act of seeing and the thing seen, the seer and the spectacle, the subject and the object, are one. We see the world piece by piece, as the sun, the moon, the animal, the tree; but the whole, of which these are shining parts, is the soul. (Ralph Waldo Emerson, 1841, p. 207)

All problems are psychological, but all solutions are spiritual. (Thomas Hora, 1986, p. 64)

Spirituality and Mental Health

Health and the sense of wholeness of being are intimately related.[2] The wholeness of being with which spirituality is concerned can be experienced in many ways. For some, it is revealed in the beauty of nature and the wonder of the physical universe; for others, it is experienced through music and the arts. Many find it in the expression of love on which families, communities, even the future of the planet, depend, while a great number seek to know the Divine through meditation, prayer and religious observance. A prime value, therefore, of introducing spirituality into mental health care is in offering a framework in which the parts may be understood in relation to the greater whole, thereby enhancing the meaning, purpose and value of life.

Over recent years there has been a steady increase in publications highlighting the spiritual dimension of mental health care (Larson et al., 2001; Koenig et al., 2012; Rosmarin and Koenig, 2020), including peer-reviewed journals such as *Mental Health, Religion and Culture* and the *Journal of Spirituality in Mental Health*, and outcome research on the value of specific spiritually informed treatment approaches for anxiety and depression (Kabat-Zinn, 2013) and substance abuse (Grim and Grim, 2019).

The spiritual dimension of psychotherapy is also gaining recognition (Stein, 1999; Schreurs, 2002; Field et al., 2005; MacKenna, 2005, 2007; Pargament, 2007; Powell,

---

[1] The author would like to record his indebtedness to Chris MacKenna, who co-authored the chapter on psychotherapy for the first edition of this book, for his textual contribution to the analysis of the poem *I AM* by John Clare.

[2] The word 'whole' shares the same root as 'healing' and 'health' (from Saxon *hāl* (healthy, safe), Middle English *hool* (healthy, unhurt), and similarly for *hel* and *heil* in High German and Old Norse.

2017a; Schuman, 2017), and since the first edition of *Spirituality and Psychiatry* (Cook et al., 2009) was published, a range of spiritually informed approaches have been developed, including *spiritually integrated cognitive behaviour therapy* (Rosmarin, 2018), *compassion-focused therapy* (Gilbert, 2010; Irons, 2019) and *forgiveness therapy* (Enright and Fitzgibbons, 2014). These specific therapies are further discussed in Chapter 14.

Of the analytical therapies, Freudian psychoanalysis has remained largely secular, although a minority of psychoanalysts have shown interest in spiritual and religious matters (Fromm, 1974; Meissner, 1984; Symington, 1994; Klein, 2003; Black, 2006; Merkur, 2013; Brown, 2019). On the other hand, Jungian analysis has traditionally valued spiritual experience (Aziz, 1990; Singer, 1995; MacKenna, 2000; Casement and Tacey, 2006).

Spirit, Soul and Ego

The Spirituality and Psychiatry Special Interest Group of the Royal College of Psychiatrists describes spirituality as 'the essentially human, personal and interpersonal dimension, which integrates and transcends the cultural, religious, psychological, social and emotional aspects of the person or is more specifically concerned with "soul" or "spirit".[3] Before further exploring the psycho-spiritual dimension of mental health care, it is helpful to introduce some working definitions of the terms being used, and to contextualise their usage, past and present.

The first term to consider is 'spirit'. Earlier civilisations believed in the existence of an animating life energy. For millennia, indigenous peoples have invoked the Great Spirit – a universal spiritual force. The Egyptians called it *ka*, the Greeks called it *pneuma* and the Romans called it *spiritus*. The Abrahamic faiths each refer to the Holy Spirit – in the Quran as denoted by the angel Gabriel who brings the word of God to humanity, in Judaism as the divine influence of God, and in the Christian Nicene Creed as 'the Lord and Giver of Life'. With small variations in meaning, spirit or its equivalent figures in the lexicon of all faith traditions.

In this chapter, 'spirit' betokens 'the limitless and unbounded consciousness that energises "all that is", both latent and manifest' (Powell, 2018, p. 73), also described as 'the sacred animating principle of Creation from which the manifest universe arises' (Powell, 2018, p. 5, footnote).

The term 'soul', on the other hand, derives from the Old English word *sawol*, meaning the spiritual or immaterial part of the human being. Whether or not a person views the soul as immortal, as used here it is understood to be the scintilla of spirit uniquely vested in each and every human being. The word itself, 'soul', resonates deeply; most people, if asked where it resides, place their hand over their heart. The humanist who thinks of the soul simply as representing the best that a person can give of him- or herself sees this accomplishment as an end in itself. Advocating a participative cosmology, the contemporary philosopher and cultural historian Richard Tarnas writes: 'the human mind is ultimately the organ of the world's own process of self-revelation. . . . Nature becomes intelligible to itself through the human mind' (Tarnas, 2010, p. 434).

---

[3] www.rcpsych.ac.uk/spirit

The term 'ego' features widely in popular parlance. It was originally defined by Freud as 'that part of the id[4] which has been modified by the direct influence of the external world' (Freud, 1923. p. 25). According to Freud, the ego obeys the 'reality principle', representing reason and common sense, concerned with adaptation to cultural norms and ensuring safety. The later school of object relations took a different view, regarding the ego as a primary structure, hence: 'The pristine personality of the child consists of a unitary dynamic ego' (Fairbairn, 1954, p. 107). Subsequently, the ego came to mean 'the part of the personality that is experienced as being oneself, which one recognises as "I"' (Rycroft, 1983, p. 39). In this chapter the term 'ego' is used to signify the conscious 'I', tasked with ensuring self-survival.

As described here, ego and soul have different agendas. The infant ego, driven at first by physiological needs (food, warmth and safety) increasingly acquires a psychological dimension. Crucial developmental steps include finding how to move and 'own' body parts, learning to distinguish 'me' from 'not-me' and, later, experiencing the physical self as a separate entity, something the child fully comprehends when discovering his or her own specular image in a mirror around the age of two.[5]

With the realisation of 'me' and 'mine' comes a new realisation, that the wider world brings not only love but also existential threat. Since the default position of the ego is self-referential, any experience of loss is to be feared – the greatest loss of all being bodily death, for the ego sees nothing beyond.

In contrast, the soul exists at the outset in a state of wonderment – the baby's mind is too unformed for anything more. However, over time, as the child matures, the soul is able to express its own innate virtues – unselfish love, compassion and wisdom. Knowing itself to exist beyond the confines of the mundane world, the soul faces loss and, importantly, death with equanimity.

Invariably, conflict arises between the self-concerns of the ego and the altruism of the soul. At best, this is a creative tension, for ego and soul are interdependent. The ego has the potential to learn from the compassion and wisdom of the soul, while the embodied ego provides the experience of human life, along with the many challenges that arise, for the advancement and enrichment of the soul as it journeys through this lifetime and beyond.[6]

The Anguish of the Poet John Clare

To illustrate the importance of the spiritual dimension, we shall begin by considering the affliction of one of the great English poets, John Clare (1793–1864). Clare was raised in an impoverished rural setting. The (then) continuing appropriation of the countryside

---

[4] Freud conceptualised the id as [containing] 'everything that is inherited, that is present at birth, that is laid down in the constitution – above all, the instincts . . .' (Freud, 1940, p. 145).
[5] The 'Stade du Miroir' described by the French psychoanalyst Jacques Lacan (1949). The importance of mirroring has since widened to include the mirroring process between mother and baby (Winnicott, 2005), the mirror test as an ethological research tool to evaluate self-recognition in higher primates and some other species, first devised by Gallup (1970) and the neurodevelopmental capacity for empathy (Stevens and Woodruff, 2018).
[6] One prominent school of esoteric teachings holds that the fundamental purpose of human life is the attainment of the 'soul-infused personality' (Bailey, 1944, p. 215).

by landowners (as a result of the Enclosure Acts) affected him deeply, since from an early age his spirituality and poetry were inspired by the countryside. To Clare's continuing distress, the income from publication of his poetry could not provide adequately for his wife and seven children. In his middle years, he began drinking heavily and suffered, it would appear, from bouts of psychotic depression. It seems the poet could find no place to rest except in the writing of poems, which continued lucid throughout his illness.

The poem *I AM*, dated 1845, was one of Clare's last. It was written in St Andrew's County Lunatic Asylum, Northampton, where Clare spent nearly all of the last 23 years of his life and where he died on 20 May 1864 (Bate, 2003). This poem of just three stanzas powerfully exemplifies the connection between Clare's mental distress and his spiritual yearning, speaking not only of his individual plight but also the suffering of all humanity, for such poetry poignantly conveys that 'what is most personal is most general' (Rogers, 1989, p. 27). Clare begins:

> I am: yet what I am, none cares or knows,
> My friends forsake me like a memory lost;
> I am the self-consumer of my woes,
> They rise and vanish in oblivious host
> Like shades in love and death's oblivion lost;
> And yet I am! and live like shadows tossed.

The first two lines powerfully convey Clare's sense of desolation and loneliness. 'I am the self-consumer of my woes' tells us that Clare feels his misery to be beyond the reach of others. The phrase 'like shades in love and death's oblivion lost' suggests there was once a time when his passions sought fulfilment in a relationship. Yet now, having lost contact with others, he is obliged to live in the solitary confinement of his own anguish. It is a measure both of Clare's isolation and of his genius that he can create a poetic form strong and supple enough to give such profound expression to his despair.

Apparently there is no one in whom Clare can confide and who might, in some measure, be able to help. The best he is able to do is to assert the fact of his existence: 'I am! and live'. However, this momentary achievement unravels in the next stanza:

> Into the nothingness of scorn and noise,
> Into the living sea of waking dreams,
> Where there is neither sense of life nor joys,
> But the vast shipwreck of my life's esteems;
> And e'en the dearest – that I loved the best –
> Are strange – nay, rather stranger than the rest.

Without a sufficient sense of self, Clare, 'like shadows tossed', is reduced to 'scorn and noise', a 'waking dream' in which there is only a sense of catastrophe (shipwreck) and estrangement from those he loved 'the best'. Finding himself in this alienated state of mind, Clare's yearning for relationship is revealed in the longing of his soul for union with God:

> I long for scenes where man has never trod,
> A place where woman never smil'd or wept;
> There to abide with my creator, God,

And sleep as I in childhood sweetly slept:
Untroubling and untroubled where I lie;
The grass below – above the vaulted sky.[7]

(Blunden and Porter, 1920, p. 240)

Given the prevalence of religious images in psychotic states of mind, from the psychiatric perspective it would be easy to pathologise Clare's spiritual *cri de coeur*. Equally, the secular psychotherapist might see it merely as the desire for regression to an infantile state.

However, it is important neither to dismiss nor to pathologise the patient's spirituality. From the psychospiritual standpoint, Clare's imagery reveals the universal need for primary relatedness of self to other. To begin with, Clare is only able to experience being in relation to himself – as the I AM. Yet he seeks to find ontological security in his relationship with the Divine Other. The effect of this is to assuage his anxiety sufficiently for the poet to put pen to paper.

Clare was an Anglican, but his introverted nature was such that he never joined in communal prayer or religious worship. Although much research associates spirituality with improved mental health (Koenig et al., 2012; Rosmarin and Koenig, 2020), some studies suggest that people who have a spiritual understanding of life in the absence of a religious framework are vulnerable to mental disorder (King et al., 2013).[8] If Clare was alive today, he might well have figured in the population studied by King.

In Clare's time, there would have been little in the way of help beyond humane shelter, so let us imagine how the poet might fare in today's world.

The Psychiatric Assessment

In order to discover what the therapeutic task may be, the psychiatrist first has to assess his or her patient in order to make a diagnosis in accordance with the International Classification of Diseases 11th Revision (ICD–11) (World Health Organization, 2020), for which detailed questioning is necessary.

A Mental State Examination (MSE) is based on an assessment of appearance, behaviour, speech, mood, affect, thought, perception, cognition and insight. Although we are in no position to make a specific diagnosis in Clare's case, it is likely that he would have been found to have a significant mental disorder for which medication and/or other physical treatments would be advised.

The MSE has more to do with systematically checking an inventory of symptoms than with establishing empathic contact with the patient. John Clare speaks for many psychiatric patients who feel that they have seen the doctor, but doubt whether the doctor has seen them: 'I am: yet what I am, none cares or knows' – the feeling of being seen, yet not seen, only serving to intensify their suffering and confusion. Further, if the psychiatrist evaluates merely on the basis of social norms, value judgements may be

---

[7] First published in the *Bedford Times* on 1 January 1848. The poem is out of copyright and in the public domain worldwide.

[8] King's study does not argue that spirituality per se leads to mental disorder. However, in the largely secular and consumerist society of today, the spiritual search for meaning and purpose can be a lonely and disquieting pursuit, especially for the burgeoning demographic of 'spiritual but not religious', who lack the community and support of a faith tradition.

made that do not take into account the unique self of the patient. This is especially likely when dealing with eccentric, creative and unusual people.

Regardless of what kind of therapy is being offered, from the outset the patient needs to feel that he or she is being sympathetically received, listened to without judgement and helped to make sense of what has gone wrong (Dixon and Sweeney, 2000). Relating empathically to the patient's personal framework of meaning and purpose is crucial here. This should include tactful exploration of his or her spiritual beliefs and values, as described in Chapter 2, which can both strengthen the therapeutic alliance[9] and help when deciding on the therapeutic approach to be taken (Culliford, 2007).

Showing sensitivity, care and concern is the hallmark of medicine as a spiritual vocation, giving the best chance of healing for mind and body.[10] No formulation of psychopathology, whether biological or psychological, should substitute for, or diminish, the recognition of a person's unique, sentient self. If someone like Clare is to be encouraged out of his or her self-isolation, it is essential to engage with the patient's inner life. The next section compares two psychotherapeutic approaches – psychoanalytic and Jungian – as they might have been offered to John Clare in later times.

Freud Revisited

How might Sigmund Freud have understood Clare's existential anguish? Freud (1911, pp. 222–223) set great store by what he called the reality principle. He also made clear his belief that 'religion is comparable to a childhood neurosis' (Freud, 1927, p. 53).

We know that Freud disavowed his own Jewish religious tradition in his aim to make a science of psychoanalysis (Bakan, 1990). Despite his attempts to remain as neutral and objective as possible, Freud's response to the free associations of his patients is likely to have influenced the flow of 'material', since the act of interpretation, however well considered, will be subtly shaped by the therapist's preconceptions. Indeed, it is possible that the secular disposition of many psychoanalysts today is a lasting reflection of Freud's avowed religious scepticism.

Faced with Clare's longing to return to an Eden-like relationship with God, and his fantasy of sleeping, childlike, in the fused embrace of mother earth and father sky, Freud would probably have assumed that he was dealing with a regression of the ego arising from a serious failure in some developmental task (Freud, 1926, pp. 241–242). Within the framework of psychoanalysis, Freud would have offered Clare the opportunity to relinquish his spiritual soliloquy in favour of more human discourse.

Psychoanalysis encourages the projection of unresolved childhood emotions on to the figure of the analyst, a process Freud called transference. Freud first used the term in 1895, in *The Psychotherapy of Hysteria*, writing that '[the patient] is transferring on to the figure of the physician the distressing ideas which arise from the content of the analysis ... through a false connection' (Breuer and Freud, 1895, p. 302).

---

[9] The 'therapeutic alliance' can be traced back to Freud (Ardito and Rabellino, 2011). The attributes needed in the therapist have been variously described as genuineness, empathy and non-possessive warmth (Truax and Carkhuff, 1967), unconditional positive regard (Rogers, 1965) and the therapist's agapeistic attitude (Lambert, 1981). (In the New Testament, the Greek word *agape* is used to refer to the love that seeks always to act in the best interest of the other.)

[10] The essence of good doctoring: 'Every time a doctor sees a patient, the patient should feel better as a result' (Lown, 1996, p. 88).

The analysis of the transference was to become a cornerstone of therapy (Racker, 1968). Freud would have endeavoured to help Clare identify such projections on to the therapist, recognising their origin and taking them back as feelings belonging to himself. This is delicate work, for there is a danger that the analyst comes to be perceived as omniscient. Given the intensity of Clare's longing for union with God, if such a transference had arisen it might have proved to become overwhelming.

Perhaps it is more likely that Clare's religious preoccupation would have resisted interpretation based on Freud's secular frame of reference, and that Clare would have perceived Freud as unsympathetic to matters spiritual. In this event, Freud would probably have concluded that Clare was not a suitable subject for psychoanalysis. Nevertheless, if therapy did make progress, there is the possibility that Freud might have enabled Clare to recover sufficiently for understanding to take the place of incoherence, and mourning for the lost object to replace the denial of loss (Freud, 1917, pp. 244–245).

Since Freud's time, psychoanalysis has developed along a number of theoretical pathways, including ego psychology, object relations theory, interpersonal psychoanalysis, self-psychology and relational psychoanalysis. A central debate has concerned the extent to which the therapist should remain a blank screen or should be a visible and human presence, rather than an object of transference.

Especially where religious or spiritual themes are to the fore, it is important to recognise that just as the patient may unconsciously project on to the figure of the therapist, so the therapist may be unaware of projections of his or her own that could prejudice the course of psychotherapy (Peteet, 2013). Freud, in first describing counter-transference, wrote that '[it arises in the analyst] as a result of the patient's influence on his unconscious feelings, and we are almost inclined to insist that he shall recognise this counter-transference in himself and overcome it' (Freud, 1910, pp. 144–145). Subsequently the term was used 'to cover all the feelings which the analyst experiences towards his patient' (Heimann, 1950, p. 81); rather than seeing countertransference as necessarily problematic, some psychoanalysts regard it as helpful in understanding the patient's internal object world. Nevertheless, the term is now most often used more generally to indicate any bias held by the therapist, whether positive or negative, that may influence the beliefs and values of the patient or distort the impartiality of the therapeutic relationship. Preconceptions of a religious or secular kind can be especially relevant here, and the psychotherapist must always keep this in mind (Lannert, 1991; Abernethy and Lacia, 1998; Meissner, 2009).

Jung Revisited

Carl Jung, Freud's former student and colleague, would also have noted the regressive nature of Clare's fantasy. However, believing as he did that conscious and unconscious processes function in a compensatory relationship, Jung is likely to have seen Clare's longing for the Divine as an attempt by his patient to engender self-healing. Specifically, it would seem that Clare's ego had taken refuge in archetypes[11] of divine nurture – the

---

[11] The term archetype refers to an inherited idea or mode of thought that has its source in the collective unconscious of humankind. Archetypes are expressed as images or personifications. Of the Imago Dei (the God image), Jung writes '[It] pervades the whole human sphere and makes mankind its involuntary exponent' (Jung, 1958. p. 417).

desire to be cradled by mother earth and by father sky – suggested by the transpersonal imagery of the poem's third stanza.

In health, these archetypes find expression in the unfolding infant–mother relationship and in the ever-widening circle of relationships that develop through childhood (Neumann, 1976). In Clare's case, however, human relationships would appear to have been abandoned, and instead, sleeping in the arms of God has the symbolic function of offering Clare both consolation and a sense of containment.

Clare's ringing words 'And yet I am' could simply be asserting that he is still alive and clinging to his identity. However, Jung, familiar with psychotic states of mind, would doubtless have heard an echo with the Hebrew name for God – YHWH, I AM THAT I AM – suggesting that Clare's unconscious is on the brink of overwhelming his ego (Jung, 1939, p. 243). Although Jung would have seen the longing for a relationship with God as entirely consistent with the capacity for loving human relationships, the problem here lies in Clare's despairing self-isolation and the compensatory solace that he seeks only from God.

How might Jung have worked with Clare's fragile ego? One possibility would have been to explore whether the fantasy of sleeping sweetly like a child, with the grass below and the sky above, could become the beginning of a process of 'active imagination' (Samuels et al., 1986) that would furnish the ingredients needed for Clare's recovery.

If it turned out that Clare adhered concretely to his fantasy, indicating that symbolic function was lost, this would suggest that a cognitive–behavioural approach rather than an analytical one should be attempted. However, if Clare could explore the symbolic meaning of his fantasy in such a way that a story began to unfold, this would suggest that a Jungian approach was suitable for him.

If psychotherapy led to a marked rise in Clare's anxiety or excitement, increasing the risk of psychotic fragmentation, psychotherapy with medication as an adjunct might be possible. Most important would be the therapist's ability to gently explore how Clare's inner and outer lives might be dynamically related, acknowledging the depth of the poet's spiritual longing while helping him to take the risk of seeking trust and intimacy in a human relationship.

Freud and Jung had many theoretical and technical differences, but each, in his own way, was devoted to his patients and would have made enormous efforts to create a containing relationship with Clare – the one thing he so conspicuously lacked. Such dedication could well have turned out to be the most powerful therapeutic factor.

Converging Pathways

Jung's analytical psychology anticipated the subsequent development of transpersonal psychology, in which the soul perspective of a larger, more meaningful reality extends beyond the confines of the personal self. However, the origins of the transpersonal approach can be traced back to William James (1842–1910), whose humane and pragmatic approach to psychology and whose lectures on religious experience given in 1901 (James, 1902/1960) set the 'gold standard' for the psychological study of religion for the next 100 years. The breadth of James' vision is evident in the following passage:

> Our normal waking consciousness, rational consciousness as we call it, is but one special type of consciousness, while all about it, parted from it by the filmiest of screens, there lie

potential forms of consciousness entirely different. We may go through life without suspecting their existence; but apply the requisite stimulus, and at a touch they are there in all their completeness. (James, 1902/1960, p. 374)

Such shifts in consciousness, in which the ego is felt to be transcended, are often accompanied by profound religious or spiritual awakening.

James maintained a down-to-earth approach to the value of religious beliefs, sympathetically evaluating a wide range of first-hand reports of religious experiences. He continued to question the ultimate source of spiritual experience, yet he was convinced that our lives are in some way continuous with a higher power which, when experienced as benign, has a demonstrably beneficial effect. In this, James anticipated the research that a century later would show the positive effects of spirituality on both physical and mental health. James concluded that, for practical purposes, belief in the chance of salvation was enough, because 'the existence of the chance makes the difference ... between a life of which the keynote is resignation and a life of which the keynote is hope' (James, 1902/1960, p. 500).

James emphasises that the patient should be helped to come to his or her own meaningful experience of subjective reality, including the healing properties of religious experience. In Clare's fervent desire, 'There to abide with my Creator, God, and sleep as I in childhood sweetly slept', the poet's need to find relief from the burdens of the mind is palpable. However, Clare has yet to find the healing that could help him to become whole, and so live to the full.

A brief account of the work of Viktor Frankl (1905–1997) is included next because his ideas form a bridge with more specifically transpersonal interventions. Frankl was a Jewish psychiatrist and psychotherapist who survived four Nazi concentration camps, in which his mother, father, brother and wife perished. Frankl's experiences formed the basis for an existential psychotherapy that he called logotherapy, founded on spirituality in the sense of humankind's 'will to find meaning' (Frankl, 1973, p. 10). This was especially important for his patients who were Holocaust survivors, and who were so damaged by trauma that they saw no point in continuing with their lives.

Three major insights inform Frankl's work: first, that we can detach from the oppression in which we may find ourselves; second, that in doing so, no matter what the outward circumstance, we are free to choose and uphold the values by which we live and die; third, that living or dying with dignity requires a framework of meaning that can embrace suffering as well as health. Frankl quotes Nietzsche's statement that 'He who knows a "why" for living will surmount almost every "how"',[12] and goes on to observe:

while the concern of most people was summed up by the question, 'Will we survive the [concentration] camp?' – for if not, then this suffering has no sense – the question which in contrast beset me was, 'Has this whole suffering, this dying, a meaning?' – for if not, then ultimately there is no sense to surviving. For a life whose meaning stands or falls upon whether one survives or not, a life, that is, whose meaning depends upon such a happenstance, such a life would not really be worth living at all. (Frankl, 1967, p. 102)

---

[12] More correctly translated as 'If we have our own why in life, we shall get along with almost any how' (Nietzsche, 1895/2016, p. 6).

Frankl's work has since influenced the development of spiritually augmented cognitive-behavioural therapy (D'Souza and Rodrigo, 2004), an approach now being used in a wide range of treatment settings (Rosmarin et al., 2019). However, Frankl is cited here because of the importance of finding meaning. It is possible that Clare's exceptional capacity to continue to write lucid poetry while otherwise incapacitated by mental illness was the poet's way of giving meaning to his suffering and, through his poetry, reaching out to humanity in the only way he could.

The larger transpersonal perspective is one that bestows on each life an enduring value that transcends death. For those who have children, there is the hope that the love shown to them will bear fruit in the fullness of their lives and for generations thereafter. For some, it is the value of service to the community and friendships, while for others there is the hope that their professional work will make a contribution, however small, to the progress of humankind. All of these share an experience fundamental to spirituality – that we belong to more than ourselves. In this regard, we could say that Clare succeeded, for he has found immortality in the enduring legacy of his consummate poetry.

Envisioning the Transpersonal

Before commenting on how a transpersonal approach may have been helpful to John Clare, a brief and selective account of transpersonal theory will be offered, concluding with examples of transpersonal psychotherapy in clinical practice.

The term 'transpersonal' is more widely known in the USA, but is not so familiar to many psychiatrists in the UK.[13] One concise and well-recognised definition of the transpersonal, sharing much with spirituality as defined earlier in this chapter, is provided by Walsh and Vaughan (1993, p. 203), namely 'experiences in which the sense of identity or self extends beyond (trans) the individual or personal to encompass wider aspects of humankind, life, psyche or cosmos'.

Set against the broad perspectives offered by William James, Carl Jung and Viktor Frankl, transpersonal psychology evolved as a California-based movement in the 1960s, a syncretism of Western philosophy, psychology and esotericism with the religious and contemplative traditions of the East. The touchstone of the therapeutic approach that subsequently evolved lies in explicitly addressing the psycho-spiritual dimension (see Washburn, 1994; Wilber, 2002; Forman, 2010; Read, 2014; Friedman and Hartelius, 2015).

Key figures in transpersonal psychology include Robert Assagioli, Abraham Maslow, Stanislav Grof and Erich Fromm, a neo-Freudian analyst who was deeply interested in Zen Buddhism. The decade of the 1960s was notable for a burgeoning interest in Eastern religions and spiritual practices, including Hinduism and Advaita Vedanta, Buddhism, Zen and Taoism, being made known to the West through the writings of D. T. Suzuki, Alan Watts, Walter Evans-Wentz, Stephen Mitchell and others. Tracing the complex epistemology of transpersonal theory, particularly with regard to its roots in the East, is beyond the scope of this chapter.[14] Here, the focus is on some of the major therapeutic contributions that have shaped the field.

---

[13] The British Psychological Society formed a Transpersonal Psychology Section in 1996, co-founded by David Fontana, Ingrid Slack and Martin Treacy.
[14] For a masterly exegesis, see Ferrer (2002).

The first one to mention is the pioneering work of the psychoanalyst Roberto Assagioli (1888–1974), who founded psychosynthesis. Assagioli identified a 'central self' positioned midway between the unconscious and what he called the 'superconscious' (Assagioli, 1965). The central self is composed purely of consciousness and will; it actively engages with the various aspects of the personality as described by Assagioli – thought, intuition, imagination, emotion-feeling, sensation and impulse-desire – yet remains separate from the personality (in contrast to Buddhism, in which, through meditation, the self is able to dis-identify with attachment and desire).

In psychosynthesis, there are two sequential therapeutic tasks. The first task is the secure integration of personality around the central self, not so different from the aim of much psychotherapy, and essential for healthy 'grounding'. The second task is to align the central self with the superconscious realm, resulting in the 'transpersonal self'. In doing so, we are led to recognise that ultimately we are all one, and with that understanding there arises a global perspective characterised by social cooperation, altruistic love and a transpersonal vision of spiritual evolution.

Abraham Maslow (1908–1970) provides an important link in the history of transpersonal psychology, and so deserves special mention. In his earlier work as a humanistic psychologist, Maslow approached the study of personality by focusing on subjective experience, free will and the innate human drive towards self-actualisation. In his seminal paper, 'A Theory of Human Motivation' (Maslow, 1943), he introduced the term 'hierarchy of needs', ranking human needs from the most basic physical level to the most advanced needs of self-actualisation, as illustrated in Fig. 6.1.

Maslow broadly described two kinds of need. There are those concerned with safety, nourishment, love, belonging, respect and self-esteem, which Maslow called 'deficiency needs' (D-needs). However, he was concerned to give equal weight to psychological well-being, with humanity aspiring naturally towards what Maslow called 'being values'

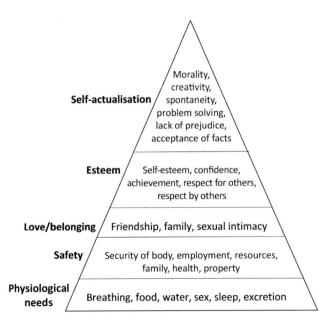

Figure 6.1 Maslow's hierarchy of needs
Image adapted from https://commons.wikimedia.org/wiki/File:Maslow%27s_hierarchy_of_needs.png and released under the GNU Free Documentation Licence by Wikimedia Commons.

(B-values). These include unity, transcendence, aliveness, uniqueness, justice, order, simplicity, goodness, beauty and truth. B-values are sustained by B-needs that are expansive – for example, the need to engage in meaningful, helpful work and service, promote justice and harmony and express one's creativity. The difference can be illustrated with a single example: the need to be loved is a D-need, and the need to love is a B-need.[15]

According to Maslow, human potential at its best is expressed by what he calls self-actualisation. This includes accurate perception of reality, comfortable acceptance of self and others, tolerance of human imperfection, living with vitality and spontaneity, being comfortable with solitude yet able to engage in deep personal relationships, and desiring to work for the benefit of humankind. Importantly, Maslow further describes mystical, ecstatic or spiritual states known as 'peak experiences' in which there is an overwhelming sense of oneness with all that is, accompanied by intense happiness that confirms the value, purpose and meaning of life.

Maslow concluded that humanistic psychology could not account for the epiphanic nature of the peak experience, and went on to become a co-founder of the school of transpersonal psychology, together with Viktor Frankl, Stanislav Grof, Anthony Sutich and others. Their work was to lay the foundation for the study of non-ordinary states of consciousness (NOSCs).

Interest in NOSCs had been aroused by Aldous Huxley's book *The Doors of Perception* (1954), in which Huxley gave a detailed account of his experimentation with mescaline. Huxley suggested that 'ordinary' consciousness was the result of the brain filtering out the awareness of information that would otherwise be overwhelming. In fact, the 'filter theory' of the mind can be traced back to the philosopher Frederic W. H. Myers in the nineteenth century, and his renowned friend and colleague William James. The concept has since been refined and elaborated with reference to quantum physics and current neuroscience (Kelly et al., 2019).

In the clinical arena, research began as early as the 1960s, when Grof started using the entheogen lysergic acid diethylamide (LSD) for therapeutic purposes. Because of alarm at the widespread recreational use of entheogens during the decade, LSD was proscribed in 1968, which led Grof to develop a breathing/sensory input programme (Holotropic Breathwork™) that could induce a comparable altered state of consciousness (Grof, 1993). Grof highlights the role of the birth experience in shaping the emotional disposition of later years, and has closely studied the relationship of psychotic breakdown to the 'spiritual emergency'. His clinical findings are reflected in the theoretical writings of Ken Wilber (1996) and linked to the Vedic concept of the chakras by the psychiatrist John Nelson (1994).

Entheogens, popularly known as psychedelics, have been known to shamanic cultures for millennia. More recently they have been the subject of anthropological fieldwork (Narby, 1998; Harner, 2005; Glass-Coffin, 2010). Yet despite attempts to re-introduce psychedelic research over several decades, it was not until 2010 that clinical trials of hallucinogens and entactogens such as MDMA (3,4-methylenedioxymethamphetamine) were able to be resumed, with promising results for post-traumatic stress disorder,

---

[15] As described here, D-needs are characteristic of the ego and B-needs are characteristic of the soul.

alcoholism and social anxiety (Sessa et al., 2019). Studies of LSD-assisted psychotherapy for the treatment of anxiety related to life-threatening diseases such as cancer have also shown striking results, with subjects reporting reduced fear of death (78%), reduced anxiety (78%) and increased quality of life (67%) (Gasser et al., 2015).

There is one last contribution to the field of transpersonal psychology that must be outlined here, namely the study of so-called paranormal phenomena. Empirical research based on nomothetic (quantitive) data has been carried out on healing (Roe et al., 2015), extrasensory perception (Radin, 2018), the near-death experience (Long, 2014; Parnia et al., 2014) and reincarnation (Stevenson, 1966, 1997; Tucker, 2014). Phenomena better suited to an idiographic (qualitative) approach include mediumship (Solomon and Solomon, 2003; Fontana, 2005), life after death (Schwartz and Simon, 2002; Kean, 2017), past-life regression (Woolger, 1999), life-between-life therapy (Newton, 1998, 2002) and spirit release therapy (Baldwin, 1995; Zinser, 2011).

Because a physicalist worldview cannot readily account for such events, there has been much scepticism voiced by mainstream science. As a result, the research findings on paranormal phenomena have, for the most part, been dismissed as 'impossible'. This may well reflect an age-old problem – the reluctance to accommodate a fundamentally different paradigm (Kuhn, 1962).[16] Yet advances in the fields of quantum non-locality (Radin, 2006; Goswami, 2012), astrophysics (Matloff, 2016) and holographic cosmology (Currivan, 2017; PhysOrg, 2017) deserve serious consideration, pointing as they do to the existence of other dimensional realms, with different rule-sets from those that structure the world we know (Carr, 2019).

Soul-Centred Psychotherapy

It will be clear that transpersonal psychology draws on a *weltanschauung* or worldview that sees all we take for 'real' as nested within a transcendent dimension, considered by many to be the birthplace of the soul. Unhappily, the wounds inflicted on the ego in the course of the human lifespan are, for some, overwhelming. However, by drawing on the wisdom and compassion of the soul – known to the human heart as unconditional love – it is possible to bring healing that enables the adversities of life to be faced with courage and hope.[17]

There is a wide range of transpersonal therapies today.[18] The case studies that follow, as practised by the author, describe soul-centred psychotherapy, an approach that directly engages the patient's spiritual reality as a powerful therapeutic tool.[19] The therapist

---

[16] A case in point: post-materialist science argues that consciousness is not epiphenomenal (a product of the brain) but primary, the brain functioning as a receiver, much as a radio converts radio waves into audible sound. This idea is not new. Max Planck, the theoretical physicist whose discovery of energy quanta won him the Nobel Prize in Physics in 1918, observed, 'I regard consciousness as fundamental. I regard matter as derivative from consciousness' (Planck, 1931, p. 17).

[17] The seventeenth-century scientist and theologian Blaise Pascal observed that 'the heart has its reasons, which reason does not know. . . . It is the heart that experiences God, and not the reason' (Pascal, 1670/2018, p. 78).

[18] These are admirably summarised by Rowan (2015) in *The Transpersonal: Spirituality in Psychotherapy and Counselling*.

[19] The therapist needs to work within the limits of his or her competence, for which the relevant clinical experience and training are necessary.

must be willing to cross the transpersonal threshold and share the reality of the patient's inner world, with trust in the healing power of the soul, and confidence that, once engaged, it will be perfectly attuned to the patient's needs.[20]

Sometimes healing begins simply by encouraging the patient to reflect in a new way on his or her experience. It is well known, for instance, that following bereavement, a person may report a visitation from the deceased, historically described in psychiatry as a hallucination. Such anomalous perceptions can be regarded not merely as statistical happenstance but as spiritually significant events, as illustrated by the following vignette[21] (Powell, 2017b, pp. 28–29):

Case study: Gareth

Gareth was referred by his general practitioner for depression.[22] He had cared for his mother during her illness with cancer, and after she died he was burdened with the memory of her suffering. When Gareth came for the second session, he said something had happened that had been a shock. One night, soon after lying down, he had clearly seen his mother standing at the end of the bed. When he rubbed his eyes and looked again, she had gone. He thought he must be going out of his mind.

Rather than just reassuring Gareth, I asked him to recall how his mother had looked. He said it was strange but she was smiling. Had she spoken? Gareth replied that nothing was said but he felt she was somehow telling him she was well and he shouldn't worry. I put to Gareth that this visit by his mother was not only nothing to be afraid of but also that it could be of great value and a comfort to him. Gareth said he was so relieved to think his mother, wherever she was, could feel well and happy again, and his mood began to lift the same day.

Freud famously wrote 'where id was, there ego shall be' (Freud, 1931, p. 80), and bringing the workings of the unconscious to light remains the aim of psychodynamic therapy to date. For some patients, however, the ego has been so badly traumatised that they lack the hope and trust needed to begin therapeutic work on the self.

At such times, the patient who can be helped to become more soul conscious will discover, surprisingly, that the essence of the self, the soul, is alive and well, unharmed by the travails of life. This is a good place to begin the work of healing, for such patients may have lost all hope of love, whether for themselves or others. Discovering that love is still very much there can be a turning point, as in the following case study:

Case study: Christine

Christine was seen for long-standing depression. Throughout childhood, she never felt valued. Academic success had temporarily bolstered her self-esteem, but later, when a

---

[20] A wide range of case studies of soul-centred therapy can be found in *Conversations with the Soul* (Powell, 2018, pp. 73–88).

[21] First published in 'The healing potential of anomalous perceptual experiences', *Journal of the Society for Psychical Research*, 2017, 81, pp. 26–31, and reproduced by kind permission of the publishers.

[22] Names given in the case studies have been changed to ensure anonymity.

personal relationship failed, this fell apart. Her emotions froze over and she became profoundly withdrawn.

Christine had described her depression as a black cave. I invited her to close her eyes, 'go inside' and report with what she could find. After some minutes, she found a pair of steel handcuffs, then a rope and an iron chain. I pressed her to go on looking. After what seemed an eternity, her expression changed to one of concern and I asked her what she had found. It was a little puppy in a dark corner. I suggested she pick it up and hold it to her. With her eyes still closed, she cradled the puppy. What could she feel? She replied that she could feel the puppy's love for her. I urged her to let her own love flow to this puppy and she began to cry. I encouraged her to find an image for her emotion and she chose a golden heart.

Rather than exploring Christine's images of pain and suffering directly, it had felt more important first to wait and see if the soul would offer a symbol of healing – in this instance, the puppy. From the psychological perspective, the puppy stood for the child Christine. She nurtured this child-self with which she had lost touch, finding she still had the capacity for love. On the transpersonal level, Christine was enabled to rediscover her soul that had been lost to view in the darkness of her childhood.

Soul-centred therapy calls for openness on the part of the therapist to whatever may arise, and preparedness to go wherever healing may need to take place, as in this next consultation:

Case study: Jan

My patient, Jan, complained of feeling depressed and 'not herself'. Taking an antidepressant had helped but she was still 'not herself'. Going into Jan's background, I learned that shortly before her symptoms started, a close friend had taken her life in Jan's home, having been staying there while my patient was away on holiday. Remembering how she had twice said she was 'not herself', I asked Jan if she had the feeling of 'someone else' when she came back home. She replied that she hadn't wanted to say in case I thought she was mad, but every time she went into the house, she had the physical sensation of her friend being right there in the room with her.

Taking this at face value, I asked Jan how she would feel about us inviting the 'spirit' of her friend to the consultation, to see if we could find out more about what was going on. Jan was willing, so I asked her to close her eyes, tune in to her friend and try letting her friend speak through her. Her friend 'came through' and went on to express deep regret at having taken her life. Suicide had solved nothing. She remained unhappy, lonely and seeking comfort. I explained that staying on was having a bad effect on my patient, and was not helping herself either. She apologised. 'If only I had known', she said, 'what I know now. I was facing the biggest challenge of my life and I went and messed it up. I feel even worse than I did before'.

I said I was sure other opportunities would be given her. She was very relieved to hear this and we talked more about her hopes for another chance at life. When she agreed that she was ready to move on, I asked her to look for 'the light'. She exclaimed 'Yes, I can see it!', and left at once. Immediately, Jan felt the burden of oppression lift from her and it did not return.

As in the case study of Gareth, when using active imagination in this way, it is not for the therapist to claim to know what is objectively 'real' – the patient can make up his or her own mind. What matters is that the narrative should be guided compassionately with a view to healing, and when this takes place, sufficient unto the day is the grace thereof.

Dreams can also be a means by which the soul brings about healing, as with the following patient:

Case study: John

John had been born into circumstances of great deprivation. Fortunately, he was saved from a life in social care by being taken in, aged four, by a neighbour, Bob, who from that time on was his father in all but name. The boy grew into a man and made good, married, had a family and moved away. Yet he often went back to see Bob, now ageing and alone but fiercely independent. Then the time came when Bob grew so frail that his neighbours had to come in and start washing and caring for him. Bob couldn't bear it. One day he got himself upstairs to the spare bedroom, lay down with his cap on his head as always, swallowed a lot of tablets and died. John was devastated at the news. He kept dreaming Bob was still alive only to wake up and find him gone, and he fell into a severe depression.

John then told me that just before attending this consultation, something had happened which had 'knocked him for six'. He had dreamed again of Bob but this was different. In the dream, he 'knew' for the first time that Bob was dead. Yet there was Bob, sitting across from him, large as life, cap on head, just the way he always sat. My patient asked him outright, 'Bob, are you dead?' Bob answered him as direct as ever, 'Yes!' His next question to Bob was 'Is there life after death?' Another emphatic 'Yes' came right back. Then he challenged Bob head on. 'Prove it to me!' Bob pulled out a book that looked like a Bible with detailed drawings in it and, sure enough, the proof was all there. Then John awoke. All day he could intensely feel Bob's presence. He found his emotions welling up and although it was very painful, he could say to me in that first meeting 'I know I'm getting better'.

This case study underlines that all healing is, ultimately, self-healing.[23] John's awareness of the forthcoming consultation evidently initiated the dream, and it only needed the occasion of sharing it to mark an important step in his recovery.

Finally, returning to our earlier reflections on John Clare, let us imagine that we are meeting with him around the time he was writing the poem *I AM*. Let us suppose that Clare is lucid, and is able and willing to converse. With the support of a therapist open to the transpersonal frame of reference, Clare could be invited to engage imaginatively with the imagery of his inner life and to begin a dialogue that would, we might hope, open him to the healing power of the soul.

Sadly, for John Clare there was no such therapeutic opportunity. For the remaining years of his life he languished in St Andrew's asylum, a great poet, bereft of his muse.

Conclusion

In recent years the spiritual dimension of mental health care has been steadily taking root and this is as it should be, for the etymology of 'psychiatry' derives from the Greek words *psyche* ('soul') and *iatros* ('healer'). Spirituality, whether implicit or explicit, is indispensable to psychiatric and psychotherapeutic best practice. Where a spiritually orientated approach is indicated, the transpersonal perspective, illustrated here by soul-centred psychotherapy, can play a unique part in harnessing the abiding spiritual resource that is our human birthright.

---

[23] 'Only what is really oneself has the power to heal' (Jung, 1917, p. 168).

References

Abernethy, A. D. and Lacia, J. J. (1998) Religion and the psychotherapeutic relationship: transferential and countertransferential dimensions. *Journal of Psychotherapy Practice and Research*, 7, 281–289.

Ardito, R. B. and Rabellino, D. (2011) Therapeutic alliance and outcome of psychotherapy: historical excursus, measurements, and prospects for research. *Frontiers in Psychology*, 2, 270.

Assagioli, R. (1965) *Psychosynthesis: A Manual of Principles and Techniques*. New York: Hobbs, Dorman & Company.

Aziz, R. (1990) *C. G. Jung's Psychology of Religion and Synchronicity*. Albany: State University of New York Press.

Bailey, A. A. (1944/1983) *Discipleship in the New Age*, Vol. 2. New York: Lucis Trust.

Bakan, D. (1990) *Sigmund Freud and the Jewish Mystical Tradition*. London: Free Association Books.

Baldwin, W. J. (1995) *Spirit Releasement Therapy: A Technique Manual*, 2nd ed. London: Headline Books.

Bate, J. (2003) *John Clare: A Biography*. London: Picador.

Black, D. M. (2006) *Psychoanalysis and Religion in the Twenty-first Century: Competitors or Collaborators?* Abingdon: Routledge.

Blunden, E. and Porter, A., eds., (1920) *John Clare: Poems Chiefly from Manuscript*. London: Richard Cobden-Sanderson Publisher.

Breuer, J. and Freud, S. (1895/1957) The psychotherapy of hysteria. In *The Standard Edition of the Complete Psychological Works of Sigmund Freud*, Vol. 2. *Studies on Hysteria* (J. Strachey, trans.). London: Hogarth Press, pp. 253–305.

Brown, R. (2019) *Groundwork for a Transpersonal Psychoanalysis: Spirituality, Relationship, and Participation*. Abingdon: Routledge.

Carr, B. (2019) Blind watchers of psi: a rebuttal of Reber and Alcock. *Journal of Scientific Exploration*, 33, 643–660.

Casement, A. and Tacey, D., eds. (2006) *The Idea of the Numinous: Contemporary Jungian and Psychoanalytic Perspectives*. Hove: Routledge.

Cook, C., Powell, A. and Sims, A., eds. (2009) *Spirituality and Psychiatry*. London: RCPsych Publications.

Culliford, L. (2007) Taking a spiritual history. *Advances in Psychiatric Treatment*, 13, 212–219.

Currivan, J. (2017) *The Cosmic Hologram: Information at the Center of Creation*. Rochester, VT: Inner Traditions.

Dixon, M. and Sweeney, K. (2000) *The Human Effect in Medicine: Theory, Research and Practice*. Abingdon: Radcliffe Medical Press.

D'Souza, R. F. and Rodrigo, A. (2004) Spiritually augmented cognitive behavioural therapy. *Australasian Psychiatry*, 12, 148–152.

Emerson, R. W. (1841/2003) The Over-Soul. In L. Ziff, ed., *Nature and Selected Essays*. New York: Penguin Books, pp. 205–225.

Enright, R. D. and Fitzgibbons, R. P. (2014) *Forgiveness Therapy: An Empirical Guide for Resolving Anger and Restoring Hope*. Washington, DC: American Psychological Association.

Fairbairn, W. R. D. (1954) Observations on the nature of hysterical states. *British Journal of Medical Psychology*, 27, 105–125.

Ferrer, J. (2002) *Revisioning Transpersonal Theory: A Participatory Vision of Human Spirituality*. Albany: State University of New York Press.

Field, N., Harvey, T. and Sharp, B., eds. (2005) *Ten Lectures on Psychotherapy and Spirituality*. London: Karnac Books Ltd.

Fontana, D. (2005) *Is there an Afterlife?* Ropley: O Books.

Forman, M. D. (2010) *A Guide to Integral Psychotherapy: Complexity, Integration, and*

Spirituality in Practice. Albany: State University of New York Press.

Frankl, V. (1967) *Psychotherapy and Existentialism: Selected Papers on Logotherapy.* New York: Simon & Schuster.

Frankl, V. (1973) *The Doctor and the Soul: From Psychotherapy to Logotherapy* London: Pelican Books.

Freud, S. (1910/1957) The future prospects of psycho-analytic therapy. In *The Standard Edition of the Complete Psychological Works of Sigmund Freud,* Vol. 11 (J. Strachey, trans.). London: Hogarth Press, pp. 139–151.

Freud, S. (1911/1966) Formulations on the two principles of mental functioning. In *The Standard Edition of the Complete Psychological Works of Sigmund Freud,* Vol. 12 (J. Strachey, trans.). London: Hogarth Press, pp. 218–226.

Freud, S. (1917/1966) Mourning and melancholia. In *The Standard Edition of the Complete Psychological Works of Sigmund Freud,* Vol. 14 (J. Strachey, trans.). London: Hogarth Press, pp. 243–258.

Freud, S. (1923/1961) The Ego and the Id. In *The Standard Edition of the Complete Psychological Works of Sigmund Freud,* Vol. 19 (J. Strachey, trans.). London: Hogarth Press, pp. 19–27.

Freud, S. (1926/1966) The question of lay analysis. In *The Standard Edition of the Complete Psychological Works of Sigmund Freud,* Vol. 20 (J. Strachey, trans.). London: Hogarth Press, pp. 183–250.

Freud, S. (1927/1966) The future of an illusion. In *The Standard Edition of the Complete Psychological Works of Sigmund Freud,* Vol. 21 (J. Strachey, trans.). London: Hogarth Press, pp. 5–56.

Freud, S. (1931/1964) Lecture 31. The dissection of the psychical personality. In *The Standard Edition of the Complete Psychological Works of Sigmund Freud,* Vol. 22 (J. Strachey, trans.). London: Hogarth Press, pp. 57–80.

Freud, S. (1940/1964) The psychical apparatus. In *The Standard Edition of the Complete Psychological Works of Sigmund Freud,* Vol. 23 (J. Strachey, trans.). London: Hogarth Press, pp. 144–147.

Friedman, H. L. and Hartelius, G., eds. (2015) *The Wiley Blackwell Handbook of Transpersonal Psychology.* Chichester: John Wiley & Sons.

Fromm, E. S., Suzuki, D. T. and DeMartino, R. (1974) *Zen Buddhism and Psychoanalysis.* London: Souvenir Press.

Gallup, G. G. (1970) Chimpanzees: self-recognition. *Science.* 167, 86–87.

Gasser, P., Kirchner, K. and Passie, T. (2015) LSD-assisted psychotherapy for anxiety associated with a life-threatening disease: a qualitative study of acute and sustained subjective effects. *Journal of Psychopharmacology,* 29, 57–68.

Gilbert, P. (2010) *Compassion Focused Therapy.* London: Routledge.

Glass-Coffin, B. (2010) Anthropology, shamanism, and alternate ways of knowing–being in the world: one anthropologist's journey of discovery and transformation. *Anthropology and Humanism,* 35, 204–217.

Goswami, A. (2012) *God Is Not Dead: What Quantum Physics Tells Us About Our Origins and How We Should Live.* Charlottesville, VA: Hampton Roads Publishing Company.

Grim, B. J. and Grim, M. E. (2019) Belief, behavior, and belonging: how faith is indispensable in preventing and recovering from substance abuse. *Journal of Religion and Health,* 58, 1713–1750.

Grof, S. (1993) *The Holotropic Mind.* New York: HarperCollins.

Harner, M. (2005) Tribal wisdom: the shamanic path. In R. Walsh and C. S. Grob, eds., *Higher Wisdom: Eminent Elders Explore the Continuing Impact of Psychedelics.* Albany: State University of New York Press, pp. 159–178.

Heimann, P. (1950) On counter-transference. *International Journal of Psychoanalysis,* 31, 81–84.

Hora, T. (1986) *Dialogues in Metapsychiatry.* Old Lyme, CT: The PAGL Foundation.

Huxley, A. (1954) *The Doors of Perception and Heaven and Hell*. London: Chatto & Windus.

Irons, C. (2019) *The Compassionate Mind Approach to Difficult Emotions: Using Compassion Focused Therapy*. London: Robinson.

James, W. (1902/1960) *The Varieties of Religious Experience: A Study in Human Nature*. London: Collins Fontana Library.

Jung, C. G. (1917/1966) *C. G. Jung: The Collected Works*, Vol. 7. *Two Essays on Analytical Psychology* (H. Read, M. Fordham and G. Adler, eds.). London: Routledge & Kegan Paul.

Jung, C. G. (1939/1977) On the psychogenesis of schizophrenia. In H. Read, M. Fordham and G. Adler, eds., *C. G. Jung: The Collected Works*, Vol. 3. *The Psychogenesis of Mental Disease*. London: Routledge & Kegan Paul, pp. 233–249.

Jung, C. G. (1958/1977) Answer to Job. In H. Read, M. Fordham and G. Adler, eds., *C. G. Jung: The Collected Works*, Vol. 11. London: Routledge & Kegan Paul, pp. 355–470.

Kabat-Zinn, J. (2013) *Full Catastrophe Living*. London: Piatkus.

Kean, L. (2017) *Surviving Death. A Journalist Investigates Evidence for an Afterlife*. New York: Three Rivers Press.

Kelly, E. F., Crabtree, A. and Marshall, P., eds. (2019) *Beyond Physicalism: Toward Reconciliation of Science and Spirituality*. Washington, DC: Rowman & Littlefield Publishers.

King, M., Marston, L., McManus, S. et al. (2013) Religion, spirituality and mental health: results from a national study of English households. *British Journal of Psychiatry*, 202, 68–73.

Klein, J. (2003) *Jacob's Ladder: Essays on Experiences of the Ineffable in the Context of Contemporary Psychotherapy*. London: Karnac Books Ltd.

Koenig, H. G., King, D. and Carson, V. B. (2012) *Handbook of Religion and Health*. Oxford: Oxford University Press.

Kuhn, T. (1962/2012) *The Structure of Scientific Revolutions*. Chicago, IL: University of Chicago Press.

Lacan, J. (1949/2006) The mirror stage as formative of the function of the I as revealed in psychoanalytic experience. In *Écrits: The First Complete Edition in English* (B. Fink, trans.). New York: W. W. Norton, pp. 75–81.

Lambert, K. (1981) *Analysis, Repair and Individuation*. London: Academic Press.

Lannert, J. L. (1991) Resistance and countertransference issues with spiritual and religious clients. *Journal of Humanistic Psychology*, 31, 68–76.

Larson, D. B., Larson, S. S. and Koenig, H. G. (2001) The patient's spiritual/religious dimension: a forgotten factor in mental health. *Directions in Psychiatry*, 21. Available at www.rcpsych.ac.uk/docs/default-source/members/sigs/spirituality-spsig/larson3.pdf (accessed 30 September 2020).

Long, J. P. (2014) Near-death experiences: evidence for their reality. *Missouri Medicine*. 111, 372–380.

Lown, B. (1996) *The Lost Art of Healing: Practicing Compassion in Medicine*. Boston, MA: Houghton Mifflin Company.

MacKenna, C. (2000) Jung and Christianity: wrestling with God. In E. Christopher and H. M. Solomon, eds., *Jungian Thought in the Modern World*. London: Free Association Books, pp. 173–190.

MacKenna, C. (2005) A personal journey through psychotherapy and religion. In N. Field, T. Harvey and B. Sharp, eds., *Ten Lectures on Psychotherapy and Spirituality*. London: Karnac Books Ltd, pp. 141–154.

MacKenna, C. (2007) The dream of perfection. *British Journal of Psychotherapy*, 23, 247–267.

Maslow, A. (1943) A theory of human motivation. *Psychological Review*, 50, 370–396.

Matloff, G. L. (2016) Can panpsychism become an observational science? *Journal of Consciousness Exploration & Research*, 7, 524–543.

Meissner, W. W. (1984) *Psychoanalysis and Religious Experience*. New Haven, CT: Yale University Press.

Meissner, W. W. (2009) Religion in the psychoanalytic relationship: some aspects of transference and countertransference. *Journal of the American Academy of Psychoanalysis and Dynamic Psychiatry*, 37, 123–136.

Merkur, D. (2013) *Relating to God: Clinical Psychoanalysis, Spirituality, and Theism*. Lanham, MD: Jason Aronson, Inc.

Narby, J. (1998) *The Cosmic Serpent: DNA and the Origins of Knowledge*. London: Victor Gollancz.

Nelson, J. (1994) *Healing the Split*. Albany: State University of New York Press.

Neumann, E. (1976) *The Child: Structure and Dynamics of the Nascent Personality*. New York: Harper and Row.

Newton, J. (1998) *Journey of Souls: Case Studies of Life between Lives*. Woodbury, MN: Llewellyn Publications.

Newton, J. (2002) *Destiny of Souls*. Woodbury, MN: Llewellyn Publications.

Nietzsche, F. (1895/2016) *Twilight of the Idols* (R. J. Hollingdale and W. Kauffmann, trans.). Scotts Valley, CA: CreateSpace.

Pargament, K. I. (2007) *Spiritually Integrated Psychotherapy*. New York: Guilford Press.

Parnia, S., Spearpoint, K., de Vos, G. et al. (2014) AWARE—AWAreness during REsuscitation—a prospective study. *Resuscitation*, 85, 1799–1805.

Pascal, B. (1670/2018) Section IV: Of the means of belief. In *Pensées (Thoughts)* (W. F. Trotter, trans.). Mineola, NY: Dover Publications.

Peteet, J. R. (2013) What is the place of clinicians' religious or spiritual commitments in psychotherapy? A virtues-based perspective. *Journal of Religion and Health*, 53, 1190–1198.

PhysOrg (2017) Study reveals substantial evidence of holographic universe. Available at https://phys.org/news/2017-01-reveals-substantial-evidence-holographic-universe.html (accessed 30 September 2020).

Planck, M. (1931) Interviews with Great Scientists: 'The Paradox of the Quantum'. *The Observer*, 25 January, p. 17.

Powell, A. (2017a) *The Ways of the Soul. A Psychiatrist Reflects: Essays on Life, Death and Beyond*. London: Muswell Hill Press.

Powell, A. (2017b) The healing potential of anomalous perceptual experiences. *Journal of the Society for Psychical Research*, 81, 26–31.

Powell, A. (2018) *Conversations with the Soul. A Psychiatrist Reflects: Essays on Life, Death and Beyond*. London: Muswell Hill Press.

Racker, H. (1968) *Transference and Countertransference*. New York: International Universities Press.

Radin, D. (2006) *Entangled Minds: Extrasensory Experiences in a Quantum Reality*. New York: Paraview Pocket Books.

Radin, D. (2018) *Real Magic: Ancient Wisdom, Modern Science, and a Guide to the Secret Power of the Universe*. New York: Harmony Books.

Read, T. (2014) *Walking Shadows: Archetype and Psyche in Crisis and Growth*. London: Muswell Hill Press.

Roe, C., Sonnex, C. and Roxburgh, E. (2015) Two meta-analyses of noncontact healing studies. *Explore*, 11, 11–23.

Rogers, C. R. (1965) *Client-Centered Therapy*. Boston, MA: Houghton Mifflin Company.

Rogers, C. R. (1989) *The Carl Rogers Reader* (H. Kirschenbaum and V. L. Henderson, eds.). Boston, MA: Houghton Mifflin Company.

Rosmarin, D. H. (2018) *Spirituality, Religion, and Cognitive-Behavioral Therapy: A Guide for Clinicians*. New York: Guilford Press.

Rosmarin, D. H. and Koenig, H. G., eds. (2020) *Handbook of Spirituality, Religion, and Mental Health*, 2nd ed. London: Academic Press.

Rosmarin, D. H., Salcone, S., Harper, D. and Forester, B. P. (2019) Spiritual psychotherapy for inpatient, residential, and intensive treatment. *American Journal of Psychotherapy*, 72, 75–83.

Rowan, J. (2015) *The Transpersonal: Spirituality in Psychotherapy and Counselling*, 2nd ed. London: Routledge.

Rycroft, C. (1983*) A Critical Dictionary of Psychoanalysis*. London: Penguin.

Samuels, A., Shorter, B. and Plaut, F. (1986) *A Critical Dictionary of Jungian Analysis*. London: Routledge & Kegan Paul.

Schreurs, A. (2002) *Psychotherapy and Spirituality: Integrating the Spiritual Dimension into Therapeutic Practice*. London: Jessica Kingsley Publishers.

Schuman, M. (2017) *Mindfulness-Informed Relational Psychotherapy and Psychoanalysis: Inquiring Deeply*. London: Routledge.

Schwartz, G. E. and Simon, W. L. (2002) *The Afterlife Experiments*. New York: Atria Books.

Sessa, B., Higbed, L. and Nutt, D. (2019) A review of 3,4-methylenedioxy-methamphetamine (MDMA)-assisted psychotherapy. *Frontiers in Psychiatry*, 10, 138.

Singer, J. (1995) *Boundaries of the Soul: The Practice of Jung's Psychology*. New York: Anchor Books.

Solomon, G. and Solomon, J. (2003) *The Scole Experiment: Scientific Evidence for Life after Death*. London: Piatkus.

Stein, S. M. (1999) *Beyond Belief: Psychotherapy and Religion*. London: Karnac Books Ltd.

Stevens, L. C. and Woodruff, C. C. (2018) *The Neuroscience of Empathy, Compassion, and Self-Compassion*. London: Academic Press.

Stevenson, I. (1966) *Twenty Cases Suggestive of Reincarnation*. Charlottesville, VA: University of Virginia Press.

Stevenson, I. (1997) *Reincarnation and Biology: A Contribution to the Etiology of Birthmarks and Birth Defects*. Vols 1 and 2. Westport, CT: Praeger Publishers.

Symington, N. (1994) *Emotion and Spirit: Questioning the Claims of Psychoanalysis and Religion*. London: Cassell.

Tarnas, R. (2010) *The Passion of the Western Mind: Understanding the Ideas That Have Shaped Our World View*. London: Pimlico.

Truax, C. B. and Carkhuff, R. R. (1967) *Towards Effective Counseling and Psychotherapy: Training and Practice*. London: Aldine Publishing Co.

Tucker, J. B. (2014) *Return to Life: Extraordinary Cases of Children Who Remember Past Lives*. New York: St Martin's Press.

Walsh, R. and Vaughan, F. (1993) On transpersonal definitions. *Journal of Transpersonal Psychology*, 25, 199–207.

Washburn, M. (1994) *Transpersonal Psychology in Psychoanalytic Perspective*. Albany: State University of New York Press.

Wilber, K. (1996) *The Atman Project: A Transpersonal View of Human Development*. Wheaton, IL: Quest Books/ Theosophical Publishing House.

Wilber, K. (2002) *Integral Psychology: Consciousness, Spirit, Psychology, Therapy*. Boston, MA: Shambhala.

Winnicott, D. W. (1967/2005) Mirror-role of mother and family in child development. In *Playing and Reality*. London: Routledge, pp. 149–159.

Woolger, R. (1999) *Other Lives, Other Selves*. New York: Bantam Books.

World Health Organization (2020) *International Classification of Diseases 11th Revision (ICD-11)*. Geneva: World Health Organization.

Zinser, T. J. (2011) *Soul-Centered Healing: A Psychologist's Extraordinary Journey into the Realms of Sub-Personalities, Spirits, and Past Lives*. USA: Union Street Press.

Intellectual Disability

Oyepeju Raji and Cristina Gangemi

Spirituality is a deeply personal experience that does not depend on being religious or belonging to a faith group. The spirit is the essence of life. The approach taken here is that spirituality is a universal dimension of human experience, being of fundamental or ultimate importance (Cook, 2004). Spirituality is about wholeness and wholesomeness, interconnection and validation; it shows that all lives have purpose and are positively influencing other lives. Each human life matters; there are no exceptions and there is no hierarchy.

Swinton (1999) defines spirituality as that aspect of human existence that gives it its 'humanness'. To deny that people with intellectual disabilities are spiritual is to devalue their human dignity, for every human being has the need to find a sense of meaning of life, a purpose and to feel he or she belongs. Other people's interpretation of what spirituality means for people with intellectual disabilities is not necessarily the same as how it is understood by people with intellectual disabilities. Gangemi et al. (2010) sought to understand this at a deeper level through participatory action research that explored the expressed spiritual and religious needs of people with intellectual disabilities. They wanted to develop a definition that was more rooted in the experience of people with intellectual disabilities. Their finding challenged the notion that there is a universal quest for a sense of meaning of life. The research showed that those with more severe cognitive difficulties who were not able to express this quest were, nonetheless, strongly spiritual. They found that spirituality is not always about a search for answers and meaning, but involves being and presence, rather than mind and ability. Their findings suggest a spirituality that is about a sense of life that is present before the ability to rationalise.

The Royal College of Psychiatrists' mental health leaflet on spirituality affirms that 'Spirituality is a central part of many cultures. It can be just as important for a person with intellectual disability, mental illness, dementia or head injury, as it is for anybody else' (Cook and Grimwade, 2021, p. 3). Hebrew Scripture declares that 'all are fearfully and wonderfully made' (Psalm 139, verse 14). Thus every human life is uniquely valuable, independent of another's perception of their 'fitness for purpose'. Each person possesses unique gifts and talents that were meant to be shared; however, it first has to be recognised that all people possess such gifts.

Beliefs About Disability Across Cultures and Ages

All human societies hold beliefs, practices and rituals for the expression of spirituality. Different spiritual belief systems ascribe different meanings to disability. Some cultures hold that people with disability are of 'lesser value', considered 'undesirable' or even feared, and different cultures deal with these attitudes and feelings in various ways. Some give spiritual explanations for disability that allow control to rest with a superior being, whereas others attempt to find a human understanding of the lives of people with a disability. Some would argue that scriptural bases of religious beliefs form the foundation for the age-old practice of exclusion that people with disabilities experience in many facets of life. Such attitudes towards disability can result in people internalising negative messages about spirituality. Beliefs about the relationship of disability to sin, adequacy of faith and miraculous healing can be challenging concepts; individuals and families wonder what they have done wrong to be 'punished' in this way, with profound psychological consequences (Treloar, 2002; African Child Policy Forum, 2014; Disability Africa, 2016). The vulnerability of people with intellectual disabilities and their dependence on carers can lead to spiritual manipulation. People without disability may look patronisingly on those with disabilities as objects of their benevolence. Others, however, appreciate that all human beings are interdependent, for no one can survive on his or her own, without the need to lean on other people for support at some stage in life.

Negative theories about the origin of intellectual disability cause stigma, and affected relatives are kept hidden to avoid embarrassment. People with intellectual disabilities are not fully accepted and have no defined roles, and in this context are excluded from the category of social beings. They are not included at social occasions, ceremonies and celebrations (Raji and Hollins, 2000; African Child Policy Forum, 2014).

Families of people with intellectual disabilities often find that their own faith, beliefs and practices play an important role in coping with their relative's impairment while dealing with social stigma and indifference. However, progress through the stages of grief over the loss of an anticipated 'non-disabled' child does not always result in acceptance, as the family wrestles with the question of whether a supernatural cause or other explanation, such as some penalty for their own past actions (e.g., 'karma'), or sin, is responsible for their predicament.

In an attempt to make sense of concepts concerning intellectual disability and mental illness, medieval Christianity sometimes explained mental disorders (including intellectual disability) as a result of the influence of the devil. Such beliefs may still be encountered in some cultures today. For example, in indigenous peoples of sub-Saharan Africa, there is still a tendency to believe in spiritual/metaphysical explanations of disability. This misconception has become rooted in cultural beliefs and traditions that include witchcraft, a curse from God, the anger of ancestral spirits, bad omens and reincarnation. Affected people are thrust out of society or, to address these problems, the person is subjected to starvation, extreme forms of violence, exorcism or even death (Stockholder, 1994; African Child Policy Forum, 2014; Disability Africa, 2016).

The first author of this chapter has observed that in parts of Nigeria, for example, affected people may be subjected to 'spiritual cleansing' and 'healing', due to this persistent belief. Christian and Islamic influences have modified the practice to some extent, but cultural traditions largely continue, giving rise to interweaving influences of spirituality, culture and science. Mpofu and Harley (2002) have described similar traditions in Zimbabwe, where the role of traditional and spiritual healers in the care of people with disabilities is formally recognised.

In many developing countries, where the science of disability is not understood at the local level, the challenges that are faced by children with disabilities are further complicated by the widespread negative attitudes, stigma and discrimination they encounter in their daily lives (African Child Policy Forum, 2014). Yet it must be conceded that segregation can arise no less in better developed and materialistic societies, where the value of a person is closely linked to their intellectual functioning and consequent economic worth.

In seventeenth-century England the introduction of the 'Poor Law' by an Act of Parliament required all parishes to establish workhouses to provide places where paupers, degenerates, people with mental illness and the 'mentally handicapped' could live. Responsibility was ascribed to parishes on the basis that people who were 'mentally defective' were viewed as morally impoverished and in need of salvation. They were also thought to be in need of education and treatment, and the first asylums were founded in the nineteenth century. This institutionalisation of people with intellectual disabilities and with mental illness continued to increase during the first half of the twentieth century, creating almost impenetrable barriers between these individuals and open society. This process laid the foundation for the organised care of people with intellectual disabilities in many parts of the world. Since then, a positive attitude towards disability has been growing (Patka et al., 2013; Benomir et al., 2016; Morin et al., 2018), although this change remains relatively slow and patchy.

Distinguishing between Mental Illness and Intellectual Disability

The development of science in the seventeenth and eighteenth centuries saw increased interest in the capabilities of the human mind, leading to a distinction between the psychological processes of people with intellectual disabilities and those of individuals who have mental illness. According to John Locke (quoted in Race, 2002, pp. 23–52), whereas the 'lunatic' had lost his or her mind and might be restored to sanity in some way, the 'idiot' had never had a mind, and what had never existed could not be artificially created, so he or she was irredeemable. Locke proposed that a person's mind is originally empty, and then develops on the basis of the senses' interpretation of experiences and the mind's reflection on those experiences. He argued that whereas people with mental illness showed normal intensity of perception but combined ideas abnormally, people with intellectual disabilities did not experience events fully.

Locke's idea that people with intellectual disabilities do not experience events fully can still be seen today in the provision of services. Dykens (2006) argues that people with intellectual disabilities have continued to be defined by their pervasive deficits, and that workers in the field of intellectual disability have traditionally focused on basic external life conditions (in relation to providing for basic needs and skills acquisition) rather than recognising strengths and positive internal states that include happiness, contentment, hope and engagement. Consequently, the experience of people with disability varies according to the social construct of disability in the culture in which they are living. In response to the uncovering of abuse of people with intellectual disabilities in 2011, NHS England devised the Transforming Care Programme (Association of Directors of Adult Social Services (ADASS), Care Quality Commission (CQC), Department of Health, Health Education England (HEE), Local Government Association (LGA) and NHS England, 2015) to ensure that people with intellectual disabilitiy and/or autism with challenging behaviours and mental health conditions were supported to live in the community with the same opportunities as everybody else. This approach has met with varying degrees of success.

Intellectual disability starts before adulthood and has a lasting effect on development, presenting with varying levels of support needs. People with intellectual disabilities can have problems accessing and engaging with formal and typical approaches to learning. Their varying and neurodiverse means of absorbing, processing and communicating information can often clash with the assumption that communication should comply with a cognitive style that overly relies on the use of the written or spoken word. Such an approach to education and communication leaves a person who experiences neurodiversity struggling with abstract concepts that are inappropriate to his or her individual learning style. Some of the 'teaching difficulties' that are encountered are thus created by the assumption of incapacity and a lack of creative approaches to education and learning. Instead, people with intellectual disability should be viewed as 'creative learners' (Gangemi and Waldron, 2018). By this we mean that learners are not measured against any difficulty that might present in accessing activities that are stereotypically created on a 'one-size-fits-all' basis. Instead, we can remain open to being amazed by the creative ways in which each unique human being finds his or her own form of creative expression. Does the phenomenon of a creative learner not provide a paradigm shift into a place of equality for all learners? Indeed, if we are all creative learners, then can we not all enjoy learning together? The psychological damage that is caused to a creative learner when they feel that they just 'do not measure up' must surely now be assigned to the past.

The disability theologian and practitioner William Gaventa, in his book titled *Disability and Spirituality*, highlighted how the abilities and needs of 'creative learners' and communicators became evident 'on the heels of legal initiatives in the rights of persons with disabilities' (Gaventa, 2018, p. 2). Consequently, in an attempt to ensure that creative learners can access their personal right to education, a critique of 'contemporary school culture ... encourages practitioners to reinvent what can and should be reinvented to realize more humane, just and democratic learning communities' (Udvari-Solner, 1997, p. 142). Thus a more inclusive and creative understanding of 'Special Educational Needs and Disability' has enabled approaches that are more empathetic towards the particular human person and his or her unique physical, spiritual and intellectual reality. Valuing diversity has led to creative approaches that enable complex ideas and requests to be understood (Gangemi et al., 2010). Where attention is paid to the whole person – body, mind and spirit – the creative learner and communicator is enabled and respected for 'who they are born to be' (Gangemi, 2018a).

Do People with Intellectual Disabilities Have a Deeper Spiritual Life?

Spirituality is not dependent on intellectual functioning, and neither is the measure of spirituality dependent on eloquence or how it is expressed. In partnership with creative communicators and learners, a research project into the realities of spirituality and religious practice for people who experience intellectual disabilities found that:

> Spirituality, in its original and more basic reality, is *presence*. It is a dialogue, being in relationship with meaningful dimensions without any word being spoken, before any rationalisation, of what is being experienced by the person, takes place. (Gangemi et al., 2010, p. 76)

> Spirituality is generally regarded as the attempt to find answers to the many questions and mysteries that we are faced with in our lives. But... would someone try to identify the number of colors in a sunset, give each one a name and separate them, in order to see that something true and beautiful is standing in front of them? Would it not be enough to just be there, present to that moment? (Tobanelli, 2013, p. 4)

Spirituality, as we can see from this research, is beyond words and may be present even in people who are in vegetative states. Swinton (1997) argues that faith and spirituality are not intellectual concepts but relational realities, and that a person's spiritual life should not be evaluated according to intellectual criteria. Finally, faith traditions believe that spirit extends beyond the physical, and that spiritual consciousness transcends the finite reality of this world.

It can be argued that freedom from intellectual preoccupation removes a barrier and allows a person to be more in touch with the spiritual. This is the case in meditation, which encourages an awareness that transcends mind and body, going beyond intellectual functioning. The more profound the intellectual disability, the less a person may be hindered by considerations of the here and now. Sulmasy (1997) reported that faith workers found that spirituality was profoundly felt with people with intellectual disabilities who were unhindered by everyday awareness, allowing the beauty of the spirit to be felt in its (pure) form. Creatively engaging with people with intellectual disabilities of varying levels of severity demonstrated such awareness. Creative engagement can be hindered by 'lack of time' in a very busy and rushed world. Therefore Swinton et al. (2013, p. 80) *made time* for the expression and revelation of the inner spirit as exemplified in this case study:

Case study: Sonia

Sonia, a young woman with Down syndrome, was electively non-verbal due to a challenging stutter. It was challenging for her because she has very rarely found anyone who would give her enough of a gap in their time to express her thoughts. She sensed people were impatient when she stuttered and so she chose not to use her voice, silenced by presumptions regarding her potential and a real lack of patience. Sonia thus became spiritually silenced by others. During one of the research activities, participants were asked 'Do you think there is something Holy amongst us'? (Swinton et al., 2013, p. 53). Using visual cues and imaginary spaces,[1] which could gather and liberate her inner voice, Sonia sensed that the researchers were committed to listening, receiving and sharing time with her. Taking a picture of a religious object from her own tradition, Sonia walked up and chose another picture of people. From somewhere within, her spirit moved and she was 'anima-ted' (Gangemi, 2020, p. 338). Her voice responded to this movement and, by her own choice, she spoke. 'It is as if people are beautiful', she shared (Swinton et al., 2013, p. 80).

Here we note the pure spirit revealed by a person who was often presumed to have little to offer, or who was often silenced by barriers of cognition. Her eloquent and embodied definition of holiness brought new meaning to beauty. The ease with which she saw and perceived beauty in 'every-Body' both adds to and challenges the formal voice of philosophers, theologians and religious leaders who, throughout time, have sought to

---

[1] The reference to visual cues and imaginary spaces is based upon the method used by the researchers, whereby a 'visual picture cue' (an open river) allows for a cognitive and sensory link to be made to the action of the researcher, as they mimed an empty space, in the shape of a river. The creative communicator was then invited to express thoughts and, in this case, the spoken word, into the 'imaginary space'.

grasp what being 'beauty-full'(Stein, 1993, p. 133) might mean. Sonia simply became a teacher to all who took the time to engage creatively in her story and with her spirit.

Opening Up the Social Model

Medical research in Western culture has concentrated on trying to identify causes of intellectual disability in a bid to eliminate or prevent it (according to the 'medical model'). However, the White Paper *Valuing People* (Department of Health, 2001) initiated a person-centred approach to the delivery of holistic care for people with intellectual disabilities, with a focus on ordinary living (the social model), which sees the person rather than the disorder. Importantly, spirituality is now being recognised as an important but often overlooked dimension of the lives of people with intellectual disabilities (Swinton, 2001a; Gangemi et al., 2010; Carter, 2016; see also the Lemos&Crane website listed under Web resources at the end of this chapter).

In the last quarter of the twentieth century, the concept of normalisation (Wolfensberger, 1972) brought people with intellectual disabilities more into mainstream society, with the aim of achieving social inclusion and with opportunities to build meaningful bonds within the community as fully accepted participants in everyday life. However, the focus has been largely on meeting the basic material needs of the service users (Sinson, 1996), and the reality is that, for some, exclusion continues to be a significant aspect of their lives. Although many secular organisations have skills in 'knowing how' to deliver services for people with intellectual disabilities, it may remain the case that there is not sufficient understanding of *why* spirituality and religious practice are important for their lives. Care providers may feel that religious communities are able to meet the spiritual and religious needs of these people, and that facilitating attendance therefore fulfils their duty of care. In turn, religious communities may *understand why* spirituality and religion are important, but may not *know how* to be more inclusive of people with intellectual disabilities (Gangemi et al., 2010; Carter and Boehm, 2019). This juxtaposition could result in lack of suitable provision, leaving the person with intellectual disability to experience a poverty of authentic access. This is a phenomenon that has been termed 'knowing *how* but not *why*, and *why* but not *how*' (Swinton et al., 2013).

Religion

Religion attends to spiritual need by providing shared rituals, narratives, symbols and guidance through scriptures, prayer and modes of social support (Dein, 2020), furthering a sense of belonging that sustains the 'self' in the construction of both personal and group identity. Yet people who cannot (verbally) communicate their 'inner world', with its hopes, dreams and needs, can miss out on this important human experience if such needs are not recognised. Studies have found that although spirituality plays a significant role in the lives of many people with intellectual disabilities, carers and support workers are often unaware of this and consequently fail to address it (Swinton, 2001b). Although the practice of religion is to some extent bound by culture, a person's ethnic or cultural background does not predict their religious or spiritual needs. Some services for people with intellectual disabilities only consider people's religious needs in line with their culture, their religion in effect being denoted by their country of origin (Hatton et al., 2004).

Although a person does not have to be religious to be spiritual, organised religion remains the most common way of understanding and expressing spirituality. Hatton et al. (2004) reported some confusion with regard to religious expression and needs of people with intellectual disabilities among paid and family carers. On a similar note, Carter and Boehm (2019) reported a striking lack of attention to the spiritual dimensions of the lives of people with intellectual and developmental disabilities in research studies. They found similar levels of reported interest in religious and spiritual activities, but only very limited involvement of this group in active participation. Scriptural interpretations with regard to disability are not consistent. An example can be found in Christian scripture on the relationship of sin to disability. Jesus on the one hand forgives sin as the means to healing a disability (Mark 2:1–12), and on the other challenges the popularly held assumption that disability was the result of sin (John 9:1–3). In Hebrew scripture, Moses commanded that extra care should be taken of the disabled (the blind) (Deuteronomy 27:18). In Islam, society is obliged to assist and respect people with intellectual disabilities (Qur'an, surah 51:19). In Hinduism, disability may be understood as the outcome of karma. A more inclusive view of disability can be found in Buddhism, where it is considered that those who are 'disabled' are not so much those with physical or intellectual impairment as those who are unable to attain spiritual enlightenment; intellectual disability itself is no hindrance to following this path. Similarly, Sikh scriptures stipulate that disability refers less to any physical or mental impairment than it does to disability of the soul, which hinders people from achieving their purpose in life (Chinvarakorn, 2006).

Evidently, theology need not discourage those with intellectual disability from joining in faith practices, and it is nothing but prejudice to suppose that people with functional impairments are disadvantaged when it comes to spiritual practice. Indeed, religious leaders and philosophers have been influential in developing a more positive view of how society should respond to people with a disability. One such example is found in the Jewish way of life, which is strongly community oriented. Bunning and Steel (2006) report models of inclusion where Jewish organisations provide culturally appropriate services to Jewish parents and children with special needs in specifically Jewish ways, to enable group identity and harness a positive sense of self. Other interdisciplinary and interfaith conversations about disability and theology are emerging in which practitioners and academics have interrogated their traditions. A theology of disability has begun to imagine how faith communities might move from exclusion to active participation (Matthews, 2013), and from inclusion to belonging (Swinton, 2012; Gaventa, 2018; Donatello, 2020).

People with disabilities, and their families, often turn to religious institutions for comfort and a sense of belonging. However, they are not always made welcome. Lack of knowledge and understanding leads to insensitivity, and congregations can be too focused on the disability rather than relating to the person. Carter (2016) reported that many congregations may struggle to move from a primary posture of 'ministry to' people with disabilities towards one that emphasises 'ministry by' people with disabilities. Indeed, religious institutions sometimes fail to create the necessary accommodation for people with disabilities, and even show covert signs of hostility towards them, possibly stemming from the most ancient of beliefs about the nature of disability.

Assessing the Spiritual Needs of People with Intellectual Disabilities

There is growing research into the significance of spirituality for people with intellectual disabilities, be it theistic, non-theistic or any combination thereof. In modern cultures, the concept of spirituality has widened beyond the confines of traditional religion to embrace what might be termed 'secular spirituality', relating to the aspect of a person that links the deeply personal to the universal, providing an understanding of one's interrelationship with nature as well as people. It includes joining with others in an appreciation of beauty, music and the creative arts, and engenders a sense of harmony. It connects all of the different pieces into a meaningful whole, with a sense of one's own place in it. Coulter (2002) considers whether it is possible to study spirituality 'scientifically' when the objective purpose and methods of science do not seem well suited to such an endeavour. The spiritual dimension, which includes love, care, acceptance and connectedness with God and others, is not easily measured (Swinton, 2004a). The advent of creative and interactive studies of spirituality and intellectual disability has challenged this 'able-ist world view'. People with intellectual disability can be enabled to shape and re-form our understanding of spirituality (Gangemi et al., 2010; Livability, 2016). We can move away from equating a person's spirituality with his or her attendance at organised religious practices where acquiescence is interpreted as participation. The belief among caregivers that spirituality is synonymous with religious practice may mean that those who do not express signs of spiritual needs in religious terms are likely to be overlooked (McSherry, 2000). Carers are more likely to address the spiritual needs of individuals if they identify themselves as spiritual. Evidence suggests that this situation may be changing.

Emerging methodology will enable the assessment of the spiritual needs and experience of people with intellectual disabilities. There is no standard 'language' of spirituality. Rather, spirituality is the sum total of all the life experiences that have helped to create a sense of being, and which can be further explored through creative studies, teachings, meetings and discussion. The danger is in operating with a verbal mindset where needs, if not expressed, are deemed absent (Raji et al., 2003). Gardner (1999) argued that people who happen to be intellectually disadvantaged may nonetheless have a rich spiritual life.

Exploration of the spiritual needs of people with intellectual disabilities calls for sensitive handling; person-centred planning puts the person at the centre of the exploration, creating an understanding of his or her internal world and not just resulting in another ticked box on the care plan.

Coping with Disability

Many factors affect the ability to cope with disability. Spiritual strategies used in coping with disability have been shown to lead to a positive outcome (Larson et al., 1993). Singer and Irvin (1989) have highlighted the effect on the lives of caregivers. They turn to clergy for support (Miltiades and Pruchno, 2002), are more likely to use prayer as a coping strategy and thus have a positive relationship with the care recipient (Wood and Parham, 1990). Spirituality can enable a person to survive bad times, to be strong and to overcome difficulties. There is a body of evidence on the positive effect of spirituality on health and coping (Treloar, 2002), and there is growing recognition that people with intellectual disabilities might benefit from spiritual support, albeit with little understanding of how (Carter and Boehm, 2019). Yet questions like 'Why me?' (Bicknell, 1983) or 'How can a good God allow this to occur?' (Baldacchino and Draper, 2001) are often asked. Hollins (1998) highlights the inability of people with disabilities to achieve acceptance or *resolution* because who they are might seem to present a burden for others. They may feel that it is their fault that they are different. People with disabilities are who they are – people and not medical conditions.

For change to occur, a culture of care, which sees the person with the disability in the light of a vulnerable need, must be replaced by an empathic culture of effective creative relationships. Spending time with the person allows for a mutual growth in understanding, fading the 'Why me?' culture into the background. Through meaningful encounters the person grows in his or her experience of self, and possible questions about blame and reparation are replaced with a knowledge of the person's meaning and value. A philosophy of being 'Because I AM' (Gangemi, 2018a) becomes the new key to an understanding of the unrepeatable nature of each and every person, and through this the language of spiritual support changes. Worth and value replace blame and punishment.

The need for such a shift in the focus of spiritual support is borne out by the many stories from parents who are traditionally the primary providers and caregivers of children with intellectual disabilities. High levels of cohesion and harmony in families positively affect the social and cognitive development of children with disabilities (Trute and Hauch, 1988). A reciprocal benefit was described by Stainton and Besser (1998), who found that families reported a positive impact of having children with intellectual disabilities. They described having an increased sense of purpose and priorities, with expanded personal and social networks and community involvement, and finding their children to be a source of joy and happiness.

Religion can play a critical role in sustaining human relationships that are strained by the everyday realities and necessities of providing and receiving care. Kaufman et al. (1990) considered that the social or spiritual aspect of religious participation had a buffering effect on parents' stress levels. On the other hand, even though religious beliefs can help family values and provide 'meaning for life' experiences (Taylor and Chatters, 1986), parents of people with disabilities do not always have positive experiences of faith communities, and feel rejected and excluded if their children are not welcome. Children and adults with intellectual disabilities may not be included in faith communities because of their behaviour (Raji et al., 2003). This can lead to segregation and isolation.

Bereavement and Grief

There are significant difficulties in understanding the reactions of people with intellectual disabilities to loss. Losing a loved one is an important spiritual experience. People with intellectual disabilities are a heterogenous group, and the greater the level of disability, the more the person's communication depends on observer interpretation. It is probably for this reason that the reaction of people with intellectual disabilities to bereavement has not been better studied. There is also a tendency to shield them from the realities of death (Raji et al., 2003; Dodd et al., 2005; McRitchie et al., 2014).

Normal grief has been extensively described (Bowlby, 1961; Parkes, 1972), and it has been suggested that it involves a progression through several non-discrete stages, which may not apply comparably to people with intellectual disabilities (McRitchie et al., 2014).

These researchers indicate that people with intellectual disabilities are more likely to experience complications during the grieving period due to factors that include issues around inclusion. Continuing, unresolved grief is a spiritual experience that is part of the lives of many people with intellectual disabilities. Swinton (2004b) found that grief, loss and a sense of disconnectedness were common phenomena among people with intellectual disabilities. Some factors that contribute to poor adjustment to loss include inhibition of the experience and expression of grief (Parkes, 1972; Oswin, 1991). Grief, if denied expression, is potentially pathological, and people with intellectual disabilities may present to services with severe emotional problems following an experience of disenfranchised grief (Hollins and Esterhuyzen, 1997). Such individuals may grieve in ways that are not understood and which may therefore be ignored, or discounted as challenging behaviour.

Funerary rituals reinforce group ties, provide cultural identity and form a source of valuable social support, which can be important in both practical and emotional terms. The exclusion of people with intellectual disabilities from these mourning customs also excludes them from valuable emotional support. Sometimes people with intellectual disabilities are not told about a death, even of a close relative. They will be sensitive to the changes around them, but are not helped to make sense of them by sharing fully in the experience. As a result, they are left bewildered and unable to play a useful part in the rituals of loss and grieving.

It is known that predictors of depression following bereavement include insecure attachment patterns in childhood (Marris, 1991) and having to adjust to a new life over which one has little control, while not understanding why things have changed. These factors are prevalent in people with intellectual disabilities. Narayanasamy et al. (2002) described a counselling approach to providing spiritual support during crisis for people with intellectual disability. This included giving time and space to build trusting relationships with a sense of security, showing love and compassion, and helping staff and other residents to achieve a sense of meaning and purpose.

Intellectual Disability and Mental Health

Over the years it has become clearer that science alone is not enough to provide a basis for understanding and caring for another human being, and psychiatrists have become interested in spirituality because of its potential benefits to mental health. Traditionally, they have had responsibility for the medical care of people with intellectual disabilities. The way in which services for people with intellectual disabilities are structured throughout the UK, and indeed Europe and North America (European Association for Mental Health in Intellectual Disability, EAMHID), continues to change. The UK has a highly specialised psychiatric service specifically for people with intellectual disabilities, steered by the Faculty of Psychiatry of Intellectual Disability at the Royal College of Psychiatrists.

Assessing the presence of mental health problems in people with intellectual disabilities is a complex process, which raises distinct theoretical questions and methodological dilemmas. Most categories of mental illness have been reported in people with intellectual disabilities (Cooper et al., 2007, 2018). There is limited evidence regarding factors that predict the presence of mental health problems in individuals with intellectual disabilities. However, there is general agreement that the rate of psychopathology in people with intellectual disabilities is substantially raised when compared with the general population, with increased vulnerability over the whole spectrum of psychopathology and especially with certain diagnostic groups, such as the autism spectrum disorders and attention deficit hyperactivity disorder (ADHD). Reported rates of psychopathology vary significantly, ranging up to 40% (Cooper et al., 2007, 2018). Psychiatric illnesses can be difficult to detect in this population, because of problems with communication and atypical presentations leading to so-called 'diagnostic overshadowing'. Most assessment techniques rely on verbal accounts and utilise parallel interviewing of both the patient (where possible) and a key informant. The higher the level of disability, the more reliant the assessor is on third-party involvement. Information about how the individual with intellectual disability regards his or her current experience is limited and often totally absent. In a chapter titled 'Remorse for being', Hollins (1998, p. 98) suggests that the 'psychological difficulties that people with disabilities might experience' (Gangemi, 2018, p. 180) due to a sense of guilt about their very existence might increase their risk of depression as well as some of the behaviours that might be challenging.

The Same Standards for Everyone?

People with intellectual disabilities who are creative communicators form a heterogeneous group, and decisions about the presence and type of mental illness are based on diagnostic criteria standardised for the general population. Costello and Bouras (2006) argued that the application of measurement techniques developed for the general population may be inappropriate in people with intellectual disabilities. There have been increasing attempts to standardise instruments for this population. However, in the absence of other evidence, these generic assessments have been extrapolated to form the basis of understanding the needs of this group of service users.

The available literature considers either the spiritual needs or the mental health needs of people with intellectual disabilities, but rarely a combination of the two. An exception is found in the publications of the L'Arche International Faith Community, which has a Christian focus.

Lack of time, uncertainty about spirituality and how to incorporate spiritual care into the role of the professional, lack of education about the spiritual dimension of people's experiences, and fear of imposing values on people have all been reported as barriers to the implementation of spiritual care for people with intellectual disabilities (Swinton, 2004b). There is a tendency simply to translate a person's spiritual experiences into the language of psychology or psychiatry, since distress may be interpreted more easily within the boundaries of a familiar psychological framework than by engaging with a spiritual paradigm (Swinton, 2001b). The attitude of carers who equate spirituality with religion may mean that, for people with intellectual disabilities, issues of secular spirituality may be missed (Gilbert and Watts, 2006). Gangemi et al. (2010) advocate encounter as a vital requirement of spiritual support, as it allows a shared experience of life and faith. The use of music, signs, symbols and kinaesthetic forms of communication can ensure that creative communicators are enabled and not dis-abled.

From such a personhood of 'we', empathy can become the primary method for living, sharing and caring with creative communicators and learners. This approach, drawn from the phenomenological wisdom of Edith Stein's *On the Problem of Empathy* (Stein, 1989), suggests that empathy can become possible when each person ('I') is considered and received in their primordial, singular and unrepeatable capacity to act and be, just as they are. Similarly, this applies to the 'you' (all that is other), in their own individual and singular way. This respect for individual experience and lived realities can give rise to a shared personhood as 'we' live and share together in the world. Empathy, over and above any danger of practising sympathetic compassion, initiates a meeting place for primordial experiences that can be shared rather than possessed or projected on to any one person's life. This, according to Stein, brings forth a 'personhood of a higher level' as we live and act as members of a whole, in a world that we share (Stein, 1989, 2002a).

Treatment Approaches for People with Intellectual Disabilities

Several treatment approaches have been demonstrated to be effective for people with intellectual disabilities who have mental health disorders. Psychopharmacology is widely used, but research on psychotherapy for people with intellectual disabilities is scarce. A number of studies have shown that psychotherapy is often effective in improving coping abilities or relieving symptoms of psychopathology. The basis of psychotherapy is similar to that for the general population, but techniques must be adapted to the developmental skills of the individual being treated (Hollins and Sinason, 2000; Banks, 2003). Psychotherapy provides a tool for finding the self and 'healing the soul', through a relationship between therapist and patient that requires a connection with another human being, highlighting shared characteristics that help to find meaning in life. There is evidence that people with intellectual disabilities have more productive and meaningful lives as a result of group therapy, which provides a shared connection with others in similar circumstances (Tomasulo, 2014).

Behaviour management programmes are widely used to modify inappropriate behaviour and teach adaptive skills. In a different approach, McGee (1993) described a combined psychotherapeutic and behaviour modification programme called 'Gentle Teaching', involving the building of a therapeutic relationship between therapist and patient that McGee refers to as 'bonding'. This technique attempts to redirect maladaptive behaviour towards meaningful human engagement.

Evidence suggests that responding to the spirituality of people with intellectual disabilities can be rewarding for clients, their families and professional carers. Research has shown that although staff experienced initial difficulty in identifying with their role, and doubted their own abilities to deliver, they discovered a sense of achievement and satisfaction when meeting clients' spiritual needs. It also led to a greater sense of cohesiveness and improved morale among staff (Montgomery, 1991; Benson and Stark, 1996; McNair and Leguit, 2000; Narayanasamy et al., 2002).

Spiritual Care and Staff Spirituality

Spirituality can enrich the working life of staff and help them to find meaningfulness in the workplace (Gilbert and Watts, 2006). Spiritual care requires provision of time that is increasingly lacking in health care, and a degree of closeness that may even be considered unprofessional. Gangemi et al. (2010) found that spiritual care is dependent on a true and honest culture of encounter – meeting the person in their wholeness becomes an imperative for practice. One viewpoint is that closeness limits objectivity in decision making. Coulter (2002) and Royce-Davis (2000) recommend that practitioners should be given the opportunity for personal exploration of spiritual issues. The absence of any training in spiritual skills (Swinton, 2001b; Gaventa, 2018, pp. 175–180) may explain why many service professionals do not emphasise spiritual needs to the same extent as other issues in mental health assessment. To provide optimal care, professionals need to understand their client's spirituality, focusing on the person, without foisting their own spiritual or religious beliefs on vulnerable individuals (Royce-Davis, 2000).

People with intellectual disabilities are valued members of society. However, they still rely heavily on 'services' to enable them to make the most of life and its meaning. Therefore, in focusing on providing efficient and effective services, it is possible to lose sight of their ordinariness and their humanity (Hart and Pettingell, 2005). Progress has been patchy and ad hoc, driven by organisational and professional goals rather than having the person with intellectual disabilities at the centre of change. This situation cannot continue. People with intellectual disabilities must have opportunities to engage in all that life has to offer, including experiences that help them to make sense of who they are and the purpose of their life here on earth.

Spiritual Care of People with Intellectual Disabilities

Issues of spirituality and faith remain a big challenge in caring for people with intellectual disabilities, especially at times of transition and during major life events. Such people require means of creative communication that get round their cognitive and linguistic difficulties. These include using simple and symbolic language, and visual cues that make abstract concepts as concrete as possible.

Religious communities in Europe and North America are becoming increasingly aware that traditional worship and rituals are inappropriate for the needs of many people with intellectual disabilities, and are finding alternative approaches that enable more meaningful participation – for example, L'Arche, SPRED (Special Religious Development), the Kairos Forum, the Livability Charity and Caritas Westminster. (For more information, see the web resources listed at the end of this chapter.) They are taking into consideration the creative ways in which people with intellectual disabilities grow in faith, concluding that strongly relational intuitive experiences are more fruitful than explanations. An empathic and deeply narrative approach has found that, when sharing one's story, empathic silence can be more profound than words.

In some parts of the world, people with intellectual disabilities face tremendous obstacles in gaining access to appropriate good-quality health care, and this is partly due to inadequate physician training (Hogg, 2001; Voelker, 2002). In the UK, education on intellectual disabilities is being provided for generic mental health professionals early on in training and through continuing professional development. Seidel (2003) reported that the European Association for Mental Health in Mental Retardation stated at its annual conference that all people with intellectual disabilities have a right to the best mental health care available to the health and social care system of any country. Training is required to enable those supporting people with intellectual disabilities to recognise and respond to their spiritual needs (Swinton, 2004a).

In the past, the lifestyles of people with mental health problems and intellectual disabilities were governed by programme models that were developed for them without their input. However, the trend today is towards a service system that is individualised and based on personal choice and satisfaction. The aim must be to supply whatever support is necessary to enable affected individuals to improve their functioning, and to help them find personal success and satisfaction in the environment of their choice. People with intellectual disabilities – creative communicators – need to be enabled to release their tacit expertise to ensure their holistic and active participation in both civil and ecclesial communities (Pope Francis, 2020). Their personal narratives should resource creative teaching in spiritual care. The focus should be on the philosophy of encounter, 'Because I AM', taking precedence over the concept of learning difficulties. Therefore a greater understanding of what spirituality looks and feels like for creative communicators must fuel effective programmes of psychiatry. Professional formation and practice need to be creative, so that multisensory, multimodal methodologies can replace narrow and hypercognitive forms of exchange.

Conclusion

People with intellectual disabilities are marginalised in society, with limited opportunity to find meaning in their lives. Their spiritual needs should be incorporated into person-centred care plans, enabling them to experience and explore their spirituality in its widest meaning. Staff need to bear in mind that spirituality is not dependent on reasoning or the ability to communicate easily, and that it transcends the bounds of ability and disability. Spirituality may not be apparent in some people because of their disability, and it is important for caregivers to find creative ways of understanding a person's tacit spiritual experience. Furthermore, care staff should be open and receptive to the spiritual experiences that people with intellectual disabilities may have, without imposing their own spiritual or religious views.

Spirituality is recognised as having a positive link to health and well-being in both preventative and restorative capacities. In developing ways of enabling people with intellectual disabilities to define their own spirituality, participatory research has shown that it is possible to move away from a verbal mindset and from the measurement of externally perceived needs, in favour of an understanding of the internal state.

Studies of the spiritual needs and experiences of people with intellectual disabilities who also have mental health needs are seriously lacking, and more research is needed on both scientific and naturalistic fronts. The emphasis should change from doing things 'to' or 'for' the person with intellectual disabilities to doing things 'with' him or her.

Beliefs inherent within the major faith traditions can act as barriers to people with disabilities. What is urgently required is an inclusiveness that welcomes those with intellectual disabilities into both religious and secular life, affirming their place of belonging as they are, *because they are*. The aim should be to speak no longer about 'them' but rather about 'us' (Pope Francis, 2020). There are ongoing developments to address these issues. Research continues to show that membership of a supportive and inclusive religious community benefits a person's mental health, and faith communities can and should be powerful sources of friendship and inclusion (Larson et al., 1997; Carter, 2016; Carter and Boehm, 2019). In the field of mental health care, spirituality extends far beyond the ambit of faith traditions (Swinton, 2004b; Gangemi et al., 2010). Available in equal measure to those with intellectual disabilities and their personal and professional carers, its inclusion in the care process can only enhance, dignify and enrich the life of people with intellectual disabilities. As equal and valued members of the human race, they are fully entitled to this.

Web Resources

Caritas Westminster: www.caritaswestminster.org.uk/services.php

European Association for Mental Health in Intellectual Disability (EAMHID): https://eamhid.eu/about-eamhid/history/ (accessed January 2021).

Kairos Forum: www.kairosforum.org

L'Arche: www.larche.org

Lemos&Crane, *Looking Together: Spiritual Beliefs and Aspirations of People with Learning Disabilities*: www.lemosandcrane.co.uk/home/index.php?id=237140&

Livability: www.livability.org.uk

SPRED: www.spred.org.uk

References

African Child Policy Forum (2014) *The African Report on Children with Disabilities: Promising Starts and Persisting Challenges*. Addis Ababa: African Child Policy Forum.

Association of Directors of Adult Social Services (ADASS), Care Quality Commission (CQC), Department of Health, Health Education England (HEE), Local Government Association (LGA) and NHS England (2015) *Transforming Care for People with Learning Disabilities – Next Steps*. London: NHS England.

Baldacchino, D. and Draper, P. (2001) Spiritual coping strategies: a review of the nursing research literature. *Journal of Advanced Nursing*, 34, 833–841.

Banks, R. (2003) Psychological treatments for people with learning disabilities. *Psychiatry*, 2, 62–65.

Benomir, A. M., Nicolson, R. I. and Beail, N. (2016) Attitudes towards people with intellectual disability in the UK and Libya: a cross-cultural comparison. *Research in Developmental Disabilities*, 51, 1–9.

Benson, L. A. and Stark, M. (1996) *Timeless Healing: The Power and Biology of Belief*. New York: Simon & Schuster.

Bicknell, D. J. (1983) The psychopathology of handicap. *British Journal of Medical Psychology*, 56, 167–178.

Bowlby, J. (1961) Processes of mourning. *International Journal of Psychoanalysis*, 42, 317–340.

Bunning, K. and Steel, G. (2006) Self-concept in young adults with a learning disability from the Jewish community. *British Journal of Learning Disabilities*, 35, 43–49.

Carter, E. W. (2016) A place of belonging: research at the intersection of faith and disability. *Review & Expositor*, 113, 167–180.

Carter, E. W. and Boehm, T. L. (2019) Religious and spiritual expressions of young people with intellectual and developmental disabilities. *Research and Practice for Persons with Severe Disabilities*, 44, 37–52.

Chinvarakorn, V. (2006) *Empowered by FAITH*. Available at www.buddhistchannel.tv/index.php?id=6,2892,0,0,1,0 (accessed January 2021).

Cook, C. C. H. (2004) Addiction and spirituality. *Addiction*, 99, 539–551.

Cook, C. C. H. and Grimwade, L. (2021) *Spirituality and Mental Health*. London: Royal College of Psychiatrists.

Cooper, S.-A., Smiley, E., Morrison, J. et al. (2007) Mental ill-health in adults with intellectual disabilities: prevalence and associated factors. *British Journal of Psychiatry*, 190, 27–35.

Cooper, S.-A., Smiley, E., Allan, L. and Morrison, J. (2018) Incidence of unipolar and bipolar depression, and mania in adults with intellectual disabilities: prospective cohort study. *British Journal of Psychiatry*, 212, 295–300.

Costello, H. and Bouras, N. (2006) Assessment of mental health problems in people with intellectual disabilities. *Israel Journal of Psychiatry and Related Sciences*, 43, 241–251.

Coulter, D. (2002) Recognition of spirituality in healthcare: personal and universal implications. In W. Gaventa Jnr., W. Gaventa and D. Coulter, eds., *Spirituality and Intellectual Disability: International Perspectives on the Effect of Culture and Religion on Healing Mind, Body and Soul*. Philadelphia, PA: Haworth Press, pp. 1–11.

Dein, S. (2020) Religious healing and mental health. *Mental Health, Religion and Culture*, 23, 657–665,

Department of Health (2001) *Valuing People: A New Strategy for Learning Disabilities for the Twenty-first Century*. London: The Stationery Office.

Disability Africa (2016) 'I thought my child was a devil'. Available at www.disability-africa.org/blog/2016/11/21/i-thought-my-child-was-a-devil (accessed December 2020).

Dodd, P., Dowling, S. and Hollins, S. (2005) A review of the emotional, psychiatric and behavioural responses to bereavement in people with intellectual disabilities. *Journal of Intellectual Disability Research*, 49, 537–543.

Donatello, V. (2020) *Nessuno escluso: i riferimenti alle persone con disabilità nel magistero e nella catecheis ecclesiale [No one excluded: in reference to people with disabilities in ecclesial, magisterium and catechetical teachings]*. Rome: Libreria Ateneo Salesiano.

Dykens, E. M. (2006) Toward a positive psychology of mental retardation. *American Journal of Orthopsychiatry*, 76, 185–193.

Gangemi, C. (2018) *Because I Am: Christian Accompaniment Through the Experience of a Pre-Birth Diagnosis of a Possible Disability: Parents' Resource*. Alton: Redemptorist Publications.

Gangemi, C. (2020) Ways of knowing God, becoming friends in time: a timeless conversation between disability, theology, Edith Stein and Professor John Swinton. *Journal of Disability & Religion*, 24, 332–347.

Gangemi, C., Tobanelli, M., Vincenzi, G., Swinton, J. (2013) *EveryBody has a Story. Enabling Communities to Meet People with Learning Disabilities and Respond Effectively to Their Expressed Spiritual and Religious Needs: A Participatory Action Research Approach*. Aberdeen: University of Aberdeen. Research report available on request from cgangemi.kairos@gmail.com

Gangemi, C. and Waldron, L. (2018) *Intellectual Disability: Caring for Yourself and Others*. Alton: Redemptorist Publications.

Gardner, H. (1999) *Intelligence Reframed*. New York: Basic Books.

Gaventa, W. (2018) *Disability and Spirituality: Recovering Wholeness*. Waco, TX: Baylor University Press.

Gilbert, P. and Watts, N. (2006) Don't mention God! *A Life in the Day*, 10, 20–25.

Hatton, C., Turner, S., Shah, R. et al. (2004) *Religious Expression: a Fundamental Human Right. The Report of an Action Research Project on Meeting the Religious Needs of People with Learning Disabilities*. London: Foundation for People with Learning Disabilities.

Hart, S. and Pettingell, J. (2005) Valuing people with learning disabilities. *Journal for the Royal Society for the Promotion of Health*, 125, 16–17.

Hogg, J. (2001) Essential healthcare for people with learning disabilities: barriers and opportunities. *Journal of the Royal Society of Medicine*, 94, 333–336.

Hollins, S. (1998) Remorse for being: through the lens of learning disability. In M. Cox, ed., *Remorse and Reparation*. London: Jessica Kingsley Publishers, pp. 95–104.

Hollins, S. and Esterhuyzen, A. (1997) Bereavement and grief in adults with learning disabilities. *British Journal of Psychiatry*, 170, 497–501.

Hollins, S. and Sinason, V. (2000) Psychotherapy, learning disabilities and trauma: new perspectives. *British Journal of Psychiatry*, 176, 32–36.

Kaufman, A. V., Campbell, V. A. and Adams, J. P. (1990) A lifetime of caring: older parents who care for adult children with mental retardation. *International Journal of Family Care*, 2, 39–54.

Larson, D., Wood, G. and Larson, S. (1993) A paradigm shift in medicine toward spirituality? *Advances*, 9, 39–49.

Larson, D., Sawyers, J. and McCullough, M. (1997) *Scientific Research on Spirituality and Health: A Consensus Report*. London: National Institute for Health and Care Research.

Livability (2016) *Share your Story: Listening to the People That Use Our Services*. Available at www.livability.org.uk/blog/disability-care/share-story-listening-service-users/ (accessed 27 January 2021).

McGee, J. (1993) Gentle teaching for persons with mental retardation: the expression of a psychology of interdependence. In R. J. Fletcher and A. Dosen, eds., *Mental Health Aspects of Mental Retardation: Progress in Assessment and Treatment*. Washington, DC: Lexington Books, pp. 350–376.

McNair, J. and Leguit, G. (2000) The local church as an agent of natural support to individuals with developmental disabilities. *Issues in Transition*, 2, 11–16.

McRitchie, R., McKenzie, K., Quayle, E., Harlin, M. and Neumann, K (2014) How adults with intellectual disability experience bereavement and grief: a qualitative exploration. *Death Studies*, 38, 179–185.

McSherry, W. (2000) *Making Sense of Spirituality in Nursing Practice*. Edinburgh: Churchill Livingstone.

Marris, P. (1991) The social construction of uncertainty. In C. M. Parkes, J. Stevenson-Hinde and P. Marris, eds., *Attachment Across the Life Cycle*. London: Routledge, pp. 77–90.

Matthews, P. (2013) *Pope John Paul II and the Apparently 'Non-Acting' Person*. Leominster: Gracewing Publishing.

Miltiades, H. B. and Pruchno, R. (2002) The effect of religious coping on caregiving: appraisals of mothers of adults with developmental disabilities. *Gerontology*, 42, 82–91.

Montgomery, C. (1991) The caregiving relationships: paradoxical and transcendent aspects. *Journal of Transpersonal Psychology*, 23, 91–105.

Morin, D., Valois, P., Crocker, G., Robitaille, C. and Lopes, T. (2018) Attitudes of health care professionals toward people with intellectual disability: a comparison with the general population. *Journal of Intellectual Disability Research*, 62, 746–758.

Mpofu, E. and Harley, D. (2002) Disability and rehabilitation in Zimbabwe: lessons and implications for rehabilitation practice in the US. *Journal of Rehabilitation*, 68, 26–40.

Narayanasamy, A., Gates, B. and Swinton, J. (2002) Spirituality and learning disabilities: a qualitative study. *British Journal of Nursing*, 11, 948–957.

Oswin, M. (1991) *Am I Allowed to Cry? A Study of Bereavement Amongst People Who Have Learning Difficulties*. London: Souvenir Press.

Parkes, C. M. (1972) *Bereavement: Studies of Grief in Adult Life*. London: Tavistock Publications.

Patka, M., Keys, C. B., Henry, D. B. and McDonald K. E., (2013) Attitudes of Pakistani community members and staff toward people with intellectual disability. *American Journal of Intellectual and Developmental Disabilities*, 118, 32–43.

Pope Francis (2020) Message of the Holy Father Francis for the International Day of Persons with Disabilities. Available at www .vatican.va/content/francesco/en/messages/pont-messages/2020/documents/papa-francesco_20201203_messaggio-disabilita .html (accessed 4 December 2020).

Race, D. G. (2002) The historical context. In D. G. Race, ed., *Learning Disability: A Social Approach*. London: Routledge, pp. 23–52.

Raji, O. and Hollins, S. (2000) Exclusion from funerary rituals and mourning: implications for social and individual identity. In J. Hubert, ed., *Madness, Disability and Social Exclusion: The Archaeology and Anthropology of 'Difference'*. London: Routledge, pp. 208–216.

Raji, O., Hollins, S. and Drinnan, A. (2003) How far are people with learning disabilities involved in funeral rites? *British Journal of Learning Disabilities*, 31, 42–45.

Royce-Davis, J. (2000) The influence of spirituality on community participation and belonging: Christina's story. *Counselling and Values*, 44, 135–142.

Seidel, M. (2003) The Declaration of Rome 2003 with regard to the promotion of interest and services for people with intellectual disabilities with mental health needs. *Journal of Policy and Practice in Intellectual Disability*, 1, 101–103.

Singer, G. H. and Irvin, L. K. (1989) Family care giving, stress and support. In *Support for Caregiving Families: Enabling Positive Adaptation to Disability*. Baltimore, MD: Paul H. Brookes Publishing, pp. 3–25.

Sinson, J. (1996) Normalisation and community integration of adults with severe mental handicaps relocated to group homes. *Journal of Developmental and Physical Disabilities*, 6, 255–270.

Stainton, T. and Besser, H. (1998) The positive impact of children with an intellectual disability on the family. *Journal of Intellectual and Developmental Disability*, 23, 57–70.

Stein, E, (1989) *On the Problem of Empathy* (W. Stein, trans.). Washington, DC: ICS Publications, p. 17.

Stein, E. (1993) *Knowledge and Faith* (V. Herder, trans.) Freiburg im Breisgau 1993, Archivum Carmelitanum Band XV of Edith Stein Werke 1993 English translation. Washington, DC: Washington Province of Discalced Carmelites.

Stockholder, J. E. (1994) Naming and renaming persons with intellectual disabilities. In M. H. Rioux and M. Bach, eds., *Disability is Not Measles: New Research Paradigms in Disability*. Toronto: Roeher Institute, pp. 153–179.

Sulmasy, D. P. (1997) *The Healer's Calling: A Spirituality for Physicians and Other Health Care Professionals*. New York: Paulist Press.

Swinton, J. (1997) Restoring the image: spirituality, faith and cognitive disability. *Journal of Religion and Health*, 36, 21–28.

Swinton, J. (1999) Reclaiming the soul: a spiritual perspective on forensic nursing. In A. Kettles and D. Robinson, eds., *Forensic Nursing and the Multidisciplinary Care of the Mentally Disordered Offender*. London: Jessica Kingsley Publishers, pp. 113–127.

Swinton, J. (2001a) *A Space to Listen: Meeting the Spiritual Needs of People with Learning Disabilities*. London: Mental Health Foundation.

Swinton, J. (2001b) *Spirituality and Mental Health Care: Rediscovering a 'Forgotten' Dimension*. London: Jessica Kingsley Publishers.

Swinton, J. (2004a) *Why Are We Here? Spirituality and the Lives of People with Learning Disabilities*. London: Mental Health Foundation.

Swinton, J. (2004b) *No Box to Tick: A Booklet for Carers and Support Workers on Meeting the Spiritual Needs of People with Learning Disabilities*. London: Mental Health Foundation.

Swinton, J. (2012) From inclusion to belonging: a practical theology of community, disability and humanness. *Journal of Religion, Disability & Health*, 16, 172–190.

Taylor, R. J. and Chatters, L. N. (1986) Church-based informal support among elderly blacks. *The Gerontologist*, 26, 637–642.

Tobanelli, M., (2013) *EveryBody Has a Story*. Unpublished paper available on request from cgangemi.kairos@gmail.com

Tomasulo, D. J. (2014) Positive group psychotherapy modified for adults with intellectual disabilities. *Journal of Intellectual Disabilities*, 18, 337–350.

Treloar, L. L. (2002) Disability, spiritual beliefs and the church: the experiences of adults with disabilities and family members. *Journal of Advanced Nursing*, 40, 594–603.

Trute, B. and Hauch, C. (1988) Building on family strength: a study of families with positive adjustment to the birth of a developmentally disabled child. *Journal of Marital and Family Therapy*, 14, 185–193.

Udvari-Solner, A. (1997) Inclusive education. In C. A. Grant and G. Ladson-Billings, eds., *Dictionary of Multicultural Education*. Phoenix, AZ: Oryx Press, pp. 141–144.

Voelker, R. (2002) Improved care for neglected population must be "rule rather than exception". *Journal of the American Medical Association*, 288, 299–301.

Wolfensberger, W. (1972) *The Principle of Normalization in Human Services*. Toronto: National Institute on Mental Retardation.

Wood, J. B. and Parham, I. A. (1990) Coping with perceived burden: ethnic and cultural issues in Alzheimer's family caregiving. *Journal of Applied Gerontology*, 9, 325–339.

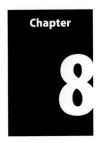

Substance Misuse and Addiction

John F. Kelly and Christopher C. H. Cook

At first glance, in the modern era of neuroscience, genomics, epigenetics and pharmacotherapies, any role for 'spirituality' in addressing the deadly serious clinical and public health problems related to substance misuse and addiction might seem at best antiquated, and at worst clinical malpractice. With lives, livelihoods and immense human suffering on the line, there should be solid reason for raising and discussing the role and impact of spirituality both in the prevention and treatment of addiction and in achieving sustained remission from it. In this chapter we argue that this is indeed so. Furthermore, we argue that a spiritual framework, especially when defined in terms of relationships, values, and meaning and purpose, can be useful for understanding the course into and out of addiction disorders, as well as for providing a conceptual language that resonates with many addiction patients and helps to engage them in treatment. First, we describe how religion and spirituality are sometimes viewed as the same, as partially overlapping or as completely distinct entities. Next we outline how religion and spirituality can provide a conceptual lens through which a useful explanatory model might be derived that may be helpful in understanding how psychiatric distress and addiction disorder evolve and remit. We then provide a historical overview of spirituality and addiction and, drawing from theoretical explications and empirical data, we consider how religion and spirituality have been found both to be a protective factor in addiction onset, and to be beneficial in helping many sufferers to achieve remission and stable recovery.

Definitions of Religion and Spirituality and Utility in Addiction Psychiatry

Religion and spirituality may be viewed as the same thing, as partially overlapping constructs or as completely distinct entities (see Chapter 1). There is a broad growing trend in many Western societies, for example, for people to identify more categorically as 'spiritual but not religious' (Mercadante, 2014). For many, spirituality is understood as placing relatively more attention on relationships, values, and meaning and purpose, whether or not any particular religious figurehead or deity is invoked. With regard to risk factors for addiction as well as recovery from it, it is these dimensions that become particularly salient and valuable. Consequently, to the extent that religion contains these 'spiritual' elements, as will be explained in more detail subsequently, both seem able to confer salubrious benefit.

A Spiritual Model of Addiction Onset and Recovery

Unlike nearly all other psychiatric disorders, substance use disorder is produced by the imbibing or consumption of something that is external to the human body, and that, when consumed, produces various combinations of pleasure and euphoria, relief from psychological angst and enhanced performance. In addition, for other well-known addiction disorders, such as gambling or sexual compulsivity, that do not involve consumption of psychoactive substances per se, the initial motivations and effects that lead into the addiction process are similar; they increase pleasure or facilitate a temporary escape from psychological pain. Because the generally positive acute beneficial effects of engaging with these substances or behaviours are almost universally experienced in the brain among all human beings, their overconsumption among a minority can be viewed by the majority as 'selfish' and 'self-indulgent', especially when the behaviour has negative externalities that cause worry or even physical harm to innocent bystanders. Although they are beyond the scope of this chapter, there are now known genetic and epigenetic modulating factors that help to explain why some individuals are much more vulnerable than others to the effects of certain substances and behaviours when they are exposed to them. This is manifested as differences in the magnitude of the experienced reward and relief on initial exposure, which in turn influence the likelihood that such exposure will lead to repetitive and increasing use, brain changes and addiction (Crabbe, 2002).

Consequently, substance use and other addiction disorders are – with the possible exception of some of the positive euphoric and energising effects of manic symptoms that can also have negative externalities – somewhat unique in the psychiatric disorder spectrum in evoking more negative moral social judgements. Indeed, these disorders generally are often found to be the most stigmatised of any psychiatric illnesses (Kelly et al., 2016, 2021) or other problems in society (Room et al., 2001). Importantly, such stigmatisation and negative moral judgements are present not only among observers, but also among sufferers themselves. This is because the disinhibiting, sedating and intoxicating properties of many commonly misused substances (e.g., alcohol, opioids) when used intensively over long periods – as they are in addiction disorders – can lead to chronic deviations from individuals' own values or moral code which, over time, can produce anxiety, guilt, shame, intense remorse, self-loathing and self-denigration. As others withdraw from the affected individual, social isolation can occur along with the deleterious shifts in values that accompany the progression of the disorder. As the substance or behaviour takes on an abnormally high priority, often becoming the central focus of daily activity (a pharmacological 'higher power'), there can be an increasing loss of meaning and purpose in the sufferer's life, as they become almost entirely consumed by the addictive cycle (e.g., obtaining the substance, using it, recovering from its effects, obtaining the substance, using it, and so on). It is because of these deviations – from what most religious and spiritual doctrines (e.g., Christianity, Islam) and social mores would view as good social and ethical conduct – that religious and social institutions often proscribe against intoxication that can lead to psychological impairment. It is also important for many suffering from addiction who want to follow a path of stable recovery to find a framework for self-forgiveness that is sufficient to alleviate the burden of shame, guilt and remorse. Many religious and spiritual frameworks provide an avenue to the achievement of such forgiveness.

With regard to recovery from addiction, the spiritual elements of social relationships, values, and meaning and purpose come back into play. In many ways the process of recovery from serious addiction disorders is one that involves exposure to, or immersion in, a supportive social network of people who can offer and model a lifestyle that is conducive to stable remission from addiction over the long term. Such social connections are successful in helping those suffering from addiction to achieve and sustain remission (e.g., Alcoholics Anonymous), and often explicitly espouse behavioural norms consistent with positive prosocial cultural mores and values. They also often facilitate a cognitive reframing of the immense suffering that has been encountered, giving it new positive meaning and purpose (e.g., 'I have learned some big lessons from my addiction', 'I survived this for a reason'), instead of what appears for many entering recovery initially to represent a random, self-inflicted and ostensibly futile experience.

Arguably, it is at these intersections of substance-induced social isolation, deviations from valued moral and ethical behaviour, and loss of meaning and purpose in life that spirituality and addiction psychiatry meet. There is overlap between these central concerns of addiction and those of many spiritual and religious traditions. Notably, the element of subjective compulsion, defined within the addiction syndrome in such a way as to include both craving and impaired control over substance-related behaviour, touches on important concerns of both Buddhist and Christian spirituality (Groves and Farmer, 1994; Groves, 1998; Cook, 2006). Because these traditions each have something important to say about the spiritual nature of addiction, it is not surprising that Christian (e.g., Celebrate Recovery), Buddhist (e.g., Refuge Recovery) and other faith-based treatment and recovery support programmes have been founded as a response to the suffering with which addiction is associated.

Sometimes any religious or spiritual discussion in relation to addiction evokes instant opposition and heated exchanges. This is because religion and spiritual frameworks are often viewed as outdated, unhelpful 'moral' or 'sin-based' explanatory models juxtaposed with our more modern understanding of addiction as a disease or disorder that radically affects the brain's structure and function (Volkow and Boyle, 2018). The description of addiction as a chronically relapsing brain disease has been shown to be one way to perhaps reduce the blame and shame that accompany addiction (e.g., Kelly et al., 2021). However, such biomedical reductionism, although compelling, belies the highly influential psychosocial contexts that facilitate entry into and out of addiction. As explained earlier, the concept of spirituality, especially when defined in terms of relationships, values, and meaning and purpose, can provide a useful explanatory framework for many, and it has been shown to make all the difference in terms of recovery for some racial and ethnic groups, such as African Americans (Kelly and Eddie, 2020).

Historical Perspective

Whatever the conceptual relationship between spirituality and addiction, history can also help to illuminate why spirituality has become entwined with addiction and addiction psychiatry. In the Western world, at least up until the end of the eighteenth century, problems such as drunkenness were not particularly distinguished from other social and moral concerns, such as theft, adultery or gluttony. As alluded to earlier, the failure to distinguish between such problems is understood as being the basis of the now dis-credited 'moral model' of addiction. However, it is doubtful that this model ever actually existed in quite the way that some people seem to imagine. Rather, 'drunkenness' was something that people were responsible for, in the same way that they were responsible for other social and personal vices. A few people were, perhaps, relative saints, but most people in society were sinners of one kind or another.

In seventeenth-century Europe, thought and belief about almost all aspects of human life began to be influenced by the intellectual movement now known as the Enlightenment. The Enlightenment emphasised reason and science as the basis for understanding human problems, thus excluding the authority of religious traditions and scriptures (see, for example, Honderich, 1995, pp. 236–237). From the late eighteenth century onwards, this movement appears to have begun to influence thinking about chronic alcohol intoxication – by far the main addiction problem of the era. In 1785, Benjamin Rush published *An Inquiry into the Effects of Ardent Spirits upon the Human Body and Mind: With an Account of the Means of Preventing, and of the Remedies for Curing Them* (Rush, 1785), and in 1804, Thomas Trotter published *An Essay, Medical, Philosophical, and Chemical, on Drunkenness and its Effects on the Human Body* (Trotter, 1804). Addiction (or 'chronic inebriety') was becoming a medical concern in addition to being a religious concern. In this context, a disease model of (alcohol) addiction became more popular, although it was rarely completely divorced from the moral model, presumably because of the negative externalities associated with intoxication and the belief that those affected were drinking voluntarily by choice, at least initially. The following quote from Trotter (1804) perhaps sums up the intersecting influence of both moral and emerging medical models of addiction (referred to here as 'evils' and 'diseases', respectively): 'Mankind, ever in pursuit of pleasure, have reluctantly admitted into the catalogue of their diseases, those evils which are the immediate offspring of their luxuries' (Trotter, 1804, Introduction, p. 1).

The disease of addiction (chronic drunkenness) was understood, in one form or another, as a disease of the will, caused by alcohol, with Trotter defining it formally as a 'disease of the mind' (Trotter, 1804).

A more biomedical framing of addiction was adopted in the twentieth century by Alcoholics Anonymous (AA), based on early AA members' understanding of addiction given to them at Charles B. Towns Hospital by its chief physician, Dr William Silkworth. It is this organisation that has had particular influence over the perception of addiction as a 'spiritual malady' in North America and Europe.

Founded in Akron, Ohio, in 1935 by two men with severe alcohol addiction, AA drew on both religious and medical sources for its understanding of alcohol addiction. The former came mainly from an entity known as the Oxford Group, an evangelical Christian movement of the time. As noted earlier, the medical framing came largely from Dr William Silkworth, the physician who treated several of the early members of AA (including its co-founder, Bill Wilson) and who later contributed a medical foreword to AA's central main text (the 'Big Book'; (Alcoholics Anonymous, 1976, pp. xxiii–xxx)). It is estimated that Silkworth treated more than 50,000 individuals who suffered from alcohol addiction during the course of his career (Kurtz, 1991, pp. 21–22). Although in the foreword to AA's 'Big Book' he offered a clinical typology based on his professional experiences that included allusions to alcohol addiction being a form of physical allergy to alcohol, he acknowledged that it was not a true allergy. He also saw very little hope for recovery, unless the alcoholic experienced what he termed an entire 'psychic change'. For this change to come about, he saw the need for 'something more than human power'

(Alcoholics Anonymous, 1976, p. xxvii). One of his most severe cases, whom he deemed to be a hopeless case, was AA's co-founder, Bill Wilson. During one of his detoxification experiences in his hospital, Bill Wilson experienced what he described as a 'spiritual awakening' that created a 'built in belief in God.' Because he had been trying to stay sober under the auspices of the Oxford Group – which had a welcoming and compassionate view of 'drunkards' – Bill Wilson believed that this was a minor miracle, and set off to help other 'drunks' who might benefit from what he had learned. Dr Silkworth's observation of this remarkable transformation and recovery was probably the reason why he allowed Bill Wilson to speak to other addicted patients at the hospital in an attempt to try to help them. That said, in much the same way as today, there was initially a great deal of scepticism about the clinical utility of a 'spiritual' approach to treating addiction. The hospital administrator, Charlie Towns, was initially very doubtful, but after observing many recoveries among 'hopeless cases' he began to support the approach that was later to become AA: 'When my head doctor, Silkworth, began to tell me of the idea of helping drunks by spirituality, I thought it was crackpot stuff, but I've changed my mind. One day this bunch of ex-drunks of yours is going to fill Madison Square Garden' (Alcoholics Anonymous, 1952, p. 136).

The founders of AA were also influenced by the work of William James, who wrote a seminal book on the psychology of religion, *The Varieties of Religious Experience* (James, 1985). Within the pages of this volume may be found many psychological accounts of religious experience, which include reference to those who struggled with alcohol addiction. The case of S. H. Hadley is recounted by James at some length (James, 1985, pp. 201–203). Hadley saw himself as a hopeless case, a 'homeless, friendless, dying drunkard', who had delirium tremens (James, 1985, p. 210). Having found himself praying in a prison cell, on his release he went to a meeting at a Mission Hall at which a man known for his work among drunkards was preaching. Responding to the call at the end of the meeting, Hadley describes how, with a breaking heart, he prayed to Jesus to help him. At this, a profound affective change came about: 'indescribable gloom' was replaced with 'glorious brightness'. Hadley concludes his account: 'From that moment till now I have never wanted a drink of whiskey, and I have never seen money enough to make me take one. I promised God that night that if he would take away the appetite for strong drink, I would work for him all my life. He has done his part, and I have been trying to do mine' (James, 1985, p. 203).

The Varieties of Religious Experience left its mark on AA. Although initially a Christian movement, it acquired a wariness of established religion that bears much of the character of James' own suspicion of doctrinal formulation and religious belief. It saw, nonetheless, a key need for spiritual transformation in recovery from alcohol addiction, and it offers a 'spiritual but not religious' transformational way of finding recovery. Indeed, although initially Bill Wilson and AA's early members believed this kind of quantum transformational change was necessary to recovery from addiction, they began to see recoveries that never involved such a sudden and dramatic shift in consciousness and outlook, but instead showed a gradual shift resulting from psychological and social change – including helping other 'drunks', which enabled people to experience a 'spiritual awakening' of the 'educational variety' (AA, Appendix II; Alcoholics Anonymous World Services, 2001) which reflected Silkworth's 'psychic change'. It is essentially a secular form of spirituality (Kurtz, 1996).

AA has since become a worldwide organisation[1] comprised of over two million members operating in more than 120,000 groups. The Twelve-Step programme, meetings and fellowship model developed by AA was adopted by numerous similar organisations seeking to help people with myriad other kinds of emotional/psychological and addiction problems, including Narcotics Anonymous (NA), Cocaine Anonymous (CA), Marijuana Anonymous (MA), Gamblers Anonymous (GA), Sex and Love Addicts Anonymous (SLAA) and Overeaters Anonymous (OA). The model also proved popular among those seeking to help families and children of those who were addicted, including AlAnon (for relatives and friends of people addicted to alcohol), Alateen (for teenage children of addicted individuals) and Families Anonymous (FA, for families of individuals addicted to any kind of drug). Furthermore, although firmly rooted as a mutual help movement, the philosophy of AA has also influenced professionally led treatment and has been adopted by both residential and community-based programmes (Cook, 1988a, 1988b). In general, all mutual-help organisations based upon the original philosophy and practices of AA, as expressed in its '12 steps', are referred to as 'Twelve-Step organisations'. Treatment programmes based upon this philosophy are often referred to as 'Twelve-Step treatment programmes' or, if they are residential in nature, as 'Minnesota Model' programmes, reflecting the original development of such treatment programmes in Minnesota in the 1940s and 1950s.

Whereas AA and its sister organisations offer a non-religious, non-denominational approach to spirituality as a pathway to recovery from addiction, various religious or faith-based organisations continue to offer different forms of spirituality anchored within their own faith traditions. Thus Christian (National Institute on Drug Abuse, 1977; Moos et al., 1978), Buddhist (Barrett, 1997), Islamic (Abdel-Mawgoud et al., 1995), Native American (Garrett and Carroll, 2000; White, 2002) and other programmes have been described, each offering their own distinctive approach to spirituality either as a response in itself, or else in combination with various secular and research-based interventions.

At the same time, mainstream healthcare provision and scientific research within the addictions field in the Western world have tended to focus on physical, social and psychological interventions that do not require, or even allude to, the need for any spiritual change. Other mutual help groups (e.g., SMART Recovery, LifeRing, Secular Organizations for Sobriety) have been established that do not require the assent to anything spiritual, even in a secular form, that is so central to AA ((Humphreys, 2004, pp. 33–93). The field of addiction treatment and recovery support services today is thus much more heterogeneous. However, the impact of the faith-based spirituality organisations has ensured that spirituality is a subject for discussion among lay people and professionals, those with their own experience of addiction and those who study the addictive behaviour of others, within treatment communities and faith communities. Spirituality has become a feature of the addictions treatment landscape.

Spirituality as a Protective Factor

Before we move on to the treatment studies, it is worth considering briefly the field of research which suggests that spirituality is a protective factor against substance misuse.

---

[1] www.alcoholics-anonymous.org.uk

Various measures of religious behaviour, religious affiliation or 'religiosity' are inversely correlated with substance use and misuse (Chamberlain and Hall, 2000, pp. 189–197; Koenig et al., 2001, pp. 189–197; Koenig, 2005, pp. 109–112; Giordano et al., 2015). In a study of 7,661 church-affiliated young people (aged 12–30 years), agreement with statements reflecting church attendance, Christian belief and spiritual practices (prayer and Bible reading) were generally found to be associated with a lower likelihood of having smoked cigarettes, drunk alcohol or used illicit drugs (Hope and Cook, 2001). However, church attendance appeared to be more important for the 12- to 16-year-olds, whereas belief and Bible reading appeared to be more important for the 17- to 30-year-olds. Perhaps for younger people, socialisation within a faith community provides protection against substance misuse, whereas for older people it is the internalisation of faith and its expression in personal spirituality that provides protection. Nevertheless, there is debate about how exactly these protective effects may operate. For example, as noted earlier, affiliation with a faith community may instill moral values that guard against substance use – especially illicit substance use – or substance misuse, because such use is explicitly forbidden or proscribed. Extending this idea, it could consequently also be the effect of conforming to the norms of the social group in which substance use or misuse is less acceptable. Furthermore, religious and spiritual traditions are associated with various measures of improved coping and mental well-being (Chamberlain and Hall, 2000, pp. 118–137; Koenig, 2005, pp. 43–81), and thus may reduce substance misuse by improving alternative coping skills or reducing perceived stress. Church-affiliated young people are often offered drugs at a rate not very different to that for other young people. Therefore, whatever the mechanism of the protective effect may be, it is not simply a case of their being hidden away from drug-using peers (Cook et al., 1997).

Measures of religiosity are clearly related to spirituality, and it would appear that spirituality is also protective against substance misuse (Zimmerman and Maton, 1992; Stewart, 2001; Leigh et al., 2005). Spirituality appears to exert a protective effect in both high- and low-risk groups (Ritt-Olson et al., 2004).

Spirituality in Substance Misuse Treatment Programmes

Spirituality may be variously understood and spiritual issues differently addressed in different kinds of treatment programmes. Broadly speaking, they can be considered in three groups: Twelve-Step spirituality, spirituality rooted in the faith traditions of faith-based organisations, and non-specific explorations of spirituality that might take place in any other treatment programmes.

Twelve-Step Spirituality

The principles adopted by Twelve-Step groups and Twelve-Step treatment programmes are summarised in the so-called '12 steps' as written down by the original founders of AA, adapted with only minor modifications by AA's sister organisations (e.g., NA, CA, AlAnon). They are expressed in the first person, reflecting their origins in the personal experiences of the early members. Table 8.1 lists these steps along with the principles generally associated with each of them.

Table 8.1. The 12 Steps of Alcoholics Anonymous[a] and the related principles involved in each step

Step		Principle
1	We admitted we were powerless over alcohol – that our lives had become unmanageable.	Honesty
2	Came to believe that a Power greater than ourselves could restore us to sanity.	Hope
3	Made a decision to turn our will and our lives over to the care of God *as we understood Him*.	Faith
4	Made a searching and fearless moral inventory of ourselves.	Courage
5	Admitted to God, to ourselves and to another human being the exact nature of our wrongs.	Integrity
6	Were entirely ready to have God remove all these defects of character.	Willingness
7	Humbly asked Him to remove our shortcomings.	Humility
8	Made a list of all persons we had harmed, and became willing to make amends to them all.	Compassion
9	Made direct amends to such people wherever possible, except when to do so would injure them or others.	Justice
10	Continued to take personal inventory, and when we were wrong promptly admitted it.	Perseverance
11	Sought through prayer and meditation to improve our conscious contact with God *as we understood Him* praying only for knowledge of His will for us and the power to carry that out.	Spirituality
12	Having had a spiritual awakening as the result of these steps we tried to carry this message to alcoholics and to practise these principles in all our affairs.	Service

[a] Alcoholics Anonymous (1977) (original emphases preserved).

The influence of the Oxford Group's spirituality is visible here, with its emphasis on personal confession and repentance of sinful acts. However, the influence of *The Varieties of Religious Experience* (James, 1985) may also be discerned in the lack of religious doctrinal language and emphasis upon God (or a 'Higher Power') as understood and experienced by the individual members of AA.

The first three steps relate to relationship, especially that with the object of addiction (in this case alcohol) over which the individual finds him- or herself powerless, and relationship with a transcendent power towards which the individual must turn for help. This transcendent or 'Higher Power' provides a subject for much debate. The explicit reference to 'God' in Steps 3, 5, 6 and 11 undoubtedly provides a reason for many a person attending AA only once or twice and then deciding that it is 'too religious'. However, in practice, all Twelve-Step groups and treatment programmes are open to people from all faiths and denominations, as well as to atheists and agnostics. 'God' is self-defined, understood by the individual according to his or her own faith beliefs, traditions, folk religion or personal notion of a higher power which is unique and meaningful to that individual. Alternatively, the 'God' aspect of the Twelve-Step programme is interpreted by many Twelve-Step members as standing for 'Group of Drunks' or 'Good Orderly Direction' – in other words, in a completely non-religious way. What is important is that a power outside of oneself is identified, from which one can obtain help. It is not so much that the member of AA has to believe in some kind of a deity (although many do) as that they need to believe that they themselves are 'not God' (Kurtz, 1991).

To use Christian terminology, Steps 4 to 9 are concerned largely with confession and repentance, but are referred to as taking and discussing a moral inventory and listing, becoming willing, and making amends to others whom the affected person may have harmed via his or her former alcohol or drug use. The concern with relationship between self and a transcendent order is anchored here in relationships with others, especially those who have been harmed by the addicted person in the course of the history of his or her addictive behaviour. It is sometimes said that the disease model offers a way of avoiding personal responsibility. In contrast, however, members of AA – at least those who work through the steps in a serious way – are engaged deeply with personal responsibility, both for what they have done and for working at their own recovery. The therapeutic outcomes of these endeavours can include enhanced self-esteem and relief from the burden of guilt and remorse for past acts, all of which can help to facilitate positivity and long-term remission (Kelly and McCrady, 2009).

Finally, Steps 10 to 12, often referred to as the 'maintenance steps', are concerned with ongoing practice and sharing with others what has been learned. It is clear that this ongoing spirituality is founded in the personal spiritual experiences of the individual. It is deemed that through 'working' the 12 steps of the programme, a 'spiritual awakening' occurs (a 'psychic change' in Silkworth's language). Such an experience might be sudden, as in the case of S. H. Hadley or Bill Wilson, or it might be gradual (of the 'educational variety'), but it is in such an experience that hope is to be found.

What does all this mean in practice? Attendance at meetings of AA and/or other Twelve-Step organisations is considered to be vital to the process. This is because the Twelve-Step principles (see Table 8.1) embodied in each step are modeled, taught, shared and observed within meetings. Also, it is at these meetings that people develop AA friendships which extend beyond the meeting format and often become a large part of attendees' social networks that help to facilitate ongoing recovery (Kelly et al., 2011, 2012). The steps are 'worked' by individual members with the assistance and guidance of a 'sponsor' – a more experienced member who acts as a mentor and guide. In general, asking whether or not a member of AA or any other Twelve-Step fellowship has a sponsor provides a good indication of whether they are actually taking the programme seriously. In fact, from a scientific standpoint, meta-analyses have shown that having a sponsor has the strongest empirical relationship to future abstinence and remission (Emrick et al., 1993).

There is an extensive literature that is supportive of Twelve-Step spirituality and recovery. A key place within this literature is held by the 'Big Book' (Alcoholics Anonymous World Services, 2001), which outlines the nature of the problem, describes the approach taken by AA in response, and provides accounts of the experiences of some of the early members. The 'Big Book' of AA is paralleled by comparable works in each of the other Twelve-Step fellowships (e.g., Narcotics Anonymous World Services, 1986). AA's other main text, *Twelve Steps and Twelve Traditions* (Alcoholics Anonymous, 1952), also contains detailed accounts of the meaning and practices involved in each of the 12 steps and outlines how a member may 'work' them in his or her life. In addition, it includes the Twelve Traditions that describe AA's organisational operational structures and recommended public relations policies.

Spirituality in the Programmes of Faith-Based Organisations

It is not possible to review here the spiritual traditions of all the world's religions. However, some examples can be given of the various connections made between the spiritualities of particular religions and the spirituality of addiction. It is also important to consider what takes place in practice in addiction treatment programmes provided by faith-based organisations, and in addiction recovery in diverse religious contexts (e.g., Ali, 2014; Groves, 2014; Loewenthal, 2014; Owen, 2014; Morjaria-Keval and Keval, 2015).

For Christianity, the problem is less in making connections between spirituality and addiction than in choosing between various possible theological understandings of what addiction is all about. At some level, there appears to be a general consensus that it is connected with 'sin' or rebellion against God, but this can mean very different things to different people. For some it implies that 'addiction is (a) sin', and for others that 'sin is addiction'. Even these two apparently similar models can result in very different approaches to helping people trapped in the labyrinth of addiction. The one appears very much like the moral model in religious clothing. The other reduces addiction to being merely an expression of the human condition, a condition of which we are all a part, and risks losing any distinctive understanding of what it is to be addicted. There are, of course, many nuances and subtleties that distinguish the ways in which these models might be expressed, such as that put succinctly by Linda Mercadante in the title of her book, *Victims and Sinners* (Mercadante, 1996).

Elsewhere, Cook (2006) has explored some of the common ground that is mapped out both by scientific studies of addiction and by some foundational Christian texts. Like Mercadante, Cook concludes that for Christian theology, grace rather than sin is central, and it is grace that (in non-theological language) the Twelve-Step programmes have also identified as vital to recovery from addiction. Grace, in Christian terms, is concerned with the relationship between God and human beings, a relationship within which God is always generously self-giving despite, and even because of, human powerlessness and self-imprisonment. Christian spirituality, like Twelve-Step spirituality, is more con-cerned with the human need to look beyond the self than with focusing on one's own faults and failings – the solution is to be found in the relationship with the Divine reality that is both deeply within human beings and also outside and beyond them.

Buddhism also finds resonance with the language of addiction. For Buddhism, concepts such as 'dependence' and 'craving' are associated with the very problems that are at the root of all human suffering (Mason-John and Groves, 2013). For instance, Groves defines craving as 'the urge or desire to obtain an experience other than the one we are experiencing at present' (Groves, 1998, p. 204). Such urges and desires can express themselves in subtle and varied ways, but they are not alien to any of us. As with Christian spirituality, we find here a reminder that the phenomenon of addiction is something that affects us all and is a part of the human condition. However, the focus is more on recognising why having the craving is unhelpful and how we may better deal with it. The answer to the latter is to be found in the development of 'skilfulness' – a quality that includes elements of wisdom, attentiveness and compassion – which enables us to view our actions and motives differently and to break away from the unhealthy motivation that is inherent within craving. In contrast to Christianity, Buddhism does not require a focus on relationship with God, but it shares a recognition that unhealthy attachments to things that are 'not God' are at the root of human suffering.

Even these two brief examples will immediately draw attention to the different ways in which faith traditions might suggest remedies for the addictive state. Thus, within the revealed monotheistic faiths – Judaism, Christianity and Islam – spirituality in the programmes offered by their associated faith-based organisations is most likely to take the form of prayer, worship and study of scripture. For Buddhist groups, spirituality might look much more like cognitive therapy (Avants and Margolin, 2004) coupled with meditation rather than prayer. Within any given faith tradition there is also a variety of approaches. For example, not all Christian programmes look alike. In some, visible reliance is placed upon secular psychological and medical techniques, with spirituality providing more of a motivating factor or rationale (see, for example, Judge, 1971). In others, exactly the opposite is true, with the emphasis entirely upon prayer, Bible study and Christian faith, and with secular therapies almost or completely absent (see, for example, Gruner, 1979).

Spirituality in Secular Treatment Programmes

Treatment programmes that follow neither a Twelve-Step design nor the spiritual tradition of a faith-based organisation might be considered 'non-spiritual'. Although a chaplain or a chaplaincy team is usually available within NHS trusts in the UK, it is very much up to the individual patient whether or not he or she takes the opportunity to talk to a chaplain about the spiritual aspects of his or her problem. It seems that patients in substance misuse services in the UK rarely take this opportunity. However, various surveys show that such patients (at least in the USA) do consider spirituality to be important (McDowell et al., 1996; Carroll et al., 2000; Arnold et al., 2002; Dermatis et al., 2004), and for some individuals this is particularly so. For example, a recent study of a nationally representative sample of recovering persons found that, compared with white Americans, black/African American individuals who self-identified as having resolved a serious alcohol or other drug problem were substantially more likely to report that religion and spirituality 'made all the difference' to their recovery (Kelly and Eddie, 2020).

There are implicit and explicit ways in which spirituality may be addressed, even within secular and medical substance misuse treatment programmes, that do not follow the traditions of a faith-based organisation or a Twelve-Step programme. It seems almost impossible to discuss problems of substance misuse without there being a spiritual dimension to the conversation, even if the word 'spirituality' is not actually used. For example, the definition of spirituality used earlier might be viewed and interpreted through a secular lens without resorting to any formal notions of spirituality. Also, a review of the body of research on addiction and spirituality (Cook, 2004), which analysed 263 publications, identified 13 common conceptual components that the authors had used to define spirituality:

1 relatedness
2 transcendence
3 humanity
4 core/force/soul
5 meaning/purpose
6 authenticity/truth

7 values
8 non-materiality
9 (non-) religiousness
10 wholeness
11 self-knowledge
12 creativity
13 consciousness.

Of these, the first two – relatedness and transcendence – were the most commonly cited (34% and 41%, respectively, of papers studied, but included in 62% and 53%, respectively, of questionnaires used to measure spirituality in addictions research). Inevitably, interventions for addiction involve considerations of relatedness, for it is the relationship with the object of addiction that is at the heart of the problem, and, as noted earlier, relationships with self and others almost inevitably suffer as a result. Transcendence, if understood in the narrower sense of the Divine or a 'Higher Power', is not integral to secular treatments for substance misuse. However, if understood in a broader sense of recognising the inadequacy of personal resources, failed previous attempts to address the problem, or of the need to accept help from others, transcendence may be considered a key premise to engaging in any helping relationship – including that offered by a substance misuse treatment service. The psychologist Abraham Maslow became famous for his 'hierarchy of needs', which outlined the human necessity of food, shelter and safety, followed on up the hierarchy by belonging, love and self-actualisation (full expression of the self) (Maslow, 1943; see Chapter 6, Figure 6.1). Interestingly, in his later years, shortly before his death, he added another level – that of 'self-transcendence' – which, although not necessarily viewed from a spiritual/religious standpoint, nevertheless reflected a notion of other-centeredness and overcoming self-limitations (Maslow, 1987).

This very brief analysis of spirituality within secular substance misuse treatment must obviously be balanced by the recognition that there are particular dynamics, including biological as well as psychological and social disturbances, which are unique to addiction and are not experienced by all human beings. However, the extent to which spirituality and addiction touch on universal aspects of the human condition – in particular our relationships with ourselves, others and the world around us – is important. It is this that creates a point of contact between therapist and service user, and it is this that offers an antidote to the stigma associated with the moral model.

There are explicit ways in which spirituality may be addressed within secular treatment programmes. For example, where cognitive–behavioural relapse prevention programmes address the need for lifestyle balance, spiritual aspects (e.g., relationships, values, meaning and purpose) as well as biological and other more common psychological and social aspects of human lifestyle can be constructively addressed (Moos, 2007). Even where plurality of faith traditions makes it difficult to address spirituality through any common understanding of religion, many NHS and other substance misuse treatment programmes allow some educational input from Twelve-Step group members, or else allow such groups to meet on their premises. This is not to suggest that such treatment programmes adopt Twelve-Step spirituality, but at least patients are afforded the opportunity to be acquainted with what these groups have to offer and to discuss concerns they may have, which can have positive benefits for engagement (Manning et al., 2012) and better clinical outcomes (Gossop et al., 2003; Kelly et al., 2020, 2021). Similarly, techniques of mindfulness and skilfulness, although associated with the Buddhist tradition, find parallels within cognitive–behavioural psychology and may be accessible to people who would not ordinarily think of themselves as interested in Buddhism. Moreover, such practices are associated with good clinical outcomes (Bowen et al., 2014).

It is also possible to introduce discussion of spirituality in a neutral way, without favouring any particular spiritual tradition, and doing so in a non-threatening and non-judgemental way can be helpful (e.g., Jackson and Cook, 2005). There is evidence that, in the UK, staff attitudes may not make this easy to do in practice (Day et al., 2005), whereas in the USA they appear to be more positive (McDowell et al., 1996; Roman and Blum, 1998; Forman et al., 2001). Staff personal awareness of their own spirituality, and the preferences and prejudices associated with this, is undoubtedly important as a first step to ensuring that service users are given the opportunity to discuss spirituality and its constituent parts (e.g., beliefs, relationships, values, meaning and purpose) during the course of their treatment.

Treatment Outcome Research

Nearly all rigorous research investigations that have examined the clinical and public health utility of spiritual/religious approaches to addiction have been conducted on Twelve-Step treatments and related involvement in AA or similar organisations (e.g., NA, CA). For example, in a systematic review of scientifically rigorous randomised controlled trials of the effects of spiritual/religious interventions on alcohol/drug use outcomes conducted by Audrey Hai and her colleagues, it was found that all of the tested spiritual/religious interventions were Twelve-Step based (Hai et al., 2019). The authors called for more rigorous studies on non-Twelve-Step spiritual/religious interventions for addiction.

The growth in rigorous spiritually oriented treatment research for addiction began in the 1990s. Given the widespread influence of AA in treatment programmes and broader society in the USA, in 1990 the US Institute of Medicine (IOM) of the National Academy of Sciences, in its published volume, *Broadening the Base of Treatment for Alcohol Problems* (Institute of Medicine, 1990), called for more research on AA, its effectiveness and its mechanisms. This legitimised serious scientific investigation into AA and related clinical treatments (i.e., Twelve-Step facilitation [TSF] treatments) that aim to link and engage addiction patients with these free community resources as a means of preventing addiction relapse. With subsequent funding from the US National Institutes of Health and the Department of Veterans Affairs Healthcare System, a flurry of high-quality research studies on comparative effectiveness and mechanisms ensued. There are now dozens of very high-quality research outcome studies that have examined the clinical and public health utility and potential benefits of providing systematic clinical linkages to AA, as well as the effects of AA involvement post treatment for alcohol and other drug use disorders. These studies have strong methodology (longitudinal, randomised/quasi-randomised design, active treatment comparison conditions, high follow-up rates and reliable/valid measures) and are published in well-regarded scientific peer-reviewed journals.

This body of work has been summarised in a Cochrane Library systematic review and meta-analysis (Kelly et al., 2020) and in other noteworthy systematic reviews (e.g., Bog et al., 2017; Hai et al., 2019). Of note, the review of the most rigorous comparative efficacy studies on the AA-oriented approaches to alcohol addiction (Kelly et al., 2020) included almost 11,000 participants across 27 trials, and examined all available clinical outcomes reported in the trials, as well as economic analyses that measured the potential for AA-based approaches to reduce healthcare costs, given that AA is available free of charge for as long as individuals want to attend.

This review found that, when compared with state-of-the-art manualised cognitive–behavioural treatments (CBTs), AA/TSF approaches were at least as effective on every outcome, with the exception of complete abstinence and remission, where AA/TSF performed substantially better. In addition, when compared with other kinds of clinical interventions, such CBTs, AA/TSF was found to substantially reduce healthcare costs while improving clinical outcomes. Thus AA/TSF was found to be as effective as or better than other existing high-quality interventions, and also to confer considerable economic savings.

Although the majority of the research has been conducted on AA/TSF approaches, there have been some high-quality research studies on TSF approaches applied to other drug use problems. These were summarised in a similar rigorous systematic review through the Campbell Collaboration, which found that compared with other clinical interventions (e.g., CBTs), TSF approaches performed at least as well if not slightly better, although the review did not report on continuous abstinence outcomes or economic analyses (Bog et al., 2017).

Of course, these studies were not direct tests of 'AA' or other Twelve-Step community-based organisations, but rather of clinical treatments that introduced patients to, educated them about, and proactively linked them with those community-based Twelve-Step organisations. Of note, however, when the proper mediational analyses were conducted (Kelly et al., 2020) to test whether the equal or better outcomes and reduced healthcare costs were in fact due to patients' greater participation in AA, it was discovered that this was indeed the case (Longabaugh et al., 1998; Litt et al., 2009; Walitzer et al., 2009). Hence, in keeping with TSF theory, one central way in which TSF clinical interventions enhance outcomes is by successfully linking patients to these free ubiquitous community resources that they can easily access in the communities in which they live. In turn, as will be outlined in more detail in the next section, AA and similar Twelve-Step organisations have been shown to confer their positive relapse prevention effects through myriad mechanisms, one of which involves increasing spiritual practices and thereby helping to reduce the risk of relapse.

In summary, on the basis of the evidence to date it would appear that treatment in programmes that incorporate spiritual ideas and practices – at least Twelve-Step-related spirituality – are just as effective as other forms of treatment. Furthermore, there is reason to believe that spirituality is positively associated with abstinence and/or length of abstinence as an outcome measure following treatment of various kinds and/or involvement in Twelve-Step mutual help groups.

Treatment Process and Mechanisms Research

Spirituality may be conceived of as either an independent (predictor) or a dependent (response) variable in treatment research. If spirituality is a universal attribute, measurable in a similar way to personality, it may prove to reflect receptiveness to treatment or to certain kinds of treatment, or it may function as a prognostic indicator. It may mediate other outcomes such as abstinence or reduced substance use (e.g., Kelly et al., 2011; Robinson et al., 2011; Tonigan et al., 2013), or it may simply be understood as reflecting a better quality of life. In addition to this, spirituality might be considered a function of treatment environment, and the spirituality of therapists (in relation to the spirituality of patients/clients) might be an important influence in treatment. These possibilities suggest complex and various ways in which spirituality could influence the treatment process, and multivariate studies of high-quality methodology will be required to unravel them.

It is also noteworthy that dozens of clinical investigations have examined the downstream mechanisms through which organisations such as AA confer benefits. This body of research (Kelly et al., 2009; Kelly, 2017) has found that these groups continue to confer benefit over time via their ability to mobilise similar kinds of psychosocial mechanisms to those that are mobilised by professionally delivered treatment services (e.g., enhancing and maintaining recovery motivation over time, boosting cognitive and behavioural relapse prevention coping skills and abstinence self-efficacy, reducing impulsivity and craving, and facilitating recovery-supportive changes in the individual's social networks). In addition, consistent with the spiritual emphasis of Twelve-Step philosophy and practices, Twelve-Step approaches are found to enhance remission and abstinence by boosting spiritual practices (Kelly et al., 2011; Robinson et al., 2011; Tonigan et al., 2013). In tests of moderated multiple mediation (Kelly et al., 2012) whereby researchers want to understand the relative importance of a set of different mediators and simultaneously examine whether these mechanisms are the same for all individuals, or whether they differ based on some other patient characteristic (e.g., addiction severity, gender, age), it has been found that spirituality is a significant mechanism of behaviour change for addiction patients with the most severe addiction problems, but not for those less severely addicted (Kelly et al., 2012). Kelly et al. (2012) surmise that individuals with more severe alcohol-related impairment may be more open to spiritual approaches or perceive a greater need for the potential benefits that such approaches offer, such as providing a framework for self-forgiveness (Robinson et al., 2011; Krentzman, 2017) and an emphasis on values and enhanced meaning and purpose (Chen, 2006).

This pattern of findings with regard to AA's efficacy and mechanisms thus suggests that TSF works by successfully linking patients to AA groups in the communities in which they live, and that AA participation in turn mobilises a variety of helpful therapeutic mechanisms, including spirituality, that help patients to remain abstinent and in remission or reduce their use and the related consequences.

A large number of additional, less scientifically rigorous studies have been published in which various measures of outcome and spirituality have been related, although they do not meet all the rigorous criteria specified by Humphreys and Gifford (2006). For further details of earlier studies, see the tables in Cook (2009).

Several other studies have looked at the ways in which spirituality has been examined in relation to the process of treatment of and/or recovery from substance misuse. The pattern of findings suggests that there is a universally positive relationship between spirituality and the treatment process, with spirituality tending to increase during treatment/recovery and/or being perceived by treatment recipients as an important part of the treatment/recovery process. However, in one study (Borman and Dixon, 1998), spirituality increased during treatment in both Twelve-Step and other types of treatment programmes. This perhaps provides a reminder that spirituality is an aspect of the treatment process that may be implicit as well as explicit, and that it deserves attention not only in explicitly spiritual approaches to treatment, but also in all forms of treatment for substance misuse.

Two further studies are worthy of further comment. A study by Chen (2006) arguably meets Humphreys and Gifford's criteria of longitudinal design, comparison groups, high follow-up rates and reliable/valid measures (Humphreys and Gifford, 2006). Attrition rates were low (28% among those attending NA and participating in a Twelve-Step course, and 26% in a group attending NA only) and valid/reliable measures were used. The study subjects were prison inmates. Therefore ultimate alcohol/drug use outcomes were not evaluated, and it remains to be seen how individuals exposed to such an intervention fare when they are released from prison. That said, the study found some noteworthy intermediate outcome benefits that are empirically associated with improvements in ultimate substance use outcomes. Specifically, those who participated in a Twelve-Step 'course' (a total of 480 hours over 6 months, providing comprehensive explanations of the 12 steps) in addition to NA attendance demonstrated a higher sense of coherence and meaning in life, and reduced anxiety, depression and hostility, over the 12-month course of the study, compared with those who did not participate in such a course.

A study by Fiorentine and Hillhouse (2000) is also of interest in terms of the light that it sheds on the treatment process. Measures of spirituality were concerned here with embracement of Twelve-Step ideology, and it is again disappointing that other more generally relevant measures were not employed. Although acceptance of Twelve-Step ideology was found to predict attendance at 12- step meetings, it was also found that acceptance of the ideology predicted abstinence independent of this. In particular, acceptance of the need for lifelong attendance at Twelve-Step meetings and the need to surrender to a 'Higher Power' were predictors of attendance, but belief that controlled drug use is not possible was predictive of abstinence (independent of attendance). However, the aspect of ideology that predicted abstinence was the idea that a return to controlled or non-problematic use would never be possible. The authors comment that their 'findings suggest that the spiritual emphasis of Twelve-Step programmes does not assist in the process of recovery' (Fiorentine and Hillhouse, 2000, p. 385). This is argued on the basis that the spiritual emphasis of the programme (which they understand only in relation to the aspects of ideology that relate directly to a 'Higher Power') must exclude some potential members. Although this may be the case, their overall conclusion regarding spirituality is highly debatable. Clearly there is a complex relationship between the component beliefs of Twelve-Step ideology, some of which might appear more immediately 'spiritual' than others, but all of which are interrelated as comprising a whole package.

A number of qualitative studies (e.g., Heinz et al., 2010; Shamsalina et al., 2014) show that individuals recovering from substance misuse believe that spirituality is an important part of the process of their recovery, and that this may take different forms, according to faith tradition, involvement with a Twelve-Step programme and other factors. The findings reveal varying understandings of what spirituality is and how it can help. These understandings generally reflect different selections, emphases upon and combinations of the 13 component concepts of spirituality discussed earlier (and described in more detail in Cook, 2004). Future research needs to more clearly identify them and examine their interrelationships and interdependence.

In summary, much has been learned about how spirituality plays a role in the change process for those suffering from addiction of various kinds. The Twelve-Step-oriented mechanisms research, which possesses strong methodological rigour, provides support for the role that salubrious changes in social networks and relationships play in helping people to achieve remission, but also for enhancing self-efficacy and coping skills, and reducing craving and impulsivity (Kelly et al., 2009; Kelly, 2017). The sophisticated multiple mediational studies and studies of moderated multiple mediation have also elucidated the notion that Twelve-Step spiritually oriented organisations confer benefit in different ways for different people over time (Kelly et al., 2012). Specifically, these organisations possess and provide access to a number of therapeutic elements from which various participants can choose in order to help them with the challenges involved in their specific stage of recovery and/or life context (Kelly, 2017). For some individuals, but not all, spirituality and spiritual practices (e.g., prayer and meditation) may play a particularly salient therapeutic role both in attracting and engaging them with treatment and recovery support programmes (e.g., black Americans; Kelly and Eddie, 2020) and in reducing the risk of relapse by providing a new sense of purpose, re-establishing a personal value system, and enabling them to engage in new meaningful relationships.

Limitations

This evidence base has several limitations. Almost all of the relevant studies were conducted in the USA, and the applicability of their findings to Europe or other parts of the world is not known. Similarly, the studies were concerned primarily with Twelve-Step spirituality. Exceptions to this include one study in which attendance at religious services predicted abstinence as a treatment outcome (Brown et al., 2004), and another in which traditional spiritual practices of Native Americans were the focus of interest (Stone et al., 2006). In many studies the faith tradition of participants was not specified, and in those where it was, the bias was almost always towards Christianity (with the exception of Stone et al., 2006). The instruments used to measure spirituality as a variable and the underlying conception of spirituality that they reflect were diverse. There remains much to be learned about how individuals themselves understand, experience and define 'spirituality', and how some people may actually change along dimensions that they themselves would not necessarily define as being 'spiritual' (e.g., relatedness, meaning and purpose in life), but others might. Qualitative research investigations of spirituality among individuals with various addiction problems reveal strong interest, complexity and richness, which thus far have not been adequately captured by existing measures. Consequently, with ever greater numbers of individuals identifying as 'spiritual but not religious', and the growth of 'spiritual' but 'not religious' organisations such as AA, there is opportunity for much research in this area for addiction scholars.

Conclusion

Spirituality and addiction are intimately related. This relationship is partly a product of the nature of the negative personal impacts as well as the negative externalities associated with alcohol and other drug use and behavioural addiction throughout history. This is especially true of the history of religious concern with the morality of substance misuse and the history of the Twelve-Step movement and its spiritual response to addiction. There also appears to be a more fundamental relationship that touches upon the very core of what it means to be a human being – the experience of being related to self, others and a wider, 'transcendent' reality, and the experiences of personal freedom and choice which are so severely compromised in the addictive state. These relationships are borne out by qualitative and quantitative research, which shows that there is an evidence base both for a protective effect of spirituality against the development of substance misuse, and also for spirituality as an important variable for study in substance misuse treatment and recovery research.

Yet, if spirituality is reduced merely to a variable of objective importance for evidence-based medicine, its true significance may be missed. It is concerned with both the objective and subjective aspects of the practice of addiction psychiatry, and with the subjectivity of what it is to be human. This is something which should draw together therapist and patient in a way that both respects and transcends the social boundaries that are defined by professional relationships.

References

Abdel-Mawgoud, M., Fateem, L. and Al-Sharif, A. I. (1995) Development of a comprehensive treatment program for chemical dependency at Al Amal Hospital, Dammam. *Journal of Substance Abuse Treatment*, 12, 369–376.

Alcoholics Anonymous (1952) *Twelve Steps and Twelve Traditions*. New York: Alcoholics Anonymous World Services.

Alcoholics Anonymous (1976) *Alcoholics Anonymous: The Story of How Many Thousands of Men and Women Have Recovered from Alcoholism*. New York: Alcoholics Anonymous World Services, Inc.

Alcoholics Anonymous (1977) *Twelve Steps and Twelve Traditions*. New York: Alcoholics Anonymous World Services, Inc.

Alcoholics Anonymous World Services (2001) *Alcoholics Anonymous: The Story of How Thousands of Men and Women Have Recovered from Alcoholism*. New York: Alcoholics Anonymous World Services.

Ali, M. (2014) Perspectives on drug addiction in Islamic history and theology. *Religions*, 5, 912–928.

Arnold, R., Avants, S. K., Margolin, A. and Marcotte, D. (2002) Patient attitudes concerning the inclusion of spirituality into addiction treatment. *Journal of Substance Abuse Treatment*, 23, 319–326.

Avants, S. K. and Margolin, A. (2004) Development of Spiritual Self-Schema (3-S) therapy for the treatment of addictive and HIV risk behavior: a convergence of cognitive and Buddhist psychology. *Journal of Psychotherapy Integration*, 14, 253–289.

Barrett, M. E. (1997) Prevention programs: Wat Thamkrabok: a Buddhist drug rehabilitation program in Thailand. *Substance Use & Misuse*, 32, 435–459.

Bog, M., Filges, T., Brannstrom, L., Jorgensen, A. and Fredriksson, M. K. (2017) Twelve-step programs for reducing illicit drug use. *Campbell Systematic Reviews*, 13, 1–149.

Borman, P. D. and Dixon, D. N. (1998) Spirituality and the Twelve steps of substance abuse recovery. *Journal of Psychology and Theology*, 26, 287–291.

Bowen, S., Witkiewitz, K., Clifasefi, S. L. et al. (2014) Relative efficacy of mindfulness-based relapse prevention, standard relapse prevention, and treatment as usual for substance use disorders: a randomized clinical trial. *JAMA Psychiatry*, 71, 547–556.

Brown, B. S., O'Grady, K., Battjes, R. J. and Farrell, E. V. (2004) Factors associated with treatment outcomes in an aftercare population. *The American Journal on Addictions*, 13, 447–460.

Carroll, J. F. X., McGinley, J. J. and Mack, S. E. (2000) Exploring the expressed spiritual needs and concerns of drug-dependent males in modified, therapeutic community treatment. *Alcoholism Treatment Quarterly*, 18, 79–92.

Chamberlain, T. J. and Hall, C. A. (2000) *Realized Religion: Relationship Between Religion and Health*, Radnor, PA: Templeton Foundation Press.

Chen, G. (2006) Social support, spiritual program, and addiction recovery. *International Journal of Offender Therapy and Comparative Criminology*, 50, 306–323.

Cook, C. C. H. (1988a) The Minnesota Model in the management of drug and alcohol dependency: miracle, method or myth? Part I. The philosophy and the programme. *British Journal of Addiction*, 83, 625–634.

Cook, C. C. H. (1988b) The Minnesota Model in the management of drug and alcohol dependency: miracle, method or myth? Part II. Evidence and conclusions. *British Journal of Addiction*, 83, 735–748.

Cook, C. C. H. (2004) Addiction and spirituality. *Addiction*, 99, 539–551.

Cook, C. C. H. (2006) *Alcohol, Addiction and Christian Ethics*. Cambridge: Cambridge University Press.

Cook, C. C. H. (2009) Substance misuse. In C. C. Cook and A. Powell, eds., *Spirituality and Psychiatry*. Cambridge: Cambridge University Press, pp. 139–168.

Cook, C. C. H., Goddard, D. and Westall, R. (1997) Knowledge and experience of drug use amongst church affiliated young people. *Drug and Alcohol Dependence*, 46, 9–17.

Crabbe, J. C. (2002) Genetic contributions to addiction. *Annual Review of Psychology*, 53, 435–462.

Day, E., Gaston, R. L., Furlong, E., Murali, V. and Copello, A. (2005) United Kingdom substance misuse treatment workers' attitudes toward twelve-step self-help groups. *Journal of Substance Abuse Treatment*, 29, 321–327.

Dermatis, H., Guschwan, M. T., Galanter, M. and Bunt, G. (2004) Orientation toward spirituality and self-help approaches in the therapeutic community. *Journal of Addictive Diseases*, 23, 39–54.

Emrick, C. D., Tonigan, J. S., Montgomery, H. and Little, L. (1993) Alcoholics Anonymous: what is currently known? In B. S. McCrady and W. R. Miller, eds., *Research on Alcoholics Anonymous: Opportunities and Alternatives*. Piscataway, NJ: Rutgers Center of Alcohol Studies, pp. 41–76.

Fiorentine, R. and Hillhouse, M. P. (2000) Drug treatment and twelve-step program participation: the additive effects of integrated recovery activities. *Journal of Substance Abuse Treatment*, 18, 65–74.

Forman, R. F., Bovasso, G. and Woody, G. (2001) Staff beliefs about addiction treatment. *Journal of Substance Abuse Treatment*, 21, 1–9.

Garrett, M. T. and Carroll, J. J. (2000) Mending the broken circle: treatment of substance dependence among Native Americans. *Journal of Counseling & Development*, 78, 379–388.

Giordano, A. L., Prosek, E. A., Daly, C. M. et al. (2015) Exploring the relationship between religious coping and spirituality among three types of collegiate substance abuse. *Journal of Counseling & Development*, 93, 70–79.

Gossop, M., Harris, J., Best, D. et al. (2003) Is attendance at Alcoholics Anonymous meetings after inpatient treatment related to improved outcomes? A six-month follow-up study. *Alcohol and Alcoholism*, 38, 421–426.

Groves, P. (1998) Doing and being: a Buddhist perspective on craving and addiction. In: P. Barker and B. Davidson, eds., *Psychiatric Nursing: Ethical Strife*. London: Edward Arnold, pp. 202–210.

Groves, P. (2014) Buddhist approaches to addiction recovery. *Religions*, 5, 985–1000.

Groves, P. and Farmer, R. (1994) Buddhism and addictions. *Addiction Research*, 2, 183–194.

Gruner, L. R. (1979) Comparative analysis of therapeutic models of using the Teen Challenge paradigm. *Cornell Journal of Social Relations*, 14, 191–211.

Hai, A. H., Franklin, C., Park, S., Dinitto, D. M. and Aurelio, N. (2019) The efficacy of spiritual/religious interventions for substance use problems: a systematic review and meta-analysis of randomized controlled trials. *Drug and Alcohol Dependence*, 202, 134–148.

Heinz, A. J., Disney, E. R., Epstein, D. H. et al. (2010) A focus-group study on spirituality and substance-user treatment. *Substance Use & Misuse*, 45, 134–153.

Honderich, T., ed. (1995) *The Oxford Companion to Philosophy*. New York: Oxford University Press.

Hope, L. C. and Cook, C. C. H. (2001) The role of Christian commitment in predicting drug use amongst church affiliated young people. *Mental Health, Religion & Culture*, 4, 109–117.

Humphreys, K. (2004) *Circles of Recovery: Self-Help Organizations for Addictions*. Cambridge: Cambridge University Press.

Humphreys, K. and Gifford, E. (2006) Religion, spirituality, and the troublesome use of substances. In W. R. Miller and K. M. Carroll, eds., *Rethinking Substance Abuse: What the Science Shows, and What We Should Do About It*. New York: Guilford Press, pp. 257–274.

Institute of Medicine (1990) *Broadening the Base of Treatment for Alcohol Problems*. Washington, DC: National Academies Press.

Jackson, P. and Cook, C. C. H. (2005) Introduction of a spirituality group in a community service for people with drinking problems. *Journal of Substance Use*, 10, 375–383.

James, W. (1985) *The Varieties of Religious Experience*. Cambridge, MA: Harvard University Press.

Judge, J. J. (1971) Alcoholism treatment at the Salvation Army: a new men's social service center program. *Quarterly Journal of Studies on Alcohol*, 32, 462–467.

Kelly, J. F. (2017) Is Alcoholics Anonymous religious, spiritual, neither? Findings from 25 years of mechanisms of behavior change research. *Addiction*, 112, 929–936.

Kelly, J. F. and Eddie, D. (2020) The role of spirituality and religiousness in aiding recovery from alcohol and other drug problems: an investigation in a national U.S. sample. *Psychology of Religion and Spirituality*, 12, 116–123.

Kelly, J. F. and McCrady, B. S. (2009) Twelve-step facilitation in non-specialty settings. In M. Galenter, ed., *Research on Alcoholism: Alcoholics Anonymous and Spiritual Aspects of Recovery*. New York: Springer, pp. 797–836.

Kelly, J. F., Magill, M. and Stout, R. L. (2009) How do people recover from alcohol dependence? A systematic review of the research on mechanisms of behavior change in Alcoholics Anonymous. *Addiction Research & Theory*, 17, 236–259.

Kelly, J. F., Stout, R. L., Magill, M., Tonigan, J. S. and Pagano, M. E. (2011) Spirituality in recovery: a lagged mediational analysis of Alcoholics Anonymous' principal theoretical mechanism of behavior change. *Alcoholism: Clinical and Experimental Research*, 35, 454–463.

Kelly, J. F., Hoeppner, B., Stout, R. L. and Pagano, M. (2012) Determining the relative importance of the mechanisms of behavior change within Alcoholics Anonymous: a multiple mediator analysis. *Addiction*, 107, 289–299.

Kelly, J. F., Saitz, R. and Wakeman, S. E. (2016) Language, substance use disorders, and policy: the need to reach consensus on an "addiction-ary". *Alcoholism Treatment Quarterly*, 34, 116–123.

Kelly, J. F., Humphreys, K. and Ferri, M. (2020) Alcoholics Anonymous and other 12-step programs for alcohol use disorder. *Cochrane Database of Systematic Reviews*, 3, CD012880.

Kelly, J. F., Greene, M. C. and Abry, A. (2021) A US national randomized study to guide how best to reduce stigma when describing drug-related impairment in practice and policy. *Addiction*, 116, 1757–1767.

Koenig, H. G. (2005) *Faith and Mental Health: Religious Resources for Healing*. West Conshohocken, PA: Templeton Foundation Press.

Koenig, H. G., McCullough, M. E. and Larson, D. B. (2001) *Handbook of Religion and Health*. New York: Oxford University Press.

Krentzman, A. R. (2017) Longitudinal differences in spirituality and religiousness between men and women in treatment for alcohol use disorders. *Psychology of Religion and Spirituality*, 9 (Suppl. 1), S11–S21.

Kurtz, E. (1991) *Not-God: A History of Alcoholics Anonymous*. Center City, MN: Hazelden.

Kurtz, E. (1996) Twelve step programs. In P. H. Van Ness, ed., *Spirituality and the Secular Quest*. New York: Crossroad Publishing Co., pp. 277–302.

Leigh, J., Bowen, S. and Marlatt, G. A. (2005) Spirituality, mindfulness and substance abuse. *Addictive Behaviors*, 30, 1335–1341.

Litt, M. D., Kadden, R. M., Kabela-Cormier, E. and Petry, N. M. (2009) Changing network support for drinking: Network Support Project two-year follow-up. *Journal of Consulting and Clinical Psychology*, 77, 229–242.

Loewenthal, K. (2014) Addiction: alcohol and substance abuse in Judaism. *Religions*, 5, 972–984.

Longabaugh, R., Wirtz, P. W., Zweben, A. and Stout, R. L. (1998) Network support for drinking, Alcoholics Anonymous and long-term matching effects. *Addiction*, 93, 1313–1333.

McDowell, D., Galanter, M., Goldfarb, L. and Lifshutz, H. (1996) Spirituality and the treatment of the dually diagnosed: an investigation of patient and staff attitudes. *Journal of Addictive Diseases*, 15, 55–68.

Manning, V., Best, D., Faulkner, N. et al. (2012) Does active referral by a doctor or Twelve-Step peer improve Twelve-Step meeting attendance? Results from a pilot randomised control trial. *Drug and Alcohol Dependence*, 126, 131–137.

Mason-John, V. and Groves, P. (2013) *Eight Step Recovery: Using the Buddha's Teachings to Overcome Addiction*. Cambridge: Windhorse.

Mercadante, L. A. (1996) *Victims and Sinners: Spiritual Roots of Addiction and Recovery*. Louisville, KY: Westminster John Knox Press.

Mercadante, L. A. (2014) *Belief Without Borders: Inside the Minds of the Spiritual but not Religious*. New York: Oxford University Press.

Maslow, A. H. (1943) A theory of human motivation. *Psychological Review*, 50, 370–396.

Maslow, A. H. (1987) *Motivation and Personality*, 3rd ed. New York: Harper & Row Publishers.

Moos, R. H. (2007) Theory-based active ingredients of effective treatments for substance use disorders. *Drug and Alcohol Dependence*, 88, 109–121.

Moos, R. H., Mehren, B. and Moos, B. S. (1978) Evaluation of a Salvation Army alcoholism treatment program. *Journal of Studies on Alcohol*, 39, 1267–1275.

Morjaria-Keval, A. and Keval, H. (2015) Reconstructing Sikh spirituality in recovery from alcohol addiction. *Religions*, 6, 122–138.

Narcotics Anonymous World Services (1986) *NA White Booklet*. Available at www.na .org/admin/include/spaw2/uploads/pdf/ litfiles/us_english/Booklet/NA%20White% 20Booklet.pdf (accessed 9 November 2010).

National Institute on Drug Abuse (1977) *An Evaluation of the Teen Challenge Treatment Program*. Bethesda, MD: National Institute on Drug Abuse.

Owen, S. (2014) Walking in balance: Native American recovery programmes. *Religions*, 5, 1037–1049.

Ritt-Olson, A., Milam, J., Unger, J. B. et al. (2004) The protective influence of spirituality and "Health-as-a-Value" against monthly substance use among adolescents varying in risk. *Journal of Adolescent Health*, 34, 192–199.

Robinson, E. A., Krentzman, A. R., Webb, J. R. and Brower, K. J. (2011) Six-month changes in spirituality and religiousness in alcoholics predict drinking outcomes at nine months. *Journal of Studies on Alcohol and Drugs*, 72, 660–668.

Roman, P. M. and Blum, T. C. (1998) Summary report (No. 3): second wave on-site results. National treatment center study. Unpublished manuscript, University of Georgia.

Room, R., Rehm, J., Trotter, R. T., Paglia, A. and Üstün, T. B. (2001) Cross-cultural views on stigma, valuation, parity, and societal values towards disability. In T. B. Üstün, S. Chatterji, J. E. Bickenbach et al., eds., *Disability and Culture: Universalism and Diversity*. Seattle, WA: Hofgrebe & Huber, pp. 247–291.

Rush, B. (1785) An inquiry into the effects of ardent spirits upon the human body and mind: with an account of the means of preventing, and of the remedies for curing them. Reprinted 1943 in *Quarterly Journal of Studies on Alcohol*, 4, 325–341.

Shamsalina, A., Norouzi, K., Fallahi Khoshknab, M. and Farhoudiyan, A. (2014) Recovery based on spirituality in substance abusers in Iran. *Global Journal of Health Science*, 6, 154–162.

Stewart, C. (2001) The influence of spirituality on substance use of college students. *Journal of Drug Education*, 31, 343–351.

Stone, R. A., Whitbeck, L. B., Chen, X., Johnson, K. and Olson, D. M. (2006) Traditional practices, traditional spirituality, and alcohol cessation among American Indians. *Journal of Studies on Alcohol*, 67, 236–244.

Tonigan, J. S., Rynes, K. N. and McCrady, B. S. (2013) Spirituality as a change mechanism in 12-step programs: a replication, extension, and refinement. *Substance Use & Misuse*, 48, 1161–1173.

Trotter, T. (1804/1988) *An Essay, Medical, Philosophical, and Chemical, on Drunkenness and its Effects on the Human Body*. London: Routledge.

Volkow, N. D. and Boyle, M. (2018) Neuroscience of addiction: relevance to prevention and treatment. *American Journal of Psychiatry*, 175, 729–740.

Walitzer, K. S., Dermen, K. H. and Barrick, C. (2009) Facilitating involvement in Alcoholics Anonymous during out-patient treatment: a randomized clinical trial. *Addiction*, 104, 391–401.

White, W. L. (2002) *The Red Road to Wellbriety: In the Native American Way*. Colorado Springs, CO: White Bison, Inc.

Zimmerman, M. A. and Maton, K. I. (1992) Life-style and substance use among male African-American urban adolescents: a cluster analytic approach. *American Journal of Community Psychology*, 20, 121–138.

Common Mental Disorders

Glòria Durà-Vilà and Simon Dein

Depression is a prevalent disorder. The 12-month prevalence of major depressive disorder worldwide is 6.6% and the lifetime prevalence is 16.2% (Kupfer et al., 2012). The disorder has a huge impact on everyday functioning, the ability to work and social relationships, it has enormous economic costs and it significantly increases the risk of suicide. Thus it is a major cause of disability worldwide (World Health Organization, 2020). Anxiety disorders are very common in developed countries. Bandelow and Michaelis (2015) note how anxiety disorders, including panic disorder with or without agoraphobia, generalised anxiety disorder, social anxiety disorder, specific phobias and separation anxiety disorder are the most prevalent mental disorders. They are associated with significant healthcare costs and a high burden of disease.

Religion plays a significant role in the lives of many people across the world (see Chapter 16). The World Gallup Poll of 143 representative populations across the world indicated that 92% of people in developing countries saw religion as being important for their lives (Crabtree and Pelham, 2009). Similarly, a Gallup Poll in 2011 in the USA indicated that 55% of American people endorsed religion as being important in their lives, and 26% stated that it was fairly important. Only 19% considered that it was not important (Newport, 2011). This chapter examines the relationship between religion, spirituality, depression and anxiety. After presenting a critical overview of studies in this area we discuss the 'Dark Night of the Soul', a time of profound sadness deeply infused with spiritual meaning, which has many similarities with depression. The final part of the chapter focuses on the clinical implications of the empirical research, particularly its implications for psychotherapy.

Before considering the empirical findings, it is important to distinguish between religion and spirituality (see Chapter 1). Both relate to the transcendent. Religion is communal, institutionalised and associated with fixed rituals and practices related to the transcendent, whereas spirituality is individualistic and reflects a sense of connectedness to a higher power, be it God or some other universal or worldly power. Spirituality is linked to a search for and discovery of the transcendent. Spirituality/religion may have different relationships with anxiety and depression. However, the extant literature points to the fact that spirituality and religion are important coping strategies in the wake of adverse life events, reducing the prevalence of mental disorders such as depression (Bonelli et al., 2012).

Studies on spirituality and common mental disorders are few and far between. Swinton (2001) found a relationship between lack of meaning and depression in a qualitative study of depressed individuals. Hodges (2002) discusses four dimensions of spirituality – meaning of life, intrinsic values, belief in transcendence and spiritual community. He asserts that each dimension demonstrates an inverse linear relationship with depression. King et al. (2013), using data from the third National Psychiatric Morbidity Study in England, found that those with a spiritual understanding of life in the absence of a religious framework were in fact more vulnerable to developing mental disorders. In this chapter we shall predominantly focus upon Christianity, although we shall briefly mention research on Islam and Judaism. We shall not specifically discuss Eastern religions.

Acedia and Depression

Glas (2003) notes how, over the past 2,000 years or so, physicians have distinguished the clinical conditions of affective or anxiety disorder from such 'normal' everyday feelings as fear, restlessness and despondency – emotions that we all experience at times in our lives. Depression and anxiety both have a conceptual history.

The relationship between religion, sin and depression has been of longstanding interest to theologians, psychiatrists and religious professionals. Scrutton (2018) notes how some Christian literature states that depression derives from sin and is a personal choice. Those who are depressed are held to lack some of the spiritual fruits that provide evidence of genuine Christian faith. They are advised to change their lifestyles, and are held to be in control of their lives. Change is within their power, and failure to implement it and 'take responsibility' is seen as sinful in itself. These views are still held by some conservative evangelical Christians in the USA and in the UK, and among Catholics (Ruiz, 1998). On these lines, many Catholic clergymen, monks and nuns argued not only that believing in God played a crucial part in keeping depression at bay, but also that depression was incompatible with having true faith in God, and they considered those who succumbed to depression as having a faith that lacked maturity and depth (Durà-Vilà, 2016, p. 151). Studies by Payne (2008, 2009) also showed that the clergy held a critical and judgemental view of those suffering from depression, considering them to be weak when facing life's adversities. Scrutton (2018) underscores the fact that we need to distinguish depression as a sin from depression as God's punishment for sin, although the two ideas often run closely together. Durà-Vilà (2016, p. 301) argues that these views would be likely to have a detrimental effect on those afflicted by depression, since they would on the one hand further accentuate their feelings of guilt and lack of self-worth, and on the other hand create obstacles to religious people's pathways to mental health care.

The term 'acedia' shares some of the characteristics of sloth, laziness, boredom and depression, but it is different to all of these. Norris (2008, p. 8) suggests that it is, at root, the 'absence of care'. Whereas sloth is a sin, acedia is not – or at least it is only a temptation to sin – and Evagrius clearly differentiated acedia from sadness (Cook, 2011, pp. 23–30). It is also referred to as the 'noonday devil', and involved low spirits or lethargy and a longing for a change in one's environment. Those suffering from it experienced an inability to motivate themselves. Its relationship to modern-day depression remains controversial (Brann, 1979; Daly, 2007). Even in medieval times it was variously seen as an unusual mental state or an atypical state of the soul.

Some religious people are reluctant to be labelled as suffering from depression, but prefer to attribute religious meaning to their distress, seeking inspiration from the experiences of sadness and desolation of mystics, many of whom left carefully written accounts of their sufferings (Álvarez, 1997). Due to psychiatry's reluctance to incorporate or relate to the religious beliefs of its religious patients – for whom a search for religious meaning and a transcendental dimension may be essential parts of their suffering – there is a danger of ending up seeing spiritual quests as pathological, diagnosing them inappropriately and offering inadequate treatment plans (Abramovitch and Kirmayer, 2003).

Religious individuals may be reluctant to take antidepressants. Various authors have argued that taking antidepressant medication may have a negative impact on people's religiosity and spiritual lives. In a paper entitled 'The Gospel according to Prozac', Barshinger et al. (1995) argue that antidepressants can trigger dilemmas and tensions in devout religious people as they are confronted by questions that challenge their beliefs. For example, what does it signify that praying and faith do not relieve depressive symptoms and antidepressants do? Perhaps even more disturbing, what does it signify when antidepressant medication seems to improve their spiritual life and experience of God? Chambers (2004), in his chapter titled 'Prozac and the sick soul', illustrates the troubling nature of this subject, describing the case of a patient who had been involuntarily admitted to the psychiatric ward because she was praying unceasingly and there were concerns that she was not able to take care of herself. Chambers reflected about the possibility of medication curing the patient of her constant praying, introducing the idea that in a different interpretative context this patient's behaviour might have been considered to be a valuable spiritual experience.

Religious Involvement and Depression

The majority of research studies indicate a protective effect of religion, and particularly religious attendance, against depression. Between 1962 and 2010 at least 444 studies have looked at the relationships between religious involvement (importance of belief, commitment and time spent involved in religious activities) and rates of depression. Of these 272 studies, 61% found a lower prevalence of depressive disorder, faster remission and/or a reduction in depressive severity in response to a religious/spiritual intervention. Only 28 studies (6%) demonstrated the opposite effect. Religious beliefs and activities may buffer the impact of adverse life events and function as potent coping strategies (Idler et al., 2003). Furthermore, the social support aspects of religious communities may protect against the development of depressive symptoms (Ellison and Levin, 1998).

Most of the studies to date on spirituality/religion and depression have been cross-sectional, with longitudinal studies being rare. Harold Koenig speculates that the potential of spirituality/religion to neutralise life stressors may prevent the onset of depression or shorten its course if it is present. Braam and Koenig (2019), in their systematic review of 152 prospective studies up to 2017, found that religiosity predicted a decrease in depressive symptoms over time. Religious struggle – a troubled relationship with a deity or religious community – on the other hand predicted greater depressive symptomatology. These results concur with the notion of negative religious coping proposed by Pargament et al. (1998). Examples might include seeing illness as a punishment from God, or being abandoned by him. Although religiosity was protective in those with psychiatric symptoms, the reverse was the case in those with physical symptoms. The authors recommend that therapists and clinicians pay close attention the role of spirituality/religion in the lives of those who are depressed and those who are predisposed to this illness.

Not all studies demonstrate positive relationships between spirituality/religion and mental health. A recent longitudinal study in the elderly indicated that public and private religious practices were not beneficial to mental health. Praying more than once daily was associated with a higher prevalence of depressive symptoms (β = 0.150, 95% CI: 0.003, 0.298) compared with individuals who never prayed. These results were adjusted for sociodemographic characteristics, physical health covariates and previous history of depression (Van Herreweghe and Van Lancker, 2020). Dein (2006) has appealed for more qualitative studies in this field in order to look at how different aspects of spirituality/religion affect individuals, and how this influences outcomes.

Faith Tradition and Depression

Although religious affiliation provides no information about levels of religiosity, it does provide information about the prevalence of depression in different faith traditions. There is evidence that people of Jewish descent and Pentecostals experience a higher prevalence of depression than other religious groups. In both cross-sectional and longitudinal studies, Jews – especially those who are not actively religious – show higher rates of depression (Kennedy et al., 1996; Levav et al., 1997). One possible explanation for these findings is selective reporting of depressive symptoms; Jews may be more likely to report depressive symptoms and to obtain help rather than resort to maladaptive coping strategies such as alcohol abuse. Rates of depression have been found to be particularly high among Jews of Eastern European descent, and genetic factors may be implicated here.

The high rates of depression among Pentecostals might result from those with pre-existing emotional problems self-selecting into Pentecostal groups, where there is a strong emphasis on overcoming emotional problems (Sethi and Seligman, 1993). Furthermore, the focus on evangelism may lead to recruitment of those in the lower socioeconomic classes who are at greater risk of depression (Koenig et al., 1994).

Non-Religious Traditions

Although there is an extensive literature linking religion to positive mental health outcomes, relatively little work has focused upon non-religious traditions, particularly atheism and agnosticism. The term 'non-religious' is an umbrella term that includes atheism, agnosticism, the spiritual but non-religious and those who have lapsed. The Pew Research Center indicates that there has been growth in the 'nones' in the USA, with the number of atheists having doubled from 2% in 2009 to 4% in 2019.[1] We cannot assume that secularity is related to higher levels of depression. Baker et al. (2018) examined a national sample of American adults and compared physical and mental health outcomes for atheists, agnostics, religiously non-affiliated theists and theistic members of organised religious traditions. Atheists expressed lower levels of psychiatric morbidity (paranoia, anxiety, obsession or compulsion) than most members of religious traditions and other secular traditions. A growing number of studies indicate that people who express strong religious beliefs and convinced atheists share positive mental health (King et al., 2013).

---

[1] www.pewresearch.org/fact-tank/2019/12/06/10-facts-about-atheists/

Two separate studies have found that both theism and atheism are correlated with lower rates of depression compared with a middle state of existential uncertainty (Riley et al., 2005). It may be the certainty rather than the type of religious belief that determines the psychological outcome. Inconsistency of belief, as seen in the agnostics and spiritual but not religious, may result in more negative psychological outcomes. Finally, recent data suggest that atheism may be associated with the restriction of displays of emotion (Burris, 2020). In this study, atheists were seen as less emotionally expressive than their religious counterparts, and were more likely to resist emotional expression, especially the expression of positive emotion.

Depression and the Dark Night of the Soul

Some religious people refer to periods of intense sadness and profound spiritual suffering as the 'Dark Night of the Soul' – an idiom that describes a spiritual process of liberation from attachments and a deepening of one's relationship with God. This term comes from the title of the sixteenth-century Spanish poem 'La noche oscura del alma,' written by the Carmelite priest St John of the Cross, which describes the arduous path travelled by the soul to reach mystical love.

Durà-Vilà (2016) conducted ethnographic research that explored the attribution of religious meaning to deep sadness among Catholic clergy and Augustinian contemplative nuns and monks. The participants used the term 'Dark Night of the Soul' to describe the experience of angst and desolation in their lives associated with profound spiritual suffering. They placed their suffering in a wider context than that offered by psychiatry and medicine in general – one that involved a connection to God and to the history of the Church, as many saints and mystics had experienced this period of spiritual angst. Many of the participating nuns, monks and priests cited specific names – such as St John of the Cross, St Teresa of Avila (also called St Teresa of Jesus), St Thérèse of Lisieux or more recent ones, such as St Teresa of Calcutta (Mother Teresa) – on whom they modelled their own experiences of the 'Dark Night', and in whose writings they found solace and hope.

Many authors have described in their works the crucial aspect of the Dark Night as giving meaning to people's lives (Font i Rodon, 1999; May, 2004; Moore, 2004/ 2011; Durà-Vilà et al., 2010; Durà-Vilà, 2016). Despite the beneficial aspects of the Dark Night, none of these authors seek to minimise the pain and suffering that accompany it. The Dark Night can be profoundly unsettling, bearing a clear resemblance to a depressive disorder, with the attendant risk of confusing the two. However, notwithstanding the similarities with depression, there is a crucial difference between them: in the Dark Night the individual never ceases to feel hope, nor does the experience ever lead to suicide. This was a common denominator in the testimonies of those undergoing the Dark Night (Cristianisme i Justicia, 1994; Font i Rodon, 1999; Durà-Vilà, 2016): it was 'their hope in the middle of their hopelessness' (Cristianisme i Justicia, 1994, p. 2). Zagano and Gillespie (2010) undertook a comprehensive analysis of Mother Teresa of Calcutta's Dark Night, arguing that despite the severity of her sadness there was no real evidence of her suffering from clinical depression, and that her profound life of prayer – no matter how arid it became – not only sustained her missionary work but also prevented her from experiencing emotional collapse.

Although the Dark Night does not lead to hopelessness, it is not devoid of risks or of deep suffering. For this reason it is important to have an accompanying personal relationship with an experienced spiritual director or confessor who can watch out for the possible dangers linked to this time of spiritual darkness – such as loss of faith and psychological morbidity – and offer spiritual guidance and companionship, and be a source of hope (Font i Rodon, 1999; Durà-Vilà, 2016).

The conceptualisation of the Dark Night of the Soul that emerged from Durà-Vilà's research made obvious the problems of the decontextualised diagnostic criteria for depression, as it would almost certainly have been considered pathological if the criteria were applied to the experiences described by the participants. Moreover, the Dark Night highlights the important part that attributing meaning to sadness plays in the way it is perceived and resolved. The participants did not see the Dark Night as a pathological phenomenon, but on the contrary they made sense of this experience in the context of their religious beliefs and faith, and were able to transform their psychological suffering into an active process of self-reflection and an opportunity for spiritual and personal growth. The Dark Night's potential to have positive consequences for the individual was one of the most fascinating aspects of the narratives provided by those who participated in Durà-Vilà's research. They described a broad range of benefits that undergoing the Dark Night could bring them, the most frequent being the resolution of inner conflicts, the 'purification' of certain negative aspects of their personalities, greater fulfilment and depth in their spiritual lives and increased compassion for those suffering around them.

Anxiety and Religion

The extant literature indicates that religion may cause anxiety just as much as it acts as a balm. Koenig et al. (1994) found that, among the baby-boomer generation, Pentecostals experienced significantly higher 6-month and lifetime rates of depressive disorder, anxiety disorder and any DSM-III disorder. The findings were highly dependent upon the types of anxiety and religion studied. Glas (2003) has argued that anxiety can be divided up into daily anxieties, anxiety disorder and existential fears, and that investigators of religion and anxiety need to distinguish between these different categories. It is important to note that, given the ubiquity of anxiety, it is surprising how little research has been conducted in this area.

Some of the work on religion and anxiety has focused on obsessive-compulsive disorder (OCD). The literature reveals mixed results, with some studies indicating positive associations (Yorulmaz et al., 2009) while other studies refute this relationship (Siev et al., 2010). One study suggests that Catholics may have a higher prevalence of OCD and experience it with greater severity (Tek and Ulug, 2001). Research suggests that 10–30% of patients with OCD have obsessive ideas about religion, and in 5% of cases their main theme is religious (Berrios and Kan, 1996). Overall, although the claim that religion predisposes to OCD has yet to be substantiated, research suggests that religion has an impact on OCD in terms of symptomatology and presentation. Finally, although religion's influence on the prevalence of OCD remains unknown, it is likely that religiosity does increase obsessional traits (Lewis and Maltby, 1994). Greenberg and Huppert (2010) have noted that religious individuals with OCD are more likely to present with scrupulosity as a primary symptom.

Although people who suffer from anxiety may deploy religion as a coping strategy, in other instances being religious may increase anxiety through threats of punishment in this life and in the afterlife. Fears of an impending apocalypse may accentuate feelings of anxiety (Koenig et al., 1994). The most commonly mentioned instances of religiously motivated pathology within the Catholic religious sample studied by Durà-Vilà (2016) were obsessive-compulsive symptomatology, scruples and guilt (when enjoying in a responsible way the healthy pleasures of life), which caused great anxiety in the individual. Intrinsic religiosity – that is, religion which is 'lived' from within – is associated with less worry and anxiety, and similarly contemplative prayer is correlated with less distress and increased security (Allport and Ross, 1967). From a Christian perspective, religiosity may heighten anxiety due to misinterpretation of certain New Testament texts which appear to say that Christians should not worry or be anxious (Cook, 2021). More recent research provides mixed results in relation to anxiety. Although some studies indicate reduced anxiety rates, others demonstrate that levels of anxiety are heightened in those who are more religious (Shreve-Neiger and Edelstein, 2004; Koenig et al., 2012). Finally, there is evidence that religiously based psychotherapies can improve anxiety to a greater degree than can secular therapy (Smith et al., 2007; Rosmarin, 2018; see Chapter 14.3).

A number of pathways have been suggested in the literature through which spirituality/religion has a positive impact on rates of depression and anxiety. They include increased social support, facilitating healthier lifestyles, less drug abuse and engendering positive emotions – such as optimism, altruism, gratitude and forgiveness – in the lives of religious individuals. In addition, religion promotes a positive worldview, places life events within a wider cosmological structure, answers some of the 'why' questions, promotes meaning, can discourage maladaptive coping and promotes other-directedness with less focus upon the self (Moreira-Almeida et al., 2006; Bonelli et al., 2012).

The Negative Impact of Spirituality/Religion on Depression and Anxiety

There is some evidence that at times spirituality/religion may have a negative impact on mental health. Not all religious beliefs and variables predict better mental health. Factors such as denomination, race, gender and types of religious coping may negatively affect the relationship between spirituality/religion and depression (Petts and Joliff, 2008). Negative religious coping (e.g., being angry with God, feeling let down by God, feeling abandoned by God), endorsing negative support from the religious community and loss of faith are all correlated with higher depression scores (Ano and Vasconcelles, 2005). As Pargament et al. (2000, p. 521) state, 'It is not enough to know that the individual prays, attends church, or watches religious television. Measures of religious coping should specify how the individual is making use of religion to understand and deal with stressors'.

A recent study on prayer by Ellison et al. (2014) indicates that prayer can ease anxiety, but this is dependent upon the personality of God that the prayer believes in. An avoidant or insecure attachment to God might result in difficulty forming an intimate relationship with him. In this study those who believed that God was distant and unresponsive were significantly more likely to demonstrate signs of anxiety-related disorders. Unanswered and unsuccessful experience of prayer may exacerbate anxiety. Finally, religious communities may engender guilt and dependency, and these may intensify feelings of anxiety. Winnell (2020) discusses the newly described religious trauma syndrome. This condition is experienced by people who are emotionally affected by leaving an authoritarian dogmatic religion and coping with the damage caused by indoctrination; symptoms include depression, anxiety, grief, loneliness and anger.

Many spiritual directors and the clergy who participated in the ethnographic study by Durà-Vilà (2016) have candidly accepted the possibility that spiritual beliefs and religious practices can turn into something harmful for the individual's mental health and well-being when religious beliefs are not well understood (due to lack of religious education of many practising people) or when religious observance becomes excessive. They considered themselves to be in an excellent position to correct these while providing pastoral and spiritual care, thus preventing religiously motivated pathology from occurring. They also argued that the church attracts individuals who are experiencing mental, physical and emotional distress, and thus people who are somewhat more susceptible to developing mental health problems.

Judaism and Common Mental Disorders

Compared with Christianity, far fewer studies have examined common mental disorders (depressive and anxiety disorders) among Jews. Apart from the research discussed earlier in this chapter on the prevalence of depression in Jews, how are specific aspects of Judaism related to anxiety and depression? Rosmarin et al. (2009) investigated the role of Jewish religiosity in anxiety, depression and happiness in a large Jewish community sample ($n = 565$). The authors included several facets of Jewish religiousness, and a theoretically based Jewish religious variable, namely trust in God. Global Jewish religiousness was unrelated to mental health functioning. However, higher levels of trust in God were associated with a reduced prevalence of anxiety and depression and with greater personal happiness, whereas inverse associations were found for mistrust in God.

In a second study, Krumrei et al. (2013) observed that trust in God and positive religious coping predicted lower levels of depressive symptoms, whereas mistrust in God and negative religious coping resulted in higher levels of depressive symptoms. These authors suggest that core beliefs about the Divine activate positive coping responses that have a positive impact on mental health.

In relation to coping, negative religious coping or 'spiritual struggles' (anger at God or religious disengagement) among Orthodox Jews have been found to increase depressive symptoms (Pirutinsky et al., 2011). The authors noted how clinical interventions should target spiritual struggles. Finally, in relation to psychological treatments, Rosmarin et al. (2019) found that cognitive–behavioural therapy was effective for anxiety and depression among Orthodox Jews.

Islam and Common Mental Disorders

Islam, a monotheistic religion based upon the teachings of the Prophet Mohammed 1,400 years ago, is the predominant religion in about 56 countries worldwide and has 1.2 billion followers (Tzeferakos and Douzenis, 2017). It is the fastest growing religion in English-speaking countries, but its impact on mental health has been under-researched (Ibrahim and Whitley, 2021).

Islamic codes of behaviour, social values and ethics enshrined in the Qu'ran and Hadith enable its followers to cope with adverse life events. Having the correct belief is a central tenet of Muslim faith. Islam engenders hope, given the fact that God is merciful: 'And never give up hope of Allah's soothing Mercy: truly no one despairs of Allah's soothing Mercy, except those who have no faith' (Quran, 12:87: Khattab, 2020). Despair has no place in Islam, since God is always in control of everything.

Despite the buffering effect of Islamic faith on adversity, rates of depression remain high in American Muslims, ranging from 27.9% to 61.9%, depending on how it is assessed (Abu-Ras and Abu-Bader, 2009; Hodge et al., 2015). It also appears that emotional disorders are prevalent in Muslims outside the USA, but there has been little research examining this specifically in Muslims (Koenig and Al Shohaib, 2017). One explanation for the findings cited earlier is that many Muslims live in relative poverty or in war-torn environments. In addition, many Muslims may experience discrimination in Western cultures, which obviously has a negative impact on mental health.

Much of the extant literature on Islam and mental health has focused on folk explanations, such as jinn possession (Fakhr El-Islam, 2008; Littlewood and Dein, 2013). There is a dearth of literature focusing on Islam and common mental disorders. However, there is evidence which suggests that people from Muslim backgrounds are more likely to deploy religious coping than are individuals from other religious groups in the UK (Barron, 2007). Another finding is that, in many parts of the world, Muslims are reluctant to seek help from mainstream psychiatric practitioners because of conflicts over explanatory models. Ibrahim and Whitley (2021) advocate that mental health practitioners should receive education in religious matters, including spiritual history taking and working with culture brokers, and that there should be greater collaboration between mental health professionals and clergy.

Spiritual Direction and Psychotherapy

The very specific aim of spiritual directors – who can be ordained or lay people – is to assist individuals in developing and deepening their personal relationship with God (May, 1982). Although the main focus of spiritual direction is on the spiritual aspects of the parishioner's life, the spiritual director is also concerned with the whole person, taking a holistic view; discussion of other issues is welcome, as they are seen as having an influence on the individual's spiritual development (Merton, 1960). It is important for the spiritual director to be skilled not only in spiritual matters but also in the psychological aspects of the self (Benner, 2002; Durà-Vilà, 2016). Spiritual directors and the clergy in the study by Durà-Vilà (2016) were found to play an important part in assisting those under their spiritual care who were battling with depression and anxiety, as they are respected, trusted and well placed at a community level, with the clergy themselves arguing that helping those who are suffering from depression and anxiety is an integral part of their pastoral care. As mentioned earlier, participants in Durà-Vilà's study attached great importance to the need to trust in an experienced spiritual director during the Dark Night in order to differentiate between a genuine Dark Night and a depressive episode, as well as offer guidance and support. The spiritual directors' own spiritual experiences equip them to fulfil a role that others could not perform to the same extent. The call felt by some clergy to become more psychologically informed and skilled is likely to derive from the deep influence that authors such as Freud, Jung, Rogers, Frankl, May and Laing, among others, have had on the Christian ministry (Nouwen, 1980; Spiegelman, 1984).

Benner (2002) offers a simple distinction between spiritual direction, which is spirit-centred, and psychotherapy, which is problem-centred. Spiritual direction and psychotherapy share similarities despite their different methods and goals. A particular case that makes the waters of distinction between psychotherapy and spiritual direction particularly murky is that of a Christian patient seeing a Christian psychotherapist. Christian psychotherapists and spiritual directors may see the goals of healing in a different light from their non-Christian counterparts (Moon, 2002). The faith of a Christian psychotherapist is likely to colour how mental health is conceptualised, thus influencing how psychotherapy is practised (McMinn and McRay, 1997).

Leaving aside the religious beliefs of the psychotherapists, Julian (1992) studied the aspects that insight-oriented psychotherapy and supportive psychotherapy had in common with spiritual direction, as well as the points of divergence among them. Being warm and empathetic are necessary skills for both the psychotherapist and the spiritual director, in order to establish a sound therapeutic relationship. Their ability to manage resistance, transference and countertransference is also essential in all three modalities. A difference noted by Julian is that for spiritual direction and supportive psychotherapy – in contrast with insight-oriented psychotherapy – the development of transference is not fostered. Regarding the criteria for selecting clients, insight-oriented psychotherapy is closer to spiritual direction: the best candidates are those who are psychologically minded, want a lasting change in themselves, have good coping skills, are able to sustain long-term close relationships and are willing and able to commit to the therapy/direction. Supportive psychotherapy may be more appropriate for those who are experiencing times of crisis, in need of emotional support or lacking the characteristics listed for insight-oriented psychotherapy and spiritual direction.

Barry and Connolly (1982) offered a key distinction between spiritual direction, psychotherapy and counselling within a Christian context, and other forms of pastoral care such as confession and preaching: the fundamental goal of spiritual direction is to assist people in developing and deepening their personal relationship with God. Sperry (2001) highlighted three areas of divergence between psychotherapy and spiritual direction – the intervention used, the aims sought and the clientele. Psychotherapists tend to use several psychotherapeutic interventions and techniques, whereas spiritual directors tend to resort to instruction through spiritual practices. The aims of psychotherapy are secular ones, such as improving functioning, decreasing symptomatology and modifying some aspects of personality; in contrast, the goals of spiritual direction are of a spiritual nature, firmly focusing on spiritual maturation and growth. Finally, the clients targeted by the two activities are also different: those seeking psychotherapy are more likely to suffer from psychopathology, whereas spiritual seekers are more likely to be relatively healthy individuals. Some might argue that another difference between spiritual directors and psychotherapists is that the former are recognised by the religious community due to their special spiritual attributes (Barry and Connolly, 1982), implying the achievement of some level of moral and spiritual superiority.

Confession

Finally, we are going to touch briefly on the parallels drawn between the Roman Catholic sacrament of confession and psychotherapy, as several authors have turned their attention to the similarities that these share. The task of easing human distress and guilt often falls upon the shoulders of the clergy and psychotherapists. Both of them deal with people's feelings of guilt, assisting them to overcome unhealthy tendencies and offering guidance towards wholeness (Worthen, 1974; Tyler, 2017). The Catholic Church believes that through the celebration of the sacramental rite of confession God grants the forgiveness of sins (Martinelli, 2009). Many religious lay people prefer it when the confessor is also open to providing an element of spiritual direction in the course of the confession (Durà-Vilà, 2016).

Jung was among the first to critically examine how the role of the priest hearing confession differed from that of the psychotherapist. The positive aspects of both disciplines were described in detail in his article 'Psychotherapists or the clergy' (Jung, 1932/1969). On the one hand, Jung considered confession to be a valuable – albeit temporary – tool for alleviating stress. He also praised the rich symbolic component of the ritual of confession, which he argued appealed to the unconscious mind, making it more accessible. On the other hand, he argued that psychotherapy did not offer moral judgements or condemnation of any behaviour, and was more objective and simpler due to its comparative lack of ritualism. Worthen (1974) believed that the interpersonal relationship established between the individual undergoing psychotherapy/confession and the psychotherapist/confessor had a key similarity in that the one-to-one interaction is needed for the process of positive change to take place. In his article 'Psychoanalysis and the cure of souls', Jung also stressed the healing nature of the colloquy carried out between the two in an atmosphere of total confidence (Jung, 1928/1969). The psychotherapist and the confessor also have in common that they are strictly bound to confidentiality.

Conclusion

In this chapter we have examined the relationships between spirituality/religion and common mental disorders, focusing on depression and anxiety. Although the overall trend is for spirituality/religion to protect against the development of these disorders, the literature is revealing more complexity than was originally supposed. Studies of these relationships need to take account of cultural and faith-based factors, and there is an urgent need for more qualitative studies in this field. The area of religious healing for these disorders, and relationships between spiritual direction and spiritually oriented therapies, have barely been explored. These are important foci for future research.

References

Abramovitch, H. and Kirmayer, L. J. (2003) The relevance of Jungian psychology for cultural psychiatry. *Transcultural Psychiatry*, 40, 155–163.

Abu-Ras, S. and Abu-Bader, S. (2009) Risk factors for depression and posttraumatic stress disorder (PTSD): the case of Arab and Muslim Americans post-9/11. *Journal of Immigrant & Refugee Studies*, 7, 393–418.

Allport, G. W. and Ross, J. M. (1967) Personal religious orientation and prejudice. *Journal of Personality and Social Psychology*, 5, 432–443.

Álvarez, J. (1997) *Mística y depresión: San Juan de la Cruz* (Mysticism and Depression: Saint John of the Cross). Madrid: Trotta.

Ano, G. G. and Vasconcelles, E. B. (2005) Religious coping and psychological adjustment to stress: a meta-analysis. *Journal of Clinical Psychology*, 6, 461–480.

Baker, J. O., Stroope, S. and Walker, M. H. (2018) Secularity, religiosity, and health: physical and mental health differences between atheists, agnostics, and non-affiliated theists compared to religiously affiliated individuals. *Social Science Research*, 75, 44–57.

Bandelow, B. and Michaelis, S. (2015) Epidemiology of anxiety disorders in the Twenty-first century. *Dialogues in Clinical Neuroscience*, 17, 327–335.

Barron, L. W. (2007) Effect of religious coping skills training with group cognitive behavioural therapy for treatment of depression. Unpublished doctoral thesis, Northcentral University.

Barry, W. A. and Connolly, W. J. (1982) *The Practice of Spiritual Direction*. New York: Seabury Press.

Barshinger, C. E., LaRowe, L. E. and Tapia, A. (1995) The Gospel according to Prozac: can a pill do what the Holy Spirit could not? *Christianity Today*, 1 August, 34–37.

Benner, D. G. (2002) *Sacred Companions: The Gift of Spiritual Friendship and Direction*. Downers Grove, IL: InterVarsity Press.

Berrios, G. E. and Kan, C. S. A. (1996) A conceptual and quantitative analysis of 178 historical cases of dysmorphophobia. *Acta Psychiatrica Scandinavica*, 94, 1–7.

Bonelli, R., Dew, R. E., Koenig, H. G. et al. (2012) Religious and spiritual factors in depression: review and integration of the research. *Depression Research and Treatment*, 2012, 962860.

Braam, A. W. and Koenig, H. G. (2019) Religion, spirituality and depression in prospective studies: a systematic review. *Journal of Affective Disorders*, 257, 428–438.

Brann, N. (1979) Is acedia melancholy? A re-examination of this question in the light of Fra Battista da Crema's *Della cognitione et vittoria di se stesso* (1531). *Journal of the History of Medicine and Allied Sciences*, 2, 180–199.

Burris, C. T. (2020) Poker-faced and godless: expressive suppression and atheism. *Psychology of Religion and Spirituality*. Advance online publication. Available at https://doi.org/10.1037/rel0000361

Chambers, T. (2004) Prozac and the sick soul. In C. Elliot and T. Chambers, eds., *Prozac as a Way of Life*. Chapel Hill: University of North Carolina Press, pp. 194–206.

Cook, C. C. H. (2011) *The Philokalia and the Inner Life: On Passions and Prayer*. Cambridge: James Clarke and Co. Ltd.

Cook, C. C. H. (2021) Worry and prayer: some reflections on the psychology and spirituality of Jesus' teaching on worry. In R. Manning, ed., *Mutual Enrichment Between Psychology and Theology*. London: Routledge, pp. 163–175.

Crabtree, S. and Pelham, B. (2009) What Alabamians and Iranians have in common: a global perspective on Americans' religiosity offers a few surprises. *Gallup News*. Available at www.gallup.com/poll/114211/alabamians-iranians-common.aspx (accessed 4 December 2013).

Cristianisme i Justicia (1994) Creer desde la Noche Oscura (I). *Testimonios. Cuadernos*, 57, 1–30.

Daly, R. W. (2007) Before depression: the medieval vice of acedia. *Psychiatry*, 70, 30–51.

Dein, S. (2006) Religion, spirituality and depression: implications for research and treatment. *Primary Care & Community Psychiatry*, 11, 67–72.

Durà-Vilà, G. (2016) *Sadness, Depression, and the Dark Night of the Soul: Transcending the Medicalisation of Sadness*. London: Jessica Kingsley Publishers.

Durà-Vilà, G., Dein, S., Littlewood, R. et al. (2010) The Dark Night of the Soul: causes and resolution of emotional distress among contemplative nuns. *Transcultural Psychiatry*, 47, 548–570.

Ellison, C. G. and Levin, J. S. (1998) The religion–health connection: evidence, theory, and future directions. *Health Education & Behaviour*, 25, 700–720.

Ellison, C. G., Christopher, G., Matt Bradshaw, K. J. et al. (2014) Prayer, attachment to God, and symptoms of anxiety-related disorders among U.S. adults. *Sociology of Religion*, 75, 208–233.

Fakhr El-Islam, M. (2008) Arab culture and mental health care. *Transcultural Psychiatry*, 45, 671–682.

Font i Rodon, J. (1999) *Religió, Psicopatologia i Salut Mental* (Religion, Psychopathology and Mental Health). Barcelona: Publicacions Abadia de Montserrat.

Glas, G. (2003) A conceptual history of anxiety and depression. In: J. A. den Boer and A. Sitsen, eds., *Handbook on Anxiety and Depression*. New York: Marcel Dekker, pp. 1–48.

Greenberg, D. and Huppert, J. D. (2010) Scrupulosity: a unique subtype of obsessive-compulsive disorder. *Current Psychiatry Reports*, 12, 282–289.

Hodge, D. R., Zidan, T. R., Husain, A. et al. (2015) Correlates of self-rated health among Muslims in the United States. *Families in Society: The Journal of Contemporary Social Services*, 96, 284–291.

Hodges, S. (2002) Mental health, depression, and dimensions of spirituality and religion. *Journal of Adult Development*, 2, 109–115.

Ibrahim, A. and Whitley, R. (2021) Religion and mental health: a narrative review with a focus on Muslims in English-speaking countries. *BJPsych Bulletin*, 45, 170–174.

Idler, E. L., Musick, M. A., Ellison, C. G. et al. (2003) Measuring multiple dimensions of religion and spirituality for health research: conceptual background and findings from the 1998 General Social Survey. *Research on Aging*, 25, 327–365.

Julian, R. (1992) The practice of psychotherapy and spiritual direction. *Journal of Religion and Health*, 31, 309–315.

Jung, C. G. (1928/1969) Psychoanalysis and the cure of souls. In *Collected Works of C. G. Jung*, Vol. 11. Princeton, NJ: Princeton University Press, pp. 348–354.

Jung, C. G. (1932/1969) Psychotherapists or the clergy. In *Collected Works of C. G. Jung*, Vol. 11. Princeton, NJ: Princeton University Press, pp. 327–347.

Kennedy, G. J., Kelman, H. R., Thomas, C. et al. (1996) The relation of religious preference and practice to depressive symptoms among 1,855 older adults. *The*

Journals of Gerontology: Series B: Psychological Sciences and Social Sciences*, 51, 301–308.

Khattab, M. (2020) *The Clear Quran*. Available at https://quran.com/12 (accessed 24 December 2020).

King, M., Marston, L., McManus, S. et al. (2013) Religion, spirituality and mental health: results from a national study of English households. *British Journal of Psychiatry*, 202, 68–73.

Koenig, H. G. and Al Shohaib, S. (2017) *Islam and Mental Health: Beliefs, Research and Applications*. North Charleston, SC: CreateSpace Publishing Platform.

Koenig, H. G., George, L. K., Meador, K. G. et al. (1994) Religious affiliation and psychiatric disorder among Protestant baby boomers. *Hospital & Community Psychiatry*, 45, 586–596.

Koenig, H. G., King, D. E. and Carson, V. B. (2012) *Handbook of Religion and Health*, 2nd ed. Oxford: Oxford University Press.

Krumrei, E. J., Pirutinsky, S. and Rosmarin, D. H. (2013) Jewish spirituality, depression, and health: an empirical test of a conceptual framework. *International Journal of Behavioral Medicine*, 20, 327–336.

Kupfer, D. J., Frank, E. and Phillips, M. L. (2012) Major depressive disorder: new clinical, neurobiological, and treatment perspectives. *Lancet*, 379, 1045–1055.

Levav, I., Kohn, R., Golding, J. M. et al. (1997) Vulnerability of Jews to affective disorders. *American Journal of Psychiatry*, 154, 941–947.

Lewis, C. A. and Maltby, J. (1994) Religious attitudes and obsessional personality traits among UK adults. *Psychological Reports*, 75, 353–354.

Littlewood, R. and Dein, S. (2013) The doctor's medicine and the ambiguity of amulets: life and suffering among Bangladeshi psychiatric patients and their families in London – an interview study – 1. *Anthropology & Medicine*, 20, 244–263.

McMinn, M. R. and McRay, B. W. (1997) Spiritual disciplines and the practice of integration: possibilities and challenges for Christian psychologists. *Journal of Psychology and Theology*, 25, 102–110.

Martinelli, R. (2009) *When and How Should I Go to Confession?* Rome: Basilica of Saints Ambrose and Charles Publications.

May, G. G. (1982) *Care of Mind, Care of Spirit: A Psychiatrist Explores Spiritual Direction.* San Francisco, CA: Harper & Row Publishers.

May, G. G. (2004) *The Dark Night of the Soul: A Psychiatrist Explores the Connection Between Darkness and Spiritual Growth.* San Francisco, CA: HarperSanFrancisco.

Merton, T. (1960) *Spiritual Direction and Meditation.* Collegeville, MN: Liturgical Press.

Moon, G. W. (2002) Spiritual direction: meaning, purpose, and implications for mental health professionals. *Journal of Psychology and Theology*, 30, 264–275.

Moore, T. (2004/2011) *Dark Nights of the Soul: A Guide to Finding Your Way Through Life's Ordeals.* New York: Avery.

Moreira-Almeida, A., Neto F. L. and Koenig, H. G. (2006) Religiousness and mental health: a review. *Brazilian Journal of Psychiatry*, 28, 242–250.

Newport, F. (2011) More than 9 in 10 Americans continue to believe in God: Professed belief is lower among younger Americans, Easterners, and liberals (online). Available at https://news.gallup.com/poll/147887/americans-continue-believe-god.aspx

Norris, K. (2008) *Acedia & Me.* New York: Riverhead.

Nouwen, H. J. M. (1980) Introduction. In K. Leech, ed., *Soul Friend: The Practice of Christian Spirituality.* San Francisco, CA: Harper & Row Publishers.

Pargament, K., Smith, B., Koenig, H. et al. (1998) Patterns of positive and negative religious coping with major life stressors. *Journal for the Scientific Study of Religion*, 37, 710–724.

Pargament, K. I., Koenig, H. G. and Perez, L. M. (2000) The many methods of religious coping: development and initial validation of the RCOPE. *Journal of Clinical Psychology*, 56, 519–543.

Payne, J. S. (2008) "Saints don't cry": exploring messages surrounding depression and mental health treatments as expressed by African-American Pentecostal preachers. *Journal of African American Studies*, 3, 215–228.

Payne, J. S. (2009) Variations in pastors' perceptions of the etiology of depression by race and religious affiliation. *Community Mental Health Journal*, 5, 355–365.

Petts, R. J. and Jolliff, A. (2008) Religion and adolescent depression: the impact of race and gender. *Review of Religious Research*, 49, 395–414.

Pirutinsky, S., Rosmarin, D. H., Pargament, K. I. et al. (2011) Does negative religious coping accompany, precede, or follow depression among Orthodox Jews? *Journal of Affective Disorders*, 132, 401–405.

Riley, J., Best, S. and Charlton, B. G. (2005) Religious believers and strong atheists may both be less depressed than existentially-uncertain people. *QJM: Monthly Journal of the Association of Physicians*, 98, 840.

Rosmarin, D. H. (2018) *Spirituality, Religion, and Cognitive-Behavioral Therapy: A Guide for Clinicians.* New York: The Guilford Press.

Rosmarin, D. H., Pirutinsky, S., Pargament, K. I. et al. (2009) Are religious beliefs relevant to mental health among Jews? *Psychology of Religion and Spirituality*, 1, 180–190.

Rosmarin, D. H., Bocanegra, E. S., Hoffnung, G. et al. (2019) Effectiveness of cognitive behavioral therapy for anxiety and depression among Orthodox Jews. *Cognitive and Behavioral Practice*, 26, 676–687.

Ruiz, P. (1998) The role of culture in psychiatric care. *American Journal of Psychiatry*, 155, 1763–1765.

Scrutton, A. P. (2018) Is depression a sin? A philosophical examination of Christian voluntarism. *Philosophy, Psychiatry, & Psychology*, 25, 261–274.

Sethi, S. and Seligman, M. E. P. (1993) Optimism and fundamentalism. *Psychological Science*, 4, 256–259.

Shreve-Neiger, A. K. and Edelstein, B. A. (2004) Religion and anxiety: a critical review of the literature. *Clinical Psychology Review*, 24, 379–397.

Siev, J., Chambless, D. and Huppert, J. (2010) Moral thought–action fusion and OCD symptoms: the moderating role of religious affiliation. *Journal of Anxiety Disorders*, 24, 309–312.

Smith, T. B., Bartz, J. and Richards, P. S. (2007) Outcomes of religious and spiritual adaptations in psychotherapy: a meta-analytic review. *Psychotherapy Research*, 17, 643–655.

Sperry, L. (2001) *Spirituality in Clinical Practice: Incorporating the Spiritual Dimension in Psychotherapy and Counseling*. Philadelphia, PA: Brunner-Routledge.

Spiegelman, J. M. (1984) Psychotherapists and the clergy: fifty years later. *Journal of Religion and Health*, 23, 19–32.

Swinton, J. (2001) *Spirituality and Mental Health Care: Rediscovering a Forgotten Dimension*. London: Jessica Kingsley Publishers.

Tek, C. and Ulug, T. B. (2001) Religiosity and religious obsessions in obsessive-compulsive disorder. *Psychiatry Research*, 10, 99–108.

Tyler, P. (2017) *Confession: The Healing of the Soul*. London: Bloomsbury.

Tzeferakos, G. A. and Douzenis, A. I. (2017) Islam, mental health and law: a general overview. *Annals of General Psychiatry*, 16, 28.

Van Herreweghe, L. and Van Lancker, W. (2020) Letter to the Editor of Public Health in response to 'Religiousness and depressive symptoms in Europeans: findings from the Survey of Health, Ageing, and Retirement in Europe'. *Public Health*, 187, 60–61.

Winnell, M. (2020) *Religious Trauma Syndrome*. Available at https://journeyfree.org/rts/ (accessed 14 November 2020).

World Health Organization (2020) *Depression*. Available at www.who.int/news-room/fact-sheets/detail/depression (accessed 4 December 2020).

Worthen, V. (1974) Psychotherapy and Catholic confession. *Journal of Religion and Health*, 13, 275–284.

Yorulmaz, O., Gençöz, T. and Woody, S. (2009) OCD cognitions and symptoms in different religious contexts. *Journal of Anxiety Disorders*, 23, 401–406.

Zagano, P. and Gillespie, C. K. (2010) Embracing darkness: a theological and psychological case study of Mother Teresa. *Spiritus: A Journal of Christian Spirituality*, 1, 52–75.

Forensic Psychiatry

Gwen Adshead

Have mercy on us, miserable offenders.
Book of Common Prayer.

Introduction

This chapter is about human spirituality in the context of forensic psychiatric services. As described by Christopher Cook (see Chapter 1), spirituality is a complex term, and I have nothing easy to offer in addition here. I start from the position that spiritual matters would seem to be those that are of significance to human existence, deeper than the temporary concerns of the everyday world. The domain of the spiritual includes consideration of non-material values and non-physical realities – accounts of faith as commitment and action, not a set of beliefs (Rohr, 2012). I have assumed here that issues of spirituality go 'deep' into human experience, and look beyond the surface to something deeper and less obvious. What lies beneath will vary from person to person, but it involves personhood, values and the meaning of our lives. What I have learned from three decades of working with offenders is that the work of making meaning of life and experience begins new every morning, and makes up the time of our life.

Forensic Psychiatry: Context and Practice

Forensic psychiatry is the practice of psychiatry with people whose mental disorders have in some way led them to act in ways that cause fear, harm and distress to others, and which often result in criminal charges. The forensic psychiatrist is therefore a general psychiatrist who works with a particular group of people at a particular time in their lives. In general, forensic psychiatrists assess, manage, treat and give opinions on people who have committed acts of violence when mentally unwell or when there are questions about their mental state at the time of the violence, or else when they have become mentally unwell after committing a violent offence, usually while in prison. Forensic psychiatrists therefore tend to work mainly with people who are usually somewhere within a criminal justice process – whether arrested, charged with an offence (usually violence), facing trial or convicted and serving a sentence.

It may surprise some readers to learn that acts of violence are a comparatively unusual way for people to break the criminal law. The commonest type of crime involves theft of another person's property, whether by stealth, fraud or occasionally force; this is most commonly the case in crimes involving drug commerce and gang violence, and although addiction is common, severe psychotic illness is rarely an issue. Forensic psychiatrists tend to be asked to assess and manage people whose violence towards others is odd, extreme or apparently driven by symptoms of mental illness. Violence towards strangers is rare, even among people with mental disorder, so when assessing future risk the relationship with the victim becomes very important. It is not too much to say that in these cases the violence is a communication to the victim, although often an incoherent one, accompanied by affects of rage, anger, fear and hatred.

Forensic psychiatry services admit people from the community, from courts and from prisons. It is well known that the UK has one of the highest prison populations in Europe; around 80,000 men and women now reside in our prisons, most of whom are there on short sentences for repeated theft and property offences, and failure to pay fines. In the range of 20–30% of the prison population (both male and female) have been convicted of serious violence towards others, and this subgroup has grown in size as increasingly lengthy sentences are given, usually in response to public cries for more punitive sentencing. For example, at the time of writing there are 60 people on whole-life tariffs, which means that they will die in prison, and it is noteworthy that there are continuing public calls for more whole-life tariffs to be imposed. There is also a large group of prisoners who are detained on indeterminate public protection orders (IPPs), who cannot be released until they have demonstrated that their risk to others has decreased. However, without help it is hard to demonstrate reduced risk, so prisoners get stuck in the system, which is highly stressful and itself leads to increased anger, distress and hopelessness. A substantial proportion of prisoners on IPPs develop serious mental health problems, often manifesting as violence towards others, paranoid symptoms and violence towards self.

Studies of prisoners in different countries have established that the prevalence of mental disorders in prisons is high (60–70%) (Fazel et al., 2016), especially substance misuse, personality dysfunction and mood disorders. Psychosis is also much more common in prisons than in the general population, which may reflect how the stress of prison life causes relapse of previous conditions, but may also indicate how psychological stress can trigger psychotic breakdowns in vulnerable people by overwhelming their capacity to manage distress (Haney, 2017). Further evidence of the stressful nature of imprisonment is provided by the high rates of suicidal ideation, suicidal behaviour and completed suicide in both male and female prisons (Favril et al., 2020). Prisoners on remand or serving sentences are therefore commonly referred to forensic services for assessment and treatment, but the UK Ministry of Justice (which oversees the management of all offenders) requires on security grounds that prisoners who become mentally unwell and require admission must be admitted to either high- or medium-secure beds. Severely mentally unwell prisoners often have to wait some time for a medium-secure bed, especially in the female prisons, and this leads to prisoners being detained in healthcare units in prison or even in segregation units because of their risk to themselves and others.

The human experience of being tried and convicted as an offender is painful and shameful for many men and women (Boyle, 1984), and the burden of imprisonment is also emotionally costly. Prisoners are socially excluded, often demeaned in the national press and on social media, and lose not only their physical freedom but also their sense of autonomy and agency. The way that detention works is that those detained often feel like children who are both disliked and punished by other 'adults', and this experience is often very close to their actual experience of childhood. A recent study of men detained in HMP Parc (Ford et al., 2019) found that 80% of prisoners had experienced one kind of childhood adversity and 47% had experienced four or more kinds of childhood adversity; such a cumulative experience is known to be associated with poor physical and mental health, which is higher than in the general population (Hughes et al., 2017). Studies of prisoners in the USA have obtained similar data. One study found that the extent to which serious, violent and chronic offenders had experienced childhood adversity predicted the degree to which they committed acts of serious violence repeatedly (Fox et al., 2015).

Forensic patients therefore tend to be a uniform group who mirror groups of violence perpetrators in the criminal justice system. They tend to be young and male with histories of antisocial states of mind and substance misuse. If they are mentally unwell they tend to be diagnosed with paranoid psychoses, and comorbidity with severe personality dysfunction and severe comorbid substance misuse is the norm. Many forensic patients struggle with borderline (emotionally unstable) personality dysfunction, which aggravates their psychotic symptoms and makes establishing interpersonal relationships with staff difficult. In urban areas, people of colour are over-represented in forensic services because they are over-represented in the criminal justice system. They include people of British-born African-Caribbean and Pakistani heritage, as well as migrants and refugees from war-torn countries. These patients may present as minorities within inpatient forensic care, which can be problematic for them, especially if English is not their first language. Women offenders are also a minority group within forensic services because so few women act violently towards others, although when they do, their violence can be highly dangerous. There are now dedicated forensic psychiatric services for women and for people with learning or developmental disabilities, but there are not enough beds to meet the demand.

The rehabilitation of these men and women is a complex process that needs to address not only recovery of good mental health but also evidence that the patient presents less risk to others. Put somewhat crudely, forensic patients have not only to feel better after treatment, but must also behave better, which means that there is a moral aspect to forensic services that is arguably not present in other psychiatric services (Adshead, 2000). Forensic services have a duty to prevent their patients from causing further harm to others, and this can lead to ethical tensions for professionals because of the potential conflict between a duty of care to the patient and a duty to protect the public.

This chapter focuses mainly on issues of spirituality within forensic psychiatric care and treatment of patients in long-stay residential secure psychiatric care. It would be beyond the scope of this chapter to address all the issues of spirituality that arise in offenders – whether at the time of arrest, while awaiting trial, at the court itself or in the first weeks and months after conviction and (usually) imprisonment. I want to pay tribute here to the important work done by colleagues in the prison chaplaincy services, as well as the NHS trust chaplaincy services that work in secure psychiatric settings. These colleagues are often 'first on the scene' after a violent offence, from a spiritual point of view, and their work is vital is reminding offenders that although one kind of earthly life is over, their spiritual life continues, and offers a way of staying connected to the values of their community and identity.

Spirituality in Forensic Psychiatry: General Comment

There is surprisingly little information about the religious affiliations of forensic patients, perhaps because this can be complex to assess in people who are acutely mentally unwell. It is not unreasonable to assume that forensic patients resemble UK prisoners, 49% of whom identify themselves as Christian and 14.6% as Muslim (Williams and Liebling, 2018); it is noteworthy that the proportion of Muslim prisoners has doubled in the last decade, and that when forensic patients seek a new religious identity, they often convert to Islam (Thomas et al., 2016). A third of prisoners have no religious affiliation, and that seems to be the case in forensic services, too, although many patients report being raised in a religious tradition of some sort.

For centuries, spirituality has been recognised as an important aspect of recovery from mental health problems, and this became more formalised with the development of the 12-Step Programme (Galanter, 2005, 2007). Spirituality as both identity and practice may assist recovery in many ways, especially with regard to coming to terms with past trauma and 'making good' bad experiences, which can be identified in what are known as 'redemption narratives' (Maruna and Ramsden, 2004; McAdams, 2006). This 'making good' process may be especially important for forensic patients whose actions have violated social norms and values and set them apart as social outcasts, and who are literally 'shunned' for their behaviour. Their experience finds parallels with practices from traditional faith discourses (especially Judaism, Christianity and Islam), whereby those people who 'sin' are condemned, judged and punished by exclusion, sometimes permanently so. The language of 'offending' and 'sin' can become intertwined, especially when patients find themselves described in the press as 'evil' or 'devilish'.

I shall describe three domains of forensic work where issues of spirituality are important. The first of these is the *medico-legal domain*, in which forensic psychiatrists give expert testimony about offenders that may have a significant impact on how both the offender and the story of the offence are seen and judged by the court. The second domain is that of *secure psychiatric care*, in which patients reside for long periods (2 to 5 years at least) in residential settings where they have to live and work with staff and fellow patients.

The final domain is one that I have called *existential forensic psychiatry*, in which the patient and forensic professionals together contemplate the patient's future, and in doing so, have to consider both his or her present and his or her past. Some of this domain includes studies of the psychological treatment of offenders, and especially what is known in the jargon as 'index offence work' – that is, the psychological work that patients do when they explore and try to understand their offence, and how they came to let themselves cause great harm, sorrow and fear to others.

Medico-Legal Work: Truth and Justice

In this section I shall focus only on expert testimony in the criminal courts, where evidence is heard and decisions made about guilt, innocence and condemnation of the accused. The individual accused may still be in shock, and will generally be advised to deny any offence and plead not guilty, even where it is obvious that they have committed the offence. The psychiatrists who assess the defendant are required to give objective testimony, which is as free from bias as it can be; for this reason, experts should generally never give expert testimony about patients for whom they are clinically responsible and with whom they have a therapeutic relationship. There are some legal and practical exemptions to this general principle. Legally, treating psychiatrists give 'expert' evidence to tribunals about whether a patient is legally detainable, and practically, the English system of healthcare provision means that it sometimes makes sense for expert evidence to be given by a psychiatrist who will treat the patient in the future, especially if they have treated him or her in the past.

The first duty of the expert is to the process of justice, and the fulfilment of that duty is attention to the truth. Norko (2018) suggests that truth is the basis for a spirituality of expert witnesses, and he discusses this further in terms of expert witness work as vocational. He describes what he calls the 'ground work' of forensic practice as empathy, compassion, presence and centring, which we might understand as mindful of the expert witness process. Norko's paper raises interesting questions about the extent to which forensic psychiatrists who give testimony in criminal trials are standing up for prosocial moral values of honesty and compassion – values which arguably the defendant has attacked by his or her offence.

The expert's testimony is also a narrative that may demonise or humanise a defendant in the eyes of the jury and judge (Griffith et al., 2010). The forensic psychiatrist therefore has a duty to ensure that he or she does not inadvertently use stigmatising stereotypes or ignore important cultural aspects of a person's identity that may be crucial to ensuring that they are seen fairly (Griffith, 1998).

There is much more to be said on this subject, which more properly falls within the literature on the ethics of expert psychiatric testimony. My point here is that the mental health professionals who work with forensic patients in prisons and secure units are members of a larger community that demands justice when one person is harmed by another. It is both ingenuous and disingenuous to claim that forensic services operate in some morally neutral zone outside the public sphere of judgement and claims to public protection. Forensic professionals are part of the social system that puts men and women in prison or in secure services, and that tension between judgement and care is psychologically active and played out from the beginning of the trial process until the person's eventual release into the community. This tension has a particular effect on the relationship between forensic staff and patients (or prisoners).

Secure Psychiatric Care: Trauma and Treatment

It is important to think about what life in a secure unit is like for patients, who can expect to live in these places for 5 years or more. For some people, this will be the first 'secure base', in the psychological sense, that they have ever had, and this is valued by many patients, contrary to stereotypes about forensic care. The regimes are therapeutic, if sometimes a little dull, and like most other residential institutions they often focus on food. Patients are informed on admission that they are there because they have a mental disorder that led them to act in high-risk ways towards others, and they are expected to work with the team to recover their mental health and show that they want to reduce their risk to others. Patients are encouraged to behave well so that they can progress, usually from an acute admission ward to a rehabilitation ward, and from there to a less secure facility or the community. Supporting recovery has been an important focus in forensic services for over a decade (Corlett and Miles, 2010; Drennan and Alred, 2013; Shepherd et al., 2016), not least because the recovery model resonates with the 'Good

Lives' model of offender rehabilitation (Barnao et al., 2016), and concepts such as 'desistance' from offending, which emphasise personal agency and narrative (Maruna, 2001).

Many patients find being a forensic patient hard at times; security is the dominant theme of most forensic milieux, and this is generally achieved (as in other custodial settings) by a small group of staff exercising power over a bigger group of residents, who tacitly agree to comply. Although there is a natural focus on physical security (walls, locks, gates, cameras, etc.) and procedural security (policies that are set both nationally and locally), staff and patients who 'live' together on a ward know full well that it is the relationships between staff and patients, patients and patients, and staff and staff that underpin safety on a ward – the kind of safety that promotes recovery. Both staff and patients together value safety, and the minority of patients in forensic units who do cause security problems are often not popular with the other patients. It is intriguing to observe how quickly patients who may well have lived highly antisocial lives become interested in living in prosocial communities that are safe for all.

I have described this concept of 'relational security' in some detail because it is relevant to how patients think about spirituality as part of their life as patients. Just as in the prisons, spirituality and faith identity are seen as vital aspects of a patient's identity, which must be respected and which may play an important part in their recovery. An early Canadian study of religious belief in forensic patients suggested that there was a positive relationship between religious belief and practice, satisfaction with life and better mental health (Mela et al., 2008). A more recent study by Glorney at al. (2019) used a qualitative method to explore forensic patients' experiences of religion and spirituality. Important themes were the relevance of spirituality and religion to recovery and personal identity, as well as prosocial engagement. Respondents also talked about how their religious beliefs supported a psychological change of mind, although some raised concerns that their faith beliefs might be pathologised as evidence of mental illness.

For many patients, their religious identity is an important aspect of their autonomy. Like other custodial institutions, forensic services often try to reduce risk by reducing patient autonomy. Patients have to seek permission to take part in many activities, and in relation to possessions and contact with others, and this dependent, supplicant position can force them into a child-like role. This is reinforced by staff often being encouraged to question patients' requests and treat what they say with a lack of seriousness, if not actual suspicion. For patients, exercising their religious freedom may be one of the few ways that they can exercise adult agency, and may explain why a substantial subgroup convert to other faiths (especially Islam) while they are inpatients (Thomas et al., 2016). Saleem et al. (2014) also note how the take-up of spiritual guidance and care is greater among Muslim forensic patients than among Christian ones, and argue that there must be proper standards and resources in the provision of a multi-faith chaplaincy in secure services.

There is another reason why it is problematic for forensic patients to be placed in child-like roles, and this is because so many forensic patients (like prisoners) have experienced trauma at the hands of parents and caregivers as children (Heads et al., 1997). The risk of unconscious re-enactments of past attachments that the patient found traumatic is high in forensic settings, where it is easy to wield authority in a tactless or even hostile manner. Some patients may fear the staff, or relate to their consultant psychiatrist as a parent, and it is not unusual for such patients to prefer to interact with the chaplain of their faith. In such cases, it is obviously vital that the chaplain maintains a dialogue with the team who are caring for the patient, and in a thoughtful and supportive way tries to help the patient to manage his or her fears and take the first steps in trust. There is of course much more to say about the pastoral care of forensic patients and prisoners (e.g., Swinton, 2013; Horner, 2019; Shaw, 2019), which is beyond the scope of this chapter and the expertise of this writer.

Existential Forensic Psychiatry: Narratives of Life After Violence

In this final section I want to explore the forensic patient's experience of being identified as an offender, and the spiritual and religious implications of this experience. It may surprise readers to learn that within the community of forensic patients there are people who have never committed an offence before the acts of serious violence that led to their trial, conviction and admission to a secure setting. For these people, their previous non-offending identity has been ripped away and they can never go back to their old identity. This is especially true for those who have killed when mentally ill, and those whose victims were close family members. For these patients, their old lives ended as surely as those of their victims, and it is not surprising that suicide rates are high in such patients (Liettu et al., 2010).

Even for patients who have long histories of violent criminality, and who have previously embraced an antisocial mindset, coming to secure psychiatric care forces them to look at their life and values. The stigma of forensic settings is well known (Williams et al., 2011; West et al., 2018), and forensic patients are often exposed to highly stigmatising accounts of who they are in newspapers and on radio and television. They are also aware of what their fellow patients have done, which can lead to conflict and anxiety. The stigma of being an offender is even embedded in the relationships with staff, who are meant to embody 'goodness' and a kind of 'moral high ground', which legitimises their authority. The sense of shame and exposure to a critical gaze can be distressing for patients, and can lead to defensive acts of hostility and belittling of care.

Forensic patients face two kinds of existential challenge – first, to come to terms with their new identity as an offender, and second, to try to redeem or rebuild a new identity that is oriented around the prosocial and literally a 'good' life. The parallels with traditional spiritual discourses from every faith are clear, yet forensic professionals are wary of making such an explicit link between 'getting better' mentally and 'becoming better' spiritually. However, the moral imperative within forensic services is stark – patients will not get freedom or privileges unless they embrace a prosocial identity and change their minds 'for the better'.

Psychological therapists who work with offenders in secure care have to be aware of the spiritual implications of what it means to come to terms with loss, trauma and fears for the future. Using concepts based on the work of McAdams (2006), Ferrito et al. (2012) explored ideas about redemption in the lives of forensic patients who had killed when mentally ill. Many respondents identified the homicide that they committed as a traumatic event for which they hoped to be forgiven and for which they wanted to make amends. A later study by the same group explored what it means for homicide perpetrators to 'come to terms' with the massive change of identity that follows a homicide, and what that might mean for their future identity (Adshead et al., 2018). We have seen patients who expressed a wish never to leave secure care because they could not envisage ever being accepted back into the general community of citizens.

The language of recovery, with its emphasis on personal narratives and agency, can be helpful to professionals who want to support patients to accept their offender identity and also 'grow' a more prosocial one. Slade (2009) suggests that narrative is at the heart of the recovery and change process in mental health, and if this is the case, it must be especially true for offenders with mental health problems. The beauty of the narrative approach is that we expect personal narratives to change over life and time, and that there may be hard 'turns in the road' (McAdams et al., 2001). Attention to narrative naturally also invites attention to language, especially the language of emotions and identity; the way we talk about our memories and experience may provide important clues about the 'security' of our mind (Hesse, 2008). The spoken word may reveal a speaker's experience of agency and choice, and also the complex relationship between their understanding of how they made the choices they did, and the judgement that is passed on their actions (Langer, 1991).

In the forensic context, narratives are not a new idea. For example, most 'quest' stories involve a transformation of the main character into a 'hero', usually after many trials and challenges (Booker, 2004). Sometimes the main protagonist becomes a hero by slaying a monster that threatens the community, and such stories have resonance for forensic patients when the 'monster' is within the protagonist – when he or she is the monster that has to be tamed and transformed, rather than destroyed. Dan McAdams' work on narrative has explored how changing the language of a troubled or tormented self into a more hopeful, generative self can lead to the verbalisation of a personal identity that uses the language of hope and possibility (McAdams, 2006).

Hope is a crucial aspect of the forensic recovery process. In fact, it may be impossible to overstate its importance when forensic patients can so easily feel overwhelmed by shame and hopelessness about the seeming impossibility of letting that shame go. Hillbrand and Young (2008) discuss the importance of hope – not just for patients, but also for staff working with patients – and practising care hopefully is another way that religious traditions link with forensic professional practice.

In previous work I have suggested that psychotherapists working with forensic patients get alongside their patients in an attempt to transform narratives of cruelty and madness into narratives of regret and hope (Adshead, 2011, 2016). The process of telling and retelling a story in the company of others and listening to their stories makes transformation possible by opening up other perspectives and other ways of seeing. It then becomes more possible to let go of a judging and shaming stance, which is so isolating, and to take up a more communal stance that emphasises what the poet William Wordsworth called 'the still sad music of humanity' (Wordsworth, 1798/2004, p. 61). Perhaps this is what the Gospel of Matthew is referring to, when Jesus advises people to 'take the beam out of your own eye' before judging the 'speck' in another's eye (Matthew 7:5), for 'how can the blind lead the blind?' (Luke 6: 39).[1]

It has been this experience of witnessing how narrative change can lead to a change in identity that has made me thoughtful about the parallels between the existential journey of the forensic patient and the spiritual journey of transformation that is common to so many faith traditions (e.g., Rohr, 2012). I have also been struck by the similarities between McAdams' account of redemption narratives as a way of making sense of bad

---

[1] Quotations are from the Bible, King James Version.

events, and the language of redemption in religious discourses – the idea of getting back something that seemed to have been lost. Finally, there are parallels between forensic psychiatry and religious discourses about judgement and 'badness' or even 'evil'. As healthcare professionals, forensic practitioners are required not to judge their patients – but, for example, to not judge a murderous assault on a small child as 'bad' seems not only implausible but also a kind of insanity in terms of the community of values to which both the patient and the professional belong. Forensic practitioners may fall back on the device of judging the sin but not the sinner, but some prefer just to look the other way and ignore the patient's offence as best they can. This turning away sounds as though it might be kind, but it risks leaving the patient alone with the enormity of what he or she has done and no companion with whom to think.

I will end this section with a reflection on kindness and compassion – 'kindness', with its roots in the word 'kin' and its emphasis on the human bonds that connect us, and compassion, with its emphasis on being with someone as they suffer, and not letting them struggle alone. Swinton (2013) has written about the importance of compassion in forensic settings and how hard this can be when one is aware that forensic patients have struggled to be compassionate to others in the past, and may continue to lack compassion for themselves. At the same time, patients and professionals alike are aware that members of the public may be outraged by expressions of compassion for people who have done dreadful things. Forensic patients are handy containers for projections of monstrousness and cruelty, and those projections may extend to staff.

Kindness is an expression of the recognition that we are more alike than we are different, and that everyone knows something about failure, getting it wrong, regretting an action or word and generally making a mess of things. In this sense, forensic practitioners can use their experiences of 'giving offence' to be kind to their patients as they struggle to achieve this new prosocial identity, to become a 'new man' (in the traditional sense of 'man' as person). It follows that those who work in forensic services may need to practise kindness and compassion not only towards their patients, but also towards themselves. The great expansion of the use of mindfulness practices in mental health in the last 20 years is potentially helpful here, although – as mindfulness practitioners know – such practices are not always easy (Witharana and Adshead, 2013).

Conclusion

I am uneasily aware that there is much more to say about spirituality and faith in forensic services, and the reader may be left unsatisfied. 'This is all very well', he or she might think, 'but what should we do to make things better? How can spirituality make people better and safer?'. My honest answer is that I do not know for certain, but I do believe that we should start with ourselves and changing our own minds so that we can be good companions on the journey for these patients. My experience has taught me that faith in people's capacity to change, and hope that they may take that first step, are essential to the practice of forensic psychiatry. A robust respect for people's capacity for cruelty is sensible, as is patience with other people's blind spots, and mine own. A sense of humour is also valuable. And in the end, all that can be said is what Julian of Norwich said: 'sin is inevitable; but all shall be well, and all shall be well, and all manner of thing shall be well' (Starr, 2014, p. 67).

References

Adshead, G. (2000) Care or custody? Ethical dilemmas in forensic psychiatry. *Journal of Medical Ethics*, 26, 302–304.

Adshead, G. (2011) The life sentence: narrative approaches to the group therapy of offenders. *Group Analysis*, 44, 175–195.

Adshead, G. (2016) Stories of transgression: narrative therapy with offenders. In C. C. H., Cook, A. Powell and A. Sims, eds., *Spirituality and Narrative in Psychiatric Practice: Stories of Mind and Soul*. London: RCPsych Publications, pp. 94–107.

Adshead, G., Berko, Z., Bose, S., Ferrito, M. and Mindang, M. (2018) Is there a murderer here? The language of agency and violence in homicide perpetrators. In J. Adlam, T. Kluttig and B. X. Lee, eds.. *Violent States and Creative States. Volume 2: Human Violence and Creative Humanity*. London: Jessica Kingsley Publishers, pp. 53–66.

Barnao, M., Ward, T. and Robertson, P. (2016) The Good Lives Model: a new paradigm for forensic mental health. *Psychiatry, Psychology and Law*, 23, 288–301.

Booker, C. (2004) *The Seven Basic Plots*. London: Continuum.

Boyle, J. (1984) *The Pain of Imprisonment*. London: Pan.

Corlett, H. and Miles, H. (2010) An evaluation of the implementation of the recovery philosophy in a secure forensic service. *British Journal of Forensic Practice*, 12, 14–25.

Drennan, G. and Alred, D. (2013) Recovery in forensic mental health settings: from alienation to integration. In *Secure Recovery: Approaches to Recovery in Forensic Mental Health Settings*. London: Routledge, pp. 1–22.

Favril, L., Yu, R., Hawton, K. and Fazel, S. (2020) Risk factors for self-harm in prison: a systematic review and meta-analysis. *The Lancet Psychiatry*, 7, 682–691.

Fazel, S., Hayes, A. J., Bartellas, K., Clerici, M. and Trestman, R. (2016) Mental health of prisoners: prevalence, adverse outcomes, and interventions. *The Lancet Psychiatry*, 3, 871–881.

Ferrito, M., Vetere, A., Adshead, G. and Moore, E. (2012) Life after homicide: accounts of recovery and redemption of offender patients in a high security hospital – a qualitative study. *Journal of Forensic Psychiatry & Psychology*, 23, 327–344.

Ford, K., Barton, E. R., Newbury, A. et al. (2019) *Understanding the Prevalence of Adverse Childhood Experiences (ACEs) in a Male Offender Population in Wales: the Prisoner ACE Survey*. Wrexham: Public Health Wales and Bangor University.

Fox, B. H., Perez, N., Cass, E. et al. (2015) Trauma changes everything: examining the relationship between adverse childhood experiences and serious, violent and chronic juvenile offenders. *Child Abuse & Neglect*, 46. 163–173.

Galanter, M. (2005) *Spirituality and the Healthy Mind: Science, Therapy, and the Need for Personal Meaning*. Oxford: Oxford University Press.

Galanter, M. (2007) Spirituality and recovery in twelve-step programs: an empirical model. *Journal of Substance Abuse Treatment*, 33, 265–272.

Glorney, E., Raymont, S., Lawson, A. and Allen, J. (2019) Religion, spirituality and personal recovery among forensic patients. *Journal of Forensic Practice*, 21, 190–200.

Griffith, E. E. (1998) Ethics in forensic psychiatry: a cultural response to Stone and Appelbaum. *Journal of the American Academy of Psychiatry and the Law*, 26, 171–184.

Griffith, E. E., Stankovic, A. and Baranoski, M. (2010) Conceptualizing the forensic psychiatry report as performative narrative. *Journal of the American Academy of Psychiatry and the Law*, 38, 32–42.

Haney, C. (2017) "Madness" and penal confinement: some observations on mental illness and prison pain. *Punishment & Society*, 19, 310–326.

Heads, T., Taylor, P. and Leese, M. (1997) Childhood experiences of patients with schizophrenia and a history of violence: a special hospital sample. *Criminal Behavior and Mental Health* 7: 117–130.

Hesse, E. (2008) The Adult Attachment Interview. In J. Cassidy and P. Shaver, eds., *Handbook of Attachment: Theory, Research, and Clinical Applications*, 2nd ed. New York: The Guilford Press, pp. 552–598.

Hillbrand, M. and Young, J. L. (2008) Instilling hope into forensic treatment: the antidote to despair and desperation. *Journal of the American Academy of Psychiatry and the Law*, 36, 90–94.

Horner, S. (2019) Through a glass darkly. In J. Fletcher, ed., *Chaplaincy and Spiritual Care in Mental Health Settings*. London: Jessica Kingsley Publishers, pp. 171–184.

Hughes, K., Bellis, M. A., Hardcastle, K. A. et al. (2017) The effect of multiple adverse childhood experiences on health: a systematic review and meta-analysis. *The Lancet Public Health*, 2, e356–e366.

Langer, L. L. (1991) *Holocaust Testimonies: The Ruins of Memory*. London: Yale University Press.

Liettu, A., Mikkola, L., Säävälä, H. et al. (2010) Mortality rates of males who commit parricide or other violent offense against a parent. *Journal of the American Academy of Psychiatry and the Law*, 38, 212–220.

McAdams, D. P. (2006) *The Redemptive Self: Stories Americans Live By*. Oxford: Oxford University Press.

McAdams, D. P., Josselson, R. and Lieblich, A., eds. (2001) *Turns in the Road: Narrative Studies of Lives in Transition*. Washington, DC: American Psychological Association.

Maruna, S. (2001) *Making Good: How Ex-Convicts Reform and Rebuild Their Lives*. Washington, DC: American Psychological Association.

Maruna, S. and Ramsden, D. (2004) Living to tell the tale: redemption narratives, shame management, and offender rehabilitation. In A. Lieblich, D. P. McAdams and R. Josselson, eds., *Healing Plots: The Narrative Basis of Psychotherapy*. Washington, DC:

American Psychological Association, pp. 129–149.

Mela, M. A., Marcoux, E., Baetz, M. et al. (2008) The effect of religiosity and spirituality on psychological well-being among forensic psychiatric patients in Canada. *Mental Health, Religion and Culture*, 11, 517–532.

Norko, M. A. (2018) What is truth? The spiritual quest of forensic psychiatry. *Journal of the American Academy of Psychiatry and the Law*, 46, 10–22.

Rohr, R. (2012) *Falling Upward: A Spirituality for the Two Halves of Life*. London: SPCK Publishing.

Saleem, R., Treasaden, I. and Puri, B. K. (2014) Provision of spiritual and pastoral care facilities in a high-security hospital and their increased use by those of Muslim compared to Christian faith. *Mental Health, Religion & Culture*, 17, 94–100.

Shaw, K. (2019) The voice of chaplaincy. In B. Winder, N. Blagden, K. Hocken et al., eds., *Sexual Crime, Religion and Spirituality*. Cham: Palgrave Macmillan, pp. 25–43.

Shepherd, A., Doyle, M., Sanders, C. and Shaw, J. (2016) Personal recovery within forensic settings – systematic review and meta-synthesis of qualitative methods studies. *Criminal Behaviour and Mental Health*, 26, 59–75.

Slade, M. (2009) *Personal Recovery and Mental Illness*. Cambridge: Cambridge University Press

Starr, M., trans. (2014) *Julian of Norwich: The Showings*. Norwich: Canterbury Press.

Swinton, J. (2013) Beyond kindness: the place of compassion in a forensic mental health setting. *Health and Social Care Chaplaincy*, 1, 11–21.

Thomas, A., Völlm, B., Winder, B. and Abdelrazek, T. (2016) Religious conversion among high security hospital patients: a qualitative analysis of patients' accounts and experiences on changing faith. *Mental Health, Religion & Culture*, 19, 240–254.

West, M. L., Mulay, A. L., DeLuca, J. S., O'Donovan, K. and Yanos, P. T. (2018) Forensic psychiatric experiences, stigma, and self-concept: a mixed-methods study. *Journal of Forensic Psychiatry & Psychology*, 29, 574–596.

Williams, A., Moore, E., Adshead, G., McDowell, A. and Tapp, J. (2011) Including the excluded: high security hospital user perspectives on stigma, discrimination, and recovery. *British Journal of Forensic Practice*. 13, 197–204.

Williams, R. J. and Liebling, A. (2018) Faith provision, institutional power, and meaning among Muslim prisoners in two English high-security prisons. In K. R. Kerley, ed., *Finding Freedom in Confinement: The Role of Religion in Prison Life*. Santa Barbara, CA: Praeger, pp. 269–291.

Witharana, D. and Adshead, G. (2013) Mindfulness-based interventions in secure settings: challenges and opportunities. *Advances in Psychiatric Treatment*, 19, 191–200.

Wordsworth, W. (1798/2004) Lines written a few miles above Tintern Abbey. In S. Gill, ed., *Selected Poems*. London: Penguin Classics.

Meditation, Prayer and Healing
A Neuroscience Perspective

Peter Fenwick and Andrew Newberg

There has been a re-evaluation since the 1980s, particularly by the medical profession, of what might be called 'spiritual medicine' – the relationship between spirituality and health. The growing number of studies of this relationship has brought widespread recognition that a spiritual component must be considered in both physical and mental illness (Koenig et al., 2012). In this chapter we shall consider some of the mechanisms underlying spiritual medicine in terms of the physiological and neurophysiological processes associated with spiritual pursuits and practices.

The Nature of Western Science

Western science is based on the rationalism of Descartes, Galileo, Locke, Bacon and Newton. Galileo defined a universe consisting of matter and energy. These 'stuffs', he said, had primary and secondary qualities. Primary qualities were those aspects of nature that could be measured, such as velocity, acceleration, weight and mass. Secondary qualities were the qualities of subjective experience, such as smell, vision, truth, beauty and love. Galileo maintained that science was the domain of primary qualities, and that secondary qualities were non-scientific: 'To excite in us tastes, odours, and sounds I believe that nothing is required in external bodies except shapes, numbers, and slow or rapid movements. I think that if ears, tongues. and noses were removed, shapes and numbers and motions would remain, but not odours or tastes or sounds' (Morton, 1997, p. 58).

Some philosophers of science have used the reductionist scheme to attempt an understanding of consciousness. Daniel Dennett, for example, argues that only what we can observe in the physical structure of the brain and its function should be included in our understanding of experience and consciousness (Dennett, 1991). This view suggests that if we understand neuronal function in its entirety, we shall then completely understand conscious experience. However, the scientific position with regard to consciousness is still very much the same as that which Sir Charles Sherrington noted 80 years ago – science: 'puts its fingers to its lips and is largely silent' (Sherrington, 1940, p. 305). Science has, to date, proved unable to formulate a comprehensive theory of consciousness.

Antonio Damasio has proposed a theory of consciousness based on an 'enchainment of precedences' – a three-layered model in which human consciousness develops from a 'protoself,' through 'core consciousness' (shared by much of the animal kingdom) to 'extended consciousness' with the emergence of an autobiographical self and giving rise to the illusion of mind–body dualism (Damasio, 2000).

The philosopher John Searle has similarly argued that mind is separate from brain, although it arises from it; it is an emergent property, but nevertheless has its own 'mind' properties. This view allows that the mind may have an effect on brain function through the brain as an independent entity (Searle, 2007).

An Expanded Understanding of Mind

A paper presented to the Royal Society by Schwartz et al. (2005) discussed John von Neumann's mathematical treatment of quantum mechanics, in which he infers two processes. Process 2 is equivalent to the old Newtonian theories of reductionist science, in which consciousness is 'made' by the brain (or is emergent, as argued by Searle), whereas Process 1 suggests that consciousness is universal and not created by or limited to individual brains.

A number of scientists and organisations now support a controversial post-Galilean view of science in which the possibility of the non-locality of consciousness, akin to the non-local influences of quantum physics, can be explored. Among these, the Galileo project of the Scientific and Medical Network, the philosophy underlying the International Association for Near-Death Studies (IANDS) and other modern societies all argue for an extension of reductionist science where non-locality is considered to be a phenomenon worthy of scientific examination.

It used to be thought that 'enlightenment' – an expanded state of mind in which the ego collapses so that the person's perception of reality is non-dual (i.e., subject and object are experienced as one) – was extremely rare and achieved only by exceptional people who had meditated in isolation for years. It is now argued that this state is not so rare, and can be triggered spontaneously after near-death experiences and other emotional traumas (Newberg and Waldman, 2016; Yaden et al., 2017). It is important to recognise this possibility as it may be confused with the psychopathology of a number of psychiatric syndromes, such as bipolar disorder or alexithymia. Jeffrey Martin (2019) describes in detail a number of different states ('locations') that finally lead to a very wide state of awakening; the Finders courses that he runs have a 70% success rate in leading to the non-dual state. Eastern mindfulness techniques, such as watching the breath and holding the mind focused, are similarly used to expand consciousness. An excellent example of this very precise observation of the mind is the Japanese Zen sesshin, which involves up to a week of concentrated mindfulness practice with no social interaction taking place. This technique has been finely honed over the years to produce an expansion of consciousness in its practitioners (Austin, 2014).

Spiritual Medicine and Healing

Spiritual medicine is an approach to healing in which verified scientific mechanisms are involved but transpersonal concepts are used. For example, in Dean Ornish's programme for reversing heart disease, meditation, group discussions and diet are all combined to produce opening of the coronary arteries and changes in the blood flow (Pischke et al., 2007). On the other hand, spiritual medicine can include examples of alleged miracles, intercessory prayer and distant healing, for which no accepted reductionist scientific mechanism can provide an explanation.

A large body of empirical research into healing has been usefully collated by Benor (2002, 2004). More recently, Roe et al. (2015, p. 11) published two meta-analyses of noncontact healing, and concluded that the 'Results suggest that subjects in the active condition exhibit a significant improvement in wellbeing relative to control subjects under circumstances that do not seem to be susceptible to placebo and expectancy effects'. Although the mechanism of the healing process remains open to question, non-locality is a consistent feature that cannot be otherwise explained.

A number of studies that have dealt with many aspects of religious and spiritual practice have shown the success of spiritual medicine. In their *Handbook of Religion and Health*, Koenig et al. (2012) look at various factors, some of which are involved in susceptibility to disease, whereas others benefit health. A number of these factors can be influenced by the behaviours that flow from an active religious faith – for example, the limitation of self-damaging behaviours such as smoking and drug and alcohol misuse, and the social support networks involved in religious belief and attendance at church services. A strong faith, positive relationships and positive thinking up-regulate the immune system, reducing the risk of cancer, improving general health and protecting the cardiovascular system.

A traditional Hawaiian conflict resolution approach known as Ho'oponopono (meaning 'to make right') has been studied by Kretzer et al. (2007), who found it enabled repentance, forgiveness and transmutation of self-image. When patients started to use this technique, their spirituality scores (on the Spiritual Orientation Inventory and the Supplementary Spirituality Questionnaire) increased and, notably, there was a significant reduction in both systolic and diastolic blood pressure.

Meditation

Spiritual techniques for raising the level of consciousness and increasing attention and focus throughout the day are found in many religious and spiritual traditions. The aims of meditation range from a simple sense of relaxation and stress relief to understanding the finest components of mind, and entering into experiences of, or union with, the Divine. Importantly, there has been a growing body of research exploring how meditation affects the brain and the rest of the body. A recent review article by Shen et al. (2020) gives a comprehensive overview of the current state of knowledge about meditation and its use in clinical practices.

Lazar et al. (2005) showed interesting brain changes in long-term meditators, which confirm the effects of habitual practised attention. They conducted a functional magnetic resonance imaging (fMRI) study of long-term meditators to test their theory that cortical thickness would change in the areas used in meditation practice. They found that the brain regions associated with attention, interoception and sensory processing, together with the prefrontal cortex and right anterior insular (used in attentional processes), were thicker in the meditators than in the controls. Importantly, older participants showed an increase in prefrontal cortical thickness compared with their matched groups, which suggested that meditation might offset age-related cortical thinning. However, it was not clear whether meditation practice had induced such changes or if there were specific predisposing brain states that enabled some individuals to engage in meditation more actively. More recent longitudinal studies have documented that meditation practices do produce significant changes by means of neuroplasticity, and that such changes are associated with improvements in cognition and emotional regulation (Newberg et al., 2010; Moss et al., 2012).

The complex set of neurophysiological processes that occur during meditation practices can differ depending on the specific elements of the practice (Newberg and Iversen, 2003). Many meditation practices involve the relaxation response, with a decrease in blood cortisol levels, pulse rate and blood pressure. There is also some reduction in the galvanic skin response. Concomitant changes in the electroencephalogram (EEG) have also been described, and some of these continue beyond the meditation sessions in long-term meditators. Other meditation practices, particularly those associated with religious traditions, can be associated with more active processes leading to an increase in activity in the sympathetic division of the autonomic nervous system, with beneficial psychological and physical effects. Here our focus will be on those practices that are typically involved in reducing stress and anxiety.

Newberg et al. (2001) published the results of a single-photon emission computed tomography (SPECT) scan study in a group of eight meditators practising a form of mantra meditation. The meditators were compared with nine controls, whose scans were part of the control group in another project. Perfusion in the left frontal lobe was enhanced during the meditation sessions, and the authors suggested that this related to a cognitive–attentional component. There was hypoperfusion of the superior parietal lobe, which they argued related to attentional processing and an altered sense of space. They also noted an increase in thalamic activity and pointed out that there was a thalamic asymmetry in the baseline of the meditators, which was different from the controls. The authors argued that these baseline changes were due to a long-term effect of the meditational practice. They also suggested that the changes in the frontal and parietal cortices during the meditation session were closely related to the positive mental states that were experienced.

Fox et al. (2014) showed that practising meditation can change brain morphology, increasing cortical thickness, grey matter volume and density. Furthermore, meditation can induce continuous changes in brain structure in the frontal cortex, sensory cortex and insula. They conducted a review and meta-analysis of 123 differences in brain morphology from 21 neuroimaging studies. Eight brain regions were found to be consistently altered in meditators, including areas key to meta-awareness, body awareness, memory consolidation and reconsolidation, self and emotion regulation, and intra- and inter-hemispheric communication. The meta-analysis suggested a global 'medium' effect size, but the authors pointed out that the methodological limitations of the study mean that further research using more rigorous methods is required to confirm the link between meditation and altered brain morphology.

Recent studies have confirmed that meditation also increases the hippocampus volume (Yang et al., 2019), as well as enhancing the cortical thickness of the prefrontal, insular and anterior cingulate cortex (Hernández et al., 2018). The change in volume of the hippocampus shows that meditation is linked to memory processes; the anterior and medial cingulate cortex, as well as the orbitofrontal cortex, are relevant to self-awareness and emotion regulation. Of note, the upper longitudinal bundle and corpus callosum are involved in both cerebral intra-hemispheric and inter-hemispheric communication.

Sperduti et al. (2012) pointed out that although there are many different forms of meditation, their common goal is to induce relaxation, regulate attention and facilitate detachment from one's thoughts, which suggests that all meditation techniques might share a core cortical network. They proposed a tentative neurocognitive model of meditation based on a quantitative meta-analysis of 10 neuroimaging studies on different meditative techniques, which showed activation of the basal ganglia, limbic system and medial frontal cortex. They suggested that the caudate nucleus, the parahippocampus and the medial prefrontal cortex are activated during meditation. The caudate nucleus and putamen participate in attention and shield irrelevant information, enabling a meditative state to be reached and maintained. The parahippocampus prevents distraction, and the medial prefrontal cortex enhances self-awareness. These activated areas may represent the core cortical network of meditation states. Moreover, there exists a dynamic process for brain activation by meditation. At the beginning of meditation, the bilateral subfrontal and temporal regions are clearly activated. As the meditation process goes deeper, this activation weakens, with the focus just on the right subfrontal cortex/right insula and the meso/epithelial layer of the right temporal lobe. This shows that the meditator experiences an initially intense self-control neural process to calm the brain, with a marked reduction in neuron activity as the depth of meditation in silence increases (Durschmid et al., 2020).

Meditation and Ageing

A number of papers describe the effects of meditation on the ageing process. Tolahunase et al. (2017) explored the impact of yoga meditation-based lifestyle on cellular ageing in healthy individuals. This prospective study looked at changes in the important biomarkers of cellular ageing in the blood. After 12 weeks there was a significant improvement in both the biomarkers of cellular ageing and the metabotropic biomarkers that influence cellular ageing via the glutamate receptor. The mean level of telomere length was increased, but was only weakly significant.

In a well-controlled study, Epel et al. (2016) compared the effects of a meditation retreat with straightforward relaxation in the retreat. They found large beneficial changes in the gene expression network, including an increase in telomerase activity, in part due to the vacation-like effect of the retreat, but also due to changes that were specific to meditation. This is an important finding, since telomerase helps to protect telomeres at the ends of chromosomes from shortening due to degradation by ageing. Progressive shortening leads to senescence and/or apoptosis (cell death). Indeed, older people with shorter telomeres have a threefold increased risk of dying from heart disease and an eightfold increased risk of dying from infection (Cawthon et al., 2003).

Conklin et al. (2018) looked specifically at the effect on telomere regulation in a 1-month residential insight meditational retreat, using meditators who were not on retreat as a control. They reported changes in telomere-related gene expression, which suggests that meditation training in a retreat setting may have positive effects on telomere regulation, which are moderated by individual differences in personality and meditation experience.

Research by Newberg et al. (2010) showed that Kirtan Kriya, a 12-minute daily mantra-based yoga practice, was associated with significant increases in resting brain function, particularly in the frontal lobes, and that these changes were associated with improvements in cognition and memory, thus reducing some effects of ageing. In addition, the study showed that there were improvements in anxiety and depression measures, suggesting that modifying frontal lobe function can help to improve emotional regulation (Moss et al., 2012).

Acevedo et al. (2016) looked at the neural mechanisms underlying meditative practices and their relationship to physical, cognitive and psychological health benefits. They compared the neural circuits implicated in meditative practices focused on present-moment awareness with those involved in active-type meditative practices combining movement (yoga), including chanting and breath practices. They suggested that mind–body practice can target the brain systems that are involved in the regulation of attention, emotional control, mood and executive cognition, and can be used to treat or prevent mood and cognitive disorders of ageing. The benefits also included improved brain function connectivity in brain systems that generally degenerate with Alzheimer's disease, Parkinson's disease and other age-related diseases.

Meditation and the EEG

An early but interesting and comprehensive EEG study by Aftanas and Golocheikine (2001) showed brain electrical changes when meditators were experiencing the Divine. The researchers examined the EEG during sahaja yoga meditation in 11 short-term meditators with 6 months' experience and 16 long-term meditators with 3–7 years' experience. They described three phases: the incoming phase, the thoughtless phase when feelings of bliss arise and dominate (this is the deepest stage of meditation, and may last for about an hour) and finally the outcome phase. The researchers were particularly interested in the correlation of electrical activity with feelings of bliss, and the difference between long-term and short-term meditators. They found that before meditation, the long-term meditators showed an increase in generalised theta activity. During the meditation session they showed high coherence (frequency correlation) of the left frontal lobe with many other brain areas. This was not seen in the short-term meditation group. The researchers also noticed a positive correlation between frontal theta power and feelings of bliss, and a negative correlation between the appearance of thoughts and frontal theta activity. This study again confirms the EEG changes in long-term meditators, and suggests that both the reduction in thoughts and the increase in feelings of bliss are related to frontal theta activity, with the left frontal lobe being very important for the higher and wider subjective mental states.

A reference paper by Kaur and Singh (2015) gives a wide-ranging review of the EEG during meditation, correlating the electrophysiological changes with different meditation practices. The authors looked at Buddhist, Zen, Chan, mindfulness, yoga and transcendental meditation, as well as other meditation practices such as paced breathing. They discuss briefly the adverse effects of meditation (increased epileptogenesis and a possible paradoxical rise in anxiety leading to disorientation and high blood pressure) and conclude that more rigorous clinical trials focusing on the use of meditation are needed. Although meditation is associated with health benefits, there are occasional reports that it may trigger or exacerbate psychotic states. Sharma et al. (2019) performed a case-based analysis of all the existing English-language case reports of psychotic disorders occurring in association with meditative practices. They concluded that although there were occasional reports of psychotic disorder arising in association with meditative practice, it was difficult to attribute a causal relationship between the two.

Braboszcz et al. (2017), in a comparison of three different types of meditation (Vipassana, Himalayan Yoga and Isha Shoonya), showed a high correlation of EEG gamma frequency between the groups.

A systematic review by Wahbeh et al. (2018) characterised the transcendental state in meditation and qualitatively described physiological and phenomenological outcomes during transcendental states (defined as being a state of relaxed wakefulness in a phenomenologically different space-time). Transcendent states were most consistently associated with slowed breathing, respiratory suspension, reduced muscle activity and EEG alpha blocking with external stimuli, and increased EEG alpha power, EEG coherence and functional neural connectivity.

Finally, several studies have explored neurotransmitter changes during meditation. An interesting positron emission tomography (PET) scan study by Kjaer et al. (2002) is, to our knowledge, the first to examine dopamine levels during meditation by using the radioactive dopamine ligand ^{11}C-raclopride. The specific meditation practice studied was yoga nidra, which is characterised by a reduced level of desire for action, giving up personal goals and loss of executive control while attending to internal sensations and withdrawing from action. The study found an increase in dopamine levels during the meditation sessions, which was particularly prominent in the ventral striatum, a nuclear complex situated deep in the brain. The subjective accounts correlated with a decrease in readiness for action and an increase in visual imagery. There was also an increase in EEG power in the theta band which correlated with the increase in dopamine levels. The paper confirms the widespread effects of meditation, and suggests that subcortical structures such as the thalamus are significantly involved. The change in dopamine levels in those structures related to movement is of particular interest, as there are many subjective reports of an alteration or improvement in movement after meditation.

In summary, there is now clear evidence that electrical changes are involved in meditation. The attention mechanisms of the dorso-lateral prefrontal cortex are prominent, as are parietal lobe changes that relate to the body image in space. Feelings of bliss and emotional changes certainly correlate with frontal theta activity, some of which will be arising from the anterior cingulate gyrus. Frontal theta also links in with specific attentional frontal lobe mechanisms. The idea of a network of areas being involved in meditation has been summarised by Lou et al. (2005).

Meditation in Clinical Practice

Orme-Johnson et al. (2006) showed the effect on the brain's response to pain in normal individuals practising transcendental meditation (TM), a mantra method of meditation. Using fMRI and applying thermally induced pain outside the meditation period, they found that 40–50% fewer voxels (small analysis areas in the pain centres) were responding to pain in the thalamus and other brain areas than in healthy matched controls. The controls then learned meditation and practised it for 5 months. When challenged with the same thermal pain stimulus outside the meditation period, this group also showed a decrease of 40–50% in the thalamus, prefrontal cortex and, marginally, in the anterior cingulate cortex. Interestingly, although there was no change in the pain intensity for the meditators, there were major reductions in the affective response to the pain, with a significant decrease in distress. This may help to explain the reduction in stress reactivity and improvements in cardiovascular disease that have been found to result from the practice of TM.

Meditation has been found to be generally helpful in those clinical conditions where high levels of arousal and anxiety are part of the pathology. Hofmann et al. (2010) analysed the effectiveness of mindfulness-based therapy for a range of psychiatric and medical conditions, and concluded that it was a promising therapy for treating anxiety and mood problems (see Chapter 14.1).

A study by Sudsuang et al. (1991) looked at Dhammakaya Buddhist meditation. The authors found that consistent meditation was related to a decrease in blood pressure, pulse rate and serum cortisol levels; these effects were not maintained if the meditation was intermittent. Jon Kabat-Zinn used mindfulness meditation (MM) to treat general anxiety or panic disorders in his Massachusetts clinic (Kabat-Zinn et al., 1992; see also Chapter 14.1). He gave an 8-week programme of weekly 2-hour sessions. These comprised a 2-hour structured class on relaxation and stress reduction each week, and in the sixth week a 7.5-hour silent meditation retreat. Overall, 20 of the 22 people involved in the study showed a significant improvement at the end of the course, and this was found to be sustained in 18 of the 22 participants at a 3-year follow-up. This study shows the significant results that may be obtained by linking meditation to group therapy. The programme was found to be such an effective way of reducing anxiety that it is now being funded by insurance companies in Massachusetts.

Zylowska et al. (2008) enrolled 24 adults and 8 adolescents with attention deficit hyperactivity disorder (ADHD) in a feasibility study of an 8-week mindfulness training programme. Pre- and post-evaluation of self-reported ADHD symptoms and test performance on tasks measuring attention and cognitive inhibition was noted, and improvements in anxiety and depressive symptoms were also observed. The researchers concluded that mindfulness training is a feasible intervention in a subset of adults and adolescents with ADHD, and may improve behavioural and neurocognitive impairments.

Reangsing et al. (2021) examined the effects of mindfulness meditation interventions (MMIs) on depression in adults over 65 years of age. They found overall that these interventions significantly improved depression, with Asians showing a greater improvement than either Europeans or North Americans. The researchers concluded that MMIs might be used as an adjunct or alternative to conventional treatment for depressed older adults.

Xue et al. (2018) found that 8 weeks of MM effectively relieves depression and anxiety emotions, and improves sleep quality. In major depressive disorder, MM can be used as an alternative therapy to medication at the maintenance stage. Meanwhile, meditation displays some adjunctive therapeutic effects in patients with severe major depressive disorder who are less effectively treated with antidepressant medication therapy (Sharma et al., 2017).

Prayer

Gardner (1983) described a number of modern miracles involving prayer that he had seen in his own medical practice. He related the case of a man in Africa who fell off a high roof and suffered potentially fatal injuries. A group gathered round the dying man to pray for his recovery. With the prayer came a change in the patient's condition and he recovered. Why, asked Gardner, were miracles of this type not more common in our own culture? He quoted the following story: 'When modern missionaries left some Gospel books behind in Ethiopia and returned many years later, they not only found a flourishing Church but a community of believers among whom miracles like those mentioned in the New Testament happened every day – because there had been no missionaries to teach that such things were not to be taken literally' (Gardner, 1983, pp. 1927–1933).

In this scientific era, how are we to conceptualise prayer? The Cochrane Committee, which reviews all double-blind randomised controlled trials, notes that proper double-blind prayer trials may be difficult to do if God is involved in the process of prayer, as 'God may not wish to comply with the conditions' of such a trial. A further methodological problem is posed by the significant background of ongoing prayer, as many churches regularly pray for the healing of the sick. Their first conclusion, after reviewing a very small sample of prayer studies, was that there was no evidence for the efficacy of prayer, although there was also no evidence against it (Roberts et al., 2009).

Prayer is a widespread practice in the USA. The 2014 US Religious Landscape Study showed that 55% of Americans pray every day (Pew Research Center, 2015). One of the early indications of the change in scientific thinking and the recognition that spiritual values could be tested by science was the publication of a paper on the first double-blind randomised controlled trial of prayer carried out in a coronary care unit (Byrd, 1988). The names of patients assigned to the active arm of the trial were sent to a prayer group, who were instructed to pray that those named would recover more quickly, have fewer complications, and so on. The results were promising. In the prayed-for group there was a fivefold reduction in the use of antibiotics, a threefold reduction in the occurrence of pulmonary oedema, fewer patients required intubation and fewer (although not significantly fewer) individuals died than in the control group. This paper became the model for a number of further studies.

Since then, there have been several high-quality double-blind randomised controlled trials of intercessory prayer. Not all of these have been positive, but many have produced some supportive evidence that prayer may be effective in healing. Harris et al. (1999) looked at 999 consecutive admissions to a coronary care unit. The patients were randomised to a group who were to be prayed for and a control group. There were no differences in coronary care and length of hospital admission, but when a coronary care unit score comprising many different variables was analysed, the patients in the group who were prayed for had a significantly lower value than those who were not prayed for. On the other hand, Aviles et al. (2001) studied 799 coronary care patients and found that prayer had no significant effect on medical outcome.

In contrast to clinical outcome studies, Ly et al. (2020) conducted a questionnaire study of 498 adults at a public university, examining their perceptions of prayer in relation to their perceptions of the efficacy of conventional medicine. The participants were asked whether their perceptions of prayer efficacy differed based on illness type, the context of prayer and whether the prayer was for oneself or someone else. Conventional medicine was perceived as more effective for alleviating health concerns overall, but participants perceived prayer as most effective when performed in a group setting for someone else. Individuals perceived prayer as more effective than conventional medicine when they reported greater religious activity, a lower health locus of control and a higher spiritual locus of control.

Does prayer help with pain relief? In a systematic review of this issue, Marta Illueca and Benjamin Doolittle evaluated a total of 411 studies, nine of which met the criteria. They concluded that 'Active prayer to God emerged as a preferred beneficial intervention for religious patients undergoing surgery or a painful procedure' (Illueca and Doolittle, 2020, p. 1), and they suggested that further research was needed to study prayer as an additional therapy for pain.

An interesting and well-referenced paper by Romez et al. (2021) describes the case of a blind girl with juvenile macular degeneration due to severe Stargardt's disease. She lost most of her central vision over the course of three months in 1959, and was declared legally blind. Her visual acuity was recorded as counting fingers in the right eye and hand motion in the left. In 1972, having been blind for over 12 years, she regained her vision instantaneously after receiving proximal intercessory prayer from her husband, who placed his hands on her head and asked God to return her sight. Her visual acuity improved to 20/100 in each eye and, when corrected, to 20/30. At the time of writing her eyesight had remained intact for 49 years. The paper reviews spontaneous healings in response to prayer, and raises the possibility of conversion syndromes, which they reject in this case. The patient's perspective is also given in the paper, and she states: 'What people need to understand is "I was blind", totally blind and attended the School for the Blind. I read Braille and walked with a white cane. ... I was blind when my husband prayed for me – then just like that – in a moment, after years of darkness I could see perfectly!' (Romez et al., 2021, p. 82).

Testing Prayer Mechanisms

The limited evidence available suggests that the attitude of the person praying is all important (Palmer et al., 2004), and that prayer is most effective when performed in a group setting for someone else (Ly et al., 2020). Furthermore, the generally accepted feeling among those who undertake prayer studies is that there is no evidence that any particular religion or faith makes any difference to the outcome. Although some studies do suggest that prayer, together with mental intent and methods of hands-on healing such as therapeutic touch, may work, much more research is needed in order to confirm these findings.

The field of prayer research contains studies that show evidence both for and against its efficacy in terms of healing. The evidence to date is that intention to heal and the way this intention is used (either as directed prayer, or as non-directed heart-centred prayer) is likely to be the most important variable, and this will then need to be tested in further research. As studies to date have predominantly come from the USA, it would be interesting to see whether European and Asian studies show a similar or different profile. Research in this field for the next decade will need to formalise and quantify methods of prayer.

Conclusion

Current research shows very clearly that practising spiritual methods such as meditation or prayer can improve mental and physical health. This chapter has demonstrated the close correlation between religious and spiritual practice and positive changes in health outcomes – what we think directly affects our health. It is therefore important for doctors to find out what their patients believe, their attitude towards faith, whether they hold any committed spiritual and/or religious beliefs and whether they participate in any supportive social structure, such as a church group. Social, religious and spiritual beliefs, when practised, can lead to an improvement in the functioning of the immune system, which may contribute to a healthier life and the possibility of an extended lifespan. Our beliefs, relationships and the way we think all have an influence on our health, and should be taken into account by any treating physician.

References

Acevedo, B. P., Fossposs, S. and Navretski, H. (2016) The neural mechanisms of meditative practices: novel approaches for healthy aging. *Current Behavioral Neuroscience Reports*, 3, 328–339.

Aftanas, L. I. and Golocheikine, S. A. (2001) Human anterior and frontal midline theta and lower alpha reflect emotionally positive state and internalised attention: high-resolution EEG investigation of meditation. *Neuroscience Letters*, 310, 57–60.

Austin, J. (2014) *Zen-Brain Horizons.* Cambridge, MA: The MIT Press.

Aviles, J. M., Whelan, S. E., Hernke, D. A. et al. (2001) Intercessory prayer and cardiovascular disease progression in a coronary care unit population: a randomized controlled trial. *Mayo Clinic Proceedings*, 76, 1192–1198.

Benor, D. J. (2002) *Spiritual Healing: Scientific Validation of a Healing Revolution.* Southfield, MI: Vision Publications.

Benor, D. J. (2004) *Consciousness, Bioenergy and Healing: Self-Healing and Energy Medicine for the Twenty-first Century.* Medford, NJ: Wholistic Healing Publications.

Braboszcz, C., Rael Cahn, B., Levy, J., Fernandez, M. and Delorme, A. (2017) Increased gamma brainwave amplitude compared to control in three different meditation traditions. *PloS One*, 12, e0170647.

Byrd, R. C. (1988) Positive therapeutic effects of intercessory prayer in a coronary care unit population. *Southern Medical Journal*, 81, 826–829.

Cawthon, R. M., Smith, K. R., O'Brien, E., Sivatchenko, A. and Kerber, R. A. (2003) Association between telomere length in blood and mortality in people aged 60 years or older. *The Lancet*, 361, 393–395.

Conklin, Q. A., King, B. G., Zanesco, A. P. et al. (2018) Insight meditation and telomere biology: the effects of intensive retreat and the moderating role of personality. *Brain, Behavior, and Immunity*, 70, 233–245.

Damasio, A. (2000) *The Feeling of What Happens: Body, Emotion and the Making of Consciousness.* London: Heinemann.

Dennett, D. (1991) *Consciousness Explained.* Boston, MA: Little, Brown and Company.

Durschmid, S., Reichert, C., Walter, N. et al. (2020) Self-regulated critical brain dynamics originate from high frequency-band activity in the MEG. *PLoS One*, 15, e0233589.

Epel, E. S., Puterman, E., Lin, J. et al. (2016) Meditation and vacation effects have an impact on disease-associated molecular phenotypes. *Translational Psychiatry*, 6, e880.

Fox, K. C. R., Nijeboer, S., Dixon, M. L. et al. (2014) Is meditation associated with altered brain structure? A systematic review and meta-analysis of morphometric neuroimaging in meditation practitioners. *Neuroscience and Biobehavioral Reviews*, 43, 48–73.

Gardner, R. (1983) Miracles of healing in Anglo-Celtic Northumbria as recorded by the venerable Bede and his contemporaries: a reappraisal in the light of twentieth century experience. *British Medical Journal*, 287, 1927–1933.

Harris, W. S., Gowda, M., Kolb, J. et al. (1999) A randomised, controlled trial of the effects of remote, intercessory prayer on outcomes in patients admitted to the coronary care unit. *Archives of Internal Medicine*, 159, 2273–2278.

Hernández, S. E., Barros-Loscertales, A., Xiao, Y. et al. (2018) Gray matter and functional connectivity in anterior cingulate cortex are associated with the state of mental silence during Sahaja yoga meditation. *Neuroscience* 371, 395–406.

Hofmann, S. G., Sawyer, A. T., Witt, A. A. and Oh, D. (2010) The effect of mindfulness-based therapy on anxiety and depression: a meta-analytic review. *Journal of Consulting and Clinical Psychology*, 78, 169–183.

Illueca, M. and Doolittle, B. (2020) The use of prayer in the management of pain: a systematic review. *Journal of Religion & Health*, 59, 681-699.

Kabat-Zinn, J., Massion, A., Kristeller, J. et al. (1992) Effectiveness of a meditation-based stress reduction program in the treatment of anxiety disorders. *American Journal of Psychiatry*, 149, 936–943.

Kaur, C. and Singh, P. (2015) EEG derived neuronal dynamics during meditation: progress and challenges. *Advances in Preventive Medicine*, 2015, 614723.

Kjaer, T. W., Bertelsen, C., Piccini, P. et al. (2002) Increased dopamine tone during meditation-induced changes of consciousness. *Cognitive Brain Research*, 13, 255–259.

Koenig, H. G., King, D. E. and Carson, V. B., eds. (2012) *Handbook of Religion and Health*. Oxford: Oxford University Press.

Kretzer, K., Davis, J., Easa, D. et al. (2007) Self-identity through Ho'oponopono as adjunctive therapy for hypertension management. *Ethnicity & Disease*, 17, 624–628.

Lazar, S., Kerr, C., Wasserman, R. et al. (2005) Meditation experience is associated with increased cortical thickness. *Neuroreport*, 16, 1893–1897.

Lou, H. C., Nowak, M. and Kjaer, T. W. (2005) The mental self. *Progress in Brain Research*, 150, 197–204.

Ly, A., Saide, A. and Richert, R. (2020) Perceptions of the efficacy of prayer and conventional medicine for health concerns. *Journal of Religion and Health*, 59, 1–18.

Martin, J. (2019) *The Finders*. Jackson, WY: Integration Press.

Morton, P. A. (1997) *A Historical Introduction to the Philosophy of Mind: Readings with Commentary*. Peterborough, Canada: Broadview Press.

Moss, A. S., Winteringm, N., Roggenkampm, H. et al. (2012) Effects of an eight-week meditation program on mood and anxiety in patients with memory loss. *Journal of Alternative and Complementary Medicine*, 18, 48–53.

Newberg, A. B. and Iversen, J. (2003) The neural basis of the complex mental task of meditation: neurotransmitter and neurochemical considerations. *Medical Hypothesis*, 61, 282–291.

Newberg, A. and Waldman, M. (2016) *How Enlightenment Changes Your Brain: The New Science of Transformation*. New York: Avery.

Newberg, A., Alavi, A., Baime, M. et al. (2001) The measurement of regional cerebral blood flow during the complex cognitive task of meditation: a preliminary SPECT study. *Psychiatry Research*, 106, 113–122.

Newberg, A. B., Wintering, N., Khalsa, D. S., Roggenkamp, H. and Waldman, M. R. (2010) Meditation effects on cognitive function and cerebral blood flow in subjects with memory loss: a preliminary study. *Journal of Alzheimer's Disease*, 20, 517–526.

Orme-Johnson, D., Schneider, R., Young, D. et al. (2006) Neuroimaging of meditation's effect on brain reactivity to pain. *Neuroreport*, 17, 1359–1363.

Palmer, R., Katerndahl, D. and Morgan-Kidd, J. (2004) A randomized trial of the effects of remote intercessory prayer: interactions with personal beliefs on problem-specific outcome and functional status. *Journal of Alternative and Complementary Medicine*, 10, 438–448.

Pew Research Center (2015) U.S. public becoming less religious: modest drop in overall rates of belief and practice, but religiously affiliated Americans are as observant as before. Available at www.pewresearch.org/religion/2015/11/03/u-s-public-becoming-less-religious/ (accessed 22 April 2022).

Pischke, C. R., Weidner, G., Elliott-Eller, M. et al. (2007) Lifestyle changes and clinical profile in coronary heart disease patients with an ejection fraction of 40% in the Multicenter Lifestyle Demonstration Project. *European Journal of Heart Failure*, 9, 928–934.

Reangsing, C., Rittiwong, T. and Schneider, J. K. (2021) Effects of mindfulness meditation interventions on depression in older adults: a meta-analysis. *Aging & Mental Health* 25, 1181–1190.

Roberts, L., Ahmed, I. and Davison, A. (2009) Intercessory prayer for the alleviation of ill health. *Cochrane Database of Systematic Reviews*, 2009, CD000368.

Roe, C. A., Sonnex, C. and Roxburgh, E. C. (2015) Two meta-analyses of noncontact healing studies. *Explore*, 11, 1550–8307.

Romez, C., Freedland, K., Zaritzky, D. and Brown, J. (2021) Case report of instantaneous resolution of juvenile macular degeneration blindness after proximal intercessory prayer. *Explore*, 17, 79–83.

Schwartz, J. M., Stapp, H. P. and Beauregard, M. (2005) Quantum physics in neuroscience and psychology: a neurophysical model of mind–brain interaction. *Philosophical Transactions of the Royal Society of London, Series B: Biological Sciences*, 360, 1309–1327.

Searle, J. R. (2007) Dualism revisited. *Journal of Physiology*, 101, 169–178.

Sharma, A., Barrett, M. S., Cucchiara, A. J. et al. (2017) A breathing-based meditation intervention for patients with major depressive disorder following inadequate response to antidepressants: a randomized pilot study. *Journal of Clinical Psychiatry*, 78, e59–e63.

Sharma, P., Mahapatra, A. and Gupta, R. (2019) Meditation-induced psychosis: a narrative review and individual patient data analysis. *Irish Journal of Psychological Medicine*. https://doi.org/10.1017/ipm.2019.47

Shen, H., Chen, M. and Cui, D. (2020) Biological mechanism study of meditation and its application in mental disorders. *General Psychiatry*, 33, e100214.

Sherrington, C. S. (1940) *Man on his Nature*. Cambridge: Cambridge University Press.

Sperduti, M., Martinelli, P. and Piolino, P. (2012) A neurocognitive model of meditation based on activation likelihood estimation (ALE) meta-analysis. *Consciousness and Cognition*, 21, 269–276.

Sudsuang, R., Chentanez, V. and Veluvan, K. (1991) Effect of Buddhist meditation on serum cortisol and total protein levels, blood pressure, pulse rate, lung volume and reaction time. *Physiology and Behaviour*, 50, 543–548.

Tolahunase, M., Sagar, R. and Dada, R. (2017) Impact of yoga and meditation on cellular aging in apparently healthy individuals: a prospective, open-label single-arm exploratory study. *Oxidative Medicine and Cellular Longevity*, 2017, Article ID 7928981.

Wahbeh, H., Sagher, A., Back, W., Pundhir, P. and Travis, F. (2018) A systematic review of transcendent states across meditation and contemplative traditions. *Explore*, 14, 19–35.

Xue, T., Li, H., Wang, M.-T. et al. (2018) Mindfulness meditation improves metabolic profiles in healthy and depressive participants. *CNS Neuroscience & Therapeutics*, 24, 572–574.

Yaden, D. B., Haidt, J., Hood, R. W., Vago, D. R. and Newberg, A.B. (2017) The varieties of self-transcendent experience. *Review of General Psychology*, 21, 143–160.

Yang, C.-C., Barrós-Loscertales, A., Li, M. et al. (2019) Alterations in brain structure and amplitude of low-frequency after eight weeks of mindfulness meditation training in meditation-naïve subjects. *Scientific Reports*, 9, 10977.

Zylowska, L., Ackerman, D. L., Yang, M. H. et al. (2008) Mindfulness meditation training in adults and adolescents with ADHD: a feasibility study. *Journal of Attention Disorders*, 11, 737–746.

Chapter 2

Religion and Spirituality in the DSM and ICD

John R. Peteet and Francis G. Lu

Introduction

In 1992 the psychiatrist and best-selling author M. Scott Peck addressed an overflowing audience at the Annual Meeting of the American Psychiatric Association (APA). There he made the case, later recorded in the epilogue of his book, *Further Along the Road Less Traveled: The Unending Journey Toward Spiritual Growth*, that American psychiatry is currently in a predicament 'because its traditional neglect of spirituality has led to five broad areas of failure: occasional, devastating misdiagnosis; not infrequent mistreatment; inadequate research and theory; an increasingly poor reputation; and limitation of psychiatrists' own personal development. Taken further these failures are so destructive to psychiatry that the predicament can properly be called grave' (Peck, 1993, p. 237).

Early History

In 1992, David Lukoff, Francis Lu and Robert Turner had proposed to the DSM-IV Task Force the inclusion of the category 'Psychoreligious and Psychospiritual Problems', which they described in a key paper titled 'Toward a More Culturally Sensitive DSM-IV: Psychoreligious and Psychospiritual Problems' (Lukoff et al., 1992). In February 1993, the Task Force recommended that the prefix 'psycho' should be dropped, and they formally established the new category of 'V62.61 Religious or Spiritual Problem (RSP)'. The 1994 DSM-IV also included the new 'Outline for a Cultural Formulation'. Then, in 1995, Robert Turner and his colleagues published a paper titled 'Religious or Spiritual Problem: A Culturally Sensitive Diagnostic Category in the DSM-IV', which argued for inclusion of this new category on the basis of the need for cultural sensitivity (Turner et al., 1995).

DSM-IV-TR, a text revision of DSM-IV, was published in 2000 (American Psychiatric Association, 2000) and contained no changes, and in 2010, Francis Lu, David Lukoff and Paul Yang proposed a revision of the category for DSM-IV, but the 2013 edition left the RSP category unchanged. However, the Outline for Cultural Formulation was revised, and a new Cultural Formulation Interview and 12 Supplemental Modules were added to help clinicians gather information for the Outline for Cultural Formulation.

The original paper by Lukoff, Lu and Turner defined psychoreligious problems as 'Experiences that a person finds troubling or distressing and that involve the beliefs and practices of an organized church or religious institution. Examples include loss or questioning of a firmly held faith, change in denominational membership, conversion to a new faith, and intensification of adherence to religious practices or orthodoxy' (Lukoff et al., 1992, pp. 676–677). By comparison, they defined psychospiritual problems as 'Experiences that a person finds troubling or distressing and that involve that person's reported relationship with a transcendent being or force. . . . Examples include near-death experience or mystical experience' (Lukoff et al., 1992, p. 677).

These definitions were intended to expand the range of psychiatric differential diagnosis to include not only purely religious or spiritual problems, but also mental disorders with religious or spiritual content, and psychoreligious or psychospiritual problems not attributable to a mental disorder. The rationale for them was fourfold: to improve diagnostic assessments when religious and spiritual issues are involved; to reduce iatrogenic harm from the misdiagnosis of psychoreligious and psychospiritual problems; to improve treatment of such problems by stimulating clinical research; and to encourage clinical training centres to address the religious and spiritual dimensions of human existence.

The 1994 edition of DSM-IV included in its Introduction a section titled 'Ethnic and Cultural Considerations', with narrative mention of cultural variations in presentation (these appear in 79 diagnostic categories), an Outline for Cultural Formulation (in Appendix I) and a Glossary of Culture-Bound Syndromes (also in Appendix I). The authors write that 'It is hoped that these new features will increase sensitivity to variation in how mental disorders may be expressed in different cultures and will reduce the possible effect of *unintended bias stemming from the clinician's own cultural background*' [italics added] (American Psychiatric Association, 1994, p. xxv).

The introductory section on 'Ethnic and Cultural Considerations' also cautioned as follows:

> Diagnostic assessment can be especially challenging when a clinician from one ethnic or cultural group uses the DSM-IV classification to evaluate an individual from a different ethnic or cultural group. A clinician who is unfamiliar with the nuances of the individual's cultural frame of reference may incorrectly judge as psychopathology those normal variations in behavior, belief, or experience that are particular to the individual's culture. (American Psychiatric Association, 1994, p. xxiv)

Biases (intended/conscious/explicit or unintended/unconscious/implicit) could concern spirituality/religion, racism, bias against immigrants/refugees, sexism, classism, ageism, homophobia or other biases.

In the section on Specific Culture Features, under the diagnosis of Brief Psychotic Disorder (298.8), clinicians are reminded to consider religion when making a differential diagnosis: 'It is important to distinguish symptoms of Brief Psychotic Disorder from culturally sanctioned response patterns. For example, in some religious ceremonies, an individual may report hearing voices, but these do not generally persist and are not perceived as abnormal by most members of the person's community' (American Psychiatric Association, 1994, p. 303).

Likewise, in the diagnosis of depersonalization disorder: 'Voluntarily induced experiences of depersonalization or derealization form part of meditative and trance practices that are prevalent in many religions and cultures and should not be confused with Depersonalization Disorder' (American Psychiatric Association, 1994, p. 488).

Religious or spiritual problems were included as V-Codes: 'Other Conditions That May Be a Focus of Clinical Attention', which are not mental disorders, but are to be coded on Axis I along with all mental disorders except the Axis II disorders. They could refer to a problem only, to an unrelated mental disorder and problem, or to a related mental disorder and problem that was 'sufficiently severe to warrant independent clinical attention' (American Psychiatric Association, 1994, p. 675).

The DSM-IV defined the code V62.89: Religious or Spiritual Problem as follows: 'This category can be used when the focus of clinical attention is a religious or spiritual problem. Examples include distressing experiences that involve loss or questioning of faith, problems associated with conversion to a new faith, or questioning of other spiritual values that may not necessarily be related to an organized church or religious institution' (American Psychiatric Association, 1994, p. 685).

APIRE

From 2000 to 2010, the American Psychiatric Institute for Research and Education (APIRE), one of three organizations affiliated with the American Psychiatric Association, provided leadership for pre-DSM-V activities. As previous APIRE workgroups had set a research agenda to provide evidence for DSM-V on culture, women, children and the elderly, the 2005–10 APIRE Workgroup on Religion and Spirituality became the tenth such workgroup (see Box 12.1). Products of the workgroup included a review of the literature for these topics concerning spiritual/religious issues, focused consideration of how to update the 'Age, Gender, and Cultural Considerations' sections to incorporate this information, and a proposed research agenda contained in the 2011 book, *Religious and Spiritual Issues in Psychiatric Diagnosis: A Research Agenda for DSM-V* (Peteet et al., 2011). This volume proposed a revised, expanded definition of a religious or spiritual problem:

> This category can be used when the focus of clinical attention is a religious or spiritual problem. *Examples include loss or questioning of faith, changes in membership, practices and beliefs (including conversion), New Religious Movements and cults, and life-threatening and terminal illness. Examples of spiritual problems include mystical experiences, near-death, psychic experiences, alien abduction experiences, meditation and spiritual practice-related experiences, possession experiences and questioning of other spiritual values that may not necessarily be related to an organized church or religious institution.* (Lukoff et al., 2011, p. 192)

Box 12.1 2005–10 APIRE Workgroup on Religion and Spirituality

Co-chairs:

    John Peteet, MD, Chair of the APA Committee on Religion, Spirituality, and Psychiatry
    Francis Lu, MD, Council on Minority Mental Health and Health Disparities

APIRE staff member support:

    William Narrow, MD, MPH

Those presenting at the APA Annual Meeting in Toronto in May 2006:

    C. Robert Cloninger, MD (Personality Disorders)
    Dan Blazer, MD (Depression)
    Gerrit Glas, MD, PhD (Anxiety and Adjustment Disorders)
    Samuel Thielman, MD, PhD (PTSD)
    Allan Josephson, MD and Mary Lynn Dell, MD (Child and Adolescent Disorders)
    Marc Galanter, MD (Substance Abuse Disorders)
    David Lukoff, PhD (Religious and Spiritual Problems)
    Francis Lu, MD (Outline for Cultural Formulation)

DSM-5

In the wake of the 2010 APIRE report, a number of modifications related to cultural considerations appeared in the 2013 DSM-5. These included changes made in the Introduction to Section I regarding 'Cultural Issues' and 'Gender Differences' (American Psychiatric Association, 2013, pp. 14–15); within Section II, in the disorder narrative sections, and in Section III, Culture-Related Diagnostic Issues (American Psychiatric Association, 2013, index, pp. 923–924), Gender-Related Diagnostic Issues, Diagnostic Criteria for Some Disorders, an expanded list of V codes, the Outline for Cultural Formulation revised from DSM-IV/DSM-IV-TR, and the new Cultural Formulation Interview. In the Appendix, a Glossary of Cultural Concepts of Distress replaced the Glossary of Culture-Bound Syndromes.

In the Introduction, the DSM-5 definition of culture was expanded to include the following: values, orientations, knowledge and practices that individuals use to understand their experiences, based on their identification with diverse groups, such as ethnic groups, faith communities, occupational groups and veterans; aspects of a person's background, experience and social contexts that may affect his or her perspective, such as geographical origin, migration, language, religion, sexual orientation, race and ethnicity; and the influence of family, friends and other community members (the individual's *social network*) on the individual's illness experience.

As an example of changes made in Section II, the section on Culture-Related Diagnostic Issues related to schizophrenia now reads:

> Cultural and socioeconomic factors must be considered, particularly when the individual and the clinician do not share the same cultural and socioeconomic background. Ideas that appear to be delusional in one culture (e.g., witchcraft) may be commonly held in another. In some cultures, visual or auditory hallucinations with a religious content (e.g., hearing God's voice) are a normal part of religious experience. . . . In certain cultures, distress may take the form of hallucinations or pseudo-hallucinations and overvalued ideas that may present as clinically similar to true psychosis but are normative to the patient's subgroup. (American Psychiatric Association, 2013, p. 103)

Also in Section II, the section on Other Conditions That May Be a Focus of Clinical Attention was now introduced as follows:

> This discussion covers other conditions and problems that may be a focus of clinical attention or that may otherwise affect the diagnosis, course, prognosis, or treatment of a patient's mental disorder. . . . A condition or problem in this chapter may be coded if it is a reason for the current visit or helps to explain the need for a test, procedure, or treatment. . . . The conditions and problems listed in this chapter are not mental disorders. Their inclusion in DSM-5 is meant to draw attention to the scope of additional issues that may be encountered in routine clinical practice and to provide a systematic listing that may be useful to clinicians in documenting these issues. (American Psychiatric Association, 2013, p. 715)

In particular, the diagnostic category V62.89 Religious or Spiritual Problem now reads: 'This category can be used when the focus of clinical attention is a religious or spiritual problem. Examples include distressing experiences that involve loss or questioning of faith, problems associated with conversion to a new faith, or questioning of other spiritual values which may not necessarily be related to an organized church or religious institution' (American Psychiatric Association, 2013, p. 725).

Parenthetically, the 2021 ICD-10-CM Crosswalk,[1] which translates DSM categories into those of the International Classification of Diseases (ICD), describes Z codes as 'factors influencing health status and contact with health services', with religious and spiritual problems listed as one example among several others of Z65.8 'Other Specified Problems Related to Psychosocial Circumstances'. These codes are billable for US medical insurance purposes, but not as the principal diagnosis, with four exceptions.

In ICD-11 the Z codes have been discontinued and the equivalent structure is 'Problems Associated with Social or Cultural Environment', located within 'Factors Influencing Health Status', where religious and spiritual considerations are less visible. Despite the case made by Abdul-Hamid (2011) for a category of religious and spiritual problems in ICD-11, perhaps similar to that in DSM, no detail is given concerning such problems, and spirituality/religion are not specifically mentioned here at all. Proposals made for ICD-11 to include information relevant to differential diagnosis between spiritual experiences and mental disorders (Moreira-Almeida and Cardena, 2011) have also not been given responses. In fact, ICD-11 includes very little reference to spirituality/religion in relation to mental disorders, apart from the fact that religious norms are mentioned in relation to prolonged grief disorder, and possession trance disorder has now been divided into two separate categories (Reed et al., 2019). In the section on symptoms, signs and abnormal clinical and laboratory findings, not elsewhere classified, religious delusions are classified as MB26.08. Under the heading of proximal risk factors for intentional self-harm, religious belief or affiliation is classified as XE98Q. The few specific references to spirituality/religion in ICD-11 thus appear to be negative and related to pathology.

The DSM-5 Outline for Cultural Formulation has several sections:

1   cultural identity of the individual
2   cultural conceptualizations of distress (cultural explanations of the individual's illness)
3   psychosocial stressors and cultural features of vulnerability and resilience (cultural factors related to psychosocial environment and functioning)
4   cultural features (elements) of the relationship between the individual and the clinician
5   overall cultural assessment (for diagnosis and care).

DSM-5 includes two versions of a Cultural Formulation Interview. The Patient version includes 16 questions (American Psychiatric Association, 2013, pp. 750–754) and the Informant version includes 17 questions (American Psychiatric Association, 2013, pp. 755–757). There are also 12 Supplementary Modules, available online,[2] which expand on each domain of the cultural formulation interview.

The Supplementary Modules contain material on assessing the patient's cultural identity, explanatory model, coping and help seeking, psychosocial stressors, social network, caregivers and level of functioning. The new Cultural Formulation Interview guides the interviewer with sample questions for introducing and probing each of these

---

[1]   https://icdlist.com/icd-10/Z65.8
[2]   www.psychiatry.org/dsm5

domains. For example, when probing for the patient's definition of the problem, the clinician might ask 'What brings you here today?' and go on to say 'Sometimes people have different ways of describing their problem to their family, friends or others in their community. How would you describe your [PROBLEM] to them?' And 'What troubles you most about your [PROBLEM]?' When eliciting the patient's understanding of causes, the clinician might ask 'Why do you think this is happening to you?', 'What do you think are the causes of your [PROBLEM]?', 'What do others in your family, friends or others in your community say are the causes of your [PROBLEM]?'

The Outline for Cultural Formulation encourages the clinician to describe the cultural constructs that influence how the individual experiences, understands and communicates his or her symptoms or problems to others. These include cultural syndromes, idioms of distress and explanatory models or perceived causes. The clinician is instructed to assess the level of severity and meaning of the distressing experiences 'in relation to the norms of the individual's cultural reference groups. Assessment of coping and help-seeking patterns should consider the use of professional as well as traditional, alternative or complementary sources of care' (American Psychiatric Association, 2013, p. 750).

The Glossary of Cultural Concepts of Distress (American Psychiatric Association, 2013, pp. 833–837) provides examples of well-studied cultural concepts of distress that illustrate the relevance of cultural information for clinical diagnosis. In replacing the DSM-IV-TR Glossary of Culture-Bound Syndromes, its examples include descriptions, DSM differential diagnoses, related categories in other cultures, and sometimes prevalence/distributions (see Table 12.1).

The Outline for Cultural Formulation calls attention both to psychosocial stressors and to cultural features of vulnerability and resilience. Stressors and supports include religion, family and other social networks that may provide support. Clinicians are instructed to evaluate the patient's level of functioning, disability and resilience in relation to the individual's cultural reference groups. Questions suggested by the Cultural Formulation Interview for eliciting these include 'Are there any kinds of support that make your [PROBLEM] better, such as support from family, friends, or others?' and 'Are there any kinds of stresses that make your [PROBLEM] worse, such as difficulties with money, or family problems?'

Table 12.1. Cultural concepts of distress

Concept	Main type	Region
Ataque de nervios	Syndrome	Latin America
Dhat syndrome	Explanation	South Asia
Khyal cap	Syndrome	Cambodia
Kunfungisisa	Idiom	Zimbabwe
Maladi moun	Explanation	Haiti
Nervios	Idiom	Latin America
Shenjing shuairuo	Syndrome	China
Susto	Explanation	Latin America
Taijin kyofusho	Syndrome	Japan

Pargament et al. (2005) provide a number of examples of Religious and Spiritual Struggles:

1 struggles with the Divine
2 anger towards God
3 concern about divine punishment
4 intrapersonal struggles
5 facing moral imperfection
6 spiritual questions and doubts
7 interpersonal struggles
8 disagreements about religious issues
9 offences by members of religious groups.

The Outline for Cultural Formulation also encourages assessment of the role of the patient's cultural identity: 'Describe the individual's racial, ethnic, or cultural reference groups' (American Psychiatric Association, 2013, p. 749), 'For immigrants and racial or ethnic minorities ... degree of involvement with both the culture of origin and the host or majority culture. ... Language abilities, preferences, and patterns of use' (American Psychiatric Association, 2013, p. 750). DSM-5 added: 'Other clinically relevant aspects of identity may include religious affiliation, socioeconomic background, personal and family places of birth and growing up, migrant status, and sexual orientation' (American Psychiatric Association, 2013, p. 750). The framework for addressing these encompasses age and generational influences, developmental and acquired disabilities, religion and spiritual orientation, ethnic and racial identity, socioeconomic status, language, sexual orientation, indigenous heritage, national origin and gender (Hays, 2016).

The Cultural Formulation Interview offers corresponding sample questions (American Psychiatric Association, 2013, p. 753):

Are there any kinds of stresses that make your [PROBLEM] worse ...? Sometimes, aspects of people's background or identity can make their [PROBLEM] better or worse. By background or identity, I mean, for example, the communities you belong to, the languages you speak, where you or your family are from, your race or ethnic background, your gender or sexual orientation, or your faith or religion.

For you, what are the most important aspects of your background or identity?

Are there any aspects of your background or identity that make a difference to your [PROBLEM]?

Are there any aspects of your background or identity that are causing other concerns or difficulties for you?'

Similarly, the Cultural Formulation Interview suggests questions about self-coping, past help-seeking, barriers and help-seeking preferences (American Psychiatric Association, 2013, pp. 753–754):

Sometimes people have various ways of dealing with problems like your [PROBLEM]. What have you done on your own to cope with your [PROBLEM]?

Often, people look for help from many different sources, including different kinds of doctors, helpers, or healers. In the past, what kinds of treatment, help, advice, or healing have you sought for your [PROBLEM]? What types of help or treatment were most useful? Not useful?

Has anything prevented you from getting the help you need? For example, money, work or family commitments, stigma or discrimination, or lack of services that understand your language or background?

Now let's talk some more about the help you need. What kinds of help do you think would be most useful to you at this time for your [PROBLEM]?

Are there other kinds of help that your family, friends, or other people have suggested would be helpful for you now?

These questions probe not only the patient's professional sources of care, but also his or her traditional, alternative or complementary sources of care, indigenous healing practices and spiritual/religious healers.

Finally, the Outline for Cultural Formulation encourages exploration of factors that influence the clinician–patient relationship:

> Identify differences in culture, language, and social status between an individual and clinician that may cause difficulties in communication and may influence diagnosis and treatment. Experiences of racism and discrimination in the larger society may impede establishing trust and safety in the clinical diagnostic encounter. Effects may include problems eliciting symptoms, misunderstanding of the cultural and clinical significance of symptoms and behaviors, and difficulty establishing or maintaining the rapport needed for an effective clinical alliance. (American Psychiatric Association, 2013, p. 750)

Clinicians are encouraged to understand their own cultural identities and development, to compare these with those of their patient, and to look for problems that might arise in the context of the encounter from either similarities or differences. Relevant considerations include the following: respect, intimacy, rapport and empathy; verbal and non-verbal communication, including the effects of limited English proficiency and health literacy on history gathering; stigma and shame; and transference and counter-transference:

> Sometimes doctors and patients misunderstand each other because they come from different backgrounds or have different expectations. Have you been concerned about this [the patient and the clinician having different backgrounds] and is there anything that we can do to provide you with the care you need? (American Psychiatric Association, 2013, p. 754)

Potential areas of matching cultural identities that could help the clinician to provide optimal care through the use of special knowledge or skills are religion/spirituality, race/ethnicity, gender, migration/acculturation, language and sexual orientation.

Overall, the cultural assessment should 'summarize the implications of the components of the cultural formulation ... for diagnosis ... as well as appropriate management and treatment intervention' (American Psychiatric Association, 2013, p. 750).

This guidance is consistent with that provided by the APA *Resource Document on Religious/Spiritual Commitments and Psychiatric Practice*: 'Psychiatrists should foster recovery by making treatment decisions with patients in ways that respect and take into meaningful consideration their cultural, religious/spiritual, and personal ideals' (American Psychiatric Association Corresponding Committee on Religion, Spirituality and Psychiatry, 2006).

The American Psychiatric Association Ethics Committee authored a 2021 Resource Document titled 'Resource Document on Ethics at the Interface of Religion, Spirituality, and Psychiatric Practice' that reinforced the use of the DSM-5 Outline for Cultural Formulation and the Cultural Formulation Interview, as well as providing additional guidance, especially concerning ethics (American Psychiatric Association Ethics Committee, 2021).

Misdiagnosis can result from any of the following: misunderstanding cultural idioms of distress, or syndromes; failure to elicit or understand explanatory models; incomplete history gathering due to an inadequate relationship; clinician bias, stereotyping or clinical uncertainty. The prevalence, course and outcome of misdiagnosis may vary with culture and gender, and risks mistreatment. Challenges in differential diagnosis include distinguishing spiritual/religious phenomena from spiritual/religious problems and from mental disorders, while recognising the possibility of concurrence.

Clinicians need to attend to both the process (negotiation and management of a plan to maximise adherence/compliance) and the content (biological, psychological and sociocultural) of treatment. Psychotherapy should: respect the patient's and family's expectations and boundaries; demonstrate empathy; consider what cultural modifications would enhance family, individual, group, supportive, skills-based (e.g., CBT) or insight-oriented approaches; incorporate possible religious or spiritual interventions based on the place of a religious or spiritual problem in the treatment plan; and take into account what therapist characteristics would facilitate or hinder treatment. Sociocultural approaches should when possible utilise cultural strengths found in the family, spiritual/religious beliefs and practices and other social networks, and should be coordinated with other systems of care, such as primary care, and faith organizations and leaders.

DSM-5-TR

There were important changes relating to cultural and social structural issues in the DSM-5 Text Revision (TR) (American Psychiatric Association, 2022). In Section I (the introduction), new sections were added on the impact of racism and discrimination on psychiatric diagnosis and how attention was paid to these issues in the DSM-5-TR, including the following relevant sentence: 'Other aspects of identity, including ethnicity, common gender, language, religion, and sexual orientation, may also be the focus and bias or stereotyping that can affect the process of diagnostic assessment' (American Psychiatric Association, 2022, p. 17).

In Section II, the Culture-Related Diagnostic Issues sections were updated with new text and references; more disorders contain these sections. The Other Conditions That May Be a Focus of Clinical Attention are now primarily Z codes instead of V codes consistent with ICD-10. There is now additional important guidance on when they may be coded as part of the diagnosis: 'A condition or problem in this chapter may be coded . . . 3) if it plays a role in the initiation or exacerbation of a mental disorder; or 4) if it constitutes a problem that should be considered in the overall management plan' (American Psychiatric Association, 2022, p. 821). The definition of Religious or Spiritual Problem remains the same as in the DSM-5, except that the code number has been changed to Z65.8

(American Psychiatric Association, 2022, p. 834).

Future Directions

The use of the 'religious or spiritual problem' category in research is a very recent development, but helpful resources are emerging for incorporating spiritual/religious considerations into culturally sensitive practice. The second edition of *The Clinical Manual of Cultural Psychiatry* (Lim, 2014) focuses on the DSM-5 Outline for Cultural Formulation. It includes video vignettes, is twice the size of the first edition, with new chapters on women, LGBT issues and religion/spirituality, and won the 2015 Creative

Scholarship Award from the Society for the Study of Psychiatry and Culture. The *DSM-5 Handbook on the Cultural Formulation Interview* (Lewis-Fernandez et al., 2016) also includes video vignettes, and a chapter on the Supplementary Module on Religion, Spirituality, and Moral Traditions.

Some of the relevant questions raised by the APIRE Workgroup for future research concern the relationship between spiritual/religious and psychopathological phenomena that may appear similar. When is anxiety an existential crisis, and when is it a symptom of a traditionally understood anxiety disorder? When are auditory hallucinations psychotic, and when are they a normal part of religious experience? Ecstatic religious experience has been confused with intoxication (now a DSM diagnosis) since biblical times (Acts 2:13). These are not mutually exclusive, and criteria are still being developed to distinguish between them (Moreira-Almeida and Cardena, 2011; see also Chapter 16 in the present volume). When is substance use abusive, and when is it normative? To answer such questions, investigators will need to develop, refine and use criteria for measuring mental and spiritual/religious health as a context within which to evaluate these phenomena. Will it be possible to identify subclinical conditions that can have both existential and emotional components (Glas, 2011)?

Secondly, the Workgroup raised questions for research on the manifestation of psychiatric disorders in religious populations. How do depression, psychosis or obsessive-compulsive disorder present differently in patients whose beliefs and practices give their symptoms particular meaning? Epidemiological research can indicate the prevalence of defining criteria within particular populations, but more focused studies are required to examine the ways in which particular faiths interpret, discourage or legitimate the expression of symptoms. For example, Thielman (2011) has pointed out the importance of interrelated cultural and worldview factors in both the development and acceptable treatment of post-traumatic stress disorder (PTSD), and Blazer (2011) has similarly emphasised the social and religious meanings of depression. This research also has obvious implications for screening and early case finding.

Thirdly, research is needed on the positive and negative effects of spirituality/religion on the course and outcome of disorders. Epidemiological research establishing associations between measures of religiosity or spiritual well-being and psychiatric symptomatology suggests that positive effects may be common. However, the mechanism of action needs to be identified – whether it involves strong beliefs, community support, mindfulness, spiritual engagement with a Higher Power, or some other factor. Studies such as that of Pargament (Harrison et al., 2001) on the implications of positive and negative religious coping have begun to explore one such factor. Studies within religious populations will be needed to distinguish and understand how other aspects of religion/spirituality assist or interfere with recovery from illness.

A fourth area in need of research is the role of spirituality/religion in developmental and personality disorders. If personality disorders can be viewed as reflecting deficiencies of virtue (Cloninger, 2011), what are the moral dimensions of their diagnosis and treatment? Are there features that can be identified across spiritual traditions that predispose to healthy or unhealthy maturation? Both Mabe et al. (2011) and Cloninger (2011) have suggested potential directions for this work.

Finally, there is a need for research on the influence of the clinician's own worldview in diagnosis and treatment planning. Given the value-laden and culturally conditioned nature of psychiatric diagnosis, when is this process most vulnerable to unwitting distortion? Blazer (2011), Cloninger (2011), Thielman (2011) and Fulford and Sadler (2011) have pointed out areas where the clinician's value commitments need to be taken into account, and Seale (2010) has provided data showing the influence of the physician's religion on treatment decisions.

Conclusion

The past three decades have seen the DSM incorporate considerations of religion and spirituality in the V-Code 'Religious or Spiritual Problem', and as elements in the Cultural Formulation Outline. The practical suggestions contained in the DSM-5's Cultural Formulation Interview go further, to facilitate comprehensive differential diagnosis and foster patient-centred treatment, consistent with the World Psychiatric Association's Position Statement on Spirituality and Religion in Psychiatry (Moreira-Almeida et al., 2016) and the APA Resource Document on Religious/Spiritual Commitments and Psychiatric Practice (American Psychiatric Association Corresponding Committee on Religion, Spirituality and Psychiatry, 2006). How psychiatry responds to Scott Peck's challenge to develop more adequate theory and research will determine how subsequent editions of the DSM engage the moral and existential as well as the cultural dimensions of religion and spirituality as important aspects of human experience.

References

Abdul-Hamid, W. K. (2011) The need for a category of 'religious and spiritual problems' in ICD-11. *International Psychiatry*, 8, 60–61.

American Psychiatric Association (1994) *Diagnostic and Statistical Manual of Mental Disorders*, 4th ed. Washington, DC: American Psychiatric Association.

American Psychiatric Association (2000) *Diagnostic and Statistical Manual of Mental Disorders*, 4th ed., text rev. Washington, DC: American Psychiatric Association.

American Psychiatric Association (2013) *Diagnostic and Statistical Manual of Mental Disorders*, 5th ed. Washington, DC: American Psychiatric Association.

American Psychiatric Association (2022) *Diagnostic and Statistical Manual of Mental Disorders*, 5th ed., text rev. Washington, DC: American Psychiatric Association.

American Psychiatric Association Corresponding Committee on Religion, Spirituality and Psychiatry (2006) *Resource Document on Religious/ Spiritual Commitments in Psychiatric Practice*. www .psychiatry.org/File%20Library/ Psychiatrists/Directories/Library-and-Archive/resource_documents/rd2006_ Religion.pdf (accessed 22 April 2022).

American Psychiatric Association Ethics Committee (2021) *Resource Document on Ethics at the Interface of Religion, Spirituality, and Psychiatric Practice*. www .psychiatry.org/getattachment/37142161-b62b-45c0-a990-4649b790d72d/Resource-Document-2021-Religion-Spirituality-and-Psychiatric-Practice.pdf (accessed 23 April 2022).

Blazer, D. G. (2011) Spirituality and depression: a background for the development of DSM-V. In J. R. Peteet, F. G. Lu and W. E. Narrow, eds., *Religious and Spiritual Issues in Psychiatric Diagnosis: A Research Agenda for DSM-V*. Arlington, VA: American Psychiatric Publishing, pp. 1–22.

Cloninger, C. R. (2011) Religious and spiritual issues in personality disorders. In J. R. Peteet, F. G. Lu and W. E. Narrow, eds., *Religious and Spiritual Issues in Psychiatric Diagnosis: A Research Agenda for DSM-V*. Arlington, VA:

American Psychiatric Publishing, pp. 151–164.

Fulford, K. W. M. and Sadler, J. Z. (2011) Mapping the logical geography of delusional and spiritual experience: a linguistic-analytic research agenda covering problems, methods and outputs. In J. R. Peteet, F. G. Lu and W. E. Narrow, eds., *Religious and Spiritual Issues in Psychiatric Diagnosis: A Research Agenda for DSM-V*. Arlington, VA: American Psychiatric Publishing, pp. 229–258.

Glas, G. (2011) Religious and spiritual issues in anxiety and adjustment disorders. In J. R. Peteet, F. G. Lu and W. E. Narrow, eds., *Religious and Spiritual Issues in Psychiatric Diagnosis: A Research Agenda for DSM-V*. Arlington, VA: American Psychiatric Publishing, pp. 79–96.

Harrison, M. O., Koenig, H. G., Hays, J. C. et al. (2001) The epidemiology of religious coping: a review of recent literature. *International Review of Psychiatry*, 13, 86–93.

Hays, P. A. (2016) *Addressing Cultural Complexities in Practice: Assessment, Diagnosis, and Therapy*, 3rd ed. Washington, DC: American Psychological Association.

Lee, R. T., Barbo, A., Lopez, G. et al. (2014) National survey of US oncologists' knowledge, attitudes, and practice patterns regarding herb and supplement use by patients with cancer. *Journal of Clinical Oncology*, 32, 4095–4101.

Lewis-Fernández, R., Aggarwal, N. K., Hinton, L., Hinton, D. E. and Kirmayer, L. J., eds. (2016) *DSM-5 Handbook on the Cultural Formulation Interview*. Washington, DC: American Psychiatric Publishing.

Lim, R. F., ed. (2014) *Clinical Manual of Cultural Psychiatry*, 2nd ed. Washington, DC: American Psychiatric Publishing.

Lukoff, D., Lu, F. and Turner, R. (1992) Toward a more culturally sensitive DSM-IV: psychoreligious and psychospiritual problems. *The Journal of Nervous and Mental Disease*, 180, 673–682.

Lukoff, D., Lu, F. G. and Yang, C. P. (2011) DSM-IV Religious and Spiritual Problems. In J. R. Peteet, F. G. Lu and W. E. Narrow, eds., *Religious and Spiritual Issues in Psychiatric Diagnosis: A Research Agenda for DSM-V*. Arlington, VA: American Psychiatric Association, pp. 171–198.

Mabe, P. A., Dell, M. L. and Josephson, A. M. (2011) Spiritual and religious perspectives on child and adolescent psychopathology. In J. R. Peteet, F. G. Lu and W. E. Narrow, eds., *Religious and Spiritual Issues in Psychiatric Diagnosis: A Research Agenda for DSM-V*. Arlington, VA: American Psychiatric Publishing, pp. 123–142.

Moreira-Almeida, A. and Cardena, E. (2011) Differential diagnosis between non-pathological psychotic and spiritual experiences and mental disorders: a contribution from Latin American studies to the ICD-11. *Revista Brasileira de Psiquiatria*, 33 (Suppl. 1), S21–S36.

Moreira-Almeida, A., Sharma, A., van Rensburg, B. J., Verhagen, P. J., and Cook, C. C. (2016) WPA Position Statement on Spirituality and Religion in Psychiatry. *World Psychiatry*, 15, 87–88.

Pargament, K. I., Murray-Swank, N. A., Magyar, G. M. and Ano, G. G. (2005) Spiritual struggle: a phenomenon of interest to psychology and religion. In W. R. Miller and H. D. Delaney, eds., *Judeo-Christian Perspectives on Psychology: Human Nature, Motivation, and Change*. Washington, DC: American Psychological Association, pp. 245–268.

Peck, M. S. (1993) *Further Along the Road Less Traveled: The Unending Journey Toward Spiritual Growth*. New York: Simon & Schuster.

Peteet, J. R., Lu, F. G. and Narrow, W. E., eds. (2011) *Religious and Spiritual Issues in Psychiatric Diagnosis: A Research Agenda for DSM-V*. Arlington, VA: American Psychiatric Publishing.

Reed, G. M., First, M. B., Cogan, C. S. et al. (2019) Innovations and changes in the ICD-11 classification of mental, behavioural and neurodevelopmental disorders. *World Psychiatry*, 18, 13–19.

Seale, C. (2010) The role of doctors' religious faith and ethnicity in taking ethically controversial decisions during end-of-life care. *Journal of Medical Ethics*, 36, 677–682.

Thielman, S. B. (2011) Religion and spirituality in the description of posttraumatic stress disorder. In J. R. Peteet, F. G. Lu and W. E. Narrow, eds., *Religious and Spiritual Issues in Psychiatric Diagnosis: A Research Agenda for DSM-V*. Arlington, VA: American Psychiatric Publishing, pp. 105–114.

Turner, R. P., Lukoff, D., Barnhouse, R. T. and Lu, F. G. (1995) Religious or spiritual problem: a culturally sensitive diagnostic category in the DSM-IV. *The Journal of Nervous and Mental Disease*, 183, 435–444.

13

Spiritual Care in the NHS

John Swinton, Sarah Mullally and Jason Roach

The issue of which healthcare system suits any given context is a matter of controversy and debate. The ongoing discussions around whether health care should be private and paid for by individuals or public and paid for by the State rumble on (King's Fund, 2019). It is not the intention of this chapter to enter into these complex social and economic discussions. We recognise the contextual nature of healthcare systems and we do not intend to hold the National Health Service (NHS) as an exemplar of good practice. It is, however, a very good example of how spirituality, spiritual care and health care are interconnected in ways that significantly affect good practice. Our aim in this chapter is to offer the NHS in the UK as a case study in how the structure and intention of a healthcare system affect the practice of spiritual care – sometimes in quite profound yet often hidden ways. Our hope is that reflection on this particular healthcare system will open up understandings and perspectives that will transfer across systems in both the private and public healthcare services in the UK and elsewhere.

What is the National Health Service?

The NHS was established on 5 July 1948 by Aneurin Bevan, the then Minister of Health within the UK government. This marked the actualisation of a vision that all UK residents should by law have the right to medical services irrespective of their ability to pay. The original intention of the NHS was to eradicate health inequalities and allow everyone access to medical care, free at the point of access. As it was stated in the Ministry of Health leaflet that was sent out to people at the inception of the NHS: 'Everyone – rich or poor, man, woman or child – can use it or any part of it. There are no charges, except for a few special items. There are no insurance qualifications. But it is not a "charity". You are all paying for it, mainly as taxpayers, and it will relieve your money worries in time of illness' (Central Office of Information, 1948, p. 1).

The NHS has a particular purpose and intention, and it is vital to recognise these if we are to understand the way in which spiritual care has developed and how it is understood and carried out within the organisation. Put slightly differently, the particular shape and form of the NHS have a significant effect on how spirituality and spiritual care are framed. To overlook the particularities of the NHS with regard to the ways in which we understand and think about spirituality and spiritual care is to risk misunderstanding spirituality, spiritual care and the particular significance it has not only for the work of the NHS, but also for the role of spirituality in any healthcare system.

In this chapter we shall begin by exploring the diverse nature of spirituality, and then focus on the way in which the NHS has developed its own way of thinking about spirituality – a way of thinking that takes its shape from the goals and intentions of the organisation. After that we shall explore what spiritual care is and what it looks like, before concluding with some reflections on some of the tensions and difficulties involved in providing spiritual care.

The Changing Nature of Spirituality: Spirituality and Religion

The UK, like most of Europe and much of the so-called Western world, is becoming increasingly secularised. Worldwide, certain forms of traditional Christian religion are finding it difficult to survive, whereas others, such as charismatic evangelical and Pentecostal churches, seem to be thriving (Diara and Onah, 2014). Likewise, other religious traditions such as Islam, although in the minority in the UK, remain important and relatively healthy. It is therefore seen to be a complicated spiritual landscape into which the NHS must speak. The complexity of the spiritual landscape is one of the reasons why, within the literature on spirituality in health care, there is a degree of consensus that it is best to separate spirituality from religion.

Spirituality

Broadly defined, spirituality is perceived as relating to issues around meaning, purpose, hope, value, desire, forgiveness and, for some people, transcendence and/or God (see Chapter 1). Within health care, these are all aspects of our humanness that can easily be overlooked or downplayed if we focus solely on developing the best technical medical remedies to address human suffering. Spirituality helps to raise our consciousness of certain aspects of illness and recovery that may otherwise go unnoticed. As such it has become the category of choice for articulating deep human experiences in ways that are not necessarily determined by any religious, philosophical or ethical framework (Cook, 2012). Traditional religions seek to answer the following questions:

- Who am I?
- Where do I come from?
- Where am I going?
- Why?

Contemporary non-religious spirituality also seeks to answer these big existential questions, but not necessarily by using religion or religious language.

Religion

Religion of course remains relevant both culturally and in terms of health care. It pertains to a set of beliefs, narratives, assumptions and worldview that are held by groups of people, around which they organise their lives and make sense of the world (Masters, 2013; see also Chapter 16). For most (but not all) religions there is belief in an all-powerful transcendent being who is involved with the world in various ways. Religion gives people's lives a certain kind of patterning and a particular interpretative framework within which they make sense of themselves, the world and the experiences that they have, including illness. Religiosity can be *intrinsic*, where it is the primary way in which an individual makes sense of the world, or *extrinsic*, where beliefs may be held very lightly and make little difference to a person's day-to-day life (Masters, 2013; see also Chapter 16). The important point for both religion and spirituality is that they provide a framework for making sense of the world. In other words, they are not just sets of beliefs, but rather they are existential maps that people use to navigate the complexities of the world (Berger, 1974). It may be the case that everybody has a spirituality, but it is not the case that everybody perceives or uses it in the same ways.

Spirituality in the NHS

In teasing out how spirituality relates to the NHS, we need to return to the basic rationale of the organisation. As already mentioned, the NHS is based on the desire that good health care should be provided free at the point of use, regardless of a person's level of income. Healthcare provision is therefore based on clinical need rather than on the ability to pay. By definition, and very importantly for current purposes, the system is designed to meet the needs of a broad range of people drawn from a highly diverse general population within which exists a variety of spiritual beliefs and needs. This observation is not particularly problematic for medicine. To do its job well, medicine in all its diverse forms must work with assumed generalities, broad-spectrum treatments and widely applicable approaches which can be effective across a broad range of different people. Within mental health care we might think, for example, of antidepressants. The same drug is given to many different people, all of whom have the same diagnosis – 'depression'. The medication here is generic in so far as it is intended to meet the same needs within a hugely diverse population. Likewise, something like cognitive-behavioural therapy is intended to work for a similarly broad range of people. Both of these approaches would differ from dynamic psychotherapy, where the nature of the treatment is inherently different and unique for each individual patient. The point here is that many forms of treatment and intervention used within the NHS are intended to meet the needs of a broad range of people. Some apply to some people and others do not, but the general principle is that treatments are generalisable. This need for general all-encompassing treatments raises important challenges for spirituality and spiritual care within the NHS.

A Universal Spirituality

Traditionally, spiritual care in the NHS was provided by clergy and/or chaplains who were clergy.[1] However, due to changes in the spiritual demographic, the secular nature of the NHS and the accompanying changing role of those disciplines traditionally assumed to be responsible for spiritual care such as chaplaincy, the type of spirituality that underpins spiritual care has changed. It is interesting to note the way in which the kind of spirituality that is outlined in much of the spirituality-in-healthcare literature is very much in line with the expectations of the institution of the NHS (Vicensi, 2019). Consider, for example, the idea that spiritual care should be for people of all faiths and none (Nolan, 2019). Such an intention is, of course, wholly appropriate. If care is for *all* people as the NHS claims, then spiritual care must also be for *all* people. Nevertheless, it is worth noting that in order for that institutional assumption – that care must be for *all* people – to be operationalised, a certain type of spirituality is required. Spirituality must

---

[1] www.britannica.com/topic/chaplain. (accessed 22 February 2021).

be perceived as *universal* and/or *generic*. The idea of universal spirituality simply means that it is assumed that everyone has a spirituality, and that it is the responsibility of the NHS to ensure that these universally present needs are met. The term 'generic' is a way of indicating the neutrality of spirituality and spiritual care (i.e., that it is not tied to any formal religious or philosophical system). The term 'generic' means something without a brand name such as Christianity, Judaism, Buddhism, Islam, and so forth. It suggests that spirituality is applicable to a broad range of people and situations. Such a universal and generic understanding of spirituality is necessary to accommodate the particularities of the NHS. Although it can be argued that spirituality has distinct qualities – meaning, purpose, hope, value, love and dignity – the actual shape, form and content of these concepts are open to whatever it might be that an individual feels is appropriate. This is not to suggest that the particularities of beliefs and religion are ignored. It is simply to note that any conversations around particularities can be difficult, as is quite well demonstrated by recent debates about whether or not psychiatrists should pray with their patients (Curlin et al., 2007; Poole and Cook, 2011). It is worth bearing in mind that although those of us who work with spirituality may think we are bringing something transformative into the system (we certainly hope we are!), it is also the case that we must shape what we bring to situations within the parameters of the implicit spirituality of the NHS. Spiritual care requires a difficult balance to be achieved between bringing new things into the NHS, and these new things being shaped, formed and perhaps re-formed as they engage with the structures and intentions of the organisation.

Therefore, to recap briefly, for something to be considered 'generic' or 'universal' it needs to be applicable to an entire group or class of people. For spirituality to be universal it needs to be something that is applicable to all people in all cultures and at all times. This form of spirituality sits neatly within the understandings and expectations of the NHS. This is an important observation with regard to the ways in which the culture and expectations of the NHS inevitably affect the understanding of spirituality that is adopted and the modes of spiritual care that are practised.

The advantage of a neutral spirituality is that carers' attention is drawn to potentially important aspects of all people which might not otherwise be on the caring agenda. In assuming that all people are in essence spiritual, irrespective of their involvement or otherwise in formal religion, certain issues are brought to the fore, such as meaning, purpose, value, hope and love. In this way the phenomenology of illness (i.e., the meanings that people ascribe to their illness experiences, which might be quite different from the medical meanings of the illness) is given priority, thereby leading to genuinely person-centred care that respects medicine and clinical practice but is not dictated solely by their explanatory frameworks. As such, a universal approach to spirituality has the potential to improve both the standard and the meaningfulness of our caring practices. This is clearly a benefit. The drawback is that the particularities of beliefs in general, and religious beliefs in particular, can (if we are not careful) be subsumed into a universal model that does not necessarily have the sensitivity to note and deal with these particularities.

Before we move on to explore the nature of spiritual care in more detail, it is worthwhile to consider a few consequences that emerge from the understanding of NHS spirituality that we have laid out thus far. Table 13.1 presents some of the implications of a universal model of spirituality for spiritual care.

Table 13.1. Options for spiritual care

Main features	Options for spiritual care
Assumed to be a universal phenomenon with biological and/or evolutionary roots (Hay, 2006)	As a universal phenomenon with a broad definition, the options for spiritual care are diverse and focused on the needs and preferences of the individual. Everyone has a spirituality and therefore everyone has spiritual needs. The pastoral task is to discover what these needs are and to seek means to fulfil them.
A search for meaning (Frankl, 1959)	The concept of 'search' usually refers to some kind of ongoing journey. People can follow well-trodden pathways established by traditional institutions, or they can construct their own distinctive pathways that have little if anything to do with established religions. This dimension assumes that all human beings have a desire to find an ultimate significance for their lives. For some this can mean God or the transcendent, but for others it will mean such things as community, family, friendships, being in touch with the environment, poetry, literature, music, and so on. Spiritual care here means ensuring that people have access to those things that lift their spirits and make life meaningful for them.
A desire for purpose	This dimension essentially means that the things that people do have a sense of moving towards a goal. So, for example, simply keeping an elderly person or someone living with dementia busy does not ensure a sense of purpose. Busyness can simply be a way of passing the time. Spiritual care that seeks to enable people to find purpose in their lives will come close to the individual, work out the kinds of things that they like to engage in, and strive to ensure that these practices are both meaningful and purposeful. Both meaning and purpose are personal rather than communal goals, which is why person-centred approaches are necessary.
An inherent desire for connectedness (Hay, 2006)	It is certainly the case that human beings are inherently relational. We become who we are as we relate to one another. These relationships can be good or bad, but either way they are deeply formative. Spiritual care here means making sure that this deep relationality is recognised and acted upon. This is a very important aspect. Loneliness is the hallmark of the lives of many elderly people, particularly people living with dementia. Ensuring that people have the opportunity to develop strong positive relationships is very important, and this is certainly captured in the emphasis on relationality within generic models of spirituality and spiritual care.
The need for love, compassion and kindness (Gilbert, 2010; Ballat et al., 2020)	This ties in very much with the emphasis on relationality. Very often it is not clear precisely what is meant by the term 'love', but it is certainly considered by some to be a significant dimension of spirituality and spiritual care.
A search for the sacred and/or the holy (Zinnbauer and Pargament, 2000)	The term 'sacred' refers not only to concepts of God and higher powers, but also to other aspects of life that are perceived to be manifestations of the divine or imbued with divine-like qualities, such as transcendence, immanence, boundlessness and that which people consider ultimate. Virtually any part of life, whether positive or negative, such as beliefs, practices, experiences, relationships, motivations, art, nature and war, can be endowed with sacred status.

Person-Centred Care

One of the advantages of a universal approach to spirituality is that it takes on the shape and form of the individual who is seeking to have his or her spiritual needs met. Within this perspective it is never appropriate for a carer to enforce his or her spirituality on an individual. Spiritual discovery is always inductive and never deductive; it always takes place from the person outwards, and never via the imposition of assumptions from 'outside'. In other words, spiritual care in the NHS is respectful and *person-centred*. Person-centred care has recently been a central focus for the Royal College of Psychiatrists (Person-Centred Training and Curriculum [PCTC] Scoping Group and Special Committee on Professional Practice and Ethics, 2018). It is a way of thinking and doing things that sees those utilising the NHS in general, and mental health services in particular, as equal partners in planning, developing and monitoring care to ensure that it meets their specific needs. We noted previously that there is a necessary ethos of generalisation within the NHS. A person-centred focus recognises this necessity but strives to develop an approach that is designed to look at the particular needs of the individual. These needs are identified, developed and negotiated between the service user and the professional who is seeking to offer support. This means looking at the individual within the context of his or her immediate experiences, wider community and broader hopes for the present and the future. It also means taking seriously service users' perspectives and developing care in dialogue, rather than imposing views on them (Raffay et al., 2016).

Patient-Centred Care

Patient-centred care seeks to replace physician-centred systems with an approach that revolves around the patient. The idea is that the patient should be involved in every aspect of his or her care. Rather than being the object of care, the patient becomes the subject of his or her own care (Stewart, 2001). This idea is important within a mental healthcare context, where it is recognised that issues of stigma, disempowerment and a loss of autonomy can profoundly affect quality of life. However, simply focusing on the individual patient is not what makes person-centred care person centred. A 'patient' cannot be understood apart from his or her community or looked at without any reference to his or her family, friends, hopes, dreams, likes, dislikes, and so on. People living with mental health challenges can only be understood as they are recognised as part of a complicated matrix of relationships within which they live, find their identity and seek happiness and fulfilment. Genuinely person-centred mental health care does not simply look at the individual – it always looks at the individual-in-their-community. People with mental health challenges are always situated within a community. Certainly mental health challenges manifest themselves within unique individuals, but they always affect and are affected by a wider community of people. The welfare of individuals is dependent on the welfare, well-being and good will of their communities. Person-centred mental health care that takes spirituality seriously requires the formation of a sense of community (professional and lay) that cares. This includes the communal environment of the hospital, the immediate community of family and friends, and the wider community within which the person is trying to live his or her life well. Spiritual care within a mental health context assumes an *assets-based approach* (Downward and Rasciute, 2020).

Assets-based approaches focus on the factors that protect and enhance people's health and well-being, and in so doing seek to improve quality of life, by drawing attention to that within a community which improves self-esteem and the ability to cope. According to this way of thinking, community is not simply understood as a geographical area. Rather it is a series of existing resources (lay and professional people and relational networks) and potential resources that, if accessed effectively, can participate positively in the development of mental health and spiritual well-being.

How Might We Think About Spiritual Care?

There have been various attempts to identify a taxonomy of spiritual needs (McSherry and Cash, 2004). To date there has been no overall consensus on exactly what a comprehensive list of spiritual needs might look like. Nevertheless, there is what we might call a 'family resemblance' between the different approaches. We have tried to capture some of the dynamics of this process in Table 13.1. These basic spiritual needs that might be addressed within the normal daily activity of healthcare include:

- the need to give and receive love
- the need to be understood
- the need to be valued as a human being
- the need for forgiveness, hope and trust
- the need to explore beliefs and values – the need to express feelings honestly
- the need to find meaning and purpose in life (Scottish Government, 2009).

Inevitably, the kind of spirituality we have been describing thus far is emergent, contextual and fluid, taking its shape and form from the particular place where people are providing care and the particularities of the experiences they are dealing with. This is important if we are to take the interdisciplinary nature of spiritual care seriously. If spiritual care is a responsibility that is shared between psychiatrists, physiotherapists, nurses, psychotherapists, chaplains and other healthcare professionals, then the context and skills that people bring will mean that the shape and form of that spiritual care will differ from place to place, sometimes quite radically. A chaplain may be present, empathic, gentle, forgiving and loving. A physiotherapist may have to be quite rough and risk inflicting physical pain in order to bring about healing. A nurse may be patient and kind as he or she seeks to alleviate the pain of those to whom he or she offers care. An occupational therapist may help an individual to develop the skills to become independent and to retain his or her autonomy and power. A psychiatrist may have to prescribe drugs that are intended to protect from harm and bring about healing, but which at the same time have very troublesome side effects that have the potential to lower the person's quality of life and sense of well-being. What does spiritual care look like when one has to advise or insist that a person has electroconvulsive therapy? What does spiritual care look like when we have to take away someone's liberty with the intention of increasing their safety and well-being? We do not say any of this flippantly or polemically. The chaplain, physiotherapist, nurse, occupational therapist and psychiatrist all desire to engage in spiritual care. However, their situations make the actual nature of spiritual care different, difficult and sometimes quite dissonant. That said, we would suggest that there are two dimensions of spiritual care that are present in all of these diverse situations, namely *love* and *presence*.

Remembering Love

The first dynamic of spiritual care that we want to draw attention to is the attitude of love. Near the beginning of Natalya Ryabova's recent powerful film *Love is Listening: Dementia Without Loneliness*, an African American woman with advanced dementia reflects on her life experience: 'I don't know where I am. I don't know where I'm going. I don't know where I've just come from. But I'm not fearful'. She pauses and looks deep into the eyes of the person she is talking to. 'Because I see all around me – I don't see a lot – but I see patience'. She looks upwards and away, and her eyes glaze over a little. 'I see gratitude. I see tolerance'. She slowly looks back towards her friend and smiles. 'I think I see love'. She smiles. 'And your face is a picture of love'.[2] (Memory Bridge, 2019). It is a very beautiful and moving scene. Even when we feel lost, uncertain about the future and unable to work out where life is going, we can still feel, see and experience love. More than that, the presence of such love can drive out fear. The experience of dementia (like that of many other conditions) can at times be frightening. We need people who will love us out of our fear and help us to find love amidst the challenges. If we know that we are loved, we need not be fearful. When we have dementia (as at all other times) we need people who will act gently, patiently, kindly, humbly, respectfully and peacefully. We need people whose lives are filled with forgiveness, honesty and integrity. We need people whose faces are a picture of love.

What Is Love?

Of course, as soon as we use the term 'love', red flags will inevitably and quite rightly be raised. We therefore need to be careful and precise about what we mean here. Throughout our lives we are tied into various modes of love. As we move through life, love changes. The love we receive from our parents is not the same as the love we find in our romantic lives. The love we find in long-term relationships shifts and changes over time and, if all goes well, we become companions as well as partners. In the final years of our lives (or in principle at any crisis point) we find ourselves being cared for by professionals. What exactly does love in a professional context look like? A little later in this chapter we shall explore the issue of professional boundaries and the risks and dangers that potentially accompany the closeness of spiritual care. Challenges are not necessarily barriers, but we do need to be clear what we mean by 'love'. The meaning of love here is quite specific: it relates to *intentionally adopting an attitude wherein we recognise the inherent value in other people, and we are genuinely glad that they are with us.* This mode of love is important in general, but is particularly important within the context of mental health, where the issues of stigma and depersonalisation are deeply significant. Mental health diagnoses are especially prone to being stigmatised (Markowits and Syverson, 2019; Krendl and Pescosolido, 2020; Violeau et al.,

---

[2] www.memorybridge.org/ (accessed 13 December 2020).

2020). Stigma occurs when the whole of a person is reduced to the size of one small part of him or her. For example, people living with schizophrenia are reduced to 'schizophrenics,' and people with bipolar disorder are rejected and alienated by the assumptions others make about their diagnosis. Stigma alienates people and makes them both feel and seem to be unloved. It is the exact opposite of the kind of love we are talking about here: *intentionally adopting an attitude wherein we recognise the inherent value of other people and we are genuinely glad that they are with us.* Stigma conveys to the person that it is *not* good that they exist, and we are *not* glad that they are here. Love reverses this dynamic by offering a dynamic of welcome and gratitude for the presence of the other (Gerrard, 1996; Natterson, 2003, see also Chapter 6). The essence of spiritual care within a mental health context is to enable people to reclaim their humanity and to feel valued, loved and cared for, and that their lives are worthwhile.

As the paradigms of business continue to be applied to the NHS, which is now being described as a 'market', 'industry' or 'sector,' with people viewed as consumers whose choice should sit at the centre of the system, there will inevitably be a challenging tension between the need for safety, professionalism, clinical compliance and financial governance on the one hand, and the 'soft,' 'dangerous' and 'risky' language of spirituality and love on the other. Nevertheless, there is a strange irony in the sense that some argue that the consumer should be at the heart of the system, while at the same time avoiding the language of the heart. The idea that love and the enablement of love might be key indicators of success within an organisation is not easily assimilated into standard business models.

We could of course simply avoid the language of love altogether. It is possible to care without loving. Imagine for a moment that you are lying in a hospital bed and a nurse comes along to care for you. He is very good at his job. You are well cared for, safe, warm, appropriately treated and comfortable. Then, for whatever reason, you come to realise that he is only caring for you because he gets paid to do so. Nothing changes in terms of the physical dimensions of care, but everything changes in terms of your relationship with him and your perspective on whether he sees you as a person or as a series of tasks. It is possible to care without love, but it is not possible to love without care. Love is an attitude – a way of looking at another person that enables us truly to see him or her – and it is necessary if our person-centred spiritual care is to be authentic and health bringing.

What Does Love Look Like?

In a recent qualitative research study that explored the faith lives of people with schizophrenia, bipolar disorder and major depression, the first author of this chapter spent three years talking with people of faith who lived with these conditions, using a phenomenological approach to try to get to the lived experience of people's faith lives (Swinton, 2020). One of the participants, Allen, recalled his experience of being diagnosed with schizophrenia. He told of how he had been having some very unusual experiences – disorientation, hearing voices and feeling that people were against him – and that eventually he had approached his doctor, who in turn had arranged an appointment with a psychiatrist. Allen spent time with the psychiatrist and was given a diagnosis of schizophrenia. His first response was disappointment. He felt that his life was over and that he had to be a patient from then onwards. He took the bus home. On the bus he met a woman whom he knew quite well; they had travelled together many times. She was welcoming towards him until he told her about his new diagnosis. When she heard that he had schizophrenia she got off the bus and they never spoke again. Allen went home. It had been a sad day for him. He told his mother that the psychiatrist had told him he was a 'schizophrenic' and that his life was basically over. His mother looked at him and said, 'Allen, you're not a schizophrenic, you are Allen, and I love you'.

This strikes us as a powerful example of what love does. It gives people back their name and upholds their dignity. The diagnosis of schizophrenia had overwhelmed Allen with a sense of hopelessness. His mother's words of love gave him back his name. Spiritual care that is truly loving, in the sense that we have outlined previously, takes diagnoses seriously but refuses to allow negative associations to shape the identity of the person who is living with difficult experiences: 'You may have challenges, but we will walk with you'.

Thinking About Presence: Resisting the Culture of Absence

The second dynamic of spiritual care that we want to draw attention to is the issue of presence. Being present is at the heart of the enterprise of spiritual care. However, being present is a complex matter. Think again about the example of the nurse carer mentioned previously, and add another dimension. All the time he is caring for you he is thinking of other things – the next task, his children, what he will do at the weekend, even what he will cook for Tuesday's supper! The nurse is in the room and physically present, but he is clearly absent in terms of noticing you *as a person*. He looks at you but cannot really see you. He is present, but he is also absent in crucial ways.

The Cultural Problem of Presence

It is worth noting that there is a general problem with presence, or rather the lack of presence, within society. How often do we see people sitting in a restaurant with each person on the phone to someone else and none of them really engaging with those who are sitting with them? They are present but clearly absent in crucial ways. The problem is that we have become used to being absent. We check our phones every 12 minutes on average during waking hours, with 7% of us admitting that we *never* turn our phones off, and 40% of us check our phones within 5 minutes of waking. Interestingly, a recent study noted that people who were distracted by emails and phone calls saw a 10-point decrease in their IQ, which was twice that found in studies on the impact of smoking marijuana (Dredge, 2018). Many of us suffer from what has been described as *continuous partial attention* (Rose, 2010), a 'condition' wherein we are constantly distracted and looking for things that we might have missed. We constantly check social media platforms such as Twitter, Facebook and Instagram to make sure that we are not missing out on something. We don't know what that something is, but we definitely don't want to miss it! We spend so much time looking around for what we have missed that we often can't see the things that are in front of us. *A lack of presence is rapidly becoming a cultural norm.* When this implicit cultural norm is transferred into a mental health setting, problems will inevitably arise. Any lack of presence that we encounter within our caring efforts is a mirror image of a wider lack of presence that significantly shapes and forms us, often unknowingly. *We live in a culture where absence has become the norm.*

Defining Presence

Presence is generally recognised as both a *quality* and an *intervention* in professional care. It is a quality in that it is a way of being with others that recognises the fullness of their humanness and seeks to be present in ways that respect that recognition. *Presence is the quality of being there for others, and the ability to understand what kinds of caring practices most enhance them as human beings.* Presence is also an intervention in so far as it is carried out in a structured and intentional way by professionals who, while recognising presence as a basic way of being with others, realise that this needs to be undertaken with integrity, competence and intentionality. We need to consciously notice what we are doing and why we are doing it. We have to actively think about what we are doing when we are present and when we are not present. The importance of presence is acknowledged within the language we use – being present, nursing presence, meaningful presence, and so on. The opposite of presence is not absence; it is avoidance and alienation. An estranged couple can sit at the same table but not be present. Likewise, a carer can be bodily with a person with mental health challenges but be totally disengaged from him or her emotionally. Presence that heals and reconciles recognises the significance of the therapeutic dimensions of caring encounters (those formal aspects of the person's care that require professional attention), but strives to develop relationships that are mutual, equal and multidimensional. Presence has a natural dimension and a learned dimension. Some people will naturally have the quality of presence, whereas others may not. However, *everyone* can be made aware of the need for presence as a quality and as an intervention.

Presence can be perceived in terms of a reciprocal and healing relationship that develops between carer and patient. Here the focus is on connection, relationality and the mutual exchange of experience. The intention is to move beyond the limitations of a 'professional relationship' (without losing the importance of boundaries, something we shall return to later), with its emphasis on distance and observation, towards a more relational approach based on mutuality, care and shared relationships. To be present is to be aware of how the other is feeling and to engage with them in ways that are compassionate, empathic, healing and therapeutic.

Problems can arise when those whom we want to be present with do not share our normal modes of communication and ways of relating. People who are deeply depressed, or who have a perspective on experience which is very different from our own, require us to recognise our own concerns and anxieties, and intentionally to strive not to allow our communicational difficulties to overrule our desire truly to be present with them. The experience of an individual living with delusions may be radically different from our normal ways of seeing the world. Nevertheless, these remain meaningful experiences for the person concerned. The temptation is to allow the idea that 'these are just symptoms' to make us less than present to the meanings and experiences that are being articulated to us. This does not mean that everything that is said is real or good. It does mean that everything that is said should be listened to, and that our bodily and psychological presence is vital if the healing power of presence is to enter into any given situation.

Of course, some degree of withdrawal is necessary for all healthy relationships. If we do not have the ability to withdraw at times, we risk becoming overwhelmed. However, when we are dealing with vulnerable people whose experiences may confuse and concern us, there is a danger that withdrawal becomes the norm. When this happens, we are tempted – consciously or unconsciously – to focus on *absence* rather than presence. Such a lack of intentional presence risks caring encounters becoming 'thin,' instrumental and task oriented, which in turn means carers may well miss important aspects of the experiences of the people to whom they are offering care. Dangerous omissions of care can occur not only consciously, by carers deliberately acting abusively, but also unwittingly by people not being present in a way that enables them to notice certain critical issues within their relationships with elderly people and/or significant problems within the culture of their working environment (Francis, 2013). An absence of presence is to a degree understandable and necessary. However, it is devastating if absence and the withdrawal of meaningful relationships become the norm. *Love and presence are the two elements that hold spiritual care together in all its complex diversity.*

Professional Boundaries

So far we have established that spiritual care within the NHS is seen to be person-centred, relational, intimate (in the sense that people have to come close and get to know one another in order to offer good spiritual care) and professional. This brings us to the crucial issue of *professional boundaries.* There is of course a real risk of overstepping boundaries when providing care in general and spiritual care in particular. We therefore need to take time to reflect on the importance of boundaries. Professional boundaries relate to the legal, ethical and structural boundaries that are designed to protect staff and clients from physical or psychological harm and to facilitate a safe working environment (Cook, 2013; see also Chapter 1). Within the context of the NHS, we might outline the parameters of professional boundaries in the following way:

- A therapeutic relationship occurs wherein a healthcare professional applies their professional knowledge, skills, talents and experience in an effort to meet the healthcare needs of patients.
- The practice of spiritual care is therapeutic in so far as it allows healthcare professionals and others to bring their skills and knowledge of spiritual issues into intentional engagement with patients, with a view to meeting their spiritual needs.
- All therapeutic relationships must ensure the protection of an individual's dignity, autonomy, privacy, respect and trust.
- Professional boundaries relate to a recognition by professionals that they are in a position of power over patients, and that they need to be aware of, monitor and take great care with the inevitable inequality of power within relationships with vulnerable people. Professional boundaries thus provide a safe space between the professional and the patient.
- Professional boundaries are set out in rules, regulations and ethical codes. Transgression of such boundaries can be dangerous, disrespectful and open to litigation.

- Crossing of professional boundaries often occurs when there is confusion between the needs of the professional and the needs of the patient.
- Respecting professional boundaries requires reflexivity and awareness – that is, an ability to recognise one's own feelings and experiences and to ensure that they are not projected, consciously or otherwise, on to the needs and expectations of patients.
- Professionals can be under-involved or over-involved with patients. Under-involvement would include ignoring patient needs, neglecting vital aspects of care and keeping a form of professional distance that makes the professional appear cold, distanced or uninterested. Over-involvement would include crossing or violating boundaries, imposing views on patients, and allowing feelings, expectations or desires to create a power imbalance between professional and patient.

These parameters of professional boundaries run across all forms of care, but can become particularly sensitive in relation to spiritual care. Concerns have been raised about certain aspects of spiritual care, such as praying with patients, doing spiritual assessments and professionals sharing about their own spirituality (Poole and Cook, 2011). As we reflect on the nature of spiritual care as understood in the ways we have outlined earlier in this chapter, we can see that the closeness of relationships and the significance of a certain kind of presence require that NHS workers closely monitor their behaviour and the impact of spiritual care on patients and others, so that the kinds of difficulties and power imbalances that have been mentioned do not become a barrier to good person-centred spiritual care and safe, secure relationships with patients.

Chaplaincy

Central to the delivery of spiritual care within the NHS is the practice of chaplaincy. It has become clear that the delivery of spiritual care is the responsibility of all NHS employees. To see the individual as a whole person, to offer him or her respect and dignity, and to take seriously his or her need for meaning, purpose, love, hope, presence and sometimes God is basic to all forms of care. Although all mental health professionals should take spirituality seriously, chaplaincy is a central aspect of spiritual care within the NHS. We might think of chaplaincy in this way:

> A chaplain is an individual who provides religious and spiritual care within an organisational setting. Although this role has evolved from within the Christian churches, the term 'chaplain' is now increasingly associated with other faith traditions. Chaplains may be qualified religious professionals, or lay people, and while religious and pastoral care might be central to their role, the increasing complexity of many large public organisations has led to an expansion in the range of their activities. (Gilliat-Ray et al., 2013, p. 5)

At an interpersonal level, the key tasks of chaplaincy are:

- to help people explore their sense of meaning and purpose in the midst of their illness experience
- to work with the meaning of diverse attitudes, beliefs, values and concerns around mental health issues
- to develop strategies to help people to discover life as worthwhile and meaningful even in the midst of mental health challenges

- to work with people's hopes, fears and concerns for themselves and others with regard to their present and future situations
- to help people to wrestle with the 'Why?' questions in relation to mental health and ill health.

At an institutional level, chaplains build bridges between the disciplines by offering spiritual care to staff and providing a vital mental health resource in stressful and sometimes difficult situations. Alongside their work with hospital staff, chaplains work with all faith groups as well as coordinating denominational activities within the healthcare context. Chaplaincy is inherently a collaborative discipline that strives to relate to and often to bring together the different dimensions of mental health care and the various disciplines that make up this aspect of the healthcare system. This cohesive role reflects the holistic nature of the practice of chaplaincy, and is a profound reminder of the wholeness of human beings and the need for that wholeness to be reflected across the board in mental health care. We might think of chaplains as the experts in spiritual care – that is, the discipline within the NHS that intentionally highlights spirituality and spiritual care as central to its professional identity. As such, chaplaincy is both an active participant in spiritual care and a vital resource for others within the NHS who wish to engage with the spiritual dimensions of their work. Chaplains are the flag bearers for spiritual care within the NHS.

Conclusion

In this chapter we have tried to outline what spirituality and spiritual care look like specifically within the context of the NHS. Spirituality is a vitally important, complex and sometimes controversial area of health care. We have tried to explore what spirituality is within the NHS, and how this feeds into the types of spiritual care that are vital for a genuinely person-centred and compassionate health service. We hope that we have managed to raise some important issues and bring clarity to several aspects of spiritual care that it is important to think clearly about. Our intention is that our contribution to this book can help all of us to care more effectively, act more compassionately and serve our patients more lovingly.

References

Ballat, J., Campling, P. and Maloney, C. (2020) *Intelligent Kindness: Rehabilitating the Welfare State*. London: Royal College of Psychiatrists.

Berger, P. L. (1974) Some second thoughts on substantive versus functional definitions of religion. *Journal for the Scientific Study of Religion*. 13, 125–133.

Central Office of Information (1948) *The New National Health Service*. London: Ministry of Health.

Cook, C. C. H. (2012) Keynote 4: spirituality and health. *Journal for the Study of Spirituality*, 2, 150–162.

(2013) Controversies on the place of spirituality and religion in psychiatric practice. In C. C. H. Cook, ed., *Spirituality, Theology and Mental Health*. London: SCM Press, pp. 1–19.

Curlin, F. A., Lawrence, R. E., Odell, S. et al. (2007) Religion, spirituality, and medicine: psychiatrists' and other physicians' differing observations, interpretations, and clinical approaches. *The American Journal of Psychiatry*, 164, 1825–1831.

Diara, B. C. and Onah, N. G. (2014) The phenomenal growth of Pentecostalism in the contemporary Nigerian society: a challenge to mainline churches.

Mediterranean Journal of Social Sciences, 5, 395.

Downward., P. and Rasciute, S. (2020) Health as an asset: enhancing personal, social and economic life. *European Journal of Public Health*, 30 (Suppl. 5), v432.

Dredge, S. (2018) Mobile phone addiction? It's time to take back control. *The Guardian* (Australian Edition). Available at www.theguardian.com/technology/2018/jan/27/mobile-phone-addiction-apps-break-the-habit-take-back-control (accessed 2 February 2020).

Francis, R. (2013) *Report of the Mid Staffordshire NHS Foundation Trust Public Inquiry*. London: Crown Publications.

Frankl, V. (1959/1984) *Man's Search for Meaning: An Introduction to Logotherapy*, 3rd ed. New York: Simon & Schuster.

Gerrard, J. (1996) Love in the time of psychotherapy. *British Journal of Psychotherapy*, 13, 163–173.

Gilbert, P. (2010) *The Compassionate Mind: A New Approach to Life's Challenges*. Oakland, CA: New Harbinger Publications.

Gilliat-Ray, S., Ali, M. and Pattison, S. (2013) *Understanding Muslim Chaplaincy*. London: Ashgate.

Hay, D. (2006) *Something There: The Biology of the Human Spirit*. London: Darton, Longman & Todd.

King's Fund (2019) Is the NHS being privatised? Available at www.kingsfund.org.uk/publications/articles/big-election-questions-nhs-privatised (accessed 22 February 2021).

Krendl, A. C. and Pescosolido, B. A. (2020) Countries and cultural differences in the stigma of mental illness: the East–West divide. *Journal of Cross-Cultural Psychology*, 51, 149–167.

McSherry, W. and Cash, K. (2004) The language of spirituality: an emerging taxonomy. *International Journal of Nursing Studies*, 41, 151–161.

Markowitz, F. and Syverson, J. (2019) Race, gender, and homelessness stigma: effects of perceived blameworthiness and

dangerousness. *Deviant Behavior*, 42, 919–931.

Masters, K. S. (2013) Intrinsic religiousness (religiosity). In M. D. Gellman and J. R. Turner, eds., *Encyclopedia of Behavioral Medicine*. New York: Springer, pp. 69–136. https://doi.org/10.1007/978-1-4419-1005-9_1585

Natterson, J. M. (2003) Love in psychotherapy. *Psychoanalytic Psychology*, 20, 509–521.

Nolan, S. (2019) Non-religious pastoral care: a practical guide. *Practical Theology*, 12, 97–99.

Person-Centred Training and Curriculum (PCTC) Scoping Group and Special Committee on Professional Practice and Ethics (2018) *Person-Centred Care: Implications for Training in Psychiatry*. College Report. London: Royal College of Psychiatrists.

Poole, R. and Cook, C. C. H. (2011) Praying with a patient constitutes a breach of professional boundaries in psychiatric practice. *British Journal of Psychiatry*, 199, 94–98.

Raffay, J., Wood, E. and Todd, A. (2016) Service user views of spiritual and pastoral care (chaplaincy) in NHS mental health services: a co-produced constructivist grounded theory investigation. *BMC Psychiatry*, 16, Article 200.

Rose, E. (2010) Continuous partial attention: reconsidering the role of online learning in the age of interruption. *Educational Technology*, 50, 41–46.

Scottish Government (2009) *Spiritual Care and Chaplaincy: Guidance on Spiritual Care in the NHS in Scotland*. Available at www.gov.scot/publications/spiritual-care-chaplaincy/pages/2/ (accessed 13 December 2020).

Stewart, M. (2001) Towards a global definition of patient centred care: the patient should be the judge of patient centred care. *British Medical Journal*, 322, 444–445.

Swinton, J. (2020) *Finding Jesus in the Storm: The Spiritual Lives of Christians with Mental Health Challenges*. London: SCM Press.

Vincensi, B. B. (2019) Interconnections: spirituality, spiritual care, and patient-centered care. *Asia-Pacific Journal of Oncology Nursing*, 6, 104–110.

Violeau, L., Dudilot, A., Roux, S. and Prouteau, A. (2020) How internalised stigma reduces self-esteem in schizophrenia: the crucial role of off-line metacognition. *Cognitive Neuropsychiatry*, 25, 154–161.

Zinnbauer, B. J. and Pargament, K. I. (2000) Working with the sacred: four approaches to religious and spiritual issues in counseling. *Journal of Counseling & Development*, 78, 162–171.

Spiritual and Religious Interventions
Introduction

Christopher C. H. Cook

As other chapters in this book have made clear, spirituality has a part to play in treatment planning in all areas of psychiatry. Patient-centred psychiatry will always properly consider the ways in which the spiritual/religious concerns of patients might have an impact upon treatment. These concerns can often be utilised to good effect, but sometimes, if they go unrecognised, they may present barriers to effective treatment. It is important to know, for example, if a patient might not take their prescribed medication because they feel that they need to trust in God, rather than in tablets. More positively, prayer, meditation and other religious practices can provide significant coping resources during the course of treatment and recovery, and it is helpful for the clinician to affirm this rather than neglect or, worse still, undermine it.

In addition to the general therapeutic milieu within which spirituality/religion can make an important contribution, certain specific interventions have evolved within psychiatry since the last decade of the twentieth century in which they play a more explicit, or central, role. Among these, Twelve-Step facilitation (TSF) (Humphreys, 1999) in the treatment of addictive disorders is probably one of the earliest examples, and is discussed in Chapter 8. TSF is a professional intervention, but its objective is to draw patients into the non-professional, mutual help programme of recovery offered by Alcoholics Anonymous and other Twelve-Step groups. In this way, patients may benefit from the spiritual programme of recovery that the Twelve-Step groups offer. Thus TSF is an 'indirectly spiritual' intervention, and is therefore in a somewhat different category to the interventions that will be discussed in this chapter.

Four specific spiritual/religious interventions will be considered, each in a separate sub-chapter authored by a leading researcher/practitioner. These interventions all incorporate both spiritual and psychological elements, and so we might call them 'psychospiritual' therapies. Alternatively, we might see them as specialised applications within a broader field of endeavour to integrate spirituality into psychotherapy more widely, as illustrated by the work of Kenneth Pargament (Pargament, 2011) and others (e.g., Hefti, 2009; Captari et al., 2018). They are all professionally led – by psychiatrists, clinical psychologists or other mental health professionals – and may be integrated into routine treatment planning (where local expertise and training allow). All have been subjected to extensive scientific research and have accumulated (or are accumulating) a significant evidence base. However, they also draw on the spiritual insights and practices of Buddhism, Christianity and other faith traditions that are accessible to people of all faiths and none, to those who consider themselves spiritual but not religious, and even to those who consider themselves neither spiritual nor religious.

Mindfulness, discussed in Chapter 14.1. is rooted in Buddhism, but shows close similarities to contemplative prayer and meditation in a number of other religious traditions, including Christianity (Knabb, 2012; Tyler, 2018). As Paramabandhu Groves explains, it forms the core component of *mindfulness-based stress reduction (MBSR)*, and is a significant component of a variety of interventions, including *acceptance and commitment therapy (ACT)* and *dialectical behaviour therapy (DBT)*. It has been widely integrated with techniques from *cognitive–behavioural therapy (CBT)*, notably in the form of *mindfulness-based cognitive therapy (MBCT)*. Mindfulness-based interventions have been applied effectively across a wide range of psychiatric disorders (Goldberg et al., 2018).

Compassion-focused therapy (CFT), as Paul Gilbert shows in Chapter 14.2, draws on cognitive therapy, Jungian analytical psychology, evolutionary psychology and neuroscience. Compassion is a central concern of many of the world's major faith traditions, including Buddhism, Islam and Christianity. Again, CFT has shown benefit across diagnostic groups. More generally, one might expect that the ability to show compassion for oneself and others would be fundamental to good healthcare delivery, yet the importance of compassion has (at least until recently) often been recognised only when it has been found to be missing (Fotaki, 2015; Gray and Cox, 2015; Sinclair et al., 2016).

A variety of approaches have been taken to integrating spirituality/religion into CBT (Rosmarin, 2018). Some of these have been developed specifically for particular religious traditions, as in the case of *transdiagnostic multiplex CBT* for Muslims (Hinton and Jalal, 2020). In Chapter 14.3, Michell Pearce provides an overview of *religiously integrated CBT (RCBT)*, including the research undertaken by her with colleagues at Duke University on a manualised approach that has been adapted for use with five major religious traditions (Christianity, Judaism, Islam, Buddhism and Hinduism).

Finally, in Chapter 14.4, Robert Enright and Jacqueline Song take a philosophical and psychological perspective on the part that forgiveness plays in the healing of various mental disorders. Two specific forms of forgiveness therapy are described – the *process model* (developed by Enright) and the *REACH model* – both of which have been subjected to extensive research. However, like compassion, forgiveness is important not so much because specific therapies have been developed within which it takes a central role, as because it can contribute to treatment planning and psychotherapy much more widely. Compassion and forgiveness have not been highlighted in traditional psychiatric therapies, but both turn out to be important considerations that can be integrated within diverse therapeutic approaches across a wide range of psychiatric disorders.

Other evidence-based therapies, which the interested reader might wish to investigate further in the literature, include *Solace for the Soul*, which is a spiritually integrated intervention for survivors of sexual abuse (Murray-Swank and Pargament, 2005), *spiritually integrated cognitive processing therapy* for moral injury (Pearce et al., 2018), pastoral care, religious counselling/psychotherapy and prayer (Koenig, 2018, pp. 255–277).

From a traditional religious perspective, some might express concern about spiritual practices being removed from their religious context and applied to secular health care, given that spirituality is not primarily concerned with the relief of symptoms but with higher aims, such as finding a transcendent purpose in life. It is about living well, though not necessarily about living comfortably. From a scientific perspective, others might well ask whether any of the original tenets of religion need to come into the picture, since the therapeutic evidence base is provided by scientific research into objective outcome criteria. Yet, for spirituality to be truly integrated into the work of psychiatry, there needs to be mutually respectful and sensitive communication across barriers and boundaries. Psychiatry has much to learn from spiritual/religious traditions, and likewise spirituality and religion can benefit from what psychiatry has to offer. The aim of the clinician, I would contend, should be to encourage collaboration by means of a fruitful and ongoing dialogue.

References

Captari, L. E., Hook, J. N., Hoyt, W. et al. (2018) Integrating clients' religion and spirituality within psychotherapy: a comprehensive meta-analysis. *Journal of Clinical Psychology*, 74, 1938–1951.

Fotaki, M. (2015) Why and how is compassion necessary to provide good quality healthcare? *International Journal of Health Policy and Management*, 4, 199–201.

Goldberg, S. B., Tucker, R. P., Greene, P. A. et al. (2018) Mindfulness-based interventions for psychiatric disorders: a systematic review and meta-analysis. *Clinical Psychology Review*, 59, 52–60.

Gray, A. and Cox, J. (2015) The roots of compassion and empathy: implementing the Francis report and the search for new models of healthcare. *European Journal for Person Centered Healthcare*, 3, 122–130.

Hefti, R. (2009) Integrating spiritual issues into therapy. In P. Huguelet and H. G. Koenig, eds., *Religion and Spirituality in Psychiatry*. Cambridge: Cambridge University Press, pp. 244–267.

Hinton, D. E. and Jalal, B. (2020) *Transdiagnostic Multiplex CBT for Muslim Cultural Groups*. Cambridge: Cambridge University Press.

Humphreys, K. (1999) Professional interventions that facilitate twelve-step self-help group involvement. *Alcohol Research & Health*, 23, 93–98.

Knabb, J. J. (2012) Centering prayer as an alternative to mindfulness-based cognitive therapy for depression relapse prevention. *Journal of Religion and Health*, 51, 908–924.

Koenig, H. G. (2018) *Religion and Mental Health: Research and Clinical Applications*. London: Academic Press.

Murray-Swank, N. A. and Pargament, K. I. (2005) God, where are you? Evaluating a spiritually-integrated intervention for sexual abuse. *Mental Health, Religion & Culture*, 8, 191–203.

Pargament, K. I. (2011) *Spiritually Integrated Psychotherapy: Understanding and Addressing the Sacred*. New York: The Guilford Press.

Pearce, M., Haynes, K., Rivera, N. R. and Koenig, H. G. (2018) Spiritually integrated cognitive processing therapy: a new treatment for post-traumatic stress disorder that targets moral injury. *Global Advances in Health and Medicine*, 7, 2164956118759939.

Rosmarin, D. H. (2018) *Spirituality, Religion, and Cognitive-Behavioral Therapy: A Guide for Clinicians*. New York: The Guilford Press.

Sinclair, S., Norris, J. M., Mcconnell, S. J. et al. (2016) Compassion: a scoping review of the healthcare literature. *BMC Palliative Care*, 15, 6.

Tyler, P. (2018) *Christian Mindfulness: Theology and Practice*. London: SCM Press.

Mindfulness

Paramabandhu Groves

Mindfulness has emerged over the last four decades as an increasingly popular therapeutic modality. Within mindfulness-based interventions (MBIs), meditation plays a central role. Contemplative practices such as meditation and prayer are a feature of many spiritual and religious traditions. Mindfulness as a therapeutic modality has its main origins in Buddhism. In addition, influences can be discerned from Hindu Neo-Vedanta and American metaphysical religion, which with its flourishing of Spiritualism, Christian Science and New Thought in the nineteenth century appears to have provided a context from which mindfulness could gain popularity in the following century (Hickey, 2019).

Buddhist Origins

'Mindfulness' is the term used to translate the Pāli word *sati*, which means something like 'presence' or 'awareness', especially awareness of the present moment (Anālayo, 2003). It is related to the verb *sarati*, meaning 'remember'. Hence there are connotations of recollecting oneself or coming back into present-moment awareness. The word *sati* is often linked with the word *sampajāna*, which means 'clearly knowing'. When put together as a compound, *satisampajāna*, the *sati* element refers to awareness of raw sensory or mental data, and the *sampajāna* element refers to the processing of that data in a wise way.

Mindfulness occurs in a number of the Buddha's principal teachings – for example, the noble eightfold path, the five spiritual faculties and the seven factors of awakening. Within the Buddhist tradition, mindfulness is an important quality to be cultivated in order to guide ethical behaviour, deepen meditation and support the development of wisdom. Key texts, such as the *satipatthāna sutta* (Ñānamoli and Bodhi, 1995), describe how to develop mindfulness of bodily sensations and the hedonic tone of experience and mental states, and then to bring to bear on this bodily and mental experience those teachings (*dhammas*) that help to bring about liberation. The *sutta* recommends developing mindfulness both through meditation, such as the mindfulness of breathing, and when going about daily life, such as by paying attention to bodily sensations when walking, sitting or lying down.

The function of mindfulness, and indeed of all Buddhist teachings, is ultimately to lead to *nibbāna* (Sanskrit: *nirvāna*) or Awakening. Although regarded as ultimately being beyond words, Awakening has been described in many different ways – including similes, images and even paradox – over the course of the two and a half millennia of the Buddhist tradition. One of the commonest ways of describing it is in terms of qualities such as wisdom and compassion. Elements of wisdom include seeing the impermanent and insubstantial nature of phenomena, which if not recognised as such and grasped will lead to suffering. The starting point of much Buddhist discourse is the nature of this suffering and how to alleviate it.

Developing Mindfulness as a Therapeutic Modality

In 1979, Jon Kabat-Zinn, a meditation practitioner and molecular biologist, set up a stress clinic at the University of Massachusetts Medical Center (Kabat-Zinn, 1990). His aim was to make the essence of the teachings of the Buddha available to a wider audience in America than might go to a Buddhist centre, especially those facing stress, pain and illness (Kabat-Zinn, 2013). He approached physician colleagues and asked them to refer to him people with physical health problems, including those with chronic pain for whom Western medicine could not offer any additional help, who might benefit from being able to better manage the mental and behavioural responses to their illness.

The course that Kabat-Zinn set up – later called mindfulness-based stress reduction (MBSR) – consisted of eight weekly sessions together with an all-day session of silent mindfulness practice. Kabat-Zinn taught mindfulness through both formal practices (sitting meditation, mindful walking, body scan and yoga exercises) and informal practices (becoming mindful, for example, of the breath, and while going about daily activities such as eating or taking a shower).

A study of patients with chronic pain who completed the course showed that two-thirds of them benefited (Kabat-Zinn et al., 1985). The benefits were maintained at a 4-year follow-up, especially for those who continued to practise mindfulness, even if only through informal practices (Kabat-Zinn et al., 1986).

The success of Kabat-Zinn's course led to growing interest in mindfulness in the USA, and the application of MBSR to other conditions. However, mindfulness did not really catch on in the UK until Zindel Segal, Mark Williams and John Teasdale developed mindfulness-based cognitive therapy (MBCT) (Segal et al., 2002). They were cognitive therapists who had been tasked with developing a maintenance form of cognitive therapy for depression, which has a high relapse rate. About 50% of people relapse after one episode of depression, and 80% after two or more episodes. The aim was to keep people well whether they had been initially treated with a psychotherapy or antidepressants, and to deliver the therapy in a group format for cost-effectiveness.

Examining the thoughts of people who are no longer depressed shows that dysfunctional attitudes are no different from those in people who have never been depressed. However, transient low mood can reactivate negative thinking and dysfunctional attitudes. In particular, a ruminative thinking style coupled with discrepancy monitoring, in which one compares one's current mental state unfavourably with others or an ideal, appears to make people vulnerable to relapsing into depression (Segal et al., 2002). When successful, standard cognitive therapy, by challenging the content of negative thoughts, leads to 'decentring', in which thoughts are seen simply as thoughts rather than as necessarily reflecting the reality to which they seem to point.

In developing a maintenance form of cognitive therapy, Segal and his colleagues aimed to help people to decentre from negative thoughts and interrupt ruminative response cycles. They approached Kabat-Zinn, initially thinking that mindfulness might be a useful adjunct to cognitive therapy techniques. However, when they were developing the new treatment, mindfulness became central. A three-centre trial conducted in

Cambridge, Bangor and Toronto randomly allocated 145 people to MBCT or treatment as usual. They found that the relapse rate in individuals with three or more episodes of depression (who represented 77% of the total sample) was reduced by about half, from 66% to 37% at one year (Teasdale et al., 2000).

From 2004, MBCT was recommended for preventing relapse in recurrent depression in guidelines published by the National Institute for Health and Care Excellence (2004). From this time the number of mindfulness studies burgeoned. To date, mindfulness has been trialled, with varying degrees of success, in most types of mental health disorders. In 2015, an All-Party Parliamentary Group advocated the use of mindfulness interventions to address mental health concerns in the areas not only of health, but also of education, the workplace and the criminal justice system (Mindfulness All-Party Parliamentary Group, 2015).

An Overview of the Content of Mindfulness Courses

The general structure of a typical mindfulness course can be considered in terms of an ABC model. A stands for developing Awareness. Enhancing awareness counteracts the tendency of the mind to wander off and drive one's behaviour without one fully recognising this, known as automatic pilot. Examples of automatic pilot include finding yourself in a room and realising that although you had meant to get something you now have no idea what it was, or planning to go to the supermarket on the way home from work and then discovering that you have missed the turn-off because your mind was elsewhere and your body had defaulted to the usual route home.

Awareness is cultivated through both formal and informal practices by paying attention to bodily sensations, thoughts and emotions. For instance, in the body scan one moves one's attention through the body, bringing awareness to sensations in different parts of the body. While one is doing this, the mind is likely to wander off (e.g., to thoughts about the past or the future, or judging what is happening). Gently noting where the mind has gone off to, one returns to the object of the meditation, in this case the sensations of the body. In doing so, one learns both to notice the tendencies of the mind, which is important for catching triggers to adverse mental states at an early point, and to step out of automatic pilot and of what are often unhelpful thinking patterns, such as rumination, by returning to the body. In addition, giving more attention to the body and the breath (e.g., in the mindfulness of breathing) develops tools that can be used in the second stage of the course.

B stands for Being with experience. Building on the foundation of the first stage of the course, 'being with' involves turning towards and staying with thoughts, emotions and bodily sensations, especially when they are difficult. When an uncomfortable mental or physical event occurs, the tendency is to want to push it away by distracting ourselves, wishing it wasn't there or feeling aversion towards it. Negative judgements about what is happening can fuel a spiral of increasingly painful mental events. Counterintuitively, 'being with' aims to turn towards the unpleasant experience without either pushing it away ('blocking') or getting completely caught up in it and overwhelmed by it ('drowning'). The qualities of attention with which one turns towards experience are those of acceptance, curiosity and kindness. This allows decentring from negative ruminative thinking and counteracts the tendency for emotional avoidance, which is thought to be involved in the maintenance of many mental health disorders (Hayes et al.,

1999). The body and the breath are of key importance in helping one to stay with a difficult experience. The body acts as a different place from which to view difficulties, rather than just think about them. Painful emotions will affect the body, and these sensations can be attended to. When the difficulty is due to painful physical sensations, attention can be focused on noticing the subtle qualities of the physical sensations, rather than becoming caught up in the overall awfulness of the experience and the narrative that goes with it. The breath can act as a gentle probe to explore physical sensations and to help to contain difficult experiences.

Finally, C stands for making wise Choices. When one is more aware of one's mental habits and no longer unthinkingly recoiling from difficulties, one is in a better position to decide how to act in a helpful and considered way. Typically in this part of the course one may draw up a list of actions that can be helpful when difficulties arise, such as calling a friend or taking a walk. Where relevant, attention is given to recognising relapse signatures and making plans to prevent relapse.

Mindfulness as a Component of Other Treatments

In addition to being used as the main form of treatment, mindfulness is sometimes used a component of other treatments. Two examples of this are dialectical behaviour therapy (DBT) and acceptance and commitment therapy (ACT). DBT was developed by Marsha Linehan for the treatment of borderline personality disorder (Linehan, 1993). She was influenced by Zen Buddhism, and used mindfulness to help with the acceptance of emotions. DBT has also been adapted for use in the treatment of substance misuse (Dimeff and Linehan, 2008).

ACT, which was developed by Stephen Hayes, did not originate from the Buddhist tradition but is rooted in relational frames theory (Hayes et al., 1999). As the name implies, there are two principal emphases – acceptance of unwanted experiences and commitment to valued directions, even in the face of difficult thoughts and emotions. The acceptance component of ACT looks very similar to mindfulness as used in MBIs (Hayes, 2007, p. 20), and ACT therapists often use mindfulness practices taken from MBIs (Forsyth and Eifert, 2007). ACT has been used for the treatment of a wide range of mental health problems.

Applications of Mindfulness-Based Approaches

Depression

MBCT was developed for reducing the risk of relapse in people who had recovered from depression. Mindfulness was initially thought to be unsuitable for people with current depression. Although mindfulness is more difficult to practise if one is depressed, more recently some work has been done to extend its use in those with current depression (Van Aalderen et al., 2012). MBCT may not be so useful in preventing episodes of bipolar disorder, although it may help to reduce comorbid symptoms such as anxiety (Perich et al., 2013).

Anxiety

The early attendees at Kabat-Zinn's stress clinic included people with anxiety disorders. A small study indicated that a mindfulness-based training programme could help to reduce symptoms of anxiety (Kabat-Zinn et al., 1992). Mindfulness may help to tackle ruminative catastrophising and assist learning to accept the uncomfortable feelings associated with anxiety.

Addiction

The MBSR and MBCT courses have been adapted for the treatment of addiction, as a course called mindfulness-based relapse prevention (MBRP) or mindfulness-based addiction recovery (MBAR) (Mason-John and Groves, 2018). Mindfulness may help to sensitise people with addictive disorders to the attentional biases that can make them vulnerable to relapse, and desensitise them to the negative affects that may trigger relapse (Breslin et al., 2002).

Eating Disorders

MBIs have been developed for a range of eating disorders, including anorexia nervosa, bulimia nervosa, binge eating and obesity. Eating is an activity that is especially likely to occur on automatic pilot, often while multi-tasking (e.g., while reading, watching television or the phone). Therefore mindfulness may help to bring more attention to the act of eating and so 'deautomatise' it. Negative affect may be a trigger to problematic eating (e.g., using eating to suppress difficult thoughts and emotions). Mindfulness may help individuals to manage these emotions without resorting to eating (Kristeller and Wolever, 2011). Early reviews suggest that this may be a promising approach (Katterman et al., 2014; O'Reilly et al., 2014).

Psychosis

In general, meditation has been thought to be contraindicated in psychosis, since it might provoke relapse, or reinforce being caught up in a delusional inner world, or simply be too difficult for someone with a psychotic illness. However, research has shown that mindfulness can be used safely in people with psychosis (Hodann-Caudevilla et al., 2020; Jansen et al., 2020).

Mindfulness may promote acceptance of psychotic phenomena and assist disengagement from them, without the need to question the validity of the content of the experience. When leading mindfulness meditation it is recommended that one keeps to shorter practices (e.g., up to 10 minutes), makes frequent comments to guide the meditation (perhaps every 30 to 60 seconds), and makes explicit reference to psychotic phenomena in order to normalise them (Chadwick, 2014).

The Evidence Base

A number of reviews of studies of mindfulness have been conducted. The efficacy of mindfulness appears to be equivalent to that of evidence-based treatments, and superior to no treatment and active controls (Goldberg et al., 2018; de Abreu Costa et al., 2019). The strongest evidence for the effectiveness of mindfulness is for its use in recurrent depression and anxiety disorders. There is also support for its use in addictions.

Piet and Hougaard (2011) concluded that MBCT produced a relative risk reduction of 34% compared with treatment as usual or placebo controls. A pre-planned subgroup analysis found a risk reduction of 43% in people with three or more episodes of depression, but no risk reduction in those with fewer episodes, thus confirming the findings of the original MBCT study and the recommendation of MBCT for treatment of recurrent depression. In addition, there is a suggestion from secondary analyses that MBCT may be more effective for those with greater vulnerability, due for example to earlier age of onset, adverse childhood conditions or less stable remission (Williams et al., 2014; Kuyken et al., 2015). A meta-analysis of its use in anxiety concluded that MBCT has an effect size for active treatment of 0.81, compared with 0.33 for treatment as usual or a waiting-list control (Hofmann et al., 2010). A review of MBIs for addictive disorders suggests that mindfulness may be best used in conjunction with treatment as usual or other active treatment (Sancho et al., 2018).

Adverse Effects

The potential adverse effects of mindfulness have not been studied fully, although case studies and observational studies have suggested a possible increased risk of suicidality, depression and negative emotions, as well as flashbacks during meditation in people with a history of trauma (van Dam et al., 2018). The aim of building increased awareness through mindfulness is likely to bring difficult mental experience to the fore, especially where this has been previously ignored by distraction or other means. If the approach of learning to be with experience (as described earlier) is not taught well or not understood by the participant, the increased awareness of painful mental contents may provoke rumination, including catastrophic thinking, and further dysphoric emotional responses, which might account for the adverse effects that have been described in studies. Adverse effects may be minimised by informed consent being based on an understanding of possible untoward effects, and by excluding individuals with current suicidality or major psychiatric disorder, unless they are in a specialised group that is targeting the particular disorder.

Neuroscience

Neuroscientific studies have shown brain changes in people who practise meditation. Larger gyrification has been found in a number of cortical regions (Luders et al., 2012), with a positive correlation between gyrification of the right anterior dorsal insula and the duration of mindfulness meditation practice. This may be associated with the ability of mindfulness to help to identify emotions through changes in body sensations (Craig, 2009). In people without training in mindfulness, strong emotions evoke an fMRI response in the right insula in association with activity in the ventromedial prefrontal cortex (vmPFC) (Farb et al., 2007). In those trained in mindfulness there is a decoupling of the association between the insula and the vmPFC, and an association of the insula with activity in the dorsolateral prefrontal cortex (dlPFC). The vmPFC is thought to be involved in self-referential activity such as rumination, whereas the dlPFC is associated with labelling emotions and being more accepting of them, leading to a down-regulation of the limbic system (Lieberman et al., 2011).

Mindfulness may have a positive impact on heart rate variability (HRV) by improving sympatho-vagal balance, with reduced sympathetic influence and increased parasympathetic influence (Nijjar et al., 2014). Greater HRV provides a more adaptive regulatory response to stress. A review of EEG studies suggests that mindfulness is associated with increased alpha and theta activity (Lomas et al., 2015). This corresponds to relaxed alertness, which may be beneficial for mental health. Mindfulness may enhance periph-eral brain-derived neurotrophic factor, which is associated with increased neuronal plasticity (Gomutbutra et al., 2020).

Mindfulness for Mental Health Professionals

Training in mindfulness has been advocated to support professionals in their work with patients. Mindfulness may promote non-judgemental acceptance and openness to experience, which in turn may foster a stronger therapeutic alliance (Razzaque et al., 2013). When a clinician is able to be with his or her own difficult emotions, he or she is more likely to be able to help patients to do the same for their distress. Mindfulness may help professionals to recognise counter-transference reactions provoked by patients (and colleagues), and to respond to them in a creative way. Instead of needing to push away and fix the patient's distress, they may be more able to connect with the patient, before working out how best to respond (Groves, 1998). Sometimes the mindful attention may itself be therapeutic, without the need for further intervention.

A number of studies suggest that medical students may benefit from training in mindfulness. Findings include an increase in empathy (Shapiro et al., 1998), a reduction in mood disturbance and a greater ability to deal with stress (Rosenzweig et al., 2003), and improved well-being during a pre-exam period (Hassed et al., 2009). Trainee therapists who participated in an MBSR course showed increased positive affect and self-compassion, which in turn correlated with increased levels of compassion for others (Shapiro et al., 2007). MBIs appear to enhance the well-being and performance of doctors, although they may struggle to make time to learn the approaches and also find it difficult to sustain them in daily life (Scheepers et al., 2020).

Is Therapeutic Mindfulness Religious, Secular or Neither?

The emergence of mindfulness as a therapeutic modality has generated considerable debate regarding its religious or secular status. Helderman (2019) has outlined some of the arguments, and notes that while some feel mindfulness is a means of smuggling Buddhism into an arena that should be wholly secular, others argue that mindfulness as a therapeutic modality is secular, with all traces of religion removed. This in turn has given rise to criticism by those who see therapeutic mindfulness as a degradation of Buddhist teaching, which threatens the purity of Buddhism. They observe that key elements of mindfulness that would be taught in a traditional Buddhist setting, such as ethics and rebirth, have been removed, while they discern other influences, such as humanistic psychotherapy, psychedelic experimentation and American transcenden-talism, which may be regarded as out of place within Buddhist practice. Stripped of its broader religious context, some have questioned whether mindfulness taught as a therapeutic modality should even be called 'mindfulness' (van Gordon and Shonin, 2019). Teachers of therapeutic mindfulness may feel under pressure from powerful institutions (e.g., medical insurance companies) to emphasise the secular nature and scientific backing of mindfulness through research studies, while also wanting to appeal to the authority of mindfulness as an ancient teaching. Some prefer to use the term 'spiritual' when discussing the origins of mindfulness, as an alternative to either 'religious' or 'secular'.

Conclusion

Regardless of the provenance of mindfulness – as religious, secular or spiritual – its popularity among the general population and its research backing from multiple studies suggest that it is more than a passing fad and likely to remain as one option for responding to mental suffering. Although debate may continue among academics regarding its religious or secular nature, the ambiguity may be advantageous for patients. For those wishing to use mindfulness practices to alleviate their suffering, it may be construed in entirely secular terms as a handy technique or as part of a spiritual journey, which they may or may not choose to see as aligned with a particular religious tradition.

References

Anālayo (2003) *Satipatthāna: The Direct Path to Realization.* Birmingham: Windhorse Publications.

Breslin, F. C., Zack, M. and McMain, S. (2002) An information-processing analysis of mindfulness: implications for relapse prevention in the treatment of substance abuse. *Clinical Psychology: Science and Practice,* 9, 275–299.

Chadwick, P. (2014) Mindfulness for psychosis. *British Journal of Psychiatry,* 204, 333–334.

Craig, A. D. (2009) How do you feel – now? The anterior insula and human awareness. *Nature Reviews. Neuroscience,* 10, 59–70.

de Abreu Costa, M., D'Alò de Oliveira, G. S., Tatton-Ramos, T. et al. (2019) Anxiety and stress-related disorders and mindfulness-based interventions: a systematic review and multilevel meta-analysis and meta-regression of multiple outcomes. *Mindfulness,* 10, 996–1005.

Dimeff, L. A. and Linehan, M. M. (2008) Dialectical behavior therapy for substance abusers. *Addiction Science and Clinical Practice,* 4, 39–47.

Farb, N. A., Segal, Z. V., Mayberg, H. et al. (2007) Attending to the present: mindfulness meditation reveals distinct neural modes of self-reference. *Social Cognitive and Affective Neuroscience,* 2, 313–322.

Forsyth, J. P. and Eifert, G. H. (2007) *The Mindfulness and Acceptance Workbook for Anxiety: A Guide to Breaking Free from Anxiety, Phobias, and Worry Using Acceptance and Commitment Therapy.* Oakland, CA: New Harbinger Publications.

Goldberg, S. B., Tucker, R. P., Greene, P. A. et al. (2018) Mindfulness-based interventions for psychiatric disorders: a systematic review and meta-analysis. *Clinical Psychology Review,* 59, 52–60.

Gomutbutra, P., Yingchankul, N., Chattipakorn, N., Chattipakorn, S. and Srisurapanont, M. (2020) The effect of mindfulness-based intervention on brain-derived neurotropic factor (BDNF): a systematic review and meta-analysis of controlled trials. *Frontiers in Psychology,* 11, 2209.

Groves, P. (1998) Doing and being: a Buddhist perspective on craving and addiction. In P. Barker and B. Davidson, eds., *Psychiatric Nursing: Ethical Strife.* London: Edward Arnold, pp. 202–210.

Hassed, C., de Lisle, S., Sullivan, G. and Pier, C. (2009) Enhancing the health of medical students: outcomes of an integrated mindfulness and lifestyle program. *Advances in Health Sciences Education,* 14, 387–398.

Hayes, S. (2007) ACT: basic and applied. In D. Chantry, ed., *Talking ACT: Notes and Conversations on Acceptance and Commitment Therapy.* Reno, NV: Context Press, pp. 9–52.

Hayes, S. C., Strosahl, K. and Wilson, K. G. (1999) *Acceptance and Commitment Therapy: An Experiential Approach to Behavior Change.* New York: The Guilford Press.

Helderman, I. (2019) *Prescribing the Dharma: Psychotherapists, Buddhist Traditions, and*

Defining Religion. Chapel Hill, NC: University of North Carolina Press.

Hickey, W. S. (2019) *Mind Cure: How Meditation Became Medicine*. New York: Oxford University Press.

Hodann-Caudevilla, R. M., Díaz-Silviera, C., Burgos-Julián, F. A. and Santed, M. A. (2020) Mindfulness-based interventions for people with schizophrenia: a systematic review and meta-analysis. *International Journal of Environmental Research and Public Health*, 17, 4690.

Hofmann, S. G., Sawyer, A. T., Witt, A. A. et al. (2010) The effect of mindfulness-based therapy on anxiety and depression: a meta-analytic review. *Journal of Consulting and Clinical Psychology*, 78, 169–183.

Jansen, J. E., Gleeson, J., Bendall, S., Rice, S. and Alvarez-Jimenez, M. (2020) Acceptance- and mindfulness-based interventions for persons with psychosis: a systematic review and meta-analysis. *Schizophrenia Research*, 215, 25–37.

Kabat-Zinn, J. (1990) *Full Catastrophe Living: Using the Wisdom of Your Body and Mind to Face Stress, Pain, and Illness*. New York: Delacorte Press.

Kabat-Zinn, J. (2013) Some reflections on the origins of MBSR, skilful means, and the trouble with maps. In J. M. G. Williams and J. Kabat-Zinn, eds., *Mindfulness: Diverse Perspectives on its Meaning, Origins and Applications*. London: Routledge, pp. 281–306.

Kabat-Zinn, J., Lipworth, L. and Burney, R. (1985) The clinical use of mindfulness meditation for the self-regulation of chronic pain. *Journal of Behavioural Medicine*, 8, 163–190.

Kabat-Zinn, J., Lipworth, L., Burney, R. and Sellers, W. (1986) Four-year follow-up of a meditation-based program for the self-regulation of chronic pain: treatment outcomes and compliance. *The Clinical Journal of Pain*, 2, 159–173.

Kabat-Zinn, J., Massion, A. O., Kristeller, J. et al. (1992) Effectiveness of a meditation-based stress reduction program in the treatment of anxiety disorders. *American Journal of Psychiatry*, 149, 936–943.

Katterman, S. N., Kleinman, B. M., Hood, M. M. et al. (2014) Mindfulness meditation as an intervention for binge eating, emotional eating, and weight loss: a systematic review. *Eating Behaviors*, 15, 197–204.

Kristeller, J. L. and Wolever, R. Q. (2011) Mindfulness-based eating awareness training for treating binge eating disorder: the conceptual foundation. *Eating Disorders*, 19, 49–61.

Kuyken, W., Hayes, R., Barrett, B. et al. (2015) Effectiveness and cost-effectiveness of mindfulness-based cognitive therapy compared with maintenance antidepressant treatment in the prevention of depressive relapse or recurrence (PREVENT): a randomised controlled trial. *The Lancet*, 386, 63–73.

Lieberman, M. D., Inagaki, T. K., Tabibnia, G. et al. (2011) Subjective responses to emotional stimuli during labelling, reappraisal, and distraction. *Emotion*, 11. 468–480.

Linehan, M. (1993) *Cognitive–Behavioral Treatment of Borderline Personality Disorder*. New York: The Guilford Press.

Lomas, T., Ivtzan, I. and Fu, C. H. Y. (2015) A systematic review of the neurophysiology of mindfulness on EEG oscillations. *Neuroscience and Biobehavioral Reviews*, 57, 401–410.

Luders, E., Kurth, F., Mayer, E. A. et al. (2012) The unique brain anatomy of meditation practitioners: alterations in cortical gyrification. *Frontiers in Human Neuroscience*, 6, 34.

Mason-John, V. and Groves, P. (2018) *Eight Step Recovery: Using the Buddha's Teachings to Overcome Addiction*. Cambridge: Windhorse Publications.

Mindfulness All-Party Parliamentary Group (2015) *Mindful Nation UK*. Available at www.themindfulnessinitiative.org/mindful-nation-report (accessed 26 April 2022).

Ñānamoli, B. and Bodhi, B., trans. (1995) Satipattāna Sutta. In *The Middle Length Discourses of the Buddha: A Translation of the Majjhima Nikāya*. Somerville, MA: Wisdom Publications, pp. 145–155.

National Institute for Health and Care Excellence (2004) *Depression: Management of Depression in Primary and Secondary Care.* Clinical Guideline [CG23]. London: National Institute for Health and Care Excellence.

Nijjar, P. S., Puppala, V. K., Dickinson, O. et al. (2014) Modulation of the autonomic nervous system assessed through heart rate variability by a mindfulness based stress reduction program. *International Journal of Cardiology*, 177, 557–559.

O'Reilly, G. A., Cook, L., Spruijt-Metz, D. et al. (2014) Mindfulness-based interventions for obesity-related eating behaviours: a literature review. *Obesity Reviews*, 15, 453–461.

Perich, T., Manicavasagar, V., Mitchell, P. B., Ball, J. R. and Hadzi-Pavlovic, D. (2013) A randomized controlled trial of mindfulness-based cognitive therapy for bipolar disorder. *Acta Psychiatrica Scandinavica*, 127, 333–343.

Piet, J. and Hougaard, E. (2011) The effect of mindfulness-based cognitive therapy for prevention of relapse in recurrent major depressive disorder: systematic review and meta-analysis. *Clinical Psychology Review*, 31, 1032–1040.

Razzaque, R., Okoro, E. and Wood, L. (2013) Mindfulness in clinician therapeutic relationships. *Mindfulness*, 2, 170–174.

Rosenzweig, S., Reibel, D. K., Greeson, J. M., Brainard, G. C. and Hojat, M. (2003) Mindfulness-based stress reduction lowers psychological distress in medical students. *Teaching and Learning in Medicine*, 15, 88–92.

Sancho, M., de Gracia, M., Rodríguez, R. C. et al. (2018) Mindfulness-based interventions for the treatment of substance and behavioral addictions: a systematic review. *Frontiers in Psychiatry*, 9, 95.

Scheepers, R. A., Emke, H., Epstein, R. M. and Lombarts, K. M. J. M. H. (2020) The impact of mindfulness-based interventions on doctors' well-being and performance: a systematic review. *Medical Education*, 54, 138–149.

Segal, Z. V., Williams, J. M. G. and Teasdale, J. D. (2002) *Mindfulness-Based Cognitive Therapy for Depression: A New Approach to Preventing Relapse*. New York: The Guilford Press.

Shapiro, S. L., Schwartz, G. E. and Bonner, G. (1998) Effects of mindfulness-based stress reduction on medical and premedical students. *Journal of Behavioural Medicine*, 21, 581–599.

Shapiro, S. L., Brown, K. W. and Biegel, G. M. (2007) Teaching self-care to caregivers: effects of mindfulness-based stress reduction on the mental health of therapists in training. *Training and Education in Professional Psychology*, 1, 105–115.

Teasdale, J. D., Segal, Z. V., Williams, J. M. G. et al. (2000) Prevention of relapse/recurrence in major depression by mindfulness-based cognitive therapy. *Journal of Consulting and Clinical Psychology*, 68, 615–623.

van Aalderen, J. R., Donders, A. R. T., Giommi, F. et al. (2012) The efficacy of mindfulness-based cognitive therapy in recurrent depressed patients with and without a current depressive episode: a randomized controlled trial. *Psychological Medicine*, 42, 989–1001.

van Dam, N. T., van Vugt, M. K., Vago, D. R. et al. (2018) Mind the hype: a critical evaluation and prescriptive agenda for research on mindfulness and meditation. *Perspectives on Psychological Science*, 13, 36–61.

van Gordon, W. and Shonin, E. (2019) Second-generation mindfulness-based interventions: toward more authentic mindfulness practice and teaching. *Mindfulness*, 11, 1–4.

Williams, J. M. G., Crane, C., Barnhofer, T. et al. (2014) Mindfulness-based cognitive therapy for preventing relapse in recurrent depression: a randomized dismantling trial. *Journal of Consulting and Clinical Psychology*, 82, 275–286.

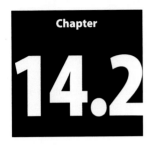

Chapter 14.2

Compassion-Focused Therapy

Paul Gilbert

Compassion and the Multi-Mind

Humans have long known that the concept of mind subsumes many different types of motivation and emotion, which at times can result in the experience of intense conflict – for example, the dilemma as to whether to put ourselves or others first. We can be very helpful to others, but are also capable of vicious cruelty and aggression (Gilbert, 2000, 2021; Plante, 2015). When we are motivated by self-focused competitiveness, our minds and bodies are organised very differently from when we wish to be helpful or show compassion. This can profoundly affect our physical and mental health (Seppälä et al., 2017).

Many spiritual traditions have highlighted the importance of cultivating compassion at the expense of self-focused motivation (Gilbert, 2009; Plante, 2015; Ricard, 2015). Yet neoliberal societies constantly stimulate self-focused competitiveness in our schools, in the field of entertainment and in career development. Such societies focus on our personal and self-focused desires to acquiring the benefits and comforts of life and wealth. The downside of this cultural norm to compete against each other increases fear of failure, a sense of inferiority, the fear of negative social comparisons, depression, self-criticism and social anxiety (Curran and Hill, 2019).

Compassion-focused therapy (CFT) is rooted in an evolutionarily informed biopsychosocial approach to mental health problems (Gilbert, 1984, 1989, 1995, 2020; Gilbert and Simos, 2022). It aims to stimulate a non-competitive motivational system with a very different physiological profile, since a compassionate approach to life changes not only our basic values but also the way our brains and minds work (Gilbert, 2014, 2020; Seppälä et al., 2017). Learning how to deal with life's setbacks from a place of compassion and understanding is entirely different from being habitually fearful of competitive failures and self-critical. The essence of all compassion-focused approaches is therefore to be sensitive to our struggles, fears, worries and setbacks, but to learn to manage them by developing a courageous, wise and caring mind when dealing with life's problems.

Bodies, Minds, Suffering and the Spiritual Quest

Mental health clinicians have always walked a fine line between the biological body, which experiences pain, suffering, decay and ultimately death, and the conscious mind, which asks spiritual questions about the meaning of all that must be endured. Humans have a degree of self-awareness that, so far as we know, animals do not possess (Byrne, 2016). We can be only too aware of our mortality and the impermanence of everything around us. The suffering inherent in this realisation is central to Buddhist psychology (Tsering, 2005). Our conscious awareness of the nature of our brief existence is also central to existential philosophy and psychotherapy. Yalom (1980) suggested that humans are constantly working with four basic issues or ultimate concerns – the reality of decay and death, the pursuit of meaning, concerns with separateness and isolation, and the issue of freedom. These are themes that recur in diagnostic consultations with psychiatrists and psychotherapists.

Some people turn to religious faith in seeking answers to these painful existential questions (Bering, 2002). Sigmund Freud argued from an atheistic perspective that belief in a god is a way of seeking comfort from a parental surrogate by projecting the need into an imagined deity. Carl Jung, however, understood the manifestation of archetypes to be representations of the *Imago Dei*, conducive to meaning making and purpose – hence the hero's spiritual quest (Ellenberger, 1970, pp. 280–281). John Bowlby, on the other hand, focused on the attachment needs of the human being, striving for a secure base and safe haven, and finding meaning primarily through relating (Bowlby, 1969, 1973, 1989).

Regardless of the various psychological explanations that have been proffered, many people turn to a god and related spiritual pursuits as the source of comfort, love and protection, and to provide a sense of meaning and connectedness (Kirkpatrick, 2005). For some, their spiritual quest leads them to use psychedelics (entheogens) that induce changes in brain chemistry. For millennia, many indigenous societies have used entheogens for this purpose (Hartogsohn, 2018; Forstmann et al., 2020). Current research suggests that such drugs can have a valuable clinical role not only because of the 'spiritual' experiences they offer, but also in the treatment of substance abuse, anxiety, depression and post-traumatic stress disorder (Garcia-Romeu et al., 2016).

One of the key spiritual experiences is related to a sense of connectedness, at times with the universe itself. Hence, given that the nature of these practices is to offer deep forms of connectedness and compassion, they are widely regarded as promoting healthy spirituality (Tagliazucchi et al., 2022). However, it is important to recognise that some forms of religion and spirituality are not like this. Indeed, any religion with a deity is vulnerable to the possibility that, based on the prevailing psychosocial context, adherents may develop a judging and punishing image of God. This destructive tendency is often found in extremist religious belief (Armstrong, 1999) and can be incredibly harmful, as in the case of the Aztecs, who believed that they could win favour with their sun god by sacrificing their own children, along with many thousands of others, mostly prisoners, defeated enemies and slaves. It is not just the fear of God's punishment that is the issue, but also how people live in fear of being watched and being judged. Far from being a historical footnote, the fear of being watched and judged affects a great number of people to this day, with profoundly negative consequences.

Compassion

Percolating through these dilemmas, there is a long tradition of philosophical and spiritual writings that highlight the value of compassion as an antidote to personal and social suffering, and to antisocial behaviour, too (Lampert, 2005; Wallace, 2007; Ricard, 2015). In addition, over the last 30 years there has been a substantial body of research on the neurophysiological, psychological and social dimensions of compassion, and on compassion training. (For reviews, see Seppälä et al., 2017; Stevens and Woodruff, 2018; Singer and Engert, 2019; Di Bello et al., 2020; Kim et al., 2020; Gilbert and Simos, 2022.) This work has been accompanied by the development of a variety of compassion training programmes and specific ways of integrating compassion training within psychotherapy (Gilbert, 2020; Gilbert and Simos, 2022).

One of the reasons for this focus on compassion is the recognition of how it emerged from the evolution of caring behaviour, particularly between parent and child (Gilbert, 1989, 2020; Porges, 2017). The reproductive strategy of animal species without attachment behaviour is to lay hundreds of eggs, of which only a very few will survive. The evolution of caring behaviour has been a fundamental game changer for life on Earth. Mammalian caring came to include providing food, thermal regulation (warmth), protection, social interaction, and brain stimulation and guidance – skills needed for survival. Bowlby (1969, 1973, 1980) identified a number of essential psychological functions, including providing the infant with a secure base from which to explore and learn, and a safe haven where the parent could assuage anxiety and thereby modulate the emotions felt by the infant.

The physiological infrastructures underpinning these dimensions of caring and compassion have been subject to considerable research over recent years. (For reviews, see Keltner et al., 2014; Brown and Brown, 2015, 2017; Mayseless, 2016; Gilbert, 2017; Seppälä et al., 2017; Stevens and Woodruff, 2018.) We know, for example, that the hormones oxytocin, endorphins and vasopressin play vital roles in the evolution of caring behaviour, both for the infant and through pair bonding with the caregiver (Carter et al., 2017). Changes to the autonomic nervous system, particularly the myelination of the parasympathetic system, led to the evolution of the tenth cranial nerve, known as the vagus nerve, which plays a significant part in the regulation of threat and the soothing function of connectedness (Porges, 2017; Stellar and Keltner, 2017). Indeed, the various physical interactions between parent and infant (e.g., touching, holding, stroking, voice tone, feeding, processes of sharing interests and ideas) all have significant and discrete physiological regulating effects (Hofer, 1994; Porges and Furman, 2011; Siegel, 2012; Cozolino, 2014; Schore, 2019). Furthermore, there is good evidence that the parasympathetic system plays a major role in prosocial behaviour, and in caring and compassion in general (Keltner et al., 2014; Petrocchi and Cheli, 2019; Di Bello et al., 2020). Hence the care-compassion motive system is linked to an endorphin–oxytocin–parasympathetic, frontal cortical integrated set of circuits that function to promote trust, affiliative behaviour and calming in face of the threat system (MacDonald and MacDonald, 2010).

This does not mean that *specific acts of compassion* involve these circuits. Di Bello et al. (2021) have published an important paper titled 'Compassion is not a benzo', in which they highlight the fact that when confronted with suffering and the desire to do something about it, the physiological activation in any specific situation depends on the context and the actions chosen. For example, the threat system can be highly activated whether one is running away from a fire or (compassionately) running towards a fire to rescue people. Each day that they go into work, clinical staff on COVID-19 wards know that they are likely to have to cope with the experience of caring for people who are dying. They are not going to be in a state of calm soothing. What is important, though, is the ability to regulate one's mind when in distress. This is fundamental to being able to pursue intentional caring behaviours in the face of distress.

From Caring to Compassion

It is clear that many species have evolved capacities for caring, particularly for their young, contingent on their underlying physiology. However, caring is not the same as compassion. The behaviour of rats looking after their pups, or birds looking after the eggs in the nest, would not be regarded as compassionate but as caring. Around a million years ago, humans began to evolve a range of cognitive competencies that facilitated capacities for reasoning, self-awareness, complex forms of empathy and language, communication and social interaction. These have given rise to what is called *knowing intentionality* (Gilbert, 2020; Gilbert & Simos, 2022). For example, lions intend to hunt their prey but not with knowing intentionality. They cannot decide to abstain from hunting because it causes suffering, or to wake up in the morning and go training in order to become better hunters. There is a major difference between doing something automatically and acting with knowing intentionality, which allows us specifically and deliberately to engage in caring behaviour. In this regard, we can define compassion as the process by which a basic motivational system such as caring is activated and guided through more high-level cognitive competencies, allowing for insight, empathy, thinking in time (knowing that one's actions will have an impact in the future), self-awareness and self-identity. This is represented in Figure 14.2.1, which depicts the process through which caring evolved with a range of (neuro)physiological systems (Seppälä et al., 2017). These can both stimulate and also recruit complex cognitive processes that give rise to courageous and wise compassion rather than automatic caring behaviours.

Although we may care for our gardens, cars and prized possessions, if they become damaged, we do not have or feel compassion for them. This is because compassion is associated with conscious suffering. What underpins compassion, therefore, is the motivation to address, prevent or relieve *suffering*. Compassion requires a sensitivity to suffering and then an awareness of what might help. It is, for the most part, a conscious 'thoughtful' experience.

This is of fundamental importance when working with mental health problems. We frequently find that a person's experience of self-criticism and shame is automatic, unintentional and unchosen, in contrast with compassion, which can be reflective, intentional and chosen. In such cases, through harnessing our wisdom and knowing intentionality, we find that fostering compassion can become an antidote to some of the more troublesome aspects of mind. This process is associated with learning mindfulness,

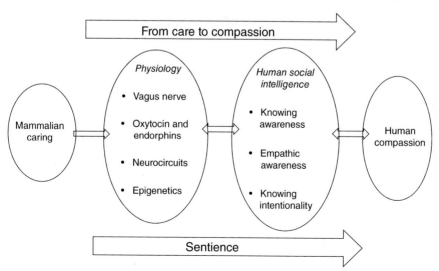

Figure 14.2.1 Process through which caring evolved.
Adapted from Gilbert (2018), with permission from the publisher.

empathy skills and body awareness skills, all guided by insight into how caring motivation systems shape us psychologically, physiologically and socially.

Compassion-Focused Therapy

Compassion-focused therapy (CFT) (Gilbert, 2000, 2009, 2010, 2020) emerged from cognitive therapy and Jungian concepts, as well as biopsychosocial and evolutionary orientation to psychopathology (Gilbert, 1989, 1998, Gilbert and Simos, 2022). It is evident that receiving cognitive therapy, people with conditions such as depression often think in ways that are congruent with the condition. Typically, depressed people hold negative views of themselves, the world and their future (Beck et al., 1979). By helping them to stand back and re-evaluate their style of thinking, cognitive therapy can help to shift them from being trapped in loops of negative thinking and feeling. However, it had been known for some time that although individuals can change how they think, this does not necessarily change how they feel (Stott, 2007).

It was while using these techniques that I first asked patients to speak aloud their self supporting and coping thoughts, using the actual voice tone in which they heard them. It was something of a surprise to find that although the content of the thought was helpful, the emotional tone of the thought was often aggressive and self-accusatory. The first task, therefore, was to help patients to generate a friendly, compassionate and empathic tone to their voiced supportive thoughts. Interestingly, many patients could not do this, and some refused to do it. Yet I also found that when patients were able to become more compassionate and empathetic towards themselves, it opened up their caring systems which at first was difficult for them.

This discovery highlights the fact that if you access any motivational system that has memories of trauma within, those traumatic memories will be re-activated. This is characteristic of basic conditioning. For example, if you enjoy going on holiday, but then on one occasion you are beaten up and need to go to hospital, when holidays are cued again, perhaps by advertising, the trauma memory may return. Similarly, a person may enjoy sexual feelings until they become a victim of rape, after which the trauma is re-activated when their sexual system is aroused. Likewise, beginning to feel caring can also activate memories of early neglect or harm and yearnings to be cared for, loved and wanted; for some patients this deep longing is too painful to bear and it triggers dissociation. Aversive memories of neglect, criticism or abuse are linked to physiological responses that run counter to caring (Lippard and Nemeroff, 2020).

One of the important challenges has been to explore how CFT can help to detoxify the caring system and overcome strong resistance to compassion. In fact there is now good evidence that fear of compassion is highly predictive of mental health problems and therapeutic outcomes (Kirby et al., 2019).

CFT uses a range of therapeutic interventions, which are designed to stimulate caring and compassion motivation systems to recruit physiological infrastructures for change. These include in particular (but not only) an endorphin–oxytocin–parasympathetic, frontal-cortical, integrated set of circuits that function to promote trust, affiliative behaviour and calming in the face of the threat (MacDonald and MacDonald, 2010; Petrocchi and Cheli, 2019). In addition, CFT teaches people how to shift to a compassionate mind state, using breathing exercises, visualisations, cognitive focusing, mentalisation, acting and behavioural practices (Gilbert and Simos, 2022). Therefore patients can practise thinking about a problem while working through different emotions, such as an anxious mind state or an angry mind state, and switching to a compassionate mind state and noticing the difference it makes (Gilbert and Basran, 2018).

One of the central concepts of CFT is that many individuals with mental health problems have a sense of disconnection from others. If we ask patients with depression, paranoid ideation, eating disorder or panic attacks whether they feel connected or alone, they nearly always answer 'alone'. In addition, many of our patients have severe problems with feelings of shame and self-criticism, which can be highly disconnecting. Indeed, shame is one of the most prominent problems for mental health care, as it results in hiding behaviour (Dearing and Tangney, 2011; Gilbert, 2007, 2011).

Vulnerability to a sense of shame, of being different and separate, not good enough, or carrying traits that are felt to lead to rejection by others, may arise from problems in childhood and a range of attachment difficulties. However, other factors arise from ways of living today that are very different from that of our ancestral hunter-gatherer past (Ryan, 2019). In those early societies, humans were integrated into caring communities and could turn not only to family but to any member of the community for support and help (Narvaez, 2017). With the advent of agriculture and the subsequent fragmentation of communities into hierarchies, and especially with the development of the present-day nuclear family (sometimes with only a single parent) that is so characteristic of industrialised society, such extended care and support is rare. Consequently, CFT commonly works with issues of disconnection and with the (often feared and avoided) underlying yearning for connection – the desire and longing to feel loved and wanted, and to have a sense of belonging. This is why compassionate mind training and genuine spirituality, which at its heart is about connectedness, and the sense of our common humanity, can be so closely linked. It is also why research into psychedelics is relevant, since these substances can bring about the emotionally profound experience of some sense of a universal connectedness (Forstmann et al., 2020; Tagliazucchi et al., 2022).

In essence, then, many mental health problems are linked to social disconnection, shame and self-criticism. The therapeutic aim is to discover the sense of connectedness, belonging, and being part of something greater than oneself which is the essence of spirituality and compassion. Psychotherapy is not just about enabling people to deal with their own thoughts – it is just as much about promoting caring connections to self and others which have profound impacts on our physiological organisation; this is a prosocial orientation that enables people to build and maintain nurturing and flourishing relationships. There is increasing evidence that this is exceptionally important for maintaining mental and physical well being (Ditzen and Heinrichs, 2014; Dedoncker et al., 2021).

Psychotherapy should not only focus on the importance of helping a person identify and live by his or her own values, if this risks becoming more self focused, narcissistic and ruthlessly self-ambitious, or seeking wealth at the expense of others. Instead, mental healthcare professionals should encourage prosocial and ethical behaviour. Failure to do so can leave patients potentially harmful to others, or lacking the capacity for social integration. As with all the great spiritual traditions, CFT emphasises the importance both of being open to receiving compassion from others and of showing compassion towards others. Furthermore, there is good evidence that in doing so, we are furthering our own mental well-being. (For reviews, see Gilbert and Simos, 2022.)

CFT in Practice

There are many practices, in different traditions, that help to develop the cultivation and strengthening of the caring and compassion motivation systems and brain states that strengthen the endorphin–oxytocin–parasympathetic, frontal-cortical, integrated set of circuits and compassion as a self-identity. First, there are practices that focus on *helping the body to support the mind*. This involves working with the autonomic nervous system, particularly supporting vagal tone and improving heart rate variability (Porges, 2017). One of the most commonly used methods involves creating an open upright posture with the shoulders back, and then slowing and deepening the breath, in particular focusing on the outbreath as a 'settling' breath. A good way to begin the practice is to breathe in for around five seconds, gently noticing the 'top' of the breath, and then gently breathe out for five seconds, while trying to ensure smoothness and regularity to the breath. This can be accompanied by practising a kindly facial expression and the genuine wish to be friendly rather than neutral or hostile. With focus on the outbreath, attention should be paid to the sensation of body and mind slowing down, and feeling slightly heavier or 'held' by the chair. Details of many such practices are available, both on the Compassionate Mind Foundation website[1] and more widely on the Internet, guiding people through different ways of working with the body. Other practices may involve yoga and chi gong.

The second set of practices focus on *helping the mind to support the body* by focusing specifically on understanding the nature of compassion. Here we invite clients to think about the key qualities of compassion and then to imagine having those qualities. We use acting techniques for people to practise thinking and behaving as if they are fully inhabiting a compassionate role (see the short video titled *Compassion for Voices*[2]). In addition, CFT orientates people to the mindful awareness that we all just find ourselves here in this life, with a body and brain built not *by us* but *for us*. No animal chooses to be the animal it is, just as no human chooses to be human, to be born male or female, or to be born into their family of origin. Therefore, rather than feeling caught up in what comes our way and the complexities of how we may respond, it is helpful to view life from a place of mindfulness. This means standing back with awareness. The compassionate position is not to identify with our built-in programmes (experienced in the form of motives, desires and emotions) but to learn to regulate them so they do not get expressed in harmful ways. We may experience anger but we do not behave aggressively; we may experience anxiety but we do not take flight except when it is appropriate. Essentially, we are discovering how to tolerate difficult emotions, while learning to *act* wisely and compassionately.

Another common practice is visualisation, where we visualise a compassionate other and initiate an imaginary set of interactions with him or her. Both the cultivation of our own compassionate mind, and dialoguing, interacting with and receiving compassion from a compassionate other are physiologically very powerful. Such is the power of imagination. Just as having a sexual fantasy will produce bodily arousal, when we fantasise about someone with whom we are angry this will stimulate our anger systems. Consequently, when we use visualisations to create compassionate interactions, the

---

[1] www.compassionatemind.co.uk
[2] www.youtube.com/watch?v=VRqI4lxuXAw

compassion systems are stimulated, and by means of neuroplasticity the regular practice of these visualisations can change our physiological pathways.

The third dimension of CFT involves *practising compassionate behaviour in daily life*, by carrying out compassionate acts – no matter how small – for others and for oneself each day. One example might be to deliberately and consciously present a friendly persona to other people when walking down the road. When people see a friendly face, it can stimulate their own affiliative systems. When we receive a friendly gesture in response to our own, we are creating a small buzz of positive emotion, both in the other people and in ourselves. Again, many such practices can be found on the Compassionate Mind Foundation website, as well as more widely on the internet.

In summary, the three key practices are using our body to support our mind, using our mind to support our body, and developing a behavioural orientation that helps us to live compassionately. The motto of the compassionate life is to live to be helpful, not harmful, to self and others.

Conclusion

This brief sub-chapter has highlighted the fact that the evolution of consciousness to the point of self-awareness opens us to special type of awareness of the suffering of life, its transient nature and the reality of loss, disease and decay. During the COVID-19 pandemic, this self-awareness has generated a renewed existential crisis for some as they reflect on the intense suffering in life. People seek comfort and search for answers to this awareness, sometimes through religion or personal spirituality and sometimes through psychotherapy. The ability to face these challenges is enhanced when there is a sense of connectedness to others, and the ability to feel physiologically stable and secure through prosocial relationships. The experience of being valued, wanted and socially connected makes a crucial contribution to mental health and is being increasingly recognised as a focus for therapy. Developing compassion for self and others is the bridge to a deep sense of interconnectedness, social belonging and social value. It is also a central theme in some spiritual quests.

References

Armstrong, K. (1999) *A History of God. From Abraham to the Present: The 4000-Year Quest for God*. London: Vintage Books.

Beck, A. T., Rush, A. J., Shaw, B. F. and Emery, G. (1979) *Cognitive Therapy of Depression*. New York: The Guilford Press.

Bering, J. M. (2002) The existential theory of mind. *Review of General Psychology*, 6, 3–24.

Bowlby, J. (1969) *Attachment and Loss, Vol. 1. Attachment*. London: Hogarth Press and The Institute of Psycho-Analysis.

Bowlby, J. (1973) *Attachment and Loss, Vol. 2. Separation, Anxiety and Anger*. London: Hogarth Press and The Institute of Psycho-Analysis.

Bowlby, J. (1980) *Attachment and Loss, Vol. 3. Loss: Sadness and Depression*. London: Hogarth Press and The Institute of Psycho-Analysis.

Bowlby, J. (1989) The role of attachment in personality development and psychopathology. In S. I. Greenspan and G. H. Pollock, eds., *The Course of Life, Vol. 1. Infancy*. New York: International Universities Press, Inc., pp. 229–270.

Brown, S. L. and Brown, R. M. (2015) Connecting prosocial behavior to improved physical health: contributions from the neurobiology of parenting. *Neuroscience and Biobehavioral Reviews*, 55, 1-17.

Brown, S. L. and Brown, R. M. (2017) Compassionate neurobiology and health. In: E. M. Seppälä, E. Simon-Thomas, S. L. Brown, M. C. Worline, L. Cameron and J. R. Doty, eds., *The Oxford Handbook of Compassion Science*. New York: Oxford University Press, pp. 159–172.

Byrne, R. W. (2016) *Evolving Insight*. Oxford: Oxford University Press.

Carter, S., Bartal, I. B and Porges, E. (2017) The roots of compassion: an evolutionary and neurobiological perspective. In E. M. Seppälä, E. Simon-Thomas, S. L. Brown, M. C. Worline, L. Cameron and J. R. Doty, eds., *The Oxford Handbook of Compassion Science*. New York: Oxford University Press, pp. 173–188.

Cozolino, L. (2014) *The Neuroscience of Human Relationships: Attachment and the Developing Social Brain*, 2nd ed. New York: W. W. Norton & Company.

Curran, T. and Hill, A. P. (2019) Perfectionism is increasing over time: a meta-analysis of birth cohort differences from 1989 to 2016. *Psychological Bulletin*, 145, 410–429.

Dearing, R. L. and Tangney, J. P. E. (2011) *Shame in the Therapy Hour*. Washington, DC: American Psychological Association.

Dedoncker, J., Vanderhasselt, M. A., Ottaviani, C. and Slavich, G. M. (2021) Mental health during the COVID-19 pandemic and beyond: the importance of the vagus nerve for biopsychosocial resilience. *Neuroscience & Biobehavioral Reviews*, 125, 1–10.

Di Bello, M. D., Carnevali, L., Petrocchi, N. et al. (2020) The compassionate vagus: a meta-analysis on the connection between compassion and heart rate variability. *Neuroscience & Biobehavioral Reviews*, 116, 21–30.

Di Bello, M., Ottaviani, C. and Petrocchi, N. (2021) Compassion is not a benzo: distinctive associations of heart rate variability with its empathic and action components. *Frontiers in Neuroscience*, 15, 617443.

Ditzen, B. and Heinrichs, M. (2014) Psychobiology of social support: the social dimension of stress buffering. *Restorative Neurology and Neuroscience*, 32, 149–162.

Ellenberger, H. F. (1970) *The Discovery of the Unconscious: The History and Evolution of Dynamic Psychiatry*. New York: Basic Books.

Forstmann, M., Yudkin, D. A., Prosser, A. M., Heller, S. M. and Crockett, M. J. (2020) Transformative experience and social connectedness mediate the mood-enhancing effects of psychedelic use in naturalistic settings. *Proceedings of the National Academy of Sciences of the United States of America*, 117, 2338–2346.

Garcia-Romeu, A., Brennan Kersgaard, B. and Addy, P. H. (2016) Clinical applications of hallucinogens: a review. *Experimental and Clinical Psychopharmacology*, 24, 229–268.

Gilbert, P. (1984) *Depression: From Psychology to Brain State*. Mahwah, NJ: Lawrence Erlbaum Associates.

Gilbert, P. (1989) *Human Nature and Suffering*. Mahwah, NJ: Lawrence Erlbaum Associates.

Gilbert, P. (1995) Biopsychosocial approaches and evolutionary theory as aids to integration in clinical psychology and psychotherapy. *Clinical Psychology and Psychotherapy*, 2, 135–156.

Gilbert, P. (1998) Evolutionary psychopathology: why isn't the mind designed better than it is? *British Journal of Medical Psychology*, 71, 353–373.

Gilbert, P. (2000) Social mentalities: internal 'social' conflict and the role of inner warmth and compassion in cognitive therapy. In P. Gilbert and K. G. Bailey, eds., *Genes on the Couch: Explorations in Evolutionary Psychotherapy*. Hove: Brunner-Routledge, pp. 118–150.

Gilbert, P. (2007) The evolution of shame as a marker for relationship security: a biopsychosocial approach. In J. L. Tracy, R. W. Robins and J. P Tangney, eds., *The Self-Conscious Emotions: Theory and Research*. New York: The Guilford Press, pp. 283–309.

Gilbert, P. (2009) *The Compassionate Mind: A New Approach to Life's Challenges*. London: Constable & Robinson.

Gilbert, P. (2010) *Compassion Focused Therapy*. London: Routledge.

Gilbert. P. (2011) Shame in psychotherapy and the role of compassion focused therapy. In R. L. Dearing and J. P. Tangney, eds., *Shame in the Therapy Hour*. Washington, DC: American Psychological Association, pp. 325–354.

Gilbert, P. (2014) The origins and nature of compassion focused therapy. *British Journal of Clinical Psychology*, 53, 6–41.

Gilbert, P. (2017) Compassion as a social mentality: an evolutionary approach. In P. Gilbert, ed., *Compassion: Concepts, Research and Applications*. London: Routledge, pp. 31–68.

Gilbert, P. (2018) *Living Like Crazy*. York: Annwyn House.

Gilbert, P. (2020) Compassion: from its evolution to a psychotherapy. *Frontiers in Psychology*, 11, 586161.

Gilbert, P. (2021) Creating a compassionate world: addressing the conflicts between *sharing and caring* versus *controlling and holding* evolved strategies. *Frontiers in Psychology*, 11, 582090.

Gilbert, P. and Basran, J. (2018) Imagining one's compassionate self and coping with life difficulties. *EC Psychology and Psychiatry*, 7, 971–978.

Gilbert, P. and Simos, G. (2022) *Compassion Focused Therapy: Clinical Practice and Applications*. London: Routledge.

Hartogsohn, I. (2018) The meaning-enhancing properties of psychedelics and their mediator role in psychedelic therapy, spirituality, and creativity. *Frontiers in Neuroscience*, 12, 129.

Hofer, M. A. (1994) Early relationships as regulators of infant physiology and behavior. *Acta Paediatrica*, 397, 9–18.

Keltner, D., Kogan, A., Piff, P. K. and Saturn, S. R. (2014) The sociocultural appraisals, values, and emotions (SAVE) framework of prosociality: core processes from gene to meme. *Annual Review of Psychology*, 65, 425–460.

Kim, J. J, Cunnington, R. and Kirby, J. N. (2020) The neurophysiological basis of compassion: an fMRI meta-analysis of compassion and its related neural processes. *Neuroscience & Biobehavioral Reviews*, 108, 112–123.

Kirby, J. N., Day, J. and Sagar, V. (2019) The 'Flow' of compassion: a meta-analysis of the fears of compassion scales and psychological functioning. *Clinical Psychology Review*, 70, 26–39.

Kirkpatrick, L. A. (2005) *Attachment, Evolution, and the Psychology of Religion*. New York: The Guilford Press.

Lampert, K. (2005) *Traditions of Compassion: From Religious Duty to Social Activism*. New York: Palgrave Macmillan.

Lippard, E. T. and Nemeroff, C. B. (2020) The devastating clinical consequences of child abuse and neglect: increased disease vulnerability and poor treatment response in mood disorders. *American Journal of Psychiatry*, 177, 20–36.

MacDonald, K. and MacDonald, T. M. (2010) The peptide that binds: a systematic review of oxytocin and its prosocial effects in humans. *Harvard Review of Psychiatry*, 18, 1–21.

Mayseless, O. (2016) *The Caring Motivation: An Integrated Theory*. Oxford: Oxford University Press.

Narvaez. D. (2017) Evolution, child raising, and compassionate morality. In P. Gilbert, ed., *Compassion: Concepts, Research and Applications*. London: Routledge, pp. 173–186.

Petrocchi, N. and Cheli, S. (2019) The social brain and heart rate variability: implications for psychotherapy. *Psychology and Psychotherapy*, 92, 208–223.

Plante, T. G., ed. (2015) *The Psychology of Compassion and Cruelty: Understanding the Emotional, Spiritual, and Religious Influences*. Santa Barbara, CA: Praeger.

Porges, S. W. (2017) Vagal pathways: portals to compassion. In E. M. Seppälä, E. Simon-Thomas, S. L. Brown, M. C. Worline, L. Cameron and J. R. Doty, eds., *The Oxford Handbook of Compassion Science*. New

York: Oxford University Press, pp. 189–202.

Porges, S. W. and Furman, S. A. (2011) The early development of the autonomic nervous system provides a neural platform for social behaviour: a polyvagal perspective. *Infant and Child Development*, 20, 106–118.

Ricard, M. (2015) *Altruism: The Power of Compassion to Change Yourself and the World*. London: Atlantic Books.

Ryan, C. (2019) *Civilized to Death: The Price of Progress*. New York: Avid Reader Press.

Schore, A. N. (2019) *Right Brain Psychotherapy*. New York: W. W. Norton & Company.

Seppälä, E. M., Simon-Thomas, E., Brown, S. L., Worline, M. C., Cameron, C. D. and Doty, J. R., eds. (2017) *The Oxford Handbook of Compassion Science*. New York: Oxford University Press.

Siegel, D. J. (2012) *The Developing Mind: How Relationships and the Brain Interact to Shape Who We Are*. New York: The Guilford Press.

Singer, T. and Engert, V. (2019) It matters what you practice: differential training effects on subjective experience, behavior, brain and body in the ReSource Project. *Current Opinion in Psychology*, 28, 151–158.

Stellar, J. E. and Keltner, D. (2017) Compassion in the autonomic nervous system: the role of the vagus nerve. In: P. Gilbert, ed., *Compassion: Concepts, Research and Applications*. London: Routledge, pp. 120–134.

Stevens, J. and Woodruff, C. C. (2018) *The Neuroscience of Empathy, Compassion, and Self-Compassion*. London: Academic Press.

Stott, R. (2007) When head and heart do not agree: a theoretical and clinical analysis of Rational-Emotional Dissociation (RED) in cognitive therapy. *Journal of Cognitive Psychotherapy*, 21, 37–50.

Tagliazucchi, E., Llobenes, L. and Gumiy, N. (2022) Psychedelics, connectedness, and compassion. In P. Gilbert and G. Simos, eds., *Compassion Focused Therapy: Clinical Practice and Applications*. London: Routledge, pp. 360–370.

Tsering, G. T. (2005) *The Four Noble Truths: The Foundation of Buddhist Thought*. Vol. 1. Somerville, MA: Wisdom Publications.

Wallace, A. B. (2007) *Contemplative Science: Where Buddhism and Neuroscience Converge*. New York: Columbia University Press.

Yalom, I. R. (1980) *Existential Psychotherapy*. New York: Basic Books.

Religiously Integrated Cognitive–Behavioural Therapy

Michelle Pearce

Introduction

The integration of religion and spirituality into health care used to be standard medical practice. Indeed, until René Descartes proposed his theory of mind–body dualism, spirituality was an integral part of health and health care. Over the last few decades, with a burgeoning of research in the field of spiritualty and health, as well as consumer demand for whole-person health care, the paradigm of health has begun to include the spirit and spirituality again. The rift between the psychological and the spiritual has also begun to mend in the realm of psychiatry and psychotherapy. Extensive reviews of empirical research have revealed that in the majority of studies, spirituality/religion has a positive and even protective effect on mental health and well-being. Research has reported a negative correlation between spirituality/religion and depression, anxiety, post-traumatic stress disorder, addiction, eating disorders and risky health behaviours, and a positive correlation with optimism, meaning and purpose, and hope (Koenig et al., 2012).

The many positive empirical associations between spirituality/religion and mental health have led researchers to ask whether integrating spirituality/religion into psychotherapy would enhance the effects of treatment for those suffering from mental health disorders. The short answer from this body of work is that explicitly integrating spirituality/religion into psychological treatment does indeed seem to be an effective treatment for psychological disorders such as depression and anxiety for religious clients, and at times is more effective than standard psychological treatment (Worthington et al., 2011; Koenig et al., 2015).

In this sub-chapter we shall examine one type of religiously integrated psychological treatment – religiously integrated cognitive–behavioural therapy (RCBT). We shall begin by describing how RCBT differs from conventional cognitive–behavioural therapy, and then briefly review the research supporting the use of this treatment, examine five of the primary tools used in this approach, and conclude by addressing some frequently asked questions about the use of RCBT in clinical practice.

What Is Religiously Integrated CBT?

Given that RCBT is an adaptation of conventional CBT, we shall begin with a brief overview of the principles and tools of CBT. Based on the work of Aaron and Judy Beck (cognitive therapy) and Albert Ellis (rational emotive therapy), CBT is a psychotherapeutic approach that integrates behavioural and cognitive principles in order to reduce negative emotional states. The theory underlying this approach is that our thoughts, emotions and behaviour are all interconnected, and therefore changing one of these components can change the other two components. Thus a therapist using CBT teaches clients how to both challenge and change unhelpful thinking styles and unhelpful behaviours in order to reduce negative emotions and increase positive emotions. CBT is a collaborative approach in which the therapist and patient work together, and it is characterised by agenda setting, eliciting patient feedback, empathetic communication, Socratic questioning, guided discovery and homework activities.

Religious CBT is based on the same theory as CBT, and it uses the same approach and style. What differs between the two approaches is the explicit use of the client's own religious beliefs, practices, teachings and values to help them to challenge and change their unhelpful cognitions and behaviours. The client's religious worldview, values and resources provide a foundation or 'standard' against which the patient can measure their thoughts and actions, allowing them to determine the truthfulness of a thought or the helpfulness of a behaviour. This provides a powerful and patient-centred way for them to shift their thinking and behaviours to line up with their belief system and to support their well-being.

Notably, it is the client's religious beliefs, values and practices, not those of the therapist, that are used in their treatment. Therapists do not engage in theological discussions or debates, nor do they impose their own religious beliefs or values on the patient. When theological issues arise, clergy are important and helpful resources for consultation and/or referrals. A manualised approach for RCBT, including therapist manuals and patient workbooks, has been developed for five major world religions – Christianity, Judaism, Islam, Buddhism and Hinduism (Pearce and Koenig, 2013; Pearce et al., 2015). The manuals provide guidance and some general information about these religions for therapists who are unfamiliar with these belief systems.

Research Support for the Use of RCBT

Intervention studies have found that integrating religious clients' spiritual/religious beliefs into therapy is at least as effective in reducing depression as is secular treatment (e.g., Propst et al., 1992; Azhar and Varma, 1995; Smith et al., 2007; Wade et al., 2007; Hook et al., 2010; Pargament et al., 2013). In a meta-analytic review of 46 spiritual intervention studies, Worthington et al. (2011) concluded that patients with spiritual beliefs who were being treated with spiritually integrated psychotherapies showed greater improvement than patients who were being treated with other psychotherapies. When compared with the same type of therapy in secular form, spiritually integrated therapies showed greater improvement on spiritual outcomes and similar improvement on psychological outcomes. Notably, in a recent survey of 989 American adults who had seen a mental healthcare provider within the last month, most (64%) reported that spirituality/religion was relevant to and improved their mental health; however, only 26% reported that the subject of their spiritual/religious beliefs was brought up by their therapist (Oxhandler et al., 2021).

Studies have also looked specifically at integrating religion into CBT. As with other religiously and spiritually integrated therapies, religiously integrated CBT (for Christians and Muslims) was found to be as effective as or more effective than conventional or control treatments for depression and anxiety (e.g., Pecheur and Edwards, 1984; Propst et al., 1992; Azhar and Varma, 1995; Razali et al., 1998; Tan, 2013; Ramos et al., 2014). Our research team conducted the largest randomised controlled trial of RCBT to date, with 132 clients with major depression (65 clients were randomised to RCBT and 67 clients to CBT) across two states using a 10-week manualised treatment with a 3-month follow-up (Koenig et al., 2015). This study revealed that RCBT was as effective as conventional CBT for the treatment of depression among the medically ill. In addition to reducing depression, RCBT and CBT also increased positive outcomes, including optimism, gratitude, generosity, and purpose and meaning in life (Koenig et al., 2014).

Primary RCBT Tools

In this section we shall examine five of the primary RCBT tools.

Renewing the Mind

Many world religions teach that our thoughts and interpretations influence our emotions and behaviour. For example, in the Christian tradition, 'metanoia' means 'change your mind' or 'change how you think', which in many versions of the Bible is translated as 'repent' (e.g., Matthew 4:17). Islam teaches this notion, too: 'Surely Allah does not change the condition of a people until they change their own condition' (Qur'an 13:11). RCBT teaches clients how to use their sacred scriptures to replace negative and inaccurate thoughts with positive thoughts that promote mental health and well-being.

Two of the methods used to renew the mind are scripture memorisation and contemplative prayer. For scripture memorisation, clients are either provided with a scripture relating to the session content (suggestions can be found in RCBT manuals) or can choose their own scripture or inspirational passage to memorise over the next week. By memorising sacred passages, clients build an 'arsenal' of positive thoughts that they can then use to challenge and change negative thinking. This is not a prescriptive activity and is not intended to lead to theological discussions or debates. Rather, it is an activity to help clients to focus their minds on positive thoughts, like planting positive seeds that produce a harvest of positive emotions.

When the scriptures or passages that the patient will memorise are chosen, several factors need to be considered. One factor is the knowledge and comfort level of the patient and therapist. Some clients and/or therapists will have a good working knowledge of scriptures in a particular tradition, from which they can select a relevant passage. This makes it easier to choose a passage each week. For those with less knowledge, a therapist might use suggestions from the RCBT manuals, or encourage the patient to search for passages on the Internet (e.g., using websites such as Bible Gateway for Christians or Quran Smart Search for Muslims) that are related to a particular topic (e.g., feeling loved by God, or gratitude).

A second important factor to consider is the context of the session material. Ideally, the patient will choose a passage that is relevant to the issue they are working on in a particular session, or that is related to their overall treatment goal. For example, a patient who is struggling with feelings of anxiety would benefit from passages related to the peace of God or the provision of God, but would be less helped by a passage on, for example, baptism or healing. Thus the patient and therapist should work together to choose a relevant passage that speaks to the heart of the client's concern.

Therapists can also teach clients how to meditate on these passages – a strategy called *contemplative prayer* that can help clients to better remember and use this type of thinking. Contemplative prayer is similar to some types of meditation, such as mantra meditation. Clients are asked to take a scripture or sacred passage and spend 5 to 10 minutes quietly reflecting on what that passage means to them. They are asked to sit quietly and enter a contemplative, prayerful state, asking themselves questions such as 'How does this speak to me?', 'What is coming up for me as I read this passage?' and 'How can I apply this to my life?' It is a time of silent reflection and listening. Clients are encouraged to have a journal with them during this time, so that they can write down any thoughts or insights that arise. This activity helps clients both to think deeply about meaningful passages and to begin to apply insights gleaned to their lives. It is also an effective way to counter depressive rumination.

Challenging Thoughts Using Religious Resources

One of the main tools used in conventional CBT is the ABCDE thought log. Clients use this tool to identify, challenge and change their unhelpful and inaccurate thinking. In Step A, which stands for Activating event, clients describe the situation in which they began to experience a negative emotion. In step B, Beliefs, clients write down the thoughts they were having during or as a result of the activating event. In step C, Consequences, clients write down what emotions they felt and behaviours they engaged in as a result of their beliefs and thoughts. In step D, Disputing beliefs, clients challenge their negative beliefs and look for evidence to support a new way of thinking. In step E, Effective new belief, clients create a new thought that will have more positive emotional and behavioural consequences.

RCBT also uses this tool, with several additions to integrate the client's religious beliefs and practices. First, as with conventional CBT, clients are introduced to categories of unhelpful thinking styles, such as 'magnification', 'all-or-nothing thinking' and 'should statements', to help them to identify which thoughts are unhelpful and why. In RCBT, a theological reflection for each style of thinking is also provided and discussed. The theological reflections ground this exercise in the client's religious tradition and worldview. Contrasting the unhelpful thinking style with their religious teaching provides another source of motivation to change negative thoughts. It can also address distorted religious beliefs, such as a misrepresentative view of a punishing God.

The following is an example of a theological reflection for the 'Fortune-Telling Error' from the Christian tradition. The Fortune-Telling Error occurs when clients jump to conclusions by anticipating that things will turn out badly. They feel convinced that their predictions are already established fact even though no one can predict the future. The following Christian theological reflection is provided for this unhelpful thinking style: 'Jesus told his followers not to be anxious about the future because he is in control and has promised to take care of them (Matthew 6:25–34). By worrying and imagining a negative future, we not only do we not improve the situation, but we also act as if we do not trust God to keep his promises' (Pearce, 2016, p. 68). Clients can use the theological reflection to better understand why this type of thinking does not line up with their value system and religious teachings. This helps them to dispute their negative thoughts.

A second addition to the RCBT thought log is the inclusion of step R, for Religious beliefs and practices, between step D (Disputing beliefs) and step E (Effective new belief). Clients are encouraged to explicitly draw upon their religious beliefs and practices as resources to help them confront and change dysfunctional beliefs. For example, clients can turn to the way they believe the world works from a religious viewpoint, looking to their sacred scriptures and religious writings, spiritual wisdom and other sources for evidence to challenge their negative beliefs. Clients are asked questions such as 'When you look at your original belief, expectation, or way of thinking about the situation, are there any beliefs or attitudes from your religious tradition that strike you as helping to generate an alternative viewpoint?' The answers that clients derive from these questions, such as supporting or negating evidence, will result in an effective new belief.

Religious Practices

RCBT uses tools for changing behaviours that contribute to depression, in addition to tools for changing cognitions. For example, most world religions encourage forgiveness, gratitude, generosity and service, all of which are behaviours that are addressed and encouraged in RCBT. Other behavioural practices that are recommended in RCBT include ongoing social contact with members of one's religious community, praying for self and others, expressing gratitude and engaging in hope-promoting, stress-reducing activities based on the spiritual concept of 'walking by faith', not by feelings. For example, in the Jewish tradition the Torah reinforces the notion that a person can use free will to engage in positive behaviours despite experiencing conflicting emotions. One of the strengths of RCBT is that it integrates CBT skills into the structure of daily spiritual activities, daily devotional practice and daily ritual. The daily behavioural practices have the potential to influence psychological skill agility (e.g., ability to readily access learned emotional regulation, thought challenging, support-seeking skills) and spiritual growth (e.g., an understanding of one's self that empowers one to overcome depression).

Religious/Spiritual Resources

Clients are encouraged to make use of the many religious/spiritual resources that they have available to them. These resources will vary by patient and religious tradition, and may include social support from or activities with members of their place of worship, conversations with religious leaders, reading religious literature, participating in religious study groups, meditation, watching religious programmes, charity work, and attending religious services or activities sponsored by religious groups, such as meditation retreats or sessions (Buddhism and Christianity), Swadhyaya activities (Hinduism) or activities in mosques (Islam).

As with all of the tools used in RCBT, this is not a prescriptive tool. Instead, clients are encouraged to access and engage with the various religious resources they have available to them. Some clients will have resources that they used to enjoy but are no longer engaging with. These individuals can benefit from encouragement to re-engage. Other clients may want to try a new religious resource, and can benefit from using brainstorming methods to enable them to find and use such a resource. Yet others may have distanced themselves from a religious resource for some reason (e.g., a disagreement with a religious leader, conflict with members of a religious community). In this case, the therapist will want to use sound clinical judgement about how to proceed (e.g., assisting the patient in finding resolution so that they are able to return to their community, helping them to find another more supportive community to join).

Involvement in a Religious Community

RCBT also encourages clients to be involved in a religious community of their choice, and to identify someone for whom they can offer support, such as someone they can pray for or spend time with. This type of involvement is different from simply seeking support from others within the religious community. Rather, supporting and caring for others offers one way for clients to live out their religious teachings. It is also likely to result in an increase in their social support (Hill and Pargament, 2003) and opportunities to engage in altruistic activities, all of which help to neutralise negative emotions (Seligman et al., 2005; Krause, 2009).

Using RCBT in Clinical Practice

What Type of Patient Might Benefit from RCBT?

RCBT is designed for religious or spiritual clients who would like to integrate their religious/spiritual beliefs into their psychological treatment. It is not appropriate for clients who are not religious or for those who do not want to integrate their faith into treatment. During the assessment and treatment-planning phase of therapy, therapists should assess their clients' religious/spiritual beliefs and practices, share with them a description of RCBT (many clients are not aware that such a treatment option exists) and determine collaboratively whether the patient would like to try this approach.

Does the Religiosity of the Therapist Matter?

The research conducted to date suggests that the religiosity of the therapist does not influence patient outcomes when administering RCBT. One study revealed that it was not the match between the client's and therapist's religiosity that was important for treatment outcomes and the therapeutic alliance, but rather the matching of the degree of religious integration with the degree of religiosity of the patient. In other words, highly religious clients did better when provided with an explicitly religiously integrated treatment (Wade et al., 2007). Another study in fact revealed that non-religious therapists who administered RCBT had better patient outcomes than did religious therapists (Propst et al., 1992).

What Resources Are Available for Learning RCBT?

Therapists who would like to use RCBT must first be well versed in conventional CBT. With this foundation, they can then learn how to sensitively, effectively and ethically integrate their client's religious beliefs and practices into the CBT model. We have developed treatment manuals and patient workbooks that provide instructions for therapists on how to do this. These materials are freely available online,[1] as is a brief introductory training video on how to conduct RCBT.[2] For those who are working with Christian clients, the author has published a book called *Cognitive Behavioral Therapy for Christians with Depression: A Practical Tool-Based Primer*, which includes

---

[1] https://spiritualityandhealth.duke.edu/index.php/religious-cbt-study/therapy-manuals
[2] https://spiritualityandhealth.duke.edu/index.php/religious-cbt-study/training-video

patient worksheets and case studies (Pearce, 2016). Some therapists will also benefit from additional training, supervision and consultation.

Conclusion

Providing culturally competent mental health care is an ethical requirement in psychiatry. Understanding how patient' religious and spiritual beliefs, values, worldview and practices influence how they both experience and recover from mental health disorders is part of culturally competent care, as is learning how to appropriately harness their religious/spiritual resources to assist in their recovery. RCBT is an empirically validated psychotherapy that has been shown to reduce symptoms of depression and anxiety and increase positive emotions (Koenig et al., 2015). The goal of RCBT is to explicitly use the client's own religious tradition as a foundation for identifying and changing unhelpful and inaccurate thoughts and maladaptive behaviours that contribute to depression. Some of the major tools of RCBT include scripture memorisation to renew one's mind, contemplative prayer, challenging of thoughts using religious teachings, engaging in religious practices (e.g., forgiveness, service, gratitude) and involvement in a religious community. This treatment approach has been developed for five major world religions – Christianity, Judaism, Islam, Buddhism and Hinduism. To provide the most effective, patient-centred and culturally sensitive care, we must work with clients from within a more holistic model – one that integrates the mind, body *and* spirit. RCBT offers one psychotherapeutic approach to doing just that.

References

Azhar, M. Z. and Varma, S. L. (1995) Religious psychotherapy as management of bereavement. *Acta Psychiatrica Scandinavica*, 91, 233–235.

Hill, P. C. and Pargament, K. I. (2003) Advances in the conceptualization and measurement of religion and spirituality: implications for physical and mental health research. *American Psychologist*, 58, 64–74.

Hook, J. N., Worthington, E. L., Davis, D. E. et al. (2010) Empirically supported religious and spiritual therapies. *Journal of Clinical Psychology*, 66, 46–72.

Koenig, H. G., King, D. E. and Benner Carson, V. (2012) *Handbook of Religion and Health*, 2nd ed. New York: Oxford University Press.

Koenig, H. G., Berk, L. S., Daher, N. et al. (2014) Religious involvement is associated with greater purpose, optimism, generosity and gratitude in persons with major depression and chronic medical illness. *Journal of Psychosomatic Research*, 77, 135–143.

Koenig, H. G., Pearce, M. J., Nelson, B. et al. (2015) Religious vs. conventional cognitive behavioral therapy for major depression in persons with chronic medical illness: a pilot randomized trial. *Journal of Nervous and Mental Disease*, 203, 243–251.

Krause, N. (2009) Religious involvement, gratitude, and change in depressive symptoms over time. *International Journal for the Psychology of Religion*, 19, 155–172.

Oxhandler, H. K., Pargament, K., Pearce, M., Vieten, C. and Moffatt, K. (2021) The relevance of religion and spirituality to mental health: a national survey of current clients' views. *Social Work*, 66, 254–264.

Pargament, K. I., Mahoney, A., Exline, J. J., Jones, J. W. and Shafranske, E. P. (2013) From research to practice: towards an applied psychology of religion and spirituality. In K. I. Pargament, A. Mahoney and E. P. Shafranske, eds., *APA Handbook of Psychology, Religion, and Spirituality: Vol. 2. An Applied Psychology of Religion and Spirituality*. Washington, DC: American Psychological Association, pp. 3–22.

Pearce, M. J. (2016) *Cognitive Behavioral Therapy for Christians with Depression: A Practical Tool-Based Primer.* West Conshohocken, PA: Templeton Press.

Pearce, M. J. and Koenig, H. K. (2013) Cognitive behavioural therapy for the treatment of depression in Christian patients with medical illness. *Mental Health, Religion & Culture,* 16, 730–740.

Pearce, M. J., Koenig, H. G., Robins, C. et al. (2015) Religiously integrated cognitive behavioral therapy: a new method of treatment for major depression in patients with chronic medical illness. *Psychotherapy,* 52, 56–66.

Pecheur, D. R. and Edwards, K. J. (1984) A comparison of secular and religious versions of cognitive therapy with depressed Christian college students. *Journal of Psychology and Theology,* 12, 45–54.

Propst, L. R., Ostrom, R., Watkins, P., Dean, T. and Mashburn, D. (1992) Comparative efficacy of religious and nonreligious cognitive–behavioral therapy for the treatment of clinical depression in religious individuals. *Journal of Consulting and Clinical Psychology,* 60, 94–103.

Ramos, K., Barrera, T. L. and Stanley, M. A. (2014) Incorporating nonmainstream spirituality into CBT for anxiety: a case study. *Spirituality in Clinical Practice,* 1, 269–277.

Razali, S. M., Hasanah, C. I., Aminah, K. and Subramaniam, M. (1998) Religious-sociocultural psychotherapy in patients with anxiety and depression. *Australian and New Zealand Journal of Psychiatry,* 32, 867–872.

Seligman, M. E., Steen, T. A., Park, N. and Peterson, C. (2005) Positive psychology progress: empirical validation of interventions. *American Psychologist,* 60, 410–421.

Smith, T. B., Bartz, J. and Richards, P. S. (2007) Outcomes of religious and spiritual adaptations in psychotherapy: a meta-analytic review. *Psychotherapy Research,* 17, 643–655.

Tan, S.-Y. (2013) Addressing religion and spirituality from a cognitive-behavioral perspective. In K. I. Pargament, A. Mahoney and E. P. Shafranske, eds., *APA Handbook of Psychology, Religion, and Spirituality: Vol. 2. An Applied Psychology of Religion and Spirituality.* Washington, DC: American Psychological Association, pp. 169–187.

Wade, N. G., Worthington, E. L., Jr. and Vogel, D. L. (2007) Effectiveness of religiously tailored interventions in Christian therapy. *Psychotherapy Research,* 17, 91–105.

Worthington, E. L., Jr., Hook, J. N., Davis, D. E. and McDaniel, M. A. (2011) Religion and spirituality. *Journal of Clinical Psychology,* 67, 204–214.

Chapter

14.4

Forgiveness Therapy

Robert D. Enright and Jacqueline Y. Song

Case study: Marvin

Marvin was only a child when his father would discipline him harshly. Now, as a middle-aged man imprisoned for life, he relates his story of abuse while a child. Every time he misbehaved, he had to crawl on his hands and knees down the long gravel driveway of the family's home, get the mail from the mailbox near the road, and crawl back again – dusty, dirty, bruised and humiliated. When he became a teenager, old enough to pick up his father's hunting rifle, he shot and killed all of his family members.

The tragedy of this story is that, had Marvin been instructed in the art of forgiveness, perhaps his rage could have been quelled sufficiently to avoid the mass murder. Had Marvin's father been schooled in the art of forgiveness, perhaps he would have found a way to forgive whoever abused him so that he did not continually displace his own anger on to his son. Had both father and son practised forgiveness, perhaps the entire family would be alive today and Marvin would not be in prison for life.

Forgiveness is important precisely because it is an antidote – perhaps the strongest antidote – to the injustices that divide, abuse and poison the inner world of those who are abused and those who perpetrate the abuse. Forgiveness is about healing and possibly reuniting. It is a cure for wounded hearts and relationships.

In this sub-chapter we shall discuss the philosophy and psychology of forgiveness as it bears on *forgiveness therapy* within the mental health professions. We shall first define what forgiveness is (its Essence in Aristotelian philosophy), next discuss that to which forgiveness points (the Final Cause in Aristotle's words, or the purpose of forgiving) and then consider the social science of forgiveness. This will include discussion of two models of forgiveness interventions, the empirical evidence for them, and the cross-cultural evidence for various forgiveness therapeutic and educational approaches.

A Philosophical Examination of What Forgiveness Is

In Plato's dialogues about Socrates' wisdom, the first question that is usually asked of any construct is 'What is it?'. Starting with an understanding of the construct is vital if we are to avoid either error in the definition or what we have called 'definitional drift' (Enright et al., 1998), in which researchers, who come after those who initiated a field of inquiry, inadvertently start to misunderstand the nature of the construct and drift away from the truth of it. In this spirit of Plato, we shall first examine what forgiveness is and then turn to a discussion of forgiveness therapy.

What Is Forgiveness?

Forgiveness is one of the moral virtues, as are justice, courage, patience and love. According to Aristotle, any moral virtue has seven characteristics (Simon, 1986). First, it is concerned with the good of human interaction. Second, the person knows that the virtue is good – this is the cognitive aspect of any moral virtue. Third, the person is motivated to effect the good towards other people – this is the affective aspect of any moral virtue. Fourth, the person practises the virtue towards others – this is the behavioural aspect, and the idea of 'practise' implies that time is needed to grow in any moral virtue. Fifth, the person is imperfect in the application of the virtues – no one attains perfection. This characteristic again suggests that time is needed if one is to grow towards the endpoint of any virtue or its perfection, even though that perfection will not be attained. Sixth, people try to be consistent in how they practise any given virtue. Seventh, people vary considerably in their ability to appropriate the virtues.

As one more philosophical foundation prior to defining forgiveness, Aristotle has instructed us that if we are to truly understand any given virtue, we need to examine it in terms of five characteristics – its Species (what it is in its Essence), its Genus (what it shares with all of the other moral virtues), its Specific Difference (how it is unique relative to the other moral virtues), its Accidents (not errors, but what is rare and still part of the virtue) and its Properties (what is important to the virtue, but not so important as to be part of its Essence) (for a more detailed discussion of these points, see Kreeft, 2018).

Forgiveness in its Essence is a moral virtue in which goodness is given to those who have offended the forgiver. Those who forgive know that they have been treated unjustly, and willingly decide to rid themselves of resentment and to offer kindness, respect, generosity and even love to the offending other person. This is the Essence of what forgiveness is (Enright and Fitzgibbons, 2015). Not all agree with this view. For example, McCullough and Hoyt (2002, p. 1556) focus their definition only on motivational aspects of forgiveness: 'forgiveness can be conceptualised as a complex of prosocial changes in one's interpersonal motivations following a transgression'. However, motivation by itself will not necessarily lead to behavioural change, or even to broader changes in thinking about who the offending person is as a person.

The Genus of forgiveness is its shared characteristic (with all of the other moral virtues) of being good to others. Its Specific Difference (again shared with all of the other moral virtues) is the forgiver's willingness to appropriate this goodness to those who have behaved unjustly towards him or her. An Accident, for example, is forgiving quickly. Although this can happen, it is not typical when the forgiver has been deeply hurt by the other. A Property of forgiving (not essential to its definition) is saying 'I forgive you' to the offending other.

Forgiveness is not about finding excuses for the other's behaviour – what happened was wrong, is wrong and always will be wrong. Forgiveness is not about forgetting, but instead remembering in new ways, without rancour. Forgiveness may or may not include reconciliation. Reconciliation is not a moral virtue, but rather it is a negotiation strategy in which two or more people come together again in mutual trust. Finally, forgiveness is not the abandonment of the quest for fairness; the forgiver does appropriate the moral virtue of justice. As Aristotle reminds us, we do not practise any given moral virtue to the exclusion of the other ones (Aristotle, 1926).

What Are the Formal and Final Causes of Forgiveness?

In understanding any phenomenon of interest, Aristotle has challenged us to ask certain questions that he called Causes. We shall discuss only two of them here – the Formal and Final Causes of forgiving. The Formal Cause is the Essence of the construct, with the question 'What is it?' as was discussed earlier. The Final Cause asks 'To what does it point or what is the goal for engaging in this virtue?'. There are at least ten Final Causes of forgiveness:

1. self-help or inner healing
2. self-improvement in character
3. helping the offending person to change the unjust behaviour
4. helping the offended person to grow in character
5. improving the relationship
6. protecting innocent others outside the family who might be the victims of displaced anger
7. protecting those within the family from displaced anger
8. protecting the community from the ravages of resentment and hatred
9. exercising forgiveness as a moral good in and of itself
10. honouring one's religious or philosophical tradition which encourages forgiving.

Patients who attend mental health services may have very different reasons for doing so. The ten reasons listed here might serve as a checklist to allow mental health professionals to discern the goals that any given patient might bring to treatment.

What Is the Purpose of Forgiveness Therapy?

Some, perhaps many, mental health professionals might say that their task is not to help a patient grow in virtue. Although forgiveness therapy can be used as a general psychotherapeutic approach, it is often used in the specific context of a person being unjustly treated by one or more others and then retaining resentment (irritability or unhealthy anger) as an effect of the unjust behaviour. The irritability can last for years because of the unfair treatment, with the subsequent emergence of anxiety or depression and other symptoms (Enright and Fitzgibbons, 2015). Learning to forgive reduces the resentment and the subsequent emergence of other symptoms, as we shall see later in this sub-chapter.

Forgiveness is always the choice of the patient. It is the task of the mental health professional to ascertain the patient's readiness for this and then to make sure that a clear understanding of forgiveness is occurring, in that it is not just about 'moving on' or accepting the situation. Before deciding whether to choose this kind of psychotherapeutic approach, the patient should explore the other issues discussed earlier in this sub-chapter regarding what forgiveness is not.

An Examination of Two Forgiveness Interventions

We shall examine here the two models of foregiveness for which the most research on validity has been undertaken, namely the process model and the REACH model.

The Process Model

The process model (Enright, 2012) consists of four *phases* of forgiveness, which incorporate the cognitive, affective and behavioural aspects of forgiveness. These phases encompass 20 units as follows:

Phase 1: Uncovering anger and hurt (8 units)

1 Denial of anger and hurt. At the start of the forgiveness process, people have sometimes suppressed the amount of hurt they have.
2 Being aware of the depth of anger and hurt. It can take time for the psychological defences of denial or repression to lessen in the patient.
3 Sometimes victims experience shame as others pass judgement on the victims, wondering what they did to deserve such negative treatment. Guilt feelings might also be present because of thoughts of revenge.
4 Energy is often depleted because of the inner resentment.
5 The forgiver sometimes ruminates about the injury, replaying it over and over again in his or her mind.
6 If the forgiver starts to compare the self with the offender, the conclusion can be that this offending person is getting away with too much injustice.
7 The forgiver may have to face permanent changes because of the injustice (e.g., ending a relationship, leaving a job).
8 The forgiver's philosophy of life may become negative (e.g., the belief that no one can be trusted).

Phase 2: Decision to forgive (3 units).

9 The forgiver realises that the previously used strategies for emotional healing are not working.
10 The person develops a willingness to explore forgiveness, including what forgiveness is and is not. This unit is important because, without a clear understanding of what forgiveness is, the patient may be going down a path in the name of forgiveness which in fact is not forgiveness. For example, if the person thinks that forgiveness is merely about moving on from the unjust situation or transcending the anger, this is not exercising forgiveness as a moral virtue.
11 The patient commits to forgive, including a homework assignment of committing to doing no harm to the one who offended.

Phase 3: Working on forgiveness (4 units).

12 The patient starts with a cognitive exploration of the person who offended. This includes the *personal perspective* (What emotional wounds has this person been carrying which led to a displacement of the discontent on to the patient?), the *global perspective* (What do the offending person and the patient share in common, such as inherent worth, uniqueness as individuals and the fact that they have both been wounded in life by others?) and, if the patient has a spiritual worldview, the *cosmic perspective* (e.g., a Jewish or Christian patient, following a reading of Genesis 1, might be asked, 'Are you and the one who hurt you both made in the image and likeness of God?').

13 As the patient explores the three cognitive perspectives about the offending person, empathy and compassion towards the other may slowly begin to emerge. Although this is part of the Essence of forgiveness, empathy and compassion may not emerge in the Existence of forgiveness within the patient, because such emotions are not under the full control of people.

14 Once the patient has started to become psychologically stronger as a result of working through units 12 and 13, the mental health professional asks him or her to consider bearing the pain of what happened so that the patient does not displace his or her discontent on to the offending person or on to unsuspecting others (Kaufman, 1984).

15 Once the patient has been strengthened by working through units 12 to 14, he or she is encouraged, but only when ready for this, to consider giving a gift to the person who offended, such as a smile or a returned phone call. This is part of the Essence of what forgiveness is, but again it need not be part of the Existence of forgiving for patients who are not ready to give a gift.

Phase 4: Deepening understanding and increasing well-being (5 units)

16 As a person suffers, there is a tendency to find meaning in that suffering (Frankl, 1959).

17 Patients often now see that they, too, have offended others, and so ask for forgiveness from those whom they have offended.

18 Patients realise that they are not alone in their forgiveness journey, and sometimes seek a companion for that journey.

19 A new purpose in life, often a motivation to assist others in their pain, emerges.

20 Improvement in psychological health is often realised, and supported by the scientific data, which we shall discuss later in this sub-chapter.

A training manual on the process model for mental health professionals is available (Enright and Fitzgibbons, 2015), as are three self-help books that can be used by patients (Enright, 2001, 2012, 2015).

The REACH model

Worthington (2020b) has developed a five-step technique of forgiveness called REACH, which is an acronym for the following:

Recall the hurt

Empathise with the one who hurt you

Altruistic gift of forgiveness, offer

Commitment to forgive, take

Hold on to the forgiveness

The five steps can be briefly described as follows:

Step 1: Recall the hurt. The patient is asked to recall the event and, even if fear or anger is present, to then try to relax in the face of this past image of unfairness. The patient is encouraged to engage in the practice of taking a deep breath and to engage in calming techniques.

Step 2: Empathise with (or step inside the shoes of) the person who offended. Dr Worthington explains that this is not necessarily to ascertain the truth of what happened, but instead to find a reasonable explanation that will allow the forgiver to let go of the negative affect. The use of what is called the 'empty-chair technique' is encouraged. The forgiver pours out his or her distress and then switches chairs and tries to explain, from the offender's viewpoint, why the injustice occurred.

Step 3: Altruistic gift of forgiveness. This includes a kindness of some sort, given to help the other person.

Step 4: Commit yourself. The commitment is the decision to forgive (decisional forgiveness). The person is encouraged to make a public commitment so that he or she is unlikely to take back the forgiveness. This can include the techniques of writing a 'certificate of forgiveness' or writing a letter of forgiveness (which is not sent) and then reading it aloud.

Step 5: Hold on to forgiveness. The techniques here include re-reading the certificate of forgiveness or the letter which was written but not sent. The point is to persevere in the decision to forgive.

Philosophical Characteristics of Forgiveness Therapy

Having described two different models of forgiveness interventions, we would like to make three philosophical clarifications about what forgiveness therapy actually is and is not.

The Difference Between Applying Forgiveness and Growing in Forgiveness

There is a difference between applying the virtue of forgiveness and growing in this virtue. For example, suppose person A is under pressure today and has an important lunch meeting with person B, who fails to show up. Person A is annoyed, forgives person B for this situation and moves on with life. This is an example of applying the virtue. Now consider person C, who was abused by her mother during her adolescent years. Person C is depressed and has low self-esteem. She cannot simply decide to forgive her mother in an hour or even in a few intervention sessions and then get on with a better life. Instead she will need time to grow, through a strong will and continual practice, to forgive her mother at a deep level. Only then will she experience the healing effects as she develops a deeper sense of forgiveness. As further clarification here, we are not suggesting that all people who experience what person C experienced should now forgive. As stated earlier, forgiveness is the patient's choice, and even the suggestion by the mental health professional would not be appropriate until the therapeutic bond has been established and the idea of forgiving seems appropriate to the professional in the current treatment context.

Forgiveness as Practising a Virtue Compared with Forgiveness as a Technique

In the above-mentioned example, person C is engaging in the process of practising a moral virtue, which requires time, practice and deepening what is offered to the offending person. At first, person C might offer a commitment to 'do no harm', which grows into a willingness to bear the pain of what happened with her mother, and eventually, over time, to being able to give a gift to her mother. In contrast, person A, who is not suffering the deep psychological effects of abuse but may need some help with overcoming her annoyance, could benefit from a short-term empty-chair technique. This could be done in one session with a good intervention outcome, but this is qualitatively different from what may be required of person C, who now is walking a path of forgiveness, and such a journey takes time.

Forgiveness as Combining All the Characteristics of a Moral Virtue Vs. Dichotomising Forgiveness into Decisional and Emotional Components

When we hear such terms as 'decisional' forgiveness and 'emotional' forgiveness, we realise that the authors who are using such terms are borrowing ideas exclusively from psychology, rather than seeing forgiveness philosophically as a whole virtue with such components – working together – as cognitive, affective and behavioural responses to the offending person. From a philosophical perspective, there are no such constructs as 'decisional' forgiveness because that is a reductionist view of what forgiveness actually is (with its focus on commitment and cognition only). This is the case because to apply cognition only when forgiving is to set aside the softened heart (compassion and even love towards an offending other person), which the philosopher North (1987) argues is essential to forgiving. As a further point about dichotomising forgiveness, the term 'decisional forgiveness' needs further clarification. Is it a cognitive or a behavioural activity? As can be seen in the REACH model, the decision (step 4) is a *cognitive activity*, yet Worthington's decisional forgiveness assessment scale has items exclusively centred on *behaviour*, or what the respondent would do when encountering the offending other person ('I will try to get back at him or her').

Clinicians also need to be careful if they focus, for example, primarily on 'emotional' forgiveness. Such a reductionistic focus might inhibit the important therapeutic process of seeing in a cognitive sense the inherent worth of the offending other, or being good to the other, which are the hallmarks or Essence of forgiveness. As a further and final point here, dichotomising forgiving into such psychological terms as 'state' and 'trait' ends up creating its own problems. Current practice (state) over time can lead to what Aristotle calls a love of the virtue (trait), and so state and trait are on a continuum for the patient – they are not completely different things. Forgiveness therapy in its accurate and fullest sense needs to encompass forgiveness in its totality, which means that psychological techniques alone and psychological splitting of forgiveness into discrete component parts (decisional/emotional or state/trait) should be avoided. Otherwise, patients may be getting either only a part of forgiveness or a distortion of forgiveness.

Forgiveness as a Focus on the Offending Person Rather Than Just Transcending a Situation

Forgiveness as a moral virtue has the following as an important quality of its Specific Difference from all other moral virtues. It is the only moral virtue in which a person willingly decides, and then acts on this insight, to be good specifically to the offending person. Not all models of forgiveness deliberately include this focus on the one who offended. For example, the model proposed by Luskin (2020) calls for transcending what happened, finding new ways to happiness, and elevating affect beyond the negative. Although all of this may be helpful to patients, from the philosophical analysis presented earlier regarding what forgiveness is, and to avoid a serious error of reductionism, a deliberate focus on the other person who acted unjustly needs to be part of the forgiveness process.

Psychological Characteristics of Forgiveness Therapy Vs. Traditional Psychotherapy

There are at least three features of forgiveness therapy, as it emerges from Aristotelian philosophy, which separate this mode of mental health intervention from all other psychotherapies. We shall consider each of these in turn.

The Focus Is Placed on the Offending Person, not on the Patient

In traditional psychotherapy, when a patient presents with certain symptoms, such as anxiety, the usual protocol is to address this symptom – its intensity, frequency and when it occurs – with approaches designed to reduce it. In contrast, the mental health professional who is offering forgiveness therapy asks the patient to focus on the other person – the person who offended – and to think about this person with a wider-angle cognitive lens than may have been the case before. The focus for the patient can be on how the other has been emotionally hurt, on how the patient and offending other share a common humanity, and what they share spiritually, depending on the patient's world-view. Yes, there is a focus on the patient, such as the strength needed to bear the pain and the heroic stance taken when giving the offending person a gift, but these emerge after the focus on the other. It should be noted that the aim of this focus is not to re-live the injurious situation (the latter is not the emphasis) but instead to better understand and to develop empathy and compassion for the other as a person.

Paradox: As One Bears the Pain, One Gets Stronger

Forgiveness therapy is in marked contrast to the use of catharsis, or the venting of anger. For example, Khoo and Adkins (2020) discuss the idea of anger expression as a psychotherapeutic approach to aid personal understanding and growth. This differs from the idea of bearing the pain, first introduced by Kaufman (1984) and Bergin (1988), which suggests that as one stands up to the pain for the sake of the one who offended, emotional healing takes place. In other words, the patient discovers strength in this and also begins to see the self in a more positive light, as one who will not displace the anger on to unsuspecting others, such as family members.

Paradox: As One Gives a Gift to the One Who Offended, It Is the One Who Was Offended Who Heals Emotionally

It seems that as the patient gives a gift to the offending person, the patient is doing all of the giving, the other is doing all of the receiving, and so the patient is placed in an unfair situation. Yet this is not about the moral virtue of justice, but instead about mercy. As the patient gives in this way, the softer emotions of compassion and empathy can further develop, thus reducing the resentment felt by the patient (Enright and Fitzgibbons, 2015).

Empirical Evidence for the Forgiveness Interventions

Four meta-analyses consistently conclude that forgiveness interventions are effective in reducing anger, anxiety and depression, and in improving hope (Baskin and Enright, 2004; Lundahl et al., 2008; Wade et al., 2014; Akhtar and Barlow, 2018). Case studies within clinical practice support the statistical observations (Enright and Fitzgibbons, 2015). Intervention studies have supported the finding that forgiveness has a significant positive effect on both mental and physical health (e.g., Hebl and Enright, 1993; Waltman et al., 2009; Lee and Enright, 2014; Ballard, 2018; Worthington, 2020a).

As one therapeutic example, Reed and Enright (2006) describe a 32-week intervention using the process model for women who have left abusive romantic relationships. The participants, who were randomly assigned to the experimental or control group, met one to one with the intervener for one hour a week. At the end of the 32-week intervention, participants in the experimental group showed less trait anxiety, depression and post-traumatic stress symptoms and a larger increase in forgiving and self-esteem than those in the control group.

Forgiveness therapy has been shown to be effective in reducing symptoms in patients with anxiety and depressive, bipolar and addictive disorders, and in reducing relationship conflicts (Enright and Fitzgibbons, 2015). This is the case when patients have been treated unjustly in the past, have residual resentment (irritability or unhealthy anger) and have not forgiven, and present with the challenges described here. Both empirical randomised experimental and control group research and case studies support this conclusion (for a summary, see Enright and Fitzgibbons, 2015).

Not all interventions are effective in the same way. For example, although the meta-analysis by Wade et al. (2014) made the claim that the process and REACH models are statistically equal in terms of their effectiveness, there is a discrepancy of time between the two research approaches. The REACH model tends to be short term (the average duration of the intervention is about 6 hours, with the maximum being 12 hours, across 18 articles; Wade et al., 2014) whereas the process model is more long term (the average duration of the intervention is about 15 hours, with the maximum being over 50 hours, across 20 articles; Hebl and Enright, 1993; Wade et al., 2014). The article by Hebl and Enright (1993) was the first forgiveness intervention article to be published, and was not reported in the study by Wade et al. (2014). Within their own contexts, these two models are successful. In addition, the process model is the only one to examine one-to-one patient and intervener interactions (see, for example, Freedman and Enright, 1996; Coyle and Enright, 1997; Reed and Enright, 2006; Lee and Enright, 2014).

Cross-Cultural Evidence

Forgiveness treatment, including forgiveness education, has been shown to be effective in Christian students in Northern Ireland (Enright et al., 2007), Muslim adolescents in Iran (Ghobari Bonab et al., 2020) and Pakistan (Rahman et al., 2018), Arab-Israeli adolescents in Israel (Shechtman et al., 2009), and also in study samples in Sierra Leone (Toussaint et al., 2010), Hong Kong (Hui and Chau, 2009), Taiwan (Wei et al., 2013) and the USA (Freedman and Enright, 1996). Forgiveness as an approach to improving mental health does not appear to be specific to participants from Western cultures.

Forgiveness and Spirituality

Patients who choose to forgive do not need to hold a particular worldview in order to engage in forgiveness therapy. Atheists, agnostics and humanists, as well as Jewish, Christian, Muslim, Buddhist, Hindu and other believers, can all engage in the activities described in the process and REACH models. Jewish and Christian patients can develop awareness of the inherent worth of the offending person and the self by a reflection on Genesis 1, which states that all people are made in the image and likeness of God, which therefore includes those who behave badly. The story of Joseph forgiving his half-brothers appears in both the Hebrew Bible (Genesis 37–45) and the Muslim Qu'ran (The Book of Joseph). The parable of the Prodigal Son in the Christian New Testament (Luke 15) presents a similar story which readers could try to model, and from which they could find motivation to forgive. The Buddhist tradition of compassion and loving-kindness can be appropriated in the context of forgiving an offending person in forgiveness therapy. A commonality across all of these belief systems is a spirituality that transcends the harm done and leads to a broader perspective on who the offending person and the forgiver are to one another.

Conclusion

Forgiveness therapy is not intended to supplant existing psychotherapeutic approaches – in fact it can be a complement to them. Yet this new form of treatment can stand alone when people present with unresolved resentment of injustices caused by others. It is important that mental health professionals first understand what forgiveness is and is not, prior to commencing forgiveness therapy with patients. They also need to give sufficient time to patients. This new and paradoxical therapy offers patients the chance to be freed from resentments that they may have been carrying for decades, and it also reduces the anxiety and depression that can emerge as a result of these pent-up feelings.

References

Akhtar, S. and Barlow, J. (2018) Forgiveness therapy for the promotion of mental well-being: a systematic review and meta-analysis. *Trauma, Violence, & Abuse*, 19, 107–122.

Aristotle (1926) *Nicomachean Ethics* (H. Rackham, trans.). Cambridge. MA: Harvard University Press.

Ballard, M. S. (2018) Integrating forgiveness therapy and the treatment of anger: a randomized controlled trial. Unpublished doctoral dissertation, University of Denver, Denver, CO.

Baskin, T. W. and Enright, R. D. (2004) Intervention studies on forgiveness: a meta-analysis. *Journal of Counseling and Development*, 82, 79–90.

Bergin, A. E. (1988) Three contributions of a spiritual perspective to counseling, psychotherapy, and behavior change. *Counseling and Values*, 33, 21–31.

Coyle, C. T. and Enright, R. D. (1997) Forgiveness intervention with post-abortion men. *Journal of Consulting and Clinical Psychology*, 65, 1042–1046.

Enright, R. D. (2001) *Forgiveness is a Choice*. Washington, DC: American Psychological Association.

Enright, R. D. (2012) *The Forgiving Life*. Washington, DC: American Psychological Association.

Enright, R. D. (2015) *8 Keys to Forgiveness*. New York: W. W. Norton & Company.

Enright, R. D. and Fitzgibbons, R. (2015) *Forgiveness Therapy*. Washington, DC: American Psychological Association.

Enright, R. D., Freedman, S. and Rique, J. (1998) The psychology of interpersonal forgiveness. In R. D. Enright and J. North, eds., *Exploring Forgiveness*. Madison: University of Wisconsin Press, pp. 46–62.

Enright, R. D., Knutson, J. A., Holter, A. C., Baskin, T. and Knutson, C. (2007) Waging peace through forgiveness in Belfast, Northern Ireland II: educational programs for mental health improvement of children. *Journal of Research in Education*, 17, 63–78.

Frankl, V. (1959) *Man's Search for Meaning.* New York: Washington Square Press.

Freedman, S. R. and Enright, R. D. (1996) Forgiveness as an intervention goal with incest survivors. *Journal of Consulting and Clinical Psychology,* 64, 983–992.

Ghobari Bonab, B., Khodayarifard, M., Geshnigani, R. H. et al. (2020) Effectiveness of forgiveness education with adolescents in reducing anger and ethnic prejudice in Iran. *Journal of Educational Psychology,* 113, 846–860.

Hebl, J. H. and Enright, R. D. (1993) Forgiveness as a psychotherapeutic goal with elderly females. *Psychotherapy,* 30, 658–667.

Hui, E. K. P. and Chau, T. S. (2009) The impact of a forgiveness intervention with Hong Kong Chinese children hurt in interpersonal relationships. *British Journal of Guidance & Counselling,* 37, 141–156.

Kaufman, M. (1984) The courage to forgive. *The Israel Journal of Psychiatry and Related Sciences,* 21, 177–187.

Khoo, G. and Adkins, B. (2020) Catharsis. In *The International Encyclopedia of Media Psychology.* Available at https://doi.org/10.1002/9781119011071.iemp0179 (accessed 26 April 2022).

Kreeft, P. (2018) *The Platonic Tradition.* South Bend, IN: St Augustine's Press.

Lee, Y.-R. and Enright, R. D. (2014) A forgiveness intervention for women with fibromyalgia who were abused in childhood: a pilot study. *Spirituality in Clinical Practice,* 1, 203–217.

Lundahl, W. B., Taylor, J. M., Stevenson, R. and Daniel, K. R. (2008) Process-based forgiveness interventions: a meta-analytic review. *Research on Social Work Practice,* 18, 465–478.

Luskin, F. (2020) Forgive for Good: Nine Steps. Available at https://learningtoforgive.com/9-steps/ (accessed 26 April 2022).

McCullough, M. E. and Hoyt, W. T. (2002) Transgression-related motivational dispositions: personality substrates of forgiveness and their links to the Big Five.

Personality and Social Psychology Bulletin, 28, 1556–1573.

North, J. (1987) Wrongdoing and forgiveness. *Philosophy,* 62, 499–508.

Rahman, A., Iftikhar, R., Kim, J. and Enright, R. D. (2018) Pilot study: evaluating the effectiveness of forgiveness therapy with abused early adolescent females in Pakistan. *Spirituality in Clinical Practice,* 5, 75–87.

Reed, G. and Enright, R. D. (2006) The effects of forgiveness therapy on depression, anxiety, and post-traumatic stress for women after spousal emotional abuse. *Journal of Consulting and Clinical Psychology,* 74, 920–929.

Shechtman, Z., Wade, N. and Khoury, A. (2009) Effectiveness of a forgiveness program for Arab Israeli adolescents in Israel: an empirical trial. *Peace and Conflict,* 15, 415–438.

Simon, Y. (1986) *The Definition of Moral Virtue.* New York: Fordham University Press.

Toussaint, L., Peddle, N., Cheadle, A., Sellu, A. and Luskin, F. (2010) Striving for peace through forgiveness in Sierra Leone: effectiveness of a psychoeducational forgiveness intervention. In A. Kalayjian and D. Eugene, eds., *Mass Trauma and Emotional Healing Around the World: Rituals and Practices for Resilience and Meaning-Making. Vol. 2. Human-Made Disasters.* Westport, CT: Praeger/ABC-CLIO, pp. 251–267.

Wade, N. G., Hoyt, W. T., Kidwell, J. and Worthington, E. (2014) Efficacy of psychotherapeutic interventions to promote forgiveness: a meta-analysis. *Journal of Consulting and Clinical Psychology,* 82, 154–170.

Waltman, M. A., Russell, D. C., Coyle, C. T. et al. (2009) The effects of a forgiveness intervention on patients with coronary artery disease. *Psychology & Health,* 24, 11–27.

Wei, N. L., Enright, R. D. and Klatt, J. S. (2013) A forgiveness intervention for Taiwanese young adults with insecure attachment. *Contemporary Family Therapy,* 35, 105–120.

Worthington, E. L., Jr. (2020a) An update of the REACH Forgiveness model to promote forgiveness. In E. L. Worthington Jr. and N. G. Wade, eds., *Handbook of Forgiveness*, 2nd ed. New York: Routledge, pp. 277–287.

Worthington, E. L., Jr. (2020b) *REACH Forgiveness of Others*. Available at www .evworthington-forgiveness.com/reach-forgiveness-of-others (accessed 26 April 2022).

The Patient Perspective

Joanna Barber

Introduction

I have been a mental health patient for 35 years and my Christian faith has always been very important to me. It gives me the hope that God has forgiven me for my failures and will even make something positive out of them. This gives me a sense of purpose in life, and helps me to accept myself and find some peace in my struggles. I have also faced problems with my religion, and it has not always been easy to find the help that I needed to tackle these. It is still a work in progress. My experiences have sparked an interest in the role of religion and spirituality in mental illness and recovery, and I am passionate about the value of spiritual care. Over the last 10 years I have become involved with some research in this field within Birmingham and Solihull Mental Health NHS Foundation Trust. The research that is in progress at present is a qualitative study exploring the process of spiritual recovery from mental illness, using semi-structured interviews with service users.

In this chapter, I am going to describe more fully what spirituality means to me and how this is linked to my own mental health. As well as using my own experiences, I shall take ideas from the experiences of other service users whom I have met along the way.[1] I am also going to share some preliminary findings from our current research study. I make no apology for combining these sources – after all, it is people's stories that first inspire research and guide its interpretation.

How Do People with Mental Health Problems Define Spirituality?

For me, spirituality is mostly defined by my religion. I know other mental health patients who are also committed to a religious faith. However, some consider themselves to be spiritual but not religious. Preliminary findings from our current study suggest that many mental health patients take ideas from a variety of religious or spiritual beliefs and develop their own individual spirituality from this. They definitely seem to prioritise their personal and individual spiritual experience.

The common theme of spirituality for mental health patients seems to be a sense of the transcendent (Starnino, 2016a). These patients talk about a deep sense of connection with an external higher power, and a connection with others or with something deep

---

[1] Many of the stories I relate in this chapter are my own. When telling those of others, I have used pseudonyms to protect their identity.

within themselves. (Jones et al., 2019). Indeed, evidence suggests that people with mental health problems tend to have a particularly acute spiritual awareness (Ouwehand et al., 2019a, 2020), whether or not they are religious.

Thus, in this chapter, when I talk about spirituality, I shall be thinking primarily of an awareness of something greater and beyond what we can experience with our physical senses. I shall include religion of any sort as just one part of this.

How Important Is Spirituality for People with Mental Health Problems?

I know I am not alone in finding spirituality very important. Scientific evidence backs this up.

- People with severe and enduring mental illness more often think of themselves as being spiritual or religious than do members of the general population (Bussema and Bussema, 2007; Russinova and Cash, 2007). In the range of 60–90% of people with a religious or spiritual belief find this important to them, with the precise figure depending on the local culture and ethnicity (Milner et al., 2020).
- Many mental health patients find that their faith is more important to them when they become unwell (Fallot, 2007).
- Studies we have conducted in Birmingham in the UK showed that over 50% of a convenience sample of 100 mental health patients of all faiths and none considered their religion or spirituality to be important to them (Barber et al., 2012, 2017).

Why Is Spirituality So Important to Service Users?

Impact of Spirituality on Mental Illness

There is no doubt that spirituality and religion can have a great impact on mental illness and recovery. This can be positive or negative. Like many in the general population, people with mental health problems often derive great strength from their spirituality or religion (Koenig, 2009; Exline, 2013). This is the experience of 'spiritual well-being'. However, for a significant minority of mental health patients, spirituality can be a source of struggle (Ellison and Lee, 2010; Zarzycka and Puchalska-Wasyl, 2020). Although such struggles are found in the general population, they are more common in people with severe mental health problems (Currier et al., 2019). For me personally, the spiritual problems that I have faced with my illness have been profound. They are not something I can just ignore – they are of crucial significance. My religion has always been important to me, even though it can seem difficult or even unhelpful at times.

Loss of Spiritual Well-Being Causes Turning to Religion or Spirituality

Mental illness can shatter lives. This may be due to the impact of mental illness on daily life and/or the result of the symptoms of the illness itself. The result is a loss of meaning, purpose and hope in life, and of a sense of identity and of connectedness with other people. These are the very qualities that a sense of spiritual well-being can be expected to provide. The preliminary results from our study suggest that this loss makes people naturally turn to some form of religion or spirituality even if they have no religious or spiritual background.

> **Case study: Philippa**
>
> Philippa is a young woman who suffered a psychotic breakdown straight after the birth of her first child. Having suffered the loss of both parents in her teenage years, she was always the one in the family who coped. To find herself unwell and in a hospital was a huge shock. Despite not having any religious background, she found herself praying to God for help. She asked to see the Christian chaplain, and found his prayers really comforting. Six months on, she prays regularly and visits a church every week to light candles.

Recovery Often Involves Rediscovery of Spiritual Well-Being

There is also a specific link between spiritual well-being and recovery from mental illness. Many qualitative studies of service user experiences agree that, for mental health patients, personal recovery means finding renewed purpose, meaning, hope, identity, empowerment and connection with others (Andresen et al., 2003; Leamy et al., 2011; Wood and Alsawy, 2018). These again are the very qualities that characterise spiritual well-being. This description of recovery is shared by people with a wide variety of diagnosed mental illnesses (De Wet et al., 2015), and is prioritised over symptom relief.

> For myself personally, finding a sense of a positive purpose and peace is what I value more than anything else for my recovery. This has always depended crucially on my Christian faith. Although I still cannot do paid work, I get great satisfaction from my voluntary work and I feel a sense of purpose from wanting to serve God in this way. I know that I am forgiven and that God even uses my mistakes.

I ask whether or not it is actually possible for people with mental health problems to find personal recovery without a positive sense of spirituality. I cannot answer this question for certain. However, from my own experiences and those of others whom I know, I suggest that spirituality or religion is the most important source of personal recovery for most people with mental health problems.

Thus there are many reasons why spirituality might be important to people with mental health problems. We shall now explore these experiences of spirituality in more detail.

How Do Service Users Experience Spiritual Problems?

I have chosen to deal with spiritual problems first because for me they are the main stumbling block to recovery. It is not possible for me to get better without addressing these. There are many different ways in which spiritual problems can be experienced (Abu-Raiya et al., 2015), and the exact nature of these experiences will be different for each person.

Loss of Spiritual Well-Being

There are so many losses associated with mental illness, many of which can involve spirituality.

When I myself first had a mental breakdown, one of the most difficult problems I encountered was the long-lasting emptiness of life. I had been a junior doctor working very long hours on the wards, and living in the hospital where I worked. Suddenly I no longer had a job, I had nowhere to live and nothing to do. Hours stretched before me and I had no goals for the future. The illness itself caused me to lose any sense of hope and motivation and to feel disconnected from the rest of the world. As someone who had a strong religious conviction from an early age, I experienced all this as having a devastating impact on my spiritual well-being.

Loss of Meaning and Purpose

A loss of meaning and purpose often involves loss of a previously meaningful role in life, perhaps the end of a successful career or the break-up of a marriage. I do not think that I personally have ever quite recovered the sense of vocation in life that I had before my breakdown.

Case study: Susan

Susan is a young woman who was formerly a professional violinist. She had a mental breakdown with severe depression and anxiety. Prior to that she had no particular faith, and her music gave her all the sense of meaning that she needed. She then found herself unable to play and as a consequence she felt that her life was completely meaningless. There followed a period of intense spiritual searching when she desperately tried many different spiritual practices. She has never found any source of meaning to replace the loss of her musical career.

Loss of Identity

A psychiatric illness can directly lead to a loss of self-identity. It can have a strong and direct impact on how people think and feel. It can disrupt one's sense of self, so that it feels as if one's very personality is under attack (Cogan et al., 2019; Davidson, 2020). For some people, becoming mentally unwell can actually be seen as a spiritual identity crisis (Guthrie and Stickley, 2008).

Case study: Lillian

Lillian is a middle-aged woman who has suffered many psychotic episodes during which her confused thoughts have caused her to question what sort of person she actually is. Formerly outgoing, with a strong Christian faith and a desire to reach out to others, she has now become reclusive and withdrawn. She says that she can no longer relate to anyone and she feels that she has nothing personally to give.

Loss of Hope

Many mental illnesses can directly result in a sense of hopelessness and despair (Barut et al., 2016). Sometimes, when mental illness becomes chronic, hope may be even more difficult to find. I always used to think that somehow eventually I would find my way back into paid work, but now I realise this is not going to happen. It is difficult to come to terms with this while retaining hope for future life. A yearning for the afterlife is a very important source of hope for many people, especially those with long-term disabling symptoms.

Case study: Abdul

Abdul is a middle-aged man who has suffered relapsing depression for many years and tried many different medications. He finds that nothing seems to work for him. He has tried many different jobs but has not been able to hold any of them down. He has taken to abusing alcohol as an escape from the mental pain. Although he has now developed physical health problems as a result of this, he says that he does not care, and that he has no hope of ever being able to live a fulfilling life.

Loss of Faith

I do not stop believing in God when I become unwell, but what I do lose is any sense of God's love. Many people have a different experience of loss of faith as part of their illness. Some lose their religious beliefs altogether. Others lose spiritual awareness. Many find it impossible to pray (Ouwehand et al., 2019b, 2020). In all these cases, a valuable coping resource is lost at the very time when it is needed.

Personal Spiritual Struggles

My personal spiritual struggles are the greatest obstacle to my recovery, and I know many others who also suffer in this way. These problems often have a spiritual component, but may also be directly linked to the illness itself. Spiritual and religious difficulties may be tangled with all kinds of mental illnesses, including depression, neuroses and psychotic illnesses (Koenig, 2009).

Anger, Despair and Guilt

Negative emotions of all sorts are commonly associated with many different mental illnesses. Anger, despair and guilt are particularly difficult to cope with in the context of spiritual or religious values.

Case study: Jane

Jane is a middle-aged woman with bipolar disorder. Every time she gets really low, she becomes quite aggressive. She then says unpleasant things to her husband – things she would normally not dream of saying. Recently she has even said that she wanted to split up with him. She is a devout Christian, and when her mood improves she cannot forgive herself for how she has behaved.

A Distorted Image of God

Many people with mental health problems believe that what is happening to them is a result of God's punishment or abandonment because of their failings (Harris et al., 2012). They fear that God is angry and unforgiving. I certainly struggle with this, and never know quite why I feel this way. From the viewpoint of a Christian faith, this indicates a distorted image of God (Exline et al., 1999).

Case study: Tracey

Tracey is a middle-aged woman with a Catholic background who was brought up to have an image of God as punitive and angry. She was constantly being told that she would rot in hell if she behaved badly. She also experienced physical abuse. Her desperation led to drug use, which was the only thing that gave her relief. She felt that, since everything she did was wrong, she would go to hell anyway, so there was no point in trying to change.

Obsessive Religious Practices

Some people with mental health problems, particularly those with severe anxiety or obsessive-compulsive disorder, can become obsessed with performing religious rituals to relieve their guilt and desire for self-punishment (Loewenthal, 2018).

This can take over their life and prevent them from moving forward towards recovery. I myself can end up reading a Bible passage or reciting liturgy over and over again, worried that I have not concentrated hard enough on it. Others experience obsessive behaviour of much greater severity.

Case study: Mohammed

Mohammed is a devout young Muslim man with obsessive-compulsive disorder who has become obsessed with reading the Quran. He feels that he must say the daily prayers at least 10 times a day, but even this does not give him any relief from his guilt and fear. He has no time for any other activities and has no social contact. Not even the Imam can help to give him any peace of mind.

Religious Perceptual Experiences as Part of a Mental Illness

Many people with a psychotic illness have hallucinations or delusions, which often have a religious content (Clarke, 2010; Cook, 2015; Powers et al., 2017; Loch et al., 2019). This religious content quite often conflicts with previously held religious or spiritual beliefs. For some people it is experienced as positive or even euphoric (Ouwehand, 2019a). For others, like myself, it can be the most intensely distressing aspect of mental illness.

Religious hallucinations are particularly distressing and frightening if they are accusatory or abusive and are apparently from divine or demonic sources. They can even be in the form of commands that may tell the sufferer to do something, such as harm him- or herself or others, which conflicts with the person's religious or spiritual values.

Case study: Margaret

Margaret is a middle-aged woman with schizophrenia and depression who repeatedly experiences hearing voices from God accusing her of committing an unforgivable sin. This concerns a sexual relationship she had with a man 20 years ago. She had actually never wanted this relationship, but thinks she upset the man involved by breaking it off. She is plagued by guilt about this and is fearful of God's judgement.

Case study: Amir

Amir is a devout young Muslim man who came to the UK to study after having been rejected by his family back in India. On hearing that his brother was unwell, he went home and brought the whole family back to the UK. However, he then felt that they were all ganging up against him again, and he experienced voices from God telling him to murder his mother. This was against his religious values, and he was in constant torment, unable to decide what to do.

Religious delusions may lead people to feel that they have special powers they can use for good or evil. Others feel possessed or controlled by spiritual forces, or even identify themselves with a particular religious figure. All of these thoughts and ideas can cause conflict with the whole idea of faith. This is intensely confusing.

Case study: Janet

Janet is a young Catholic woman with chronic schizophrenia who often has visions of snakes, which she believes are being caused by a witch doctor. She thinks these snakes are attacking her spirit. This makes her extremely frightened, and she feels unable to challenge or control them in any way. She is constantly praying to the Virgin Mary for relief from these frightening experiences, which she does not get.

Another problem faced by people who are experiencing hallucinations or delusions concerns their interpretation of their unusual experiences. Many people have a kind of dual explanation. In a study of people with bipolar disorder (Ouwehand et al., 2020), 46% thought that their experiences were spiritual, 15% thought they were induced by their illness and 42% thought they were both spiritual and pathological. The others were uncertain. I definitely have this problem. Certain things remain in the back of my mind even when I may be quite well, and remembering, accepting and understanding what to dismiss as illness can be difficult.

Spiritual Problems Arising from Relationships with Others

Lack of Understanding by Faith Communities

Stigma Around Mental Health Problems

Sometimes just having a diagnosis of mental health problems is considered a weakness by a faith community. Any experiences that have religious content, such as feeling demon possessed, can be viewed by a faith community as a spiritual problem and the person almost blamed for their experience (Fallot, 2007).

> **Case study: Lucy**
>
> Lucy had an episode of hypomania while attending a church service 30 years ago. During the episode, she blasphemed and behaved rather inappropriately. Since then, she has been ostracised by that church community. People have even crossed the road rather than meet her face to face. After all these years she still feels unable to attend the church, and no one from the church has ever come to visit her. She even has problems going out in case she might meet one of them.

Experiences of Faith Healing

The experience of a mental health breakdown leads many people to ask for prayers for healing from their faith community. Although prayers for healing can be very helpful and inspiring, sometimes there is no relief of symptoms after such attempts. This can cause guilt, confusion and disillusionment for the person involved (Tuffour, 2020).

Lack of Understanding by Mental Health Services

Sometimes mental health patients feel that their spiritual experiences are not taken seriously by mental health staff. They resent the assumption that these experiences are just part of the illness (Milner et al., 2020). This situation leads to a sense of rejection and is a highly damaging source of mistrust in the therapeutic relationship.

> **Case study: Clare**
>
> Clare is a middle-aged Baptist woman who keeps seeing images of devils, which she thinks she should warn others about. She thinks she has special powers to defeat these devils. She feels that her experiences have been dismissed by the medical professionals, who

have simply told her she is ill and will have to take medication. She refuses to take it, and has ended up being sectioned multiple times. She has now completely lost trust in all the clinical staff.

Experience of Double Stigma

Some mental health patients experience double stigma (Dein et al., 2012). Not only do they feel rejected by their faith community, but also they cannot trust the medical staff to help them with their spiritual problems.

In my own life, after experiencing an apparently unsuccessful healing ministry, I felt a sense of rejection and left the church thinking that it was all my own fault. After this, having struggled on my own for several years, I then found myself in hospital, where my difficult religious struggles were pathologised as illness. There was no help available to resolve this dilemma. I did not feel able to talk to anyone about these problems for many years.

Importance of Internal Conflict

Perhaps one of the most distressing aspects of all these spiritual problems is the internal conflict involved. Constantly wondering whether you are responsible for the spiritual problems that you face can lead to feelings of great unease, guilt and distress. Some people oscillate uncomfortably between various interpretations of their own experiences. I suggest that this really perpetuates mental illness. When people blame themselves for their problems, and repeatedly doubt the validity of their own thoughts, this becomes a painful vicious circle that blocks recovery.

How Do Service Users Experience a Positive Sense of Spirituality?

Although spiritual problems in mental illness can be very serious, the majority of people with mental health problems have a much more positive experience (Milner et al., 2020).

For myself, since spiritual well-being is a necessary feature of my recovery, when I relapse I need to rediscover this, so that I can move forward once more.

A Comfort in Acute Suffering

Some people in the acute stage of a mental illness can immediately find solace in their spirituality (Ouwehand et al., 2019b). I know people who find that prayer helps them to cope at such times, and I look up to them as inspiring examples.

When I was first hospitalised, one of the other patients had bipolar disorder and was extremely depressed. She was a very committed Christian and before her hospital admission had been attending an evangelical church. Although the thought of suicide was appealing to her at the time, she hung on to the idea that God had a plan for her life, and she took comfort in this belief and prayed for God's help. She actually reached out to me despite her own distress. I confided in her long before I managed to trust any clinical staff.

A Tool for Persevering Towards Recovery
The Importance of Religion

For some people, practising a religious faith is an important part of recovery. Indeed, in our current study, religion of some sort often seems to provide the motivation to begin the recovery journey. Religious practices, including personal prayer, reading scriptures and attending services, may all be important (Jones et al., 2019; Tuffour, 2020), giving meaning and hope. The familiarity may be comforting. Sometimes faith communities help by offering crucial understanding, acceptance and social support, walking with the person and holding hope for him or her (Heffernan et al., 2016).

Case study: Emma

Emma is a young woman now recovering from a psychotic depressive episode. She has left the high-powered job that had allowed her no time or energy to practise her Christian faith. She has begun to read her Bible again, prioritise personal prayer and attend church services. Her church community has been supportive. She says that returning to practising her faith has been by far the most helpful thing for her recovery journey.

Although I have felt alienated from the church in general in the past, I have now joined another church. It is a very tolerant church, accepting everyone without question, and I feel that I belong there. People look out for each other. Someone phones me every couple of weeks for a chat. Nobody tries to 'fix' me, and I no longer feel I have to be 'cured'. This faith community has really helped me in my recovery journey.

The Importance of Personal Spirituality

I have been struck by how many people in our current study seem to gain great strength and motivation from personal spiritual practices. These may not be specific to any particular religion. They include personal prayer, meditation, mindfulness and enjoying nature, art or music. All can feed into a sense of spiritual well-being and thus promote recovery. Here are a few specific examples.

- Many people pray to God on their own even though they do not go near a church. They find this a comfort, and some seem to trust God in their troubles more profoundly than many who practise a religion.

Case study: Abbas

Abbas is a young man with schizophrenia who feels unable to sincerely practise the Muslim faith in which he was brought up. However, the most important thing that keeps him going in life is personal prayer. Recently he has been successful in finding paid employment, which he believes is an answer to his prayers and a confirmation of God's love and acceptance. He feels he is definitely on the road to recovery.

Case study: Edith

Edith is an elderly woman who has suffered from anxiety and depression for many years. There are now problems in her family, one of whom is in prison. She also has her own physical health difficulties. Even though she does not identify with a religious faith, she has always coped by constantly repeating a short prayer acknowledging the greatness of God. A variety of medications have proved unhelpful. Her prayers are her best medicine.

- For some people, going into a church and lighting a candle can be a therapeutic and meaningful thing to do. It can be experienced as tapping into a higher power, which people find comforting and inspiring.

Case study: Sally

Sally is a young woman who has suffered with postnatal depression and is still struggling. Every time she passes by a church, she goes in to light a candle in memory of her grandfather, to whom she was very close. Although she would say she has no faith and does not pray, she still finds this very comforting and feels that it has definitely helped her to move towards recovery.

- Many people find a spiritual connection by being outside connecting with nature.

Case study: Kathleen

Kathleen is a young woman who is constantly plagued by severe anxiety. She finds some relief by going out walking, when she seems to feel a particular connection to trees. This can give her a special sense of God's presence, which can last for half an hour or more. At those times, all of her anxieties seem to melt away.

Case study: Eileen

Eileen is an elderly woman with crippling anxiety and depression who finds great solace in walking in a forest she knows. She is in awe of the beauty she sees around her there, with the birds, flowers and trees. If she goes quietly on her own, she finds that her unbearable sense of trauma actually passes. She describes this relief as a huge burden being lifted.

- Many people find meditation a great help for tuning in to something greater than this world. Although it takes perseverance to learn this technique, some people say that it can still the mind like nothing else, and ease inner conflicts and pain. Some individuals can meditate for hours every day. Others go regularly to meditate in a group with other people, enjoying the discipline and structure involved.

Case study: Matthew

Matthew is an elderly man with psychotic depression which has been experiencing remissions and relapses for 20 years. Recently he has found strength by attending a Buddhist centre for meditation in a group that lasts for several hours, at least three times a week. He finds this is the only thing that gives him relief from the mental torture of his long-term depressed state.

- Some people find spiritual inspiration in the arts, music or literature.

I myself play the violin, and the power of music in my own life and recovery has been huge. Listening to music has always been a spiritual experience for me, comforting and soothing my soul. When I play, I sometimes feel I am expressing feelings that cannot be described in words. It can make me feel closer to God. When I play for or with other people, I am sometimes moved by a sense of deep spiritual connection with them, much closer than if I was talking with them. For me, then, music can be a spiritual tool that helps me with my recovery.

Spirituality in the Longer Term

Even if it does not appear to help in the short term, spirituality can be a powerful source of psychological well-being over a period of time (Huguelet et al., 2011; Huguelet, 2016; Jones et al., 2019), whether or not ongoing symptoms are present. It can be helpful both when it involves a specific religion and when it is a more individual experience. For some it involves coping with long-term disability, and for others it is a protracted journey towards a new and highly satisfying life.

Coping with Adversity

For people with long-term and disabling symptoms, practising a religion can be a lifeline that gives structure and meaning to life. A faith community can also provide invaluable long-term support and acceptance.

> **Case study: Nadeem**
>
> Nadeem is a middle-aged man with chronic schizophrenia. After suffering a breakdown at university, he has had to accept a life with disabling symptoms and being unable to fulfil any of his dreams. He cannot even manage voluntary work and is profoundly depressed. However, his religious faith gives him the motivation to keep going. A devout Muslim, he says his prayers every day, goes to the Mosque every week and feels supported there. Despite all of his troubles he has great confidence in the goodness of Allah, and he looks forward with hope to the afterlife.

Spiritual Growth

Many people work through their spirituality and religion over a period of time, and experience positive spiritual growth (Forrester-Jones, 2018; Ouwehand et al., 2019b). Our current study suggests that a new lifestyle can be adopted, persevering with helpful spiritual practices and self-care. I personally have met many mental health patients who have taken up new and more fulfilling jobs even though they now earn less money than before. This has been inspired by spiritual well-being and a desire to help people. Some even consider their new life to be better than their life before their illness (Ouwehand et al., 2020).

> **Case study: Jonathan**
>
> Jonathan, a middle-aged businessman with recurrent depression, was really inspired by the cheerfulness and thankfulness of people in an African country he visited, where so many were starving and all were impoverished. As a result, he took up Buddhism, changed his lifestyle completely and is now working to set up a charity to help these people. He feels that he has been spiritually guided to do these things. Despite ongoing struggles, he says that his life has been transformed.

> **Case study: Bridget**
>
> Bridget, a woman in her forties, has struggled with a personality disorder and drug addiction for many years. She has now found new hope by taking up a job as a peer support worker in her local mental health trust. This has given her new meaning in life, and she says that she has never felt happier.

How Do Mental Health Service Users Experience Spiritual Care?

There is much evidence that mental health service patients are desperate for help with spiritual issues (Raffay et al., 2016). I personally have been greatly helped by spiritual care over the years. It has been the most important thing in helping me to find recovery. I really do think that it is possible for most people with mental health problems to discover spiritual well-being with the right help, even if, as is the case for me, some long-term support is also needed.

The Importance of Narrative

Spiritual care is based on listening, talking and relationship. Putting spiritual experiences in a narrative context is the best way to understand their significance to the individual concerned (Cook et al., 2016). Many mental health patients feel the need to share their whole story in order to explain how spirituality is important to them in their life now. This helps them to make sense of things, own their experiences and establish a spiritual identity. Sometimes re-working parts of the story in a more helpful light can be valuable. In all stages of spiritual care, it is therefore necessary to hear the full story rather than focusing solely on current issues.

For myself, the sense of failing God that I have struggled with for many years cannot be understood without knowing how I felt called by God to be a missionary from a very young age. When I was forced to admit that I was not even going to make it to work as a doctor, the sense of letting God down was profound. This has been a huge source of guilt for me. I have had to painfully learn that God can use me even in my current situation.

Planning Spiritual Care

Who Does It?

Although the Spiritual Care Team are the experts at providing this care, all staff members should be ready to help, depending on the preferences of the individual patient (Barber et al., 2015). Sometimes crucial spiritual support can even be given by staff members who are not officially part of the clinical team.

I personally remember being in a single room in a hospital after having been sectioned. Those were some of the most lonely days I have ever experienced. I felt that I could not trust the nurses who occasionally came in to check on me. I thought they would just lock me away for ever. However, the cleaner came in twice daily, and kept saying to me 'Don't worry, things will get better, God will get you through'. Her reassurance at this time was very precious.

Some patients want to speak to a minister of the appropriate faith. For such individuals a referral to the Spiritual Care Team should be offered. Other people request a visit from the minister or leader of their local faith community. However, many patients just want to discuss their spirituality with clinical staff, especially when decisions about treatment are being made and they want their spiritual needs to be recognised and addressed within their clinical treatment plan (Cook et al., 2011; Cook, 2012). In order to identify the right person, it is important that discussions about spiritual issues are raised as part of the initial history taking (Koenig, 2015; Payman, 2016; see also Chapter 2).

Whoever actually provides spiritual care, the principles of best practice are the same and should follow a person-centred individual approach. Within mental health services, patients tend to lose control in so many ways that it is really important to allow personal control over spiritual care. The process involves a detailed spiritual assessment, the collaborative development of an individual plan and the delivery of care as agreed.

The Spiritual Assessment

If the subject is raised respectfully, many mental health patients are keen to talk about their spirituality (Huguelet et al., 2011). The first priority is the establishment of a trusting and non-judgemental relationship (Gomi et al., 2014), within which people may share things that they have not told any other staff member. The spiritual assessment has been described in more detail in Chapter 2 of this book.

I personally had many secrets I was ashamed about, and it took me many months to develop trust in a mental health chaplain. When I finally did, the unconditional acceptance I received from this person was a huge source of comfort and relief for me.

During the assessment, both spiritual problems and spiritual strengths must be identified. Broadly describing spiritual problems in terms of spiritual loss or spiritual struggles is also helpful for planning the best approach for the individual concerned.

Formation of a Spiritual Care Plan

The formation of an individualised care plan should be patient led. There are three basic approaches to spiritual intervention, any combination of which can be used to help to construct a care plan (Barber et al., 2015). The first involves giving support and encouragement during a process of spiritual searching (spiritual loss). The second involves trying to deal with religious conflicts and specific spiritual problems (spiritual struggles). The third involves providing spiritual resources and support for the positive spiritual beliefs and practices that may already be of help to a particular individual. These three approaches can be used in parallel, in any order and in varying proportions, depending on the needs of the individual.

Addressing Spiritual Problems

Problems That Involve Loss of Spiritual Well-Being

Some people may have never had any sort of spiritual belief before. Others may want to take stock and find a new lifestyle that involves a new spiritual direction. For all these people, exploring different faiths and spiritual approaches with a spiritual care advisor may be helpful. For others, help may be required to re-connect with a previous spiritual conviction. In such cases, talking this through with the appropriate faith chaplain can be very helpful.

> **Case study: Ann**
>
> Ann is a young woman who has been struggling to find meaning in her life since she was 11. She has no religious background and does not know where this search comes from. So far she has not been able to identify with any religion, although she considers herself spiritual. Over many years she has been persistently told that her problems are due to mental illness. She does not agree. She is now finding help to explore a spiritual framework for her life, which is helping her far more than anything else to move forward with her recovery.

Problems That Involve Religious or Spiritual Struggles

There are several approaches that can be helpful here. For these, the authority of a minister as a representative of a particular faith can be especially important.

Dealing with Guilt

It is important to recognise and challenge false or excessive guilt, particularly when sufferers are blaming themselves for their problems. Other people may have a more appropriate sense of guilt. For them, the assurance of forgiveness is crucial. Sometimes, confession and absolution within a religious framework is helpful. Reminding someone of their positive qualities, skills and strengths is also very important.

Reassurance

Simple reassurance can be very powerful in the following situations:

- when the person feels that God has abandoned them
- when the person feels that there is no hope
- when the person is in fear of God's judgment and feels that he or she cannot be forgiven
- when the person feels anger towards God for what has happened to him or her
- when the person feels that his or her illness is a punishment from God
- when the person is upset, disillusioned and feels blamed because prayers for healing or even exorcism have apparently not been answered.

Personally, when I have wondered why prayers for healing do not appear to have been answered, and I have felt completely cut off from God, reassurance about God's love and forgiveness from a minister has been crucial.

Correcting Misunderstandings

Matters of doctrine are complex, as different faiths and spiritual beliefs vary so much in their philosophy and values. However, some people have an unhelpful understanding that actually contradicts the established doctrine of their particular faith. Talking this through can certainly help.

I personally have very often worried that I have committed an unforgivable sin and therefore cannot be forgiven. Having explored this problem with a chaplain, I now understand that the very fact that I worry about it and regret it deeply means that I cannot have done such a thing. My conviction is fundamentally flawed! I am now more able to challenge these thoughts when they inevitably occur.

Tackling Unhelpful Perceptual Experiences

This relates to tackling delusions and hallucinations that have a religious content. It can be helpful to try to distinguish these from truly spiritual problems. However, this may be impossible. What is considered truly religious varies according to culture and personal religiosity before illness, and there is probably a continuous spectrum between this and the pathological (Cook, 2015). Nevertheless, input from a chaplain can be very helpful. The following points, all of which I have found helpful, have been suggested to me by chaplains and ministers I have known over the years:

- Distressing and damaging religious experiences, by definition, do not come from a Divine power.
- The Devil tells lies.
- The Divine must be always greater than anything evil, and certainly greater than ourselves. Focusing on a Divine power can thus help us to have control over such experiences.

- If experiences are partly symptoms of illness, this possibility can be gently explored. For some people this can be help them to reject the experiences, or at least to gain control of them.

When Spiritual Problems Are Related to Other People

If people are facing stigma or discrimination from a faith community then it might be possible for them to be reconciled by using a chaplain as an advocate.

When patients feel that their spiritual or religious beliefs are not taken seriously by clinical staff, or that they are dismissed as illness, merely being given the opportunity to discuss this is important. Sometimes a chaplain can attend a multidisciplinary team meeting to give the service user's viewpoint (Dein et al., 2010).

When people experience double stigma from their faith community and from mental health staff, it is essential that this is shared with someone who can understand. It is a painful experience that may take a long time to resolve.

The Importance of Longer-Term Support

I do not think I am entirely alone in experiencing recurrent spiritual conflict. This has been described by one of the participants in our current study as walking on a tightrope. I identify with this concept. For such people, continued spiritual reassurance and help is necessary to help them to navigate their recovery journey.

People Who Already Have a Positive Experience of Spirituality

It is especially important to build on a person's existing positive spirituality with some simple spiritual support. If they have a faith, they should be encouraged to practise it in whatever way is right for them. They might want to attend religious services or to engage in private prayer. For some, input from a specific faith chaplain can be very inspiring. Many people really appreciate being prayed for. Several of the participants in our current study did not even know that the Spiritual Care Team existed, and wished that they had been given the opportunity to be referred to them.

Case study: Mandy

Mandy is a young woman with a personality disorder who was sectioned for several weeks and is a very committed Christian. She had turned away from her faith after prayers for healing did not seem to have helped her, but when she was feeling at rock bottom on the hospital ward she turned back to it and was searching for help to practise her faith again. She had no idea that a Spiritual Care Team existed in the NHS trust. She would have given anything to be able to talk to a chaplain at that time.

Other people may not want to see a chaplain. However, they may still want to practise their spirituality, and should be encouraged and facilitated to do so in their own way, perhaps by going to light a candle in a church or chapel, being creative with music or art, or taking a walk and enjoying nature.

During my own stays in hospital, it might have been helpful if I had been proactively encouraged to play my violin. I do not think anyone realised how important it is to me. Of course, I would have struggled to even try to play it at that stage, but a little encouragement could perhaps have gone a long way.

Over a longer period of time, spiritual support can promote spiritual growth and greatly facilitate recovery. I have benefited from informal support that I have received from ministers in the church which I now attend. Making such support more routinely and readily available could transform lives.

Implications for Clinical Care

Spiritual care as a part of routine clinical care aims to help people to resolve their spiritual problems and find a renewed sense of positive meaning and purpose, with peace, hope and joy.

There are many reasons why a spiritual dimension to care is needed.

- Many patients experience a spiritual loss associated with their mental illness.
- For some patients there seems to be an actual spiritual component to their illness, which suggests that trying to tackle this directly will give the best outcome.
- A sense of spiritual well-being is directly related to the experience of personal recovery.
- Many patients actually want to discuss spiritual issues.
- Qualitative evidence suggests that spiritual care does indeed facilitate mental health recovery (Cook, 2012; Amerongen-Meeuse et al., 2018; Forrester-Jones et al., 2018).
- Spiritual struggles can be transformed into spiritual growth and then be a powerful resource for facilitating recovery (Starnino, 2016b). For some, life will then be more meaningful than it ever was before their illness.

Because of all this, it is well worth investing in good-quality spiritual care within mental health services. There need to be a sufficient members of the Spiritual Care Team to respond to demand on their services.

The many clinical staff who provide spiritual care need to be given adequate resources. Mental healthcare professionals are less likely to have a religious faith or spiritual awareness than service users themselves (Dein et al., 2010; Milner et al., 2020) and therefore need suitable training in spiritual issues (Cook, 2011). Likewise, faith leaders should be trained in understanding mental health problems.

This is a specialist field. Neither a faith leader nor a member of the clinical team is fully equipped to deal with these issues on their own, and a collaborative approach is needed.

Conclusion

Spiritual issues are closely related to mental illness. Loss of spiritual well-being is frequently associated with mental health problems, and its rediscovery can define personal recovery. Spiritual awareness can ease the burden of mental distress and facilitate recovery. However, spirituality can cause problems. In this chapter we have considered the disparate ways in which spirituality may be experienced by people with mental health problems, and how these people can best be helped to find positive inspiration from their spirituality.

It is clear that the interaction of spirituality and mental illness is highly complex and poorly understood. The many different positive and negative aspects of spiritual experience can each occur to a different extent in any one individual. We cannot make a spiritual 'diagnosis'. If we are to understand, we need to listen to each individual patient's spiritual experiences within the context of their full story, so that appropriate help can be given.

I personally was unable to move forward in my recovery until I made some sense of some of my experiences by talking them through with a chaplain. Although I still have periods of darkness, and need repeated assurance of God's forgiveness, I have an underlying sense of purpose. I boldly say that my faith often gives me hope, peace – and sometimes even joy. And there are times when being prayed for by a chaplain can bring peace in a way that no psychiatric medicine has the power to do.

References

Abu-Raiya, H., Pargament, K. I. and Exline, J. J. (2015) Understanding and addressing religious and spiritual struggles in health care. *Health & Social Work*, 40, e126–e134.

Amerongen-Meeuse, J. C, Schaap-Jonker, H., Schuhmann, C. et al. (2018) The "religiosity gap" in a clinical setting: experiences of mental health care consumers and professionals. *Mental Health, Religion & Culture*, 21, 737–52.

Andresen, R., Oades, L. and Caputi, P. (2003) The experience of recovery from schizophrenia: towards an empirically validated stage model. *Australian and New Zealand Journal of Psychiatry*, 5, 586–594.

Barber, J. M., Parkes, M., Parsons, H. and Cook, C. C. H. (2012) Importance of spiritual well-being in assessment of recovery: the Service-user Recovery Evaluation (SeRvE) scale. *The Psychiatrist*, 36, 444–450.

Barber, J. M., Parkes, M. and Wilson, C. (2015) *Handbook of Spiritual Care in Mental Illness*. Birmingham: Spiritual Care Team, Birmingham and Solihull Mental Health NHS Foundation Trust.

Barber, J. M., Parsons, H., Wilson, C. A. and Cook, C. C. H. (2017) Measuring mental health in the clinical setting: what is important to service users? The Mini-Service user Recovery Evaluation scale (Mini-SeRvE). *Journal of Mental Health*, 26, 530–537.

Barut, J. K., Dietrich, M. S., Zanoni, P. A. et al. (2016) Sense of belonging and hope in the lives of persons with schizophrenia. *Archives of Psychiatric Nursing*, 30, 178–184.

Bussema, E. F. and Bussema, K. E. (2007) Gilead revisited: faith and recovery. *Psychiatric Rehabilitation Journal*, 30, 301–305.

Clarke, I. (2010) *Psychosis and Spirituality: Consolidating the New Paradigm*, 2nd ed. Chichester: John Wiley & Sons.

Cogan, N. A., Schwannauer, M. and Harper, S. (2019) Recovery and self-identity development following a first episode of psychosis. *Journal of Public Mental Health*, 18, 169–179.

Cook, C. C. H. (2011) The faith of the psychiatrist. *Mental Health, Religion & Culture*, 14, 9–17.

Cook, C. C. H. (2012) Pathway to accommodate patients' spiritual needs. *Nursing Management*, 19, 33–37.

Cook, C. C. H. (2015) Religious psychopathology: the prevalence of religious content of delusions and hallucinations in mental disorder. *International Journal of Social Psychiatry*, 61, 404–425.

Cook, C. C. H., Powell, A. E., Sims, A. and Eagger, S. (2011) Spirituality and secularity: professional boundaries in psychiatry. *Mental Health, Religion & Culture*, 14, 35–42.

Cook, C. C. H., Powell, A. and Sims, A. (2016) *Spirituality and Narrative in Psychiatric Practice: Stories of Mind and Soul*. London: RCPsych Publications.

Currier, J. M., Foster, J. D., Witvliet, C. et al. (2019) Spiritual struggles and mental health outcomes in a spiritually integrated inpatient program. *Journal of Affective Disorders*, 249, 127–135.

Davidson, L. (2020) Recovering a sense of self in schizophrenia. *Journal of Personality*, 88, 122–132.

Dein, S., Cook, C. C. H., Powell, A. and Eagger, S. (2010) Religion, spirituality and mental health. *The Psychiatrist*, 34, 63–64.

Dein, S., Cook, C. C. H. and Koenig, H. G. (2012) Religion, spirituality, and mental health: current controversies and future directions. *Journal of Nervous and Mental Disease*, 200, 852–855.

De Wet, A., Swartz, L. and Chiliza, B. (2015) Hearing their voices: the lived experience of recovery from first-episode psychosis in schizophrenia in South Africa. *International Journal of Social Psychiatry*, 61, 27–32.

Ellison, C. G. and Lee, J. (2010) Spiritual struggles and psychological distress: is there a dark side of religion? *Social Indicators Research*, 98, 501–517.

Exline, J. J. (2013) Religious and spiritual struggles. In K. I. Pargament, J. J. Exline and J. Jones, eds., *APA Handbook of Psychology, Religion, and Spirituality. Vol. 1: Context, Theory, and Research.* Washington, DC: American Psychological Association, pp. 459–476.

Exline, J. J., Yali, A. M. and Lobel, M. (1999) When God disappoints: difficulty forgiving God and its role in negative emotion. *Journal of Health Psychology*, 4, 365–379.

Fallot, R. D. (2007) Spirituality and religion in recovery: some current issues. *Psychiatric Rehabilitation Journal*, 30, 261–270.

Forrester-Jones, R., Dietzfelbinger, L., Stedman, D. and Richmond, P. (2018) Including the 'spiritual' within mental health care in the UK, from the experiences of people with mental health problems. *Journal of Religion and Health*, 57, 384–407.

Gomi, S., Starnino, V. R. and Canda, E. R. (2014) Spiritual assessment in mental health recovery. *Community Mental Health Journal*, 50, 447–453.

Guthrie, T. and Stickley, T. (2008) Spiritual experience and mental distress: a clergy perspective. *Mental Health, Religion & Culture*, 11, 387–402.

Harris, J. I., Erbes, C. R., Engdahl, B. E. et al. (2012) Religious distress and coping with stressful life events: a longitudinal study.

Journal of Clinical Psychology, 68, 1276–1286.

Heffernan, S., Neil, S., Thomas, Y. and Weatherhead, S. (2016) Religion in the recovery journey of individuals with experience of psychosis. *Psychosis*, 8, 346–356.

Huguelet, P. (2016) Spiritual meaning in life and values in patients with severe mental disorders. *Journal of Nervous and Mental Disease*, 204, 409–414.

Huguelet, P., Mohr, S., Betrisey, C. et al. (2011) A randomized trial of spiritual assessment of outpatients with schizophrenia: patients' and clinicians' experience. *Psychiatric Services*, 62, 79–86.

Jones, S., Sutton, K. and Isaacs, A. (2019) Concepts, practices and advantages of spirituality among people with a chronic mental illness in Melbourne. *Journal of Religion and Health*, 58, 343–355.

Koenig, H. G. (2009) Research on religion, spirituality, and mental health: a review. *Canadian Journal of Psychiatry*, 54, 283–291.

Koenig, H. G. (2015) Religion, spirituality, and health: a review and update. *Advances in Mind and Body Medicine*, 29, 19–26.

Leamy, M., Bird, V., Le Boutillier, C. et al. (2011) Conceptual framework for personal recovery in mental health: systemic review and narrative synthesis. *British Journal of Psychiatry*, 199, 445–452.

Loch, A. A., Elder, L. F., Hortêncio, L. et al. (2019) Hearing spirits? Religiosity in individuals at risk for psychosis—results from the Brazilian SSAPP Cohort. *Schizophrenia Research*, 204, 353–359.

Loewenthal, K. M. (2018) The OCD – religion package: might it relate to the rise of spirituality? *Mental Health, Religion & Culture*, 21, 123–130.

Milner, K., Crawford, P., Edgley, A., Hare-Duke, L. and Slade, M. (2020) The experiences of spirituality among adults with mental health difficulties: a qualitative systematic review. *Epidemiology and Psychiatric Sciences*, 29, e34.

Ouwehand, E., Braam, A. W., Renes, J. et al. (2019a) Prevalence of religious and spiritual experiences and the perceived influence thereof in patients with bipolar disorder in a Dutch specialist outpatient center. *Journal of Nervous and Mental Disease*, 207, 291–299.

Ouwehand, E., Zock, H. T. H., Muthert, H. J. K., Boeije, H. and Braam, A. W. (2019b) "The awful rowing toward God": interpretation of religious experiences by individuals with bipolar disorder. *Pastoral Psychology*, 68, 437–462.

Ouwehand, E., Braam, A. W., Renes, J. W., Muthert, H. J. K. and Zock, H. T. (2020) Holy apparition or hyper-religiosity: prevalence of explanatory models for religious and spiritual experiences in patients with bipolar disorder and their associations with religiousness. *Pastoral Psychology*, 69, 29–45.

Payman, V. (2016) The importance of taking a religious and spiritual history. *Australasian Psychiatry*, 24, 434–436.

Powers, A. R., Kelley, M. S., Corlett, P. R. et al. (2017) Varieties of voice-hearing: psychics and the psychosis continuum. *Schizophrenia Bulletin*. 43, 84–98.

Raffay, J., Wood, E. and Todd, A. (2016) Service user views of spiritual and pastoral care (chaplaincy) in NHS mental health services: a co-produced constructivist grounded theory investigation. *BMC Psychiatry*, 16, 200–211.

Russinova, Z. and Cash, D. (2007) Personal perspectives about the meaning of religion and spirituality among persons with serious mental illness. *Psychiatric Rehabilitation Journal*, 30, 271–284.

Starnino, V. R. (2016a) Conceptualizing spirituality and religion for mental health practice: perspectives of consumers with serious mental illness. *Families in Society*, 97, 295–304.

Starnino, V. R. (2016b) When trauma, spirituality, and mental illness intersect: a qualitative case study. *Psychological Trauma: Theory, Research, Practice, and Policy*, 8, 375–383.

Tuffour, I. (2020) 'There is anointing everywhere': an interpretative phenomenological analysis of the role of religion in the recovery of Black African service users in England. *Journal of Psychiatric and Mental Health Nursing*, 27, 352–361.

Wood, L. and Alsawy, S. (2018) Recovery in psychosis from a service user perspective: a systematic review and thematic synthesis of current qualitative evidence. *Community Mental Health Journal*, 54, 793–804.

Zarzycka, B. and Puchalska-Wasyl, M. (2020) Can religious and spiritual struggle enhance well-being? Exploring the mediating effects of internal dialogues. *Journal of Religion and Health*, 59, 1897–1912.

Chapter 16

Religion and Religious Experience

Christopher C. H. Cook

For most people worldwide, religion has inherently positive connotations. For many it is the very source of life, providing meaning, purpose and hope. For such people it is impossible to talk about their spirituality without talking about its religious context. Religion is widespread and popular, and is flourishing around the world. It has even been suggested that it is a 'fundamental characteristic of humankind' (Johnson et al., 2013, p. 9).

For a minority worldwide, religion is deeply unattractive, perhaps even perceived as a source of harm, and concerned with dogma, ritual, hierarchy and institutions; it is restricting and life denying. For some who self-identify as spiritual but not religious, spirituality is even understood as the opposite of religion; spirituality is 'not religion'. Among those for whom religion has negative connotations, psychiatrists have featured prominently. For Freud, religious beliefs were indemonstrable and illusory beliefs arising from wish fulfilment, and he foresaw a future in which they would fall away in the face of science and reason (Dufresne, 2012). Following in this negative tradition, mental health professionals have typically been less religious than their patients, creating a so-called religiosity gap between psychiatrists and their patients (Cook, 2011) and making mutual understanding more difficult in relation to religious matters.

Ironically, given Freud's predictions, it is science that is now providing evidence to support the contention that religion is good for mental health (Koenig et al., 2020). However, the social and biological sciences are not the only contributors to the debate. The human sciences more widely, the medical humanities and theology and religious studies all have a contribution to make. This chapter will therefore draw broadly from these disciplines in considering the nature of religion as relevant to psychiatry.

Religions

Religion may mean different things to different people, at least in part, because of the amazing diversity that it displays. There are seven or eight major global religions, usually understood to include Christianity, Islam, Judaism, Hinduism and Buddhism, among others (but with some disagreement as to exactly which religions should be included in the list) (see Figure 16.1). There are approximately 10,000 different religions in total around the world (Johnson et al., 2013, p. 9). There are also people who do not identify with any religious tradition, including both agnostics and atheists. This group has always been statistically in a minority, but the numbers of non-religionists around the world have fluctuated over the course of the last century.

Religious diversity is evident within religious traditions as well as between them. Christians divide broadly into Catholic, Protestant and Orthodox, with over half of all

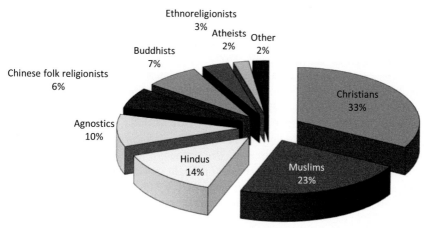

Figure 16.1 Adherents of world religions in 2010.
Data from Johnson et al. (2013, p. 10).

Christians worldwide identifying as Catholic, but there are also other groups (e.g., Coptic) and there is diversity within each of the main groups (especially among different Protestant denominations). Approximately 86% of the world's Muslims identify as Sunni, but there are also Shi'a, Sufi and other schismatic groups. Hinduism, which is the third largest and the oldest major world religion, has no shared doctrine, no historical founder and an immense pantheon of gods, with a wide variety of devotion to one or more of these divinities.

Notwithstanding all of this diversity, there are certain 'family resemblances' between religions (Asma, 2018, p. 8). Most religions provide social cohesion and a sense of identity. They involve belief in a transcendent order, usually including a personal God, or gods (although Buddhism, Daoism and Confucianism are exceptions to this), and convey expectations of communication with this order in prayer and meditation. They provide sacred stories, or narratives, of human origins, of creation and salvation within which the lives of their followers are contextualised. They prescribe rituals and ceremonies, often involving sacred objects of some kind, and moral norms. They engender strong feelings and emotions, such as love, joy, awe, reverence and gratitude, but also guilt, fear and anxiety. Many (but again not all) have sacred texts or scriptures.

These family resemblances may have contributed to the research base which (generally, and with some dissension) is now interpreted as showing that 'religion' is good for mental health. However, we must keep in mind that individual religions are very different from one another, and much more research is needed to investigate the diverse ways in which, for example, Christianity, Islam and Buddhism contribute to mental well-being.

What is Religion?

We all know what religion is until we come to try to define it. For academics in the humanities, especially in departments of theology or religious studies, religion is understood as a complex concept that is all but impossible to define. It is a Western European concept, with its roots in colonialism, and it often carries Protestant Christian theological preconceptions (Hanegraaff, 2016; Bowker, 2018, pp. 1–38).

Attempts to find a definition that avoids cultural or theological preconceptions tend to broaden the scope of the discussion. For example, one influential approach has been that of the anthropologist Clifford Geertz, who argues that religion is concerned with symbolic understanding of the nature and meaning of human existence, and that these symbolic systems have powerful effects upon moods and motivations (Geertz, 1993). Symbolic meanings can be very important in psychiatry, especially when they become embedded in psychopathology, or in dynamic psychotherapeutic approaches to the interpretation of thoughts and dreams. Unfortunately, the usefulness of Geertz's approach is limited by its inclusion of systems of thought that are not usually considered to be religious, such as humanism or Marxism. At the same time, it does not easily include religions, such as Quakerism, within which symbols are not considered significant (Harrison, 2006).

On a more pragmatic level, a religion is effectively defined by its followers (Johnson et al., 2013, pp. 139–140). It is what they devote themselves to, it is what they identify with, and so it is relatively easy in research (or in clinical practice) simply to ask people how they self-identify in religious terms. A religion can also be defined in terms of what it is about – its beliefs, doctrines, rituals and scriptures (see, for example, Bowker, 2007). This allows comparisons between religious systems of thought, but is less helpful in clinical practice, where the need is to know what the individual patient actually believes, rather than what is doctrinally prescribed by any religious leader, formulary or institution.

In contrast to any focus on beliefs and practices (sometimes referred to as an essentialist approach), functionalist approaches to religion seek to identify social utility (Asma, 2018, pp. 8–9). Religions promote social cohesion and a system of shared values, they confer a sense of identity and they assist in the human quest for meaning and purpose. Religions address the dynamics of interpersonal forgiveness and reconciliation. They also provide a means for relieving sorrow and grief, and for managing desires and emotions (Asma, 2018). Much psychological and psychiatric research has therefore focused on functionalist, rather than essentialist, understandings of religion.

There has thus been a move among some scholars and practitioners to shift the discussion away from religion and towards concepts such as worldview, or systems of meaning (Taves, 2018). Worldviews draw attention to fundamental questions that people ask, and the human search for meaning and purpose that religions facilitate. Freud believed that everyone had a worldview, or Weltanschauung, and that these fell into two basic types, which we might consider as the 'spiritual' and the 'scientific' (Nicholi, 2004). However, it is neither necessary nor helpful to see worldviews in such crude terms (which were, in any case, influenced strongly by Freud's own scientific worldview). The idea of worldviews has been taken up by some psychiatrists. For example, it can provide a helpful approach to assessment (Josephson and Wiesner, 2004), drawing attention to the way in which the worldview of the psychiatrist may influence that assessment. Alison Gray (who also provides a helpful map of worldviews in relation to religion) draws attention to their relevance in diagnosis and treatment (Gray, 2011).

Religion in Psychiatric Research

Scientists need clear definitions for their research variables. Spirituality is conspicuously lacking in this regard. There is no widely agreed definition, and spirituality is hopelessly confounded with the outcome variables that it purports to influence. In contrast, Harold Koenig asserts, religion has much to offer; it is 'a unique construct whose definition is generally agreed upon by researchers in the field' (Koenig et al., 2012, p. 37). Thus he urges that healthcare research should focus on religion, not spirituality (Koenig, 2008). How is it that Koenig finds religion so easy to define, in contrast to the many scholars of religious studies who agree only that it is all but impossible to define?

Although he acknowledges that religion is multidimensional, and that research design should take account of this, Koenig understands religion as fundamentally related to the transcendent: 'Religion involves beliefs, practices, and rituals related to the transcendent, where the transcendent is God, Allah, HaShem, or a Higher Power in Western religious traditions, or to Brahman, manifestations of Brahman, Buddha, Dao, or ultimate truth/reality in Eastern traditions' (Koenig et al., 2012, p. 45).

The central focus of this definition, on the transcendent, unfortunately just moves the argument from one term that is difficult to define to another (Smart, 1998, p. 12; Cook, 2013). However, the specific dimensions of religion that Koenig suggests should be studied do not focus directly on this. Instead, they include such things as religious affiliation, religious beliefs, religious experiences, religious knowledge, prayer, attendance at religious services, and so on. These, he asserts, are 'conceptually distinct and separate' both from each other and from 'other psychological and social constructs' (Koenig et al., 2012, pp. 45–46). These 'dimensions of religion' are actually various aspects of religiosity, rather than religion, a consideration to which I shall return later. It is also not completely clear that they are in fact completely conceptually distinct from each other or (at least sometimes) from other psychological constructs.

Religious beliefs and religious knowledge, for example, are conceptually different, but not necessarily distinct and separate from each other. Delusional religious beliefs may be distinguishable from other religious beliefs, but such distinctions are on a continuum (Van Os et al., 2000) and not categorically or conceptually separate. The difference between religious delusions and other delusions, similarly, may be dimensional rather than categorical. Religious delusions seem to be held with particular intensity, and may therefore be relatively resistant to cognitive–behavioural therapies (Appelbaum et al., 1999).

Contrast Koenig's approach with that of Ann Taves, a professor of religious studies: 'Given that religion, religious, and religions are Western folk concepts, that their meaning is unstable and contested, and that they cannot be defined so as to specify anything uniquely, we need to consider broader, more generic ways of characterizing the sorts of things that interest us as scholars of religion' (Taves, 2011, p. 58). It may well be that the things that interest scholars of religion are not the same as the things that interest psychiatrists (and we might enquire as to whether or not they should, in fact, be interested in the same or different things). However, Taves goes on to suggest that we should consider religion as one particular example of things that are considered 'special'. 'Special things', things that are set apart in some unique way, are not amenable to commodification. They cannot be reduced to other things – for example, to monetary value or, I would add, operationalised research variables. Things that are set apart in this way are protected by various taboos. Among the kinds of special things that Taves considers are 'ideals' – things that are perfect or complete in some way. Transcendence falls into this category (along with reality, truth, good, etc.). Other special things include anomalous experiences (perceptions or feelings), which suggest the presence of an anomalous agent and thus grab the attention of the person concerned. According to Taves, special things may be understood as the 'building blocks' of religion.

According to Taves, religious practices are not dimensions of religion (as Koenig proposes) but rather they are aids to reaching a special goal, and therefore constitute 'special paths'. Taves' approach thus side-steps the need to define religion, and avoids the problem of the very different ways in which particular religions conceptualise the transcendent.

It would be helpful to research in psychiatry, I would suggest, if we acknowledged that religion is not easy to define, and that concepts such as 'transcendence' draw us into consideration of the diversity of religion rather than things held in common. A broader category, such as the 'specialness' that Taves proposes, allows us to focus more upon the common experiences of religious (and sometimes non-religious) people in widely differing cultural contexts. It also draws attention to the fact that it is not 'religion' that psychiatric researchers are actually measuring, but rather the practices – or special paths – which people adopt in pursuit of their religious aspirations.

Religion Around the World

The way in which religion will be viewed in psychiatry, and the influence that it will have upon clinical practice, depend very much upon geography, and upon the cultural context and background of both patient and psychiatrist. An understanding of a global view of religion in the world today is therefore important as the context of psychiatric practice. This will be particularly true for readers of this chapter who come from different countries, but is also important for practitioners in culturally diverse cities such as London, New York or Paris. The same religion can look very different in different parts of the world.

Much of the research on religion and psychiatry has been conducted in the Western world, and especially in Europe and North America. This has produced a selective focus on particular religious traditions, and especially on Christianity. Christianity is the largest world religion, numerically speaking, and is also the largest religion on five continents (see Figure 16.1 and Figure 16.2). However, over the course of the last century there has been a global shift of Christianity from the Northern to the Southern Hemisphere. In 1910, 80% of Christians lived in the global north, but by 2010 more than 60% lived in the global south (Johnson et al., 2013, pp. 12–16). Psychiatric research has focused on Christianity in a Western cultural context, whereas most Christians today live in the Southern Hemisphere.

Like Christianity, Islam is a truly global religion and over the last century there has been rapid growth of the Muslim population in Europe, North America and Africa (Johnson et al., 2013, pp. 16–23). Although traditionally Muslim countries in the Middle East continue to have a high proportion of Muslims in their populations, Indonesia now has more Muslims in its population than any other country in the world.

Asia, and particularly India, is home to most of the world's Hindus. However, there has been rapid growth in the Hindu population in North America and Europe over the

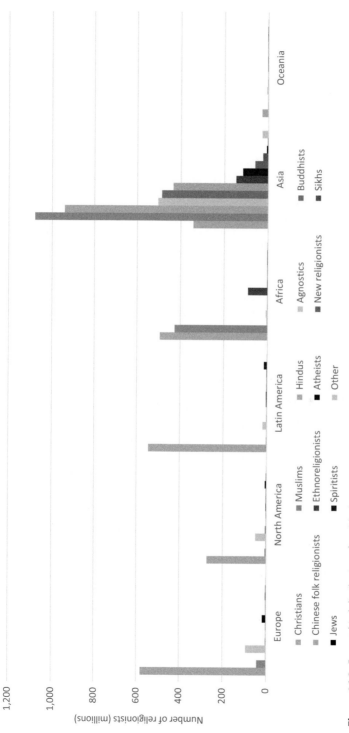

Figure 16.2 Geographical distribution of world religions in 2010.
Data from Johnson et al. (2013, pp. 344–345).

last century (Johnson et al., 2013, pp. 23–26). Asia remains the most religiously diverse continent on the planet. Only in Asia do Christians find themselves, overall, a minority religious group.

The influence of religion on the presentation of psychiatric disorders, and on the practice of psychiatry, may thus be expected to be very different according to the country (examples are shown in Figure 16.3) or even the city in which one lives. This is important not only because of the influence of the majority religion upon culture, ethics and norms, but also because of the struggles inherent in being part of a religious minority (Marks et al., 2019). Although it may be easy in some places to see the global context as irrelevant, by virtue of the great homogeneity of religious belonging (e.g., in Islamic Saudi Arabia or Christian North Carolina), there is hardly any corner of the world today in which there are not some religious minority groups. No clinician can afford to be unaware of the implications of this for psychiatric practice.

New Religionists

New religions, founded after 1800, include a variety of offshoots of traditional religions as well as various syncretistic combinations of Christian and Eastern religions. They include such groups as Baha'i, Theosophy, Rastafarians, Hare Krishna, the Unification Church ('Moonies') and Scientology (notable for its antagonism towards psychiatry). However, there are literally thousands of such movements, and almost 1.8 billion new religionists, worldwide.

Although new religions are concentrated predominantly in Asia (with an especially large number in Japan), more than 1.6 million new religionists were to be found in the USA in 2010, and Australia and the UK ranked fourth and seventh, respectively, in terms of growth in numbers of new religionists between 1910 and 2010 (Johnson et al., 2013, pp. 41–47). There is some debate as to where the boundaries lie between new religions and cults, with sociologists tending to prefer to talk about 'new religions' rather than 'cults', or 'new religious movements', thus blurring the boundaries and avoiding implicit value judgements. However, some new religions are more 'world affirming' and others are more 'world denying', with some being more clearly associated with the potential to cause psychological harm than others, and so the distinction is probably a helpful one for psychiatrists to maintain (see Chapter 17).

Non-Religionists

The vast majority of the non-religious in the world today live in China (unless one argues that Communism is a religion), not in North America or Europe. Nonetheless, agnosticism (taken for this purpose to include all those who are uncertain and unaffiliated, as well as agnostics in the strict sense; see Glossary) accounts for almost 10% of the world's population. In 1910, 80% of the world's agnostics and atheists lived in the global north; by 2010, 75% were to be found in Asia (Johnson et al., 2013, p. 41).

If religion is difficult to define then, by the same token, so is non-religion (Taves, 2018). Given that many non-religionists have strongly held worldviews, they may in fact have more in common with some religionists than they do with those who might be described as existentially indifferent. This is important in clinical practice. The patient who says 'I am neither spiritual nor religious' may in fact have strongly held worldviews that have a direct impact on his or her sense of well-being.

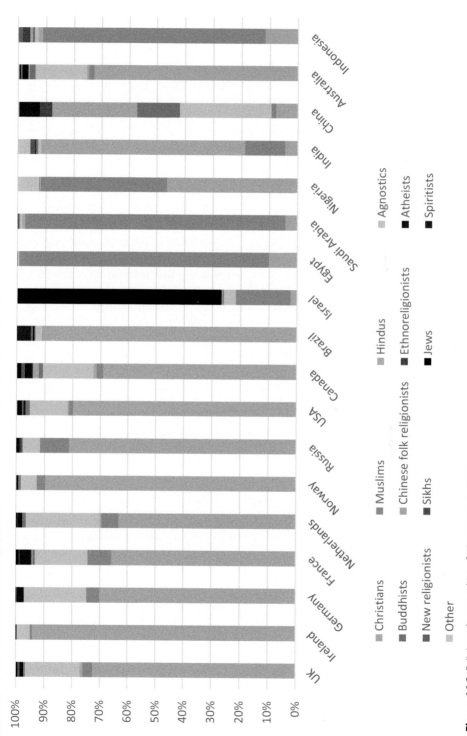

Figure 16.3 Religious demographics of 18 countries in 2010.
Data from Johnson et al. (2013, pp. 337–345).

Religiosity

The research literature is beset by diverse and different understandings of religiosity (Hackney and Sanders, 2003). Worse still, the term is rarely defined and is often confused with religion. In the minds of some, religiosity has a negative connotation, referring to excessive or ostentatious ways of being religious. In practice, in scientific research, it refers to operationalised, quantitative measures of individual differences in religiousness or religious commitment. Whereas religion is concerned with human groups, religiosity represents a shift of focus to the individual (Glock and Stark, 1965, pp. 18–19). Measures of religiosity are often characterised as being concerned with religion; they are actually concerned with religious forms of spirituality.

There are many ways in which religiosity may be measured (e.g., Hill and Hood, 1999; Büssing, 2019a, 2019b), and many (if not all) of these reflect particular preconceptions about what religion is, or what is important about religion. The diversity of measures can be grouped together to reflect different dimensions of religiosity which, ideally or theoretically, could be measured and compared across different world religions and cultures. In their influential book, *Religion and Society in Tension*, Charles Glock and Rodney Stark identified five core dimensions of religiosity within which 'all of the many and diverse manifestations of religiosity prescribed by the different religions of the world can be ordered': experiential, ideological, ritualistic, intellectual and consequential (Glock and Stark, 1965, p. 20).

More recent research has proliferated the categories. Thus, for example, Koenig identifies 17 dimensions of religiosity:

Religious affiliation
Religious belief
Public religious practices
Private religious practices
Religious salience (subjective religiousness)
Religious motivation
Religious well-being
Religious coping
Religious history
Religious support
Religious experience
Religious attachment
Religious giving
Religious knowledge
Religious seeking, striving or quest
Religious growth/development
Religious commitment (Koenig, 2018, pp. 25–33).

Religiosity may thus be measured in very different ways in different research studies, and each of these has its clinical correlate. It is unlikely that any clinician could routinely ask about all of these, nor are they all covered within standard approaches to assessing spirituality (see Chapter 2).

Koenig (2011, pp. 215–216) has also proposed a simpler three-dimensional categorisation derived from the consensus of an interdisciplinary panel: organisational religiosity (frequency of religious attendance and other group activities), non-organisational religiosity (prayer, scripture reading, viewing/listening to religious media) and religious importance or salience (subjective religiousness, religious importance, intrinsic religious motivation). However one groups the measures currently available, it is clear that much of the research is highly selective and that the choice of measures may well influence the findings. The most commonly used scales have measured religious orientation/motivation, but two multi-dimensional scales (Duke University Religion Index and the Brief Multidimensional Measure of Religiosity and Spirituality) have become popular over the last 20 years, as has the Religious Commitment Inventory (Koenig, 2018, pp. 35–37).

In a meta-analysis by Hackney and Sanders (2003), 'institutional religiosity' (broadly similar to Koenig's 'organisational' dimension) was found to produce the weakest (and only negative) correlations with mental health. 'Ideology' (including attitudes, salience of beliefs and fundamentalism) and 'personal devotion' (including intrinsic religiosity, emotional attachment to God, devotional intensity and colloquial prayer) produced the strongest correlations.

Similarly, clinicians may be predisposed (in the interests of saving time, if for no other reason) to ask selective questions which are likely to elicit an incomplete picture of the religiosity of any given patient. This raises the important matter of which initial questions to ask in the context of a busy clinic or ward situation, and how to prioritise the subsequent enquiry in the light of the initial responses to these questions. (For further exploration of these issues, see Chapter 2.)

For researchers and clinicians alike there is a danger that the religiosity of the individual is presumed to conform to the social expectations of the (idealised) religion or institution. In fact, the 'lived religion' of ordinary people is much messier than this. It does not necessarily conform to the definitional boundaries of academia or religious hierarchies. People draw sometimes contradictory ideas and practices from various religious traditions, and traditions change over time. Lived religion is embodied, especially when it comes to matters of health and healing, and it concerns the whole person – body, mind and spirit (McGuire, 2008).

Religious and Spiritual Struggles

Religion may, in many ways, be supportive of good mental health, and the brief review of the literature in Chapter 1 would appear to support this contention. However, religion can also present challenges and difficulties that non-religious people do not experience, and these may sometimes be a source of distress. Empirical research attention was initially drawn to such experiences by Kenneth Pargament and his colleagues (Pargament et al., 1998), who identified a negative form of religious coping involving beliefs concerning punishment by God, religious/spiritual discontent, attributions of demonic influence, and questioning whether or not God was able/willing to influence the situation. There is now good evidence that negative religious coping is associated with poor mental health, but the strength of evidence for a causal relationship (i.e., that negative religious coping causes poor mental health) is less clear. It remains possible (and in some specific clinical circumstances may be very likely) that poor mental health causes negative religious coping (Koenig, 2018, pp. 181–200).

In the Religious and Spiritual Struggles Scale developed by Julie Exline and her colleagues (Exline et al., 2014), six domains of struggle are identified:

Divine – including anger or disappointment with God, understanding God as the cause of the struggle, religious fear/guilt and an unstable relationship with God.

Demonic – attributions of negative events to demonic influence, and beliefs or concerns that evil spirits are attacking the individual.

Interpersonal – difficult interpersonal relationships with religious people/institutions and/or conflict with these people over religious issues.

Moral – wrestling with religious moral norms; worry or guilt over perceived offences/transgressions.

Doubt – doubts and questions about spiritual/religious beliefs.

Ultimate meaning – failure to perceive meaning in life.

A relatively small literature addresses the question of whether or not various interventions are effective in reducing negative religious coping, and the findings are mixed. Although there are positive outcomes in a number of studies, it is not clear that interventions directed specifically at negative religious coping are any more effective than other spiritual/religious treatments, nor is it clear that any of these interventions are superior to standard cognitive–behavioural therapy or pharmacotherapy (Koenig, 2018, pp. 194–200).

As an example of this literature, in a study by Bowland et al. (2012) of older, Christian, female trauma survivors, an 11-session group intervention allowed participants to explore their spiritual histories and their spiritual needs and struggles, and to develop a recovery strategy. At the end of the intervention the treatment group had significantly lower levels of depression, anxiety and physical symptoms compared with the control group, and this was maintained at 3-month follow-up. In another study, by Gibbel et al. (2019), a nine-session spiritually integrated intervention produced better spiritual and psychological outcomes in a small group ($n = 9$) of patients with mental illness compared with controls.

Avoidance of spiritual struggles seems to be associated with higher levels of depression and anxiety (Dworsky et al., 2016). Spiritual and religious struggles are therefore matters that the clinician should – at the very minimum – be able and willing to discuss with a patient, and such evidence as is available would suggest that such discussions are indeed beneficial.

The area of spiritual struggles that has proved most controversial has been that labelled by Exline and her colleagues as the demonic. In a study of 343 psychiatric outpatients in Switzerland (selected on the basis of the importance of religion to them from a larger group of 536 patients), predominantly from a Protestant Christian background, 37.6% believed that their problems might be caused by evil spirits, and 30.3% sought help through prayers for deliverance and exorcism. The patients' psychiatric symptoms were not improved by these interventions (Pfeifer, 1994, 1999).

There have been reports of harm caused to patients with dissociative identity disorder who were subjected to exorcism, with adverse effects on both spiritual and mental health being observed (Bowman, 1991; Fraser, 1993). However, there have also been reports of positive outcomes (Bull et al., 1998), and professional opinion in the field is divided (Rosik, 2003).

Similar phenomena do occur within other religious traditions and cultures, but the differences between traditions are significant, and it is not clear that these parallel phenomena are necessarily to be viewed as 'struggles' in quite the same way. For example, within Spiritism the practice of disobsession, or spirit release treatment, seeks to remove harmful spiritual influences exerted by spirits ('obsessors') upon an individual. The nature of the obsessors as understood in such treatments is very different (less unambiguously 'evil') from that of demons as understood in Christian practices of exorcism or deliverance. The understanding of disobsession in clinical practice is more fully integrated with the biopsychosocial model, and anecdotal reports suggest that there is a good outcome for patients suffering from depression (Moreira-Almeida and Lotufo Neto, 2005; Lucchetti et al., 2012, 2015).

Similarly, within Spiritualism, mediums score well on measures of psychological well-being, and are not distressed by their experiences of encounters with spirits (Roxburgh and Roe, 2011, 2014).

Religious Experience

Religious experience can be understood in a variety of different ways. At one extreme, all of the experiences of a religious person might be understood as 'religious' experiences in some way or another. At the opposite end of the spectrum, the term might be reserved for unusual or especially intense experiences such as conversion experiences, visionary experiences or mystical experiences. For William James, in his classic work titled *The Varieties of Religious Experience*, religious experience was understood to be somewhere in between these two extremes in terms of relationship with the divine: 'Religion ... shall mean for us the feelings, acts, and experiences of individual men in their solitude, so far as they apprehend themselves to stand in relation to whatever they may consider the divine' (James, 1902, p. 31).

James' definition has been very influential, and it helpfully presents religious experience as a relational affair – between the believer and a transcendent reality. However, it characterises religion as a very individual affair, whereas, for the psychiatrist, there is ample evidence that it has an important social dimension. James also showed a strongly Western bias in the accounts of experiences that he included.

Scales of religious experience used in scientific research over the last 50 years or more also show a bias in the kinds of experience to which they attend. For example, Edwards' Religious Experience Questionnaire (REQ) (Hill and Hood, 1999, pp. 218–220) refers to experiences of God (such as awareness of love or anger towards God), private prayer in 'places other than church' and prayer as 'like I'm having a conversation with a close friend'. The Religious Experience Episodes Measure (REEM), developed initially by Hood (Hill and Hood, 1999, pp. 220–224), takes as its benchmark 15 first-person experiences drawn from *The Varieties of Religious Experience* and then asks respondents to compare their experiences with these. In their Index of Core Spiritual Experiences (INSPIRIT), Kass et al. (1991) take a step towards making their questionnaire more accessible to people from diverse religious and spiritual perspectives, by asking respondents to use their own definition of 'God'. Questions involve such things as how religious the respondent is, the amount of time spent in religious practices, experience of the 'presence' of God, and the opportunity to choose on a scale of 1 to 7 between contrasting images of God (e.g., Father vs. Mother).

The REQ would seem likely to work best for Christian respondents, although it might be adapted to other monotheistic faiths, and it focuses on everyday experiences. The REEM is heavily shaped by selected examples drawn from William James' research over a century ago, almost all of a more mystical and less everyday variety. INSPIRIT is a little more receptive to readers from diverse religious traditions, but it also has a much more inclusive approach to 'experience', taking in such things as self-assessed importance of religion, religious practices, experiences of presence, and mental images of God. Religious experiences – at least in the research context – thus include a diverse spectrum of practices, affects, perceptions and beliefs.

The search for a scale that is completely culture-free and unbiased is likely always to be elusive, and this is not necessarily a bad thing, although it may complicate any attempt at comparison of religious experiences between different traditions. The more important issue for psychiatry is the study within traditions of experiences associated with psycho-pathology. Spiritual, mystical and religious experiences overlap with experiences that psychiatrists might diagnose as pathological.

Religious Experience, Psychopathology and Psychiatric Diagnosis

David Lukoff proposed that the overlap between mystical experiences and psychotic states may be understood as including two possible diagnostic categories: 'mystical experiences with psychotic features' and 'psychotic disorders with mystical features', which could be distinguished on the grounds of various features indicative of a likely positive prognosis (good pre-episode functioning, acute onset, stressful precipitants, and positive exploratory attitude) (Lukoff, 1985).

Like Lukoff, others have proposed criteria that purportedly enable differential diagnosis between spiritual experience and mental disturbance. For example, de Menezes and Moreira-Almeida (2009) propose nine such criteria:

1 lack of suffering
2 lack of functional impairment
3 short duration/sporadic frequency
4 critical attitude to the experience
5 compatibility with cultural background
6 absence of comorbidities
7 control over the experience
8 personal growth
9 other-directedness.

Some would place more emphasis than these authors do on phenomenology (Sims, 1992), whereas others have suggested that traditional psychiatric phenomenology is not helpful and that the emphasis should be on values and beliefs (Jackson and Fulford, 1997).

For Sims, the important distinction to be made is that between form and content. He gives the example of a man whose belief was that he was 'at war with the Evil one' (Sims, 1992, p. 43). Because the form of the belief demonstrated the characteristics of a delusion, and an associated auditory hallucination spoke the man's thoughts out loud, Sims is clear that the diagnosis is one of schizophrenia. The religious content of the belief is thus a secondary consideration. Indeed, many Christians might – in a general sense –

believe that they are 'at war' with evil. However, the definition of delusion is controversial, and we now know that auditory verbal hallucinations are experienced by people without a diagnosis of schizophrenia (Cook. 2018, p. 7). The form of psychopathology alone is not always an easy or reliable indicator of psychopathology.

Jackson and Fulford, in contrast to Sims, argue that psychopathology is not a reliable test of the distinction between psychosis and spiritual experience. Rather, the distinction depends upon the values and beliefs of the person concerned. In their study, 15 cases were selected from an archive of 1,000 accounts of spiritual experience on the basis of evidence of possible delusions or hallucinations, absence of psychiatric treatment, good social functioning and geographical proximity to the research centre. In this highly selected (and presumably very unusual) sample, evidence of psychopathology was, unsurprisingly, present. However, the individuals concerned valued their experiences, identified them as spiritual and were not incapacitated by them. The authors do not finally offer specific guidance on how to distinguish between spiritual and pathological experiences. However, they do emphasise the need to understand psychopathology as 'embedded' within the values and beliefs of the person concerned.

In this context, the nine criteria (listed earlier in this chapter) offered by Menezes and Moreira-Almeida are potentially helpful when assessing any particular patient. They do not include psychopathology within their list and one might argue, *pace* Jackson and Fulford, that this is a significant omission. In many cases, exactly as Sims argues, the form of psychopathology may provide helpful pointers towards a diagnosis. However, Menezes and Moreira-Almeida do show awareness of what Jackson and Fulford would call 'embeddedness'. Spiritual/religious experiences have to be assessed in the context of impact on functioning, cultural background, a broadly holistic understanding of well-being ('personal growth') and the impact on relationships with others.

However, there are a number of problems with the approach taken by Menezes and Moreira-Almeida. First, and importantly, the criterion 'lack of suffering', which is given pride of place in their list, does not adequately nuance the relationship between suffering and spiritual/religious experiences. Although the authors note that 'the initial stages of a religious or spiritual experience can be accompanied by great personal suffering', they go on to suggest that this 'can be overcome as the individual progresses in the comprehension and control of his experience'. Given that many of the most profound spiritual and religious experiences have been forged through suffering (e.g., Julian of Norwich or John of the Cross; see 'Dark Night Experiences' entry in the Glossary), and that neither spirituality nor religion guarantees that suffering can be avoided or 'overcome' (depending on exactly what is meant by this word), this is not a helpful indicator of pathology. Indeed, it may be likely to lead to misclassification rather than help with diagnosis.

Secondly, it is now clear that many psychotic-like experiences (including some that are spiritual/religious) are identifiable in the general population among people who are functioning well and not in need of help from psychiatric services (Heriot-Maitland et al., 2012). Valid distinctions in psychopathology, if they can be made at all, may depend upon quantitative rather than qualitative differences (Johns and Os, 2001).

Thirdly, and most importantly of all, such an approach is prejudicial towards people suffering from mental disorders. Why may someone not be mentally ill *and* have a valid spiritual/religious experience? In support of this last contention, recent qualitative research suggests that patients may indeed have important and meaningful religious experiences during the course of episodes of mania (Ouwehand et al., 2018; Ouwehand, 2020).

Where does this leave the psychiatrist when assessing those patients who assert that they are not ill and that they have had a meaningful and valuable spiritual/religious experience? Although it might seem highly problematic and difficult to assess, the most important message here must be that it is not a matter to be ignored or avoided simply because it is 'too difficult'. Complex assessments of this kind are a part of what psychiatry is all about, and, I would argue, the literature does give us grounds for saying some things with confidence.

First, Sims is right. Psychopathology is important, and if we neglect to do a thorough mental state examination we run the risks of failing to properly understand the experiences of our patients, and missing signs of mental disorder. However, it is not all about psychopathology.

Secondly, therefore, Jackson and Fulford are right. Psychopathology does not always help us to distinguish the pathological from the spiritual/religious, and mental phenomena are embedded within the beliefs and values of our patients. If we do not assess these, we fail to understand what is really important – both to our patients, and for our own work as diagnosticians.

As Menezes and Moreira-Almeida have pointed out, there is a bigger picture to consider and we need to view our patients' experiences from a variety of different angles. However, speaking personally, I do not like the idea of 'differential diagnosis' being applied to spiritual experience. This seems a much too medical approach, which risks alienation and misunderstanding between patient and clinician, and implies an either/or dichotomy which is not helpful. The making of a diagnosis is a core task for the psychiatrist, but every patient, whatever their diagnosis (or lack of one), has to be able to make sense of their experiences within their spiritual/religious tradition or worldview. It is the task of the psychiatrist to assist in this process, and not to undermine it.

In summary, religious experiences may be diverse in frequency, form, content and significance. Their relationship to psychopathology is complex, but this complexity is not well characterised on the basis of binary distinctions between clinical vs. non-clinical, or spiritual vs. pathological. Experiences, including experiences of illness, can be spiritually and religiously meaningful, and psychiatry needs to take care to tread carefully on this sacred ground.

Hearing Voices

Recent research on voice hearing (auditory verbal hallucinations) is particularly illuminating with respect to these problems. Although voice hearing is traditionally associated with major mental illness, it is now known that many people in the general population hear voices (De Leede-Smith and Barkus, 2013). The main distinction between clinical and non-clinical groups appears to be in terms of the negative content and emotional valence of the voice. Those who hear distressing voices are more likely to be diagnosed as suffering from mental disorder. However, both groups are more likely to have experienced childhood trauma, with odds ratios ranging from two to seven times the rate observed in healthy controls (Daalman et al., 2012). A history of suffering per se therefore does not distinguish between the groups (Cook, 2018, pp. 185–186).

Voice hearing is also associated with spiritual/religious practices (Dein and Littlewood, 2007; Luhrmann, 2012; Dein and Cook, 2015), at least within the Christian tradition (and probably also within other religious traditions, although research on other traditions is currently, with some exceptions, largely lacking). A recent qualitative study of spiritually significant voices, in a predominantly Christian sample in the UK, showed evidence of phenomenological similarity with voices traditionally considered to be evidence of mental disorder, even though most of the respondents did not report a psychiatric diagnosis (Cook et al., 2020). It also showed that content and context were important to understanding the significance of the voice. Thus, for example, some religious voices are heard only at times of crisis, whereas others may be ongoing experiences associated with either positive or negative affect. Most of the voices reported in this study were benevolent, but some were understood as evil. Similarly, spiritually significant voices may be identified within other religious traditions – for example, voices attributed to djinn by Muslims (Blom and Hoffer, 2012) and disincarnate spirits in Spiritualism (Powell and Moseley, 2020).

Conclusion

Returning to our starting point, what may we conclude in relation to the importance of religion for psychiatry?

Amidst the diversity of the world's religious traditions, certain 'family resemblances' may be identified – concerns for social cohesion, identity, sacred narratives and a way of life constructed around a relationship, in ritual, prayer or meditation, with the transcendent. Religions are concerned with such things as meaning and purpose in life, which are also important for psychiatry, but religions address these concerns with very different systems of symbols, vocabularies and practices from those in psychiatry. The potential for misunderstanding between psychiatrists and their religious patients is therefore great.

Although clinicians will not wish to become immersed in academic arguments about the definition of 'religion', psychiatric research has focused unduly on easily operationalised research variables, and thus an emphasis on various kinds of religiosity at the expense of understanding what is at the heart of religion. Psychiatric research attends to what Taves would call the 'special paths' that lead to the ultimate goals of religion, rather than giving attention to the 'special things' that constitute those goals.

There is a certain irony in that many religions, in practice, appear to be very concerned about the special paths that people take, even though it is ultimately only the special things that matter. Disentangling all of this – for example, in a case of obsessive-compulsive disorder – can be complicated, and such tasks are often best worked on by collaboration between a psychiatrist and a mental health chaplain or faith leader.

Psychiatry, as clinical practice and as science, has understandably tended to focus on its own goal of mental well-being, but this is not the ultimate end towards which religions look. Of course, it does depend upon how psychiatrists define mental well-being (Cook, 2020), but generally such definitions have not explicitly included spiritual or religious well-being. A clinical understanding of the religious goals and aspirations of patients is sometimes essential (and often helpful) in service of the contextualisation of psychopathology, and the possibility of a treatment plan that is owned by both patient and psychiatrist.

Among the special paths that patients take which psychiatrists should be particularly concerned about are various forms of religious and spiritual struggles and other (unusual or distressing) religious experiences. Struggling is not necessarily a sign of ill health. Indeed, in a spiritual/religious context, struggles may be a sign of well-being, even if they are sometimes associated with psychiatric symptomatology. Anger with God, conflict with religious authorities, worry and guilt, doubt or questions about meaning may all have positive and/or negative connotations, and their significance for diagnosis cannot be properly understood out of context. Similarly, beliefs about demonic affliction, or about the significance of hallucinatory voices, can only be properly understood in their social, cultural and religious context. A patient-centred approach, which takes into account – and values – the richness of religious narrative and tradition, is essential.

The bewildering diversity of religions is certainly a challenge to research, but it is also a challenge in clinical practice. The clinical art should surely be the ability to find out what are the 'special things' – the symbols and systems of meaning – towards which any particular patient desires to move. The paths that they take, although important, are not the primary concerns of religion. However, the good psychiatrist needs to show a sympathetic ability to be conversant both about the paths that people take (their particular forms of religiosity) and the special things towards which they orientate their lives. This does not require an encyclopaedic knowledge of religions. It requires an ability to engage in meaningful and curious conversation about the lived religion of the individual patient in his or her wider social, cultural and religious context.

Spiritual/religious experience is not merely another option on the list of differential diagnoses. It is a domain of enquiry that needs particular and careful attention in its own right. Patients rarely present to mental health services unless they (or others) are suffering in some way, but suffering may also be a sign of spiritual well-being and does not always require a medical diagnosis.

References

Appelbaum, P. S., Robbins, P. C. and Roth, L. H. (1999) Dimensional approach to delusions: comparison across types and diagnoses. *American Journal of Psychiatry*, 156, 1938–1943.

Asma, S. T. (2018) *Why We Need Religion*. Oxford: Oxford University Press.

Blom, J. D. and Hoffer, C. B. M. (2012) Djinns. In J. D. Blom and I. E. C. Sommer, eds., *Hallucinations: Research and Practice*. New York: Springer, pp. 235–247.

Bowker, J. (2007) *Beliefs That Changed the World*. London: Quercus.

Bowker, J. (2018) *Religion Hurts: Why Religions Do Harm as Well as Good*. London: SPCK.

Bowland, S., Edmond, T. and Fallot, R. D. (2012) Evaluation of a spiritually focused intervention with older trauma survivors. *Social Work*, 57, 73–82.

Bowman, E. S. (1991) Clinical and spiritual effects of exorcism in fifteen patients with multiple personality disorder. *Dissociation*, 6, 222–238.

Bull, D. L., Ellason, J. W. and Ross, C. A. (1998) Exorcism revisited: positive outcomes with dissociative identity disorder. *Journal of Psychology and Theology*, 26, 188–196.

Büssing, A., ed. (2019a) *Measures of Spirituality/ Religiosity (2018)*. Basel: MDPI.

Büssing, A., ed. (2019b) *Measures of Spirituality/ Religiosity: Description of Concepts and Validation of Instruments*. Basel: MDPI.

Cook, C. C. H. (2011) The faith of the psychiatrist. *Mental Health, Religion & Culture*, 14, 9–17.

Cook, C. C. H. (2013) Transcendence, immanence and mental health. In C. C. H. Cook, ed., *Spirituality, Theology & Mental Health: Multidisciplinary Perspectives*. London: SCM, pp. 141–159.

Cook, C. C. H. (2018) *Hearing Voices, Demonic and Divine: Scientific and Theological Perspectives*. London: Routledge.

Cook, C. C. H. (2020) Mental health and the Gospel: Boyle Lecture 2020. *Zygon*, 55, 1107–1123.

Cook, C. C. H., Powell, A., Alderson-Day, B. and Woods, A. (2020) Hearing spiritually significant voices: a phenomenological survey and taxonomy. https://doi.org/10.1136/medhum-2020-012021.

Daalman, K., Diederen, K. M., Derks, E. M. et al. (2012) Childhood trauma and auditory verbal hallucinations. *Psychological Medicine*, 42, 2475–2484.

De Leede-Smith, S. and Barkus, E. (2013) A comprehensive review of auditory verbal hallucinations: lifetime prevalence, correlates and mechanisms in healthy and clinical individuals. *Frontiers in Human Neuroscience*, 7, 367.

De Menezes, A. and Moreira-Almeida, A. (2009) Differential diagnosis between spiritual experiences and mental disorders of religious content. *Revista de Psiquiatria Clínica*, 36, 69–76.

Dein, S. and Cook, C. C. H. (2015) God put a thought into my mind: the charismatic Christian experience of receiving communications from God. *Mental Health, Religion & Culture*, 18, 97–113.

Dein, S. and Littlewood, R. (2007) The voice of God. *Anthropology & Medicine*, 14, 213–228.

Dufresne, T., ed. (2012) *The Future of an Illusion: Sigmund Freud*. Ontario: Broadview.

Dworsky, C. K. O., Pargament, K. I., Wong, S. and Exline, J. J. (2016) Suppressing spiritual struggles: the role of experiential avoidance in mental health. *Journal of Contextual Behavioral Science*, 5, 258–265.

Exline, J. J., Pargament, K. I., Grubbs, J. B. and Yali, A. M. (2014) The Religious and Spiritual Struggles Scale: development and initial validation. *Psychology of Religion and Spirituality*, 6, 208–222.

Fraser, G. A. (1993) Exorcism rituals: effects on multiple personality disorder patients. *Dissociation: Progress in the Dissociative Disorders*, 6, 239–244.

Geertz, C. (1993) Religion as a cultural system. In C. Geertz, ed., *The Interpretation of Cultures: Selected Essays*. New York: Fontana, pp. 87–125.

Gibbel, M. R., Regueiro, V. and Pargament, K. I. (2019) A spiritually integrated intervention for spiritual struggles among adults with mental illness: results of an initial evaluation. *Spirituality in Clinical Practice*, 6, 240–255.

Glock, C. Y. and Stark, R. (1965) *Religion and Society in Tension*. Chicago, IL: Rand McNally & Company.

Gray, A. J. (2011) Worldviews. *International Psychiatry*, 8, 58–60.

Hackney, C. H. and Sanders, G. S. (2003) Religiosity and mental health: a meta-analysis of recent studies. *Journal for the Scientific Study of Religion*, 42, 43–55.

Hanegraaff, W. J. (2016) Reconstructing "religion" from the bottom up. *Numen*, 63, 576–605.

Harrison, V. S. (2006) The pragmatics of defining religion in a multi-cultural world. *International Journal for Philosophy of Religion*, 59, 133–152.

Heriot-Maitland, C., Knight, M. and Peters, E. (2012) A qualitative comparison of psychotic-like phenomena in clinical and non-clinical populations. *British Journal of Clinical Psychology*, 51, 37–53.

Hill, P. C. and Hood, R. W. (1999) *Measures of Religiosity*. Birmingham, AL: Religious Education Press.

Jackson, M. and Fulford, K. W. M. (1997) Spiritual experience and pychopathology. *Philosophy, Psychiatry, & Psychology*, 4, 41–65.

James, W. (1902) *The Varieties of Religious Experience: A Study in Human Nature*. New York: Longmans, Green & Co.

Johns, L. C. and Os, J. V. (2001) The continuity of psychotic experiences in the general population. *Clinical Psychology Review*, 21, 1125–1141.

Johnson, T. M., Grim, B. J. and Bellofatto, G. A. (2013) *The World's Religions in Figures: An Introduction to International Religious Demography*. Oxford: Wiley-Blackwell.

Josephson, A. M. and Wiesner, I. S. (2004) Worldview in psychiatric assessment. In A. M. Josephson and J. R. Peteet, eds., *Handbook of Spirituality and Worldview in Clinical Practice*. Washington, DC: American Psychiatric Publishing, pp. 15–30.

Kass, J. D., Friedman, R., Leserman, J., Zuttermeister, P. C. and Benson, H. (1991) Health outcomes and a new index of spiritual experience. *Journal for the Scientific Study of Religion*, 30, 203–211.

Koenig, H. G. (2008) Concerns about measuring "spirituality" in research. *Journal of Nervous and Mental Disease*, 196, 349–355.

Koenig, H. G. (2011) *Spirituality and Health Research: Methods, Measurements, Statistics, and Resources*. West Conshohocken, PA: Templeton Press.

Koenig, H. G. (2018) *Religion and Mental Health: Research and Clinical Applications*. London: Academic Press.

Koenig, H. G., King, D. E. and Carson, V. B., eds. (2012) *Handbook of Religion and Health*. New York: Oxford University Press.

Koenig, H. G., Al-Zaben, F. and Vanderweele, T. J. (2020) Religion and psychiatry: recent developments in research. *BJPsych Advances*, 26, 262–272.

Lucchetti, A. L., Peres, M. F., Vallada, H. P. and Lucchetti, G. (2015) Spiritual treatment for depression in Brazil: an experience from Spiritism. *Explore (NY)*, 11, 377–386.

Lucchetti, G., Aguiar, P. R., Braghetta, C. C. et al. (2012) Spiritist psychiatric hospitals in Brazil: integration of conventional psychiatric treatment and spiritual complementary therapy. *Culture, Medicine and Psychiatry*, 36, 124–135.

Luhrmann, T. M. (2012) *When God Talks Back*. New York: Knopf.

Lukoff, D. (1985) The diagnosis of mystical experiences with psychotic features. *Journal of Transpersonal Psychology*, 17, 155–181.

McGuire, M. B. (2008) *Lived Religion: Faith and Practice in Everyday Life*, Oxford: Oxford University Press.

Marks, L. D., Dollahite, D. C. and Young, K. P. (2019) Struggles experienced by religious minority families in the United States. *Psychology of Religion and Spirituality*, 11, 247–256.

Moreira-Almeida, A. and Lotufo Neto, F. (2005) Spiritist views of mental disorders in Brazil. *Transcultural Psychiatry*, 42, 570–595.

Nicholi, A. M. (2004) Introduction: definition and significance of a worldview. In A. M. Josephson and J. R. Peteet, eds., *Handbook of Spirituality and Worldview in Clinical Practice*. Washington, DC: American Psychiatric Publishing, pp. 3–12.

Ouwehand, E. (2020) *Mania and Meaning: A Mixed Methods Study into Religious Experiences in People with Bipolar Disorder: Occurrence and Significance*. Groningen: Faculty of Theology & Religious Studies, University of Groningen.

Ouwehand, E., Muthert, H., Zock, H., Boeije, H. and Braam, A. (2018) Sweet delight and endless night: a qualitative exploration of ordinary and extraordinary religious and spiritual experiences in bipolar disorder. *International Journal for the Psychology of Religion*, 28, 31–54.

Pargament, K. I., Smith, B. W., Koenig, H. G. and Perez, L. (1998) Patterns of positive and negative religious coping with major life stressors. *Journal for the Scientific Study of Religion*, 37, 710–724.

Pfeifer, S. (1994) Belief in demons and exorcism in psychiatric patients in Switzerland. *British Journal of Medical Psychology*, 67, 247–258.

Pfeifer, S. (1999) Demonic attributions in nondelusional disorders. *Psychopathology*, 32, 252–259.

Powell, A. and Moseley, P. (2020) When spirits speak: absorption, attribution, and identity among spiritualists who report 'clairaudient' voice experiences. *Mental Health, Religion & Culture*, 23, 841–856.

Rosik, C. H. (2003) Critical issues in the dissociative disorders field: six perspectives from religiously sensitive practitioners. *Journal of Psychology and Theology*, 31, 113–128.

Roxburgh, E. C. and Roe, C. A. (2011) A survey of dissociation, boundary-thinness, and psychological wellbeing in Spiritualist mental mediumship. *Journal of Parapsychology*, 75, 279–299.

Roxburgh, E. C. and Roe, C. A. (2014) Reframing voices and visions using a spiritual model. An interpretative phenomenological analysis of anomalous experiences in mediumship. *Mental Health, Religion & Culture*, 17, 641–653.

Sims, A. C. P. (1992) Symptoms and beliefs. *Journal of the Royal Society of Health*, 112, 42–46.

Smart, N. (1998) *The World's Religions*. Cambridge: Cambridge University Press.

Taves, A. (2011) Special things as building blocks of religions. In R. A. Orsi, ed., *The Cambridge Companion to Religious Studies*. Cambridge: Cambridge University Press, pp. 58–83.

Taves, A. (2018) What is nonreligion? On the virtues of a meaning systems framework for studying nonreligious and religious worldviews in the context of everyday life. *Secularism & Nonreligion*, 7, 9.

Van Os, J., Hanssen, M., Bijl, R. V. and Ravelli, A. (2000) Strauss (1969) revisited: a psychosis continuum in the general population? *Schizophrenia Research*, 45, 11–20.

Pathological Spirituality

Nicola Crowley and Gillie Jenkinson

'Pathological spirituality' is, on one level, a misnomer and a contradiction in terms. The quality of spirituality, for the purposes of this book (see Chapter 1), is by definition the opposite of pathological dysfunction and disease, though it does embrace an approach to suffering.

The Jonestown massacre in the jungle of Guyana in 1978, the deadly Sarin nerve gas attacks in the Tokyo underground by Aum Shinrikyo in 1995, the terrorist attacks by suicide bombers of 9/11 in the USA in 2001 and the 7 July bombings in the UK in 2005, various reports of sexual abuse in the Church of England and the Catholic Church, and the successful case against Keith Raniere and NXIVM in 2020, all illustrate, in different contexts, how pathological and harmful spiritual values can be when a group's beliefs and doctrines take precedence over human health and well-being.

This chapter explores the potential for spiritual beliefs, practices and experiences to become pathological, and considers aspects of psychological control that are used in the fields of religion and spirituality to cause harm.

Path or Pathology?

The past 100 years have witnessed immensely destabilising changes within our society, including the emergence in early 2020 of the novel coronavirus that caused the COVID-19 pandemic. With traditionally cohesive social structures such as the church and the family unit already losing their former status (Murray, 2004), we saw new social 'lock-down' measures introduced on a global scale, restricting people from freely meeting in person, and requiring the use of face coverings. This in turn necessitated an increased reliance on technology (with its capacity operating beyond most people's understanding) together with increased exposure to mainstream, alternative and social media, each working to its own algorithms. The ways in which this is likely to deeply affect humanity remain to be seen.

It is these sorts of psychosocial disruptors that can disturb one's healthy sense of reality, and which can both consciously and unconsciously affect human decision making and behaviour. It is therefore during these times of uncertainty that individuals are particularly vulnerable to the influence of pathological or high-demand or cultic groups using 'push and pull factors' (Vergani et al., 2018) to subtly influence thoughts, emotions and behaviour.

'Information disease' (Conway and Siegelman, 2005) is a category of disorders relating to the lasting changes of mind and personality that may be brought on by, among other things, reckless or excessive use of popular spiritual and personal growth practices. In addition, during the last decade this personal growth has been intensified by the unregulated use of 'medicine' (psilocybin, ayahuasca and other hallucinogenic drugs) for spiritual 'journeys' with enthusiastic but largely untrained and unregulated 'spiritual guides' (Pollan, 2019). In parallel with this there has been a resurgence of medical interest in these compounds (Carhart-Harris and Goodwin, 2017) but, as this chapter will demonstrate, our Western cultural background and education have often not prepared us to safely navigate this challenging new territory.

Seeking a clearly guided path that promises relief from suffering, answers important existential questions and offers some form of self-improvement or self-transformation feels necessary to many. The advent of psychoanalysis in the twentieth century, with its own controversial dismissal of religious or mystical experience as merely regressive, and the subsequent evolution of numerous different schools of psychology and psychotherapy, together with the New Age movement and popular psychology self-help books, each provide a different perspective on what it is to be human. When, however, does adherence to a spiritual, religious or therapeutic path lead to pathologically dehumanising or even life-threatening consequences?

Healthy Vs. Pathological Spirituality

A distinction needs to be made between those spiritual practices and beliefs that foster the healthy development of a person within his or her community and those that have been incorporated into a person's lifestyle and subsequently cause harm to him or her or to others.

The issue of harm is complex. Almendros et al. (2013) note that some groups (including religious and spiritual groups) may be positive in certain respects, display sect-like (or cult-like) characteristics in other respects and be innocuous in yet other respects.

Rather than attempting to classify groups as 'good' or 'bad' or 'harmful' or 'not harmful', and their beliefs as 'true' or 'false', it can be helpful to envisage a continuum with a critical point beyond which a group can progress to become harmful if it takes its beliefs and/or practices to the extreme (Chambers et al., 1994; Kendall, 2006). Figure 17.1 illustrates this point.

Battista (1996) describes pathological spirituality by exploring two concepts – spiritual defences and offensive spirituality.

Spiritual Defences

Spiritual defences are spiritual beliefs that prevent a person from expressing his or her actual embodied emotional self. They include. for example:

- submission to 'the other', or to authority, rationalised as 'the spiritual'
- the quality of humility
- inability to develop intimacy in relationships, rationalised as God being the primary and only necessary relationship in life
- failure to deal with interpersonal or sexual needs, rationalised as ascetic practice
- failure to deal with the practical materialistic aspect of life, rationalised as 'God will provide'.

Spiritual defences enable a 'spiritual bypass' – a premature transcendence of personal pain and suffering and denial of the real substance of a grounded life that, if it was not

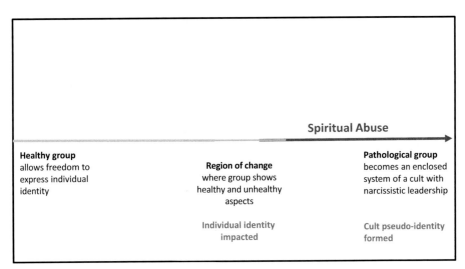

Figure 17.1 Continuum of group dynamics from healthy to pathological.

ignored, could instead be viewed as the 'ore' (Hillman, 2004) which if forged on the 'anvil of life' can shape our development and yield valuable qualities.

Offensive Spirituality

This refers to an individual's assertion of him- or herself as spiritually developed, as a means of constraining another person. It is the narcissistic use of a spiritual persona or spiritual identification (Battista, 1996). The narcissistic misuse of both spiritual and psychoanalytic principles has been addressed by cultural critics (Frank and Frank, 1993; Masson, 1994; Raubolt, 2006; Shaw, 2013). Failure to recognise this quality in gurus, leaders and influencers can be a serious pitfall for those on the path of psychospiritual exploration.

False Spiritual Teachers or Gurus

Anthony Storr defines a guru as a teacher who 'claims special knowledge of the meaning of life, and therefore feels entitled to tell others how life should be lived' (Storr, 1996, p. xi). He differentiates between 'morally superior individuals [who] exist [with] integrity, virtue and goodness . . . beyond the reach of most of us' (Storr, 1996, p. xii) and self-appointed experts who promise their followers new ways of self-development and new paths to salvation. The latter tend to demonstrate narcissistic and/or sociopathic personality traits.

Storr observes that guru types tend to have experienced isolated childhoods. They possess a limited capacity to form friendships, tend to be elitist and anti-democratic, and are often intolerant of criticism. They hold their belief systems with unshakeable conviction and this certainty, together with their persuasiveness, adds to their charisma. Eileen Barker states that 'Almost by definition, charismatic leaders are unpredictable, for they are bound neither by traditions nor rules; they are not answerable to other human beings' (Barker, 1989, p. 13). Shaw notes that such leaders often use power to 'intimidate, seduce, coerce, belittle and humiliate others' (Shaw, 2013, p. 47).

Unshakeable convictions may follow a period of chaotic suffering in the guru's life, thus giving meaning to it. They may have experienced a period of mental illness, involving paranoia or grandiosity. Regardless of whether their experience fulfils psychiatric diagnostic criteria, the essential question remains: is their behaviour harmful to others or not? Deikman (1983) asserts that a teacher who is guilty of financial or sexual exploitation represents a drastic failure of responsibility that disqualifies him or her from any special consideration. Examples of grandiose and paranoid cult leaders include the convicted NXIVM cult leader Keith Raniere (Zeiders and Devlin, 2020, p. 105) and the sex offender 'John of God' (Nogueira, 2019). The former Anglican bishop and sex offender Peter Ball was the founder of a monastic community (the Community of Glorious Ascension), where practices included sexual abuse of men and boys, hidden from public view (Independent Inquiry into Child Sexual Abuse, 2019), and which was little more than an abusive and harmful cult.

Harmful Groups

The beneficial aspects of belonging to a group, religious or otherwise, are well recognised in psychological and sociological literature. It is a matter of moral, ethical, religious, political and sometimes clinical opinion whether the influences of being part of a particular group have, or have not, been good for the individual and hence for society.

Definitions of groups that may be harmful derive from different epistemologies, and can be ambiguous, pejorative and controversial (Barrett, 2001; Langone, 2007). Attempts to define and understand them lead to polarisation of views (Jenkinson, 2016; Lalich, 2004). Although there have been numerous attempts to define harmful spiritual groups, here we shall consider the following categories from the cultic studies field:

- cults
- sects
- new religious movements (NRMs)
- charismatic groups.

Cults

It has been estimated that there are around 5,000 potentially harmful cultic groups in the USA (Matthews and Salazar, 2014) and 800–1,500 NRMs operating in the UK (INFORM, personal communication, 12 January 2016). Some of these are 'abusive cults', although because of the hidden nature of abuse (Herman, 1992) it is virtually impossible to ascertain how many 'abusive cults' exist.

There are numerous definitions of cults – dictionary, anthropological, theological, psychological (definitions which describe the effects of cult involvement on the psychosocial well-being of individuals and their families) and sociological (definitions which tend to view behaviour as it occurs in social interactions with a group or a movement). Jenkinson (2016, p. 82) has adapted the psychological definitions of a cult proposed by Langone (1993) and Lifton (1999) as follows:

> An abusive cult is a group or movement that to a significant degree:
>
> A Exhibits great or excessive devotion to some person, idea, or thing.
> B Uses a thought-reform programme to persuade, control, and socialise members (i.e. to integrate them into the group's unique pattern of relationships, beliefs, values, and practices).

C Systematically induces states of psychological dependency in members.

D Displays a combination of quest from the seeker below, and exploitation from the leadership above, usually economic or sexual, in order to advance the leadership's goals.

E Engenders an 'us' and 'them' mentality, fear and rejection of the world outside the group.

F Causes psychological harm to members, their families and the community, including children.

G Ill treatment or impairment of children's health (mental or physical) or development (physical, intellectual, emotional, social or behavioural) attributable to lack of adequate parental care or control.

H May be abusive throughout or in a particular geographical location or sub-section of the organisation.

Stein (2017, pp. 15–21) has defined and expanded on five dimensions of a totalist group or cult as follows:

1 leadership (as charismatic and authoritarian)
2 structure (as closed, hierarchical, yet insecure)
3 ideology (closed and exclusive)
4 process ('brainwashing')
5 outcomes (exploitation and deployability of followers).

At the extreme, the term 'destructive cult', sometimes called 'doomsday cult' (Singer, 2003), can be used to refer to any group that becomes potentially deadly, including quasi-religious groups that have intentionally killed people (Lifton, 1999).

Crowley (2020) notes that the first two decades of the twenty-first century have been characterised by numerous violent terror attacks, also involving suicides of the perpetrators and the deaths of many others. These terror attacks have reportedly been mostly carried out by terrorist groups who are thought to be motivated by a religious ideology (in this case, scholars argue that this is the ideology of the 'Salafi-jihad' rather than the religion of Islam; Moghadam, 2008) and apparently acting under the direction of a so-called self-appointed religious authority (Hassan and Shah, 2019). Clear parallels between types of destructive cults and terrorist groups have been discussed in the literature (Rodríguez-Carballeira et al., 2011), with one evidence-based historical qualitative meta-analysis concluding that ISIS meets the criteria for being an apocalyptic 'death' cult (Barron and Maye, 2017). This underlines the importance of recognising the characteristics of cultic groups, and how they can develop across different political, religious and cultural belief systems, causing immense personal and collective harm.

There are also many religious groups, new and old, that are not cults as defined here. A group should not be assumed to be a cult simply because it exhibits one or two of the above-mentioned features.

Sects

A sect is generally viewed as 'a separate, exclusive entity, with abstract ideas, existing within another, larger religious organisation' (Reber and Reber, 2001, p. 656).

New Religious Movements

Jenkinson (2016) notes that the term 'new religious movement' (Barker, 1989) was adopted by sociologists of religion in the 1970s to refer to a religious faith or an ethical, spiritual or philosophical movement of recent origin that is not part of an established faith tradition. The term was coined in an attempt to 'neutralise' the label (Brockway and Rajashekar, 1987; Barker, 1989). The fact that groups labelled cults or NRMs may not have a religious basis, but may be political, scientific, alien-orientated or emphasise personal growth, such as psychotherapeutic and human potential movements, contributes to the complexity (Barker, 1996; Healy, 2011) and confusion. Added to this are those groups that are not 'new' but have been in existence since the early twentieth century or earlier, and those that formed within already established mainstream churches, such as the Nine O'Clock Service in Sheffield (Howard, 1996) – a cult which, unusually, evolved within a mainstream Church of England church. An NRM is nevertheless defined as a group or movement that 'has taken its rise in the past 150 years and remains extant' (Chryssides, 2016, p. 17), is primarily religious and operates apart from the dominant culture in which it is located. It seeks adherents from the host culture, but may originate from another culture. The important point is that it is set apart from the dominant culture, at least initially (Healy, 2011, p. 3). Psychologists and clinicians have generally avoided the NRM label. (For further discussion, see Chapter 16.)

Charismatic Groups

The model of the charismatic group has been developed by Galanter (1989), who uses this term to describe modern cults and zealous self-help movements. He proposes that members of charismatic groups are characterised by the following psychological elements:

- a shared belief system
- a high level of social cohesiveness
- strongly influenced by the group's behavioural norms
- impute charismatic (or sometimes divine) power to the group or its leadership (Galanter, 1989, p. 5).

Galanter asserts that charismatic groups, including some therapy groups, can relieve certain aspects of psychopathology, as well as precipitate psychiatric symptoms.

Harmful Vs. Healthy groups

Religious, spiritual and therapy groups can be positive and life-affirming or inherently authoritarian and manipulative. Some key differences are listed in Table 17.1.[1]

Group dynamics are powerful and can exert considerable influence on their members' psychiatric status (Galanter, 1990). Certain therapy groups have been described as applying orthodox methods of psychological treatment in an unorthodox and ill-directed manner (Singer, 2003). Professionals and non-professionals alike have been involved in such groups (Temerlin and Temerlin, 1982, 1986). Some psychoanalysts have commented on the cult-style aspects of psychoanalytic training and institutes (Kernberg, 1986; Masson, 1994; Raubolt, 2006; Shaw, 2013).

---

[1] We thank Ian Haworth of the Cult Information Centre, UK for his kind permission to reproduce the tables.

Table 17.1. Comparison of healthy religious/spiritual and potentially harmful cult-style groups[a]

Healthy religious/spiritual group	Potentially harmful cult-style group
Conversion or 'worldview shift' (Lalich, 2004)	Coercion or 'coercive persuasion conversion' (Lalich, 2004)
Commitment freely chosen	Commitment via psychological force
Between individual and God	Between individual and group
Empowers members	Disempowers members
Increases discernment	Decreases discernment
Unconditional love for members	Conditional love for members
Recognises and values the family	Alienates members from the family
Growth and maturing of members	Regression and stunting of members
Individual uniqueness	Cloned personalities
Happiness and fulfilment	Artificial 'high'
Unity	Uniformity
Truth leads to experience	Experience becomes 'truth'
Accountability of leadership	No accountability of leadership
Questioning encouraged	Questioning discouraged
Honesty prevails	The end justifies the means
Does not hide behind fronts	Hides behind fronts

[a] Adapted from Haworth (2001).

Frank and Frank (1993) take the view that all psychotherapies are a vehicle for influence and persuasion. Indeed they define psychotherapy as a form of influence, characterised by a healing agent, 'typically a person trained in a socially sanctioned method of healing believed to be effective by the sufferer', 'a sufferer who seeks relief from the healer' and 'a healing relationship' in which the healer 'tries to bring about relief of symptoms' (Frank and Frank, 1993, p. 2). Their definition of psychotherapy therefore encompasses Western psychotherapy, the placebo effect in medicine, religio-magical healing (including religious revivalism), the activity of cults, thought reform and brainwashing. They refer to the power imbalance in the therapeutic encounter, and comment that 'in long term therapy, the patient and therapist progressively shape each other's behaviour, with the patient increasingly fulfilling the therapist's expectations' (Frank and Frank, 1993, p. 176).

The reality is usually less unbalanced, but there is a warning here for the spiritual, religious, psychiatric and psychotherapeutic professions to be aware of the inherent power imbalance, and to avoid causing harm. The key differences between healthy and potentially harmful therapeutic approaches are listed in Table 17.2.

Some Descriptions of Cult Dynamics

Terms such as 'conversion', 'brainwashing', 'thought reform', 'coercive persuasion', 'mind control techniques' and 'snapping' are all attempts to describe psychological methods employed by cult-style groups to recruit and maintain new members.

Table 17.2. Key differences between healthy and potentially harmful therapeutic groups[a]

Healthy therapeutic group	Potentially harmful, cult-style therapy group
Rehabilitates	Debilitates
Objectives: goals agreed by client	Objectives: therapist or leader's goals
Promotes healthy relationships with others	Fosters alienation from others
Aim: independence of client	Aim: dependence of member
Psychologically enables the client	Psychologically disables the member
Questioning encouraged	Questioning discouraged
Decision making ability enhanced	Decision making ability impaired
Therapist accountable	Cult leader not accountable
Qualifications recognized by outside body	Self-appointed
Fees agreed in advance	Fees often inflated once member fully involved
For benefit of client	For benefit of leader
Does not hide behind fronts	Hides behind fronts

[a] Adapted from Haworth (2001).

Conversion or Worldview Shift

It is widely recognised that conversion to a religious faith is, for many, deeply significant, life-enhancing and can bring with it a huge sense of relief (Storr, 1996).

The term is used here in a broader sense. Lalich (2004) notes that conversion is typically thought of as a process of religious change, but that it also takes place in social contexts, such as changing political views. She notes that conversion is a process by which a person develops a new perspective on life, that external pressure may or may not be present, and that the process may be sudden or gradual. Again, it occurs on a continuum. Conversion may, in some cases, be genuine despite external pressure or coercion.

Lalich (2004, p. 15) has adopted the term 'worldview shift' to describe the internal change that takes place as a person adopts this new perspective (the term is not restricted to religious settings). If the worldview shift has taken place within a coercive environment (a 'coercive persuasion conversion'), the initial sense of relief at 'having found the answer', which is associated with a kind of personal freedom, may also result in a loss of sense of self and the development of the cult pseudo-personality (Lalich, 2004; Jenkinson, 2008, 2016).

Brainwashing Theories

'Brainwashing' is a popular term that was coined in 1951 by the journalist Edward Hunter, and is a loose translation of the Chinese phrase *hsi nao*, meaning 'washing the brain'. It describes the process by which individuals captured in the Korean War and in Communist China could quickly reverse their allegiance and confess to fictional war crimes (Lifton, 1989; Hassan, 2000).

Thought Reform

Robert Jay Lifton, who studied this process, noted that the term 'brainwashing' quickly 'developed a life of its own' (Lifton, 1989, p. 3), sometimes causing fear at one end of the continuum or ridicule at the other. He noted that the term is 'far from precise with a questionable usefulness' (Lifton, 1989, p. 4). To describe the process of conversion from one ideology to another, Lifton preferred to use the term 'thought reform'. He describes eight psychological components that are used to create the 'totalist' environment in which this takes place (Lifton, 1989, pp. 419–537):

1   milieu control – the control of the environment, information and communication
2   mystical manipulation – the manipulation of experiences that appear spontaneous but in fact were planned and orchestrated in order to elevate the leader
3   demand for purity – the world is viewed in all or nothing terms and the members are constantly exhorted to conform to the ideology of the group and strive for perfection
4   confession – sins, as defined by the group, are to be confessed either to a personal monitor or publicly to the group
5   sacred science – the group's doctrine or ideology is considered to be the ultimate 'truth', beyond all questioning or dispute
6   loading the language – the group interprets or uses words and phrases in new ways that the outside world does not understand, which results in 'thought stopping' and restricts critical thinking
7   doctrine over person – the doctrine takes precedence over the member's well-being, and the member's personal experience is subordinated to the sacred science and any contrary experiences must be denied or reinterpreted to fit the ideology of the group
8   dispensing of existence – the group has the prerogative to decide who has the right to exist and who does not, sometimes taken literally.

Lifton (1999) later came to believe that thought reform could be accomplished without physical coercion (as was the case with Korean and Chinese prisoners of war), and acknowledged that it is used in some cults (Lifton, 2019). There is some evidence of this type of psychosocial conditioning in the training of terrorists and suicide bombers (Stahelski, 2005; Lalich and Tobias, 2006), and, as already mentioned, there are clear parallels between destructive cults and terrorist groups (Rodríguez-Carballeira et al., 2011).

Coercive Persuasion

There are other perspectives on 'brainwashing'. One is the socio-psychological analysis conducted by Edgar Schein following his study of American civilians who were indoctrinated as Chinese prisoners of war (Schein, 1961). He described this as 'coercive persuasion'. Schein asserted that the essence of coercive persuasion is to produce ideological and behavioural changes in a fully conscious, mentally intact individual. The psychologist Margaret Singer has adapted these theories and applied the term 'co-ordinated programs of coercive influence and behavioural control' (Ofshe and Singer, 1986, p. 4) to the practices of certain religious, spiritual or other types of groups.

Mind Control Techniques

Mind control techniques are strategies designed to manipulate another person's thoughts, feelings and behaviour, within a given context over a period of time, resulting in a relatively greater gain for the manipulator than for those being manipulated (Zimbardo, 1993). Examples include hypnosis, sleep deprivation and control of diet, peer group pressure, rejection of old values, financial commitment, forbidding questioning and fear (Haworth, 2001; Hassan, 2015).

Snapping

Conway and Siegelman (2005, p. 6) applied the term 'snapping' to describe the phenomenon of 'sudden, drastic alteration of personality in all its many forms', precipitated specifically by intentional manipulation by others. Their research concluded that this phenomenon was more than a superficial alteration of behaviour or belief, and that it could bring about deeper 'organic' changes in awareness and personality structure.

Who Joins or Is Recruited?

There is no one particular type of person who joins or is recruited into a harmful religion or cult (Lalich and Tobias, 2006). Individual vulnerability factors, such as being friendly, obedient, altruistic and malleable, are a more accurate predictor than personality type. The individual may be vulnerable to recruitment simply because they are at a transition point in their life, bereaved, slightly depressed, lonely (Singer, 2003) or merely in the wrong place at the wrong time (Langone, 2007). Most individuals become involved in a religious or spiritual practice or group in the hope that it will be life-enhancing, but the extent of the premeditated deception applied by these groups is underestimated. Some groups mask their true intention, using deceitful recruitment techniques (Martin, 1993) and grooming practices in order to increase membership.

Research increasingly refers to those joining cults in adulthood as 'first generation' and those who spend all or part of their childhood in a cult as 'second generation' (Kendall, 2006) or 'born and or raised'. A further 'multi-generation' category has been identified (Aebi-Mytton, 2018, 2021), with grandparents and even great grandparents having been born into one of the older groups. The individual has little exposure to culture outside the group. An example of this would be the Amish, usually considered to be a sect rather than a cult.

Psychiatric Intervention

Occasionally, a psychiatrist or psychotherapist will be asked to help someone who has recently left a cult, or be told that the patient under his or her care has been under the influence of such a group. The patient may present with symptoms of anxiety, depression and a dissociative state, perhaps with psychotic symptoms, or be described by their friends or relatives as having completely changed in terms of their personality. It may also be the case that a person with psychosis talks about being damaged or chased by a cult. Some cults continue to threaten former members after they have left, so this information may need to be verified (Singer, 2003).

The following four case studies are compositions based on real clinical situations. All names and identifying details have been changed to protect anonymity.

Case study: Taylor

Born and raised in a cult, recovering from and re-engaging with spiritual practice
Taylor is a 44-year-old married woman, of Anglo-Native American (Cherokee) descent, originally from the southern states of America. She was born into a religious group that was later exposed as a cult in the 1970s. This group held a mixture of fundamentalist, charismatic, Christian teaching and pseudo-Christian views, along with ideas from other sources. It included teaching on the need to 'crucify the shadow' and that there would be

'a second coming of Jesus'. It predicted 'the tribulation' (a 7-year period during which a world religious–political leader called the Anti-Christ takes power), 'Armageddon' (a terrible war provoked by the Anti-Christ in which most people on earth will die) and 'The Rapture' (a miraculous event when Christ will descend from the heavens and save 144.000 believers).

Taylor's mother was a member of the group, but her father lived away from it. He was a highly intelligent man, 'a genius' in mathematics, a recluse who lacked some social skills, but who Taylor describes as gentle in nature. She describes her mother as a beautiful, strong, impassioned woman, who had spiritual gifts such as prophetic dreaming and the ability to speak in tongues, but who also had a dark, violent side to her nature.

Ritualistic abuse occurred on a regular basis. At the age of 5, Taylor took part in a staged 'live judgement day'. The right-hand side of the room was cast as heaven with cult members, including her mother, dressed in white, singing to beautiful angelic music. The other side was cast as hell, with people dressed as Satan moving to loud demonic music. Her aunt was painted white, lying as if dead in a coffin, waiting for resurrection. Her uncle was cast as God, directing cult members to one side or the other. Taylor and her little brother were cast over to the devil's side. She remembers her little brother screaming hysterically, wanting to be with his mother. The children were indoctrinated with the fact that they were part of the devil from then on.

Sunday school lessons consisted of learning from a book called Lucifer. There were hundreds of demonic names associated with each of the negative emotions, which needed to be rote learned and chanted. Anger was not thought to come from the self, but was thought to be given in spirit from the devil.

Rebuke circles were common events, when the person thought to be full of demons would be surrounded by cult members dancing, speaking in tongues, singing in rapture and touching them to force out the devil. Taylor was defiant, and disagreed that she was the devil. She was beaten so severely that her whole face and body would be covered in welts, and she remembers looking at herself in the mirror and shouting to the adults 'Now I am like Jesus'.

She was also sexually abused in the cult by one of its elders and two of her brothers. Her source of refuge was her father's home outside the cult. Sexual abuse was a regular occurrence there, too, by both her father and her grandfather, but the environment and experience of it was much less violent, so she preferred it to the cult environment.

By the time she was 12, she was so full of anger and murderous rage that she declared that if any man ever touched her again she would kill them. She was believed, and the abuse stopped. After this she started to experience nightmares full of terrifying, violent, dark and erotic material, and severe panic attacks that lasted up to 30 minutes at a time, at least three times a day, which lasted for years.

She left the cult at the age of 14 – the age when parents were no longer deemed responsible for the souls of their children. She survived in the outside world. Soon afterwards, the group was exposed as a cult in a local newspaper.

Part of Taylor's recovery has involved working on connecting with her spirituality without dissociating from her body. The practice of martial arts has been useful in this regard. In her recovery she has also needed to recognise felt emotions such as joy and anger, and to disentangle these from the alternative demonic or spiritual names attached to them in her psyche. She has had to learn to recognise emotions as coming from herself. This also meant that later in her recovery she had to accept that the dark negative energies which she naturally experiences are also from within her. This was especially hard, as her early survival of the cult had involved defying her elders' projections that she was a demon. As a mature woman she has been able to work on integrating both sides of herself at a deep level.

For the vast majority of the time that she spent in the cult, both she and the other cult members were in various altered states of consciousness, 'as if we were all hypnotised'. Traumatic memories from that time were stored at that altered level of consciousness, and were barely accessible in everyday normal waking consciousness. Straight-talking therapy therefore provided vital containment and support, but it was not able to touch and hence adequately process the unconscious, damaging material in her psyche, which was driving her agoraphobic symptoms and 'emotional seizures'.

Taylor has since engaged in well-run shamanic and breath-work practices. These processes have allowed her to access this material in a safe setting with the guidance of a qualified practitioner, and as a result her symptoms have completely abated. She currently has a strong psychotherapeutic and spiritual focus in her life. She works as a mental health professional within the psychiatric system, drawing upon her experience working with indigenous cultures, as well as her own training in shamanic and breath-work techniques.

Case study: Steve

Anxiety, quasi-psychotic thoughts and dissociation

At the age of 15, Steve became involved in a pseudo-Buddhist group that promoted the idea of enlightenment. He had been seduced into the group by an older woman whom he recalled had stared at him in a strange and powerful way, exerting a hypnotic effect on him, and he had fallen in love with her. He later discovered that the founding leader of the group was homosexual and was himself persuaded over time that he was in fact homo-sexual, although he had never previously had sexual inclinations towards men. He was traumatised by the cult leader, who had homosexual sex with him when he was just over the age of consent. This act, apparently necessary for 'enlightenment,' was essentially non-consensual, but Steve complied due to subtle threats that non-compliance would lead to expulsion from the group and therefore loss of enlightenment.

Part of the group practice would involve long periods of time meditating, chanting and rocking back and forth. At irregular intervals someone would stand at a microphone giving out very loud injunctions to 'surrender to the Buddha', via the cult leader.

Steve left the group when he was in his mid-twenties, and had considerable problems readjusting to mainstream life. He sought specialist help for his panic attacks and episodes of feeling 'spaced out'. Because he had spent long periods of time effectively in a dissoci-ated state, he was now struggling to focus his mind and critical faculties.

During the therapeutic intervention it was noted that some of his ideas sounded rather paranoid; for example, he was convinced that the group was out to kill him and he remembered someone mentioning turning him into a suicide bomber. He remembered veiled threats about what would happen to him if he left the group. He also expressed some bizarre ideas, that people are really reptiles, which his group had believed along with more classic Buddhist beliefs. He believed he had a reptile living within him, and he said he could see the reptile eyes blinking inside others.

Steve was calmly helped to recall as much as he could in a non-judgemental atmos-phere. His fears relating to threats to his safety and that of others, from this apparently peace-loving Buddhist group, were taken seriously. He was encouraged to challenge the more bizarre ideas by using cognitive techniques, including critical thinking and reasoning.

His levels of dissociation and the bizarre ideas with which he had been indoctrinated began to lessen as he adjusted to the 'real' world. He had a supportive family and was slowly able to normalise back into a functional day-to-day routine.

Case study: Gina/Martha

Cult pseudo-identity

By her mid-twenties, Gina had become disillusioned with being a teacher and was disenchanted with her local church. She heard about a new radical Christian community that had started up a few miles away and although she had heard it was a bit 'wacky', and knew little about it, she felt that there would be no harm in going along and seeing what it was like.

She quickly became involved with the community, drawn in by their apparent genuineness, caring and desire to see her join. The leader was attractive, charismatic and seemed to think she was special.

Gina visited increasingly often, not fully listening to her gut feeling that perhaps it was too good to be true, yet not seeing anything that she felt should put her off. She spent a good deal of time in groups reading the Bible and being taught new ways of interpreting it. This included a teaching that you must leave your family and friends to show commitment to 'God'. She decided to leave her flat and job and to give all of her time to the community. Her family and friends were very concerned about this, but Gina didn't care as her new friends were pushing her to 'lay down her life for Christ' and to 'surrender' herself for the work of the community. She was excited about being accepted into this special group of people. They suggested that she should change her name to Martha to show her commitment to God and to them. She felt more connected to them than ever.

After being a member for some months she was asked to cook the evening meal, but politely declined as she was busy. The demeanour of her new 'friend' suddenly changed. She became cold, hard and chastised her. Gina/Martha was shocked by this sudden change. She could barely comprehend it and became confused. Initially, she felt a spark of anger, but quickly turned this anger against herself for questioning in the first place. This incident was followed by a period of silence towards her from members of the group. Gina/Martha soon learned that if she complied she would feel accepted, and if she did not comply she would receive similar rebukes and silences.

One Sunday, Gina/Martha went for a walk and came back 'full of the joys of spring'. The leader told her to make some breakfast, and she immediately felt resentful and let him know with a small huff that she did not want to. He insisted, so she complied. When the community met for their worship meeting later that day, Gina/Martha was received with chilling coldness, and was told that God was angry with her for her 'bad attitude' and that they wanted to talk to her privately. She was filled with dread. Later, they told her that God would reject her if she did not change her attitude. Gina/Martha was deeply shocked by this and was shaking and frightened. From that time Gina became Martha in actuality. She became quiet, serious and religious, complying fully with the beliefs and practices of her new 'family'. She dressed differently, wore her hair differently and had no more contact with her own family.

Not long afterwards, she was told that God wanted new members to join the community, and although at one time Gina would have questioned 'going out and dragging people in', and would have absolutely refused to do so, at some level Martha remembered the anger and shock of being rebuked, which had happened unpredictably many more times, and she complied. She was told that any tactics were sanctioned in order to bring people in. She was assigned to bring men into the group. Martha understood the implications and Gina was truly buried deep within. Martha believed that sleeping with men in order to 'convert them' and obeying without question was the work of God.

Gina's personality was profoundly altered by this experience. She had grown up in a middle-class, well-adjusted family, done well at school, and as a young woman she had enjoyed partying, travelling and generally having fun. She had had a few boyfriends and had slept with one of them, but since then she had felt that she wanted to wait until she was in a long-term, stable relationship before she slept with anyone again.

After she left the group, Gina said 'Martha was "born" in order to become the person they expected me to be: hating my parents, rejecting all outside the community, and doing things I would never have done before – I was a stranger to myself. Martha is still present in me, and her voice is different to mine'.

Gina's therapist understood that she had developed a 'cult pseudo-identity' that was compliant with the cult, and informed her that this usually happens after an abusive cult experience. Her therapist held in mind the fear that Gina had been under and adopted a gentle, non-challenging, empowering stance with her. Gina was helped to recall what she was like before her time in the community, and she began a process of remembering and reconnecting with her pre-cult identity.

Her therapist encouraged her to get in touch with her family and old friends again, and to think carefully about what she wanted to wear, how she wanted to arrange her hair and what she wanted to eat, in order to assist this process. She was encouraged to use critical thinking and to challenge the way the Bible and her belief in God had been used to control her, including finding other ways of interpreting the Bible. Gina's family were supportive, and learned as much as they could about harmful and abusive cults. They supported Gina financially for several months as she had no savings; the cult had taken all of her money, and she struggled with dependency issues. In time, she began to reconnect with her pre-cult identity, although her therapist could sometimes see her 'floating' between the two personas.

Gina talked of how ashamed she felt about having had sex with men to bring them into the group. Her therapist explained to her that within the coercive belief system of the community it made sense (Lalich, 2004). This helped to normalise her feelings and to disarm her feelings of shame. She suffered traumatic reactions, such as nightmares and flashbacks, and these were worked with, again in the context of helping Gina to under-stand the cult control and helping her to ground herself in the reality that she had been abused. (Adapted from Jenkinson, 2008.)

Case study: Kent

Born and raised in a cult, recovering from abuse and finding authentic self

Kent was born and raised in a Bible-based community. His parents met in the group when they were in their early twenties, and were chosen for each other by the leadership. They moved into a community house together and worked for the group, without pay or pension. When Kent was born his parents had to abdicate responsibility for him, so any adult was able to have input into his life, discipline him or look after him. He lived in various community houses throughout his childhood.

When Kent was 6, he was assigned a 'caring brother' who was specifically responsible for his upbringing alongside his parents, and who shared a dormitory with him and other young boys. He was sexually abused by this 'caring brother' numerous times, and although he told his parents, they did not believe that this 'brother' would do such things. Kent felt utterly alone and terrorised for several years until his parents were moved to another community house.

The group was constantly recruiting vulnerable individuals off the streets, promising to take care of them and heal them of their mental and physical problems. When Kent was 14, a man in his forties joined the community house where he lived. This man had been in prison for murder and was a drug addict. The community leaders believed that God would miraculously heal this new recruit of his drug addiction if they prayed for him. This was in effect an unmonitored detox, as he came off the drugs 'cold turkey'. They told Kent he should watch, to frighten him off ever taking drugs. Kent was horrified and deeply shocked by what he saw. After that time he had nightmares, became deeply depressed and decided that he would leave as soon as he possibly could.

At the age of 17, Kent told the leadership of his community house, and his parents, that he was leaving. They were deeply upset and warned him that God would not be able to protect him from Satan outside the confines of the group. They warned him that it would be difficult for him to return.

When Kent left, he was shunned and ostracised by the group and he felt utterly lost. He had attended mainstream school but had always felt 'weird' and different to the other children. This feeling increased after leaving the group, as he struggled to find a way forward. Fortunately, unbeknown to the group, he had made a friend at school and he moved into accommodation with this friend who helped him to find manual work – something he had learned in the group.

In time, Kent realised that he loved sports (an activity he was not allowed to do in the group), and he started training and eventually became a gym coach. Although Kent had left the group physically, he struggled with memories of the years of spiritual, physical and sexual abuse and he sought therapy. He was relieved when he learned there was therapy available that could address the cult issues specifically, and as he began to understand the dynamics in the cultic group in which he grew up, he began to leave psychologically. He also realised it was not his fault that things had gone so terribly wrong, and he began to heal. He had very little contact with his parents, because they were resistant to acknowledging the level of abuse that Kent had suffered, and did not want to face the fact that they had brought their son up in a cult and as such had dedicated their lives to something that was so abusive.

Post-Cult Psychopathology

Marlene Winell proposes the theoretical concept of 'religious trauma syndrome' (RTS). She states that 'the teachings and practices of a restrictive religion can be toxic and create lifelong mental damage' (Winell, 2017, p. 611). Leaving can result in serious problems for the individual, including losing social support and needing to reconstruct their life. Very often the leaver has been taught to fear the outside world and may lack the skills needed to adjust to normal life. Winell notes four key areas of dysfunction that result from RTS:

- cognitive (resulting in confusion, difficulty with decision making and critical thinking, identity confusion)
- affective (resulting in anxiety, panic attacks, depression, suicidal ideation, anger, grief, guilt, loneliness, lack of meaning)
- functional (sleep and eating disorders, nightmares, sexual dysfunction, substance abuse, somatisation)

- social/cultural (rupture of family and social networks, employment issues, financial stress, problems acculturating, interpersonal dysfunction) (Winell, 2017, p. 611).

Leaving a harmful religion or cult-style group is therefore often a traumatic experience. The way individuals leave may have an impact on their recovery process. They may walk away, be expelled (Singer, 2003), leave by means of an intervention by an ethical 'cult-exit counsellor' (Giambalvo, 1995) or leave when their parents leave the cult (Kendall, 2006).

Other psychological problems that result from membership of a harmful religion or cult-style group include increased social dependency and decreased autonomy (Walsh and Bor, 1996), cult-induced attachment disorders where the individual's natural attachments are cut off and turned towards the group and the leader in a form of 'trauma bonding' (Stein, 2017), high degrees of dissociation (Martin et al., 1992) and significant adjustment difficulties (McKibben et al., 2000).

In addition to these specific findings, there is wide agreement between a number of authors and researchers concerning general post-cult characteristics and symptoms, including persistent emotional states such as shame, guilt, fear and cognitive deficiencies, dependence, conformity, difficulty in decision making, cult-induced phobias, anxiety and panic attacks, depression, dissociation, derealisation, depersonalisation, complex post-traumatic stress disorder (including persistent nightmares) and psychotic symptoms (Langone, 1993; Martin, 1993; Hassan, 2000; McKibben et al., 2000; Singer, 2003; Conway and Siegelman, 2005; Lalich and Tobias, 2006; Lalich and McLaren, 2018). Individuals have also attempted suicide, developed eating disorders and been rendered mute following traumatic cult experiences (Tylden, 1995).

Kendall (2006) examined whether the indications of harm and/or benefits were different for people who became part of an 'extremist authoritarian sect' (i.e., a cult) as adults (first generation), compared with those who spent all or part of their childhood in a cult (second generation). She compared their scores on psychological distress scales in adulthood as well as childhood experiences, and concluded that the second generation had higher scores in adulthood for psychological distress than the samples of either first-generation former members or those who had spent no time in a cult.

The term 'cult pseudo-identity' describes the phenomenon whereby a person's identity has been distorted or altered, and as a result a different cult persona now overlays their authentic self (Jenkinson, 2016). However, less well studied is how particular forms of environmental stress can disrupt the normally integrative function of identity. A pseudo-identity can be generated by particular types of external stress in a person who may have previously been free of any signs or symptoms of personality malfunction (Jenkinson, 2008; 2016; Jenkinson, 2008; West and Martin, 1996). There can be an abrupt switching back and forth between behaviours characteristic of the two identities, with the new identity primarily reflecting the new situational forces and requirements within the cult. Lalich (2004) suggests that the authentic identity fades into the background, whereas the cult identity emerges and becomes stronger: 'The cult member undergoes the development of a personality that stands for, and with, the newly adopted worldview and its practices. Total and unquestioning commitment requires a new self' (Lalich, 2004, p. 19).

In 1979, John Clarke from Harvard Medical School testified before a special committee of the Vermont State Senate that was investigating 'the effects of some religious cults on the health and welfare of their converts'. In his statement he cited the known health hazards, both physical and psychological, and concluded: 'The fact of a personality shift in my opinion is established. That this is a phenomenon basically unfamiliar to the mental health profession I am certain of. The fact that our ordinary methods of treatment don't work is also clear, as are the frightening hazards to the process of personal growth and mental health' (Conway and Siegelman, 2005, p. 78).

Diagnosis

In terms of making a diagnosis it is therefore relevant to know whether a person's symptoms are induced by the cult-style group or religion, so as to enable their appropriate treatment and care. Both the ICD-11 (World Health Organization, 2020) and DSM-V (American Psychiatric Association, 2013) diagnostic classification manuals describe post-traumatic stress disorders (PTSD), dissociative disorders including *dissociative identity disorder (DID)*, and stress-related disorders, all of which may form primary diagnoses. Of specific relevance is the inclusion in DSM-V of 'Other Specified Dissociative Disorder' (Diagnostic Criteria – Code 300.15), which is described under point 2 as 'identity disturbance due to prolonged and intense coercive persuasion: Individuals who have been subjected to intense coercive persuasion (e.g., brainwashing, thought reform, indoctrination while captive, torture, long-term political imprisonment, recruitment by sects/cults or by terror organisations) may present with prolonged changes in, or conscious questions of, their identity.'

Also of relevance to psychiatrists working with people who present with severe mental disturbance is the work of Lacter and Lehman (2018), who have devised guidelines to assist with the differential diagnosis between schizophrenia and ritual abuse/mind control traumatic stress. Based on their clinical experience and preliminary validation studies, they describe this as a 'culture-bound condition, uniquely born out of the subculture of isolation, torture, religious indoctrination, and coercive programming, inherent in ritual trauma and mind control, understandable only in that context' (Lacter and Lehman, 2018, p. 115).

Controversy surrounds the area of ritual abuse. The term broadly includes 'any organised abusive practice that furthers the abuser group's ideology' (Lacter and Lehman, 2018, p. 86). 'False memory syndrome' adherents consider ritual abuse to be an unfounded 'moral panic' (Noll, 2014; Katchen, 2018; Raschke, 2018), despite the fact that a significant body of psychological literature supports the existence of 'ritualistic abuse' as distinct from other kinds of abuse (Noblitt and Noblitt, 2018).

If the existence of ritual abuse is accepted or confirmed, it would be expected to cause the symptoms of trauma and dissociation specific to this type of abuse. DID, a diagnosis that is often associated with ritual abuse, is in turn one of the more controversial psychiatric diagnoses (Ofshe, 1992; Reinders, 2008; Radcliffe and Rix, 2019).

Despite being challenged by a 'discourse of disbelief' (Holland, 2001), specialist psychological therapy has been developed for survivors of ritualistic abuse (Sinason, 1994; Miller, 2018; Sinason et al., 2018) as distinct from the post-cult counselling modality (described later in this chapter). There is an ever growing body of clinical research and survivor testimonies (Spring, 2016) indicating that 'structural dissociation' (van der Hart et al., 2006), 'fragmented selves' (Fisher, 2017) and a diagnosis of DID are helpful in providing a gateway to strategies for integration (Boon et al., 2011) and healing of the dissociated 'parts'. Mental health professionals therefore need to be aware that claims of extreme abuse in the context of complex psychiatric symptoms, including psychotic symptoms, need to be accompanied by irrefutable counter-evidence before a primary diagnosis of a psychotic disorder such as schizophrenia is made (Kurz, 2016).

Treatment

Psychiatric and psychotherapeutic help is unlikely to be of benefit to ex-cult members unless the full history and context of their cult involvement are known and understood (Martin, 1993; Singer, 2003).

The latest research shows that specialist psychotherapy for all ex-cult members and for those who have left a harmful religion requires a phased approach if recovery is to occur (Jenkinson, 2016, 2019). The phases can be described as follows:

Phase 1 The potential ex-member needs to leave physically. They also need to begin the process of understanding what happened in the cult, and this can lead to them beginning to leave psychologically.

Phase 2 This phase encompasses the need for a cognitive understanding of the cult dynamics and experience. It entails focused psychoeducation to support the ex-member to tell their story while they begin to see more clearly what the cult did to them. This enables them to undo indoctrinated teachings, beliefs and practices that now compromise their autonomy.

Phase 3 This is the emotional healing phase when the ex-member can focus on shame, grief, loss, complex PTSD, and family-of-origin issues for first-generation survivors.

Phase 4 By this stage the ex-member is in touch with their authentic identity, and has got rid of the cult pseudo-identity. They may exhibit signs of post-traumatic growth (Joseph, 2011; Tedeschi and Calhoun, 2004) and are able to move on with their life.

The phases may need to be revisited if the individual encounters a new issue that has not been previously addressed, or if an old issue triggers memories of time in the cult or spiritually abusive setting.

In addition to these phases, specialist counselling for second- and multi-generation cult survivors needs to acknowledge their different and unusual needs. They will have no, or very little, experience outside the cult, and may need a wide range of practical as well as psychological support in order to integrate into the very different and alien world outside the cult (Van Eck Duymaer Van Twist, 2015; Lalich and McLaren, 2018).

Conclusion

The post-modern world is characterised by a search for meaning in the midst of the breakdown of traditional structures and beliefs. Many people are exploring new ideas and are being attracted to a wide range of wellness and spiritual approaches. Amid this chaos a significant number will fall victim to false gurus and pathological spirituality.

Mind-altering techniques exert their influence along a continuum, but when used in an environment where there is an imbalance of power, they may cause harm. Groups that use techniques such as 'brainwashing', 'persuasive coercion', 'thought reform' and 'mind control' may be damaging to individuals, their communities and society at large. When such techniques are used, spiritual beliefs, practices and experiences may become pathological.

Psychiatry must therefore be prepared to understand the potent effects of 'pathological spirituality' not only on the mindset of individuals but also, from the cultic studies' perspective, on the dynamics within groups. Only then can psychiatrists hope to recognise the signs and help those involved in the most effective way.

References

Aebi-Mytton, J. (2018) A narrative exploration of the lived experience of being born, raised in, and leaving a cultic group: the case of the Exclusive Brethren. DPsych Thesis, Middlesex University/Metanoia Institute.

Aebi-Mytton, J. (2021) "That's not me": an exploration of first, second and multi-generation adult leavers. *ICSA Today*, 12, 6–13.

Almendros, C., Eichel, S. K. D., Giambalvo, C. et al. (2013) Dialogue and cultic studies: why dialogue benefits the cultic studies field. *ICSA Today*, 4, 2–7.

American Psychiatric Association (2013) *Diagnostic and Statistical Manual of Mental Disorders*, 5th ed. Washington, DC: American Psychiatric Association.

Barker, E. (1989) *New Religious Movements: A Practical Introduction*. London: HMSO.

Barker, E. (1996) New religions and mental health. In D. Bhugra, ed., *Psychiatry and Religion*. London: Routledge, pp. 125–137.

Barrett, D. V. (2001) *The New Believers: Sects, 'Cults' and Alternative Religions*. London: Cassell.

Barron, B. and Maye, D. (2017) Does ISIS satisfy the criteria of an apocalyptic Islamic cult? An evidence-based historical qualitative meta-analysis. *Contemporary Voices: St Andrews Journal of International Relations*, 8, 18–33.

Battista, J. R. (1996) Offensive spirituality and spiritual defences. In W. Scotton, A. B. Chinnen and J. R. Battista, eds., *Textbook of Transpersonal Psychiatry and Psychology*. New York: Basic Books, pp. 250–260.

Boon, S.. Steele, K. and van der Hart, O. (2011) *Coping with Trauma-Related Dissociation: Skills Training for Patients and Their Therapists*. New York: W. W. Norton & Company.

Brockway, A. R. and Rajashekar, P. J. (1987) *New Religions and the Churches*. Geneva: World Council of Churches.

Carhart-Harris, R. L. and Goodwin, G. M. (2017) The therapeutic potential of psychedelic drugs: past, present, and future. *Neuropsychopharmacology*, 42, 2105–2113.

Chambers, W. V., Langone, M. D., Dole, A. A. and Grice, J. W. (1994) The Group Psychological Abuse Scale: a measure of the varieties of cultic abuse. *Cultic Studies Journal*, 11, 88–117.

Chryssides, G. D. (2016) *Jehovah's Witnesses: Continuity and Change*. Abingdon: Ashgate Publishing.

Conway, F. and Siegelman, J. (2005) *Snapping: America's Epidemic of Sudden Personality Change*, 2nd ed. New York: Stillpoint Press.

Crowley, N. (2020) Perspectives from front-line exit-workers and exit-counsellors on what helps individuals leave cults and radical extremist groups: a thematic analysis. Unpublished MSc thesis, University of Salford.

Deikman, A. J. (1983) The evaluation of spiritual and utopian groups. *Journal of Humanistic Psychology*, 23, 8–19.

Fisher, J. (2017) *Healing the Fragmented Selves of Trauma Survivors: Overcoming Internal Self-Alienation*. New York: Routledge.

Frank, J. D. and Frank, J. B. (1993) *Persuasion and Healing: A Comparative Study of Psychotherapy*, 3rd ed. Baltimore, MD: The Johns Hopkins University Press.

Galanter, M. D. (1989) *Cults: Faith, Healing and Coercion*. Oxford: Oxford University Press.

Galanter, M. D. (1990) Cults and zealous self-help movements: a psychiatric perspective. *American Journal of Psychiatry*, 147, 543–551.

Giambalvo, C. (1995) *Exit Counseling: A Family Intervention*. Bonita Springs, FL: American Family Foundation.

Hassan, S. (2000) *Releasing the Bonds: Empowering People to Think for Themselves*. Newton, MA: Freedom of Mind Resource Center.

Hassan, S. (2015) *Combating Cult Mind Control*, 3rd ed. Newton, MA: Freedom of Mind Resource Center.

Hassan, S. and Shah, M. J. (2019) The anatomy of undue influence used by terrorist cults and traffickers to induce helplessness and trauma, so creating false identities. *Ethics, Medicine and Public Health*, 8, 97–107.

Haworth, I. (2001) *Cults: a Practical Guide*. London: Cult Information Centre.

Healy, J. P. (2011) Involvement in a new religious movement: from discovery to disenchantment. *Journal of Spirituality in Mental Health*, 13, 2–21.

Herman, J. L. (1992) *Trauma and Recovery: From Domestic Abuse to Political Terror*. London: Pandora.

Hillman, J. (2004) *A Terrible Love of War*. New York: The Penguin Press.

Holland, S. (2001) *The Politics and Experience of Ritual Abuse: Beyond Disbelief*. Buckingham: Open University Press.

Howard, R. (1996) *The Rise and Fall of the Nine O'Clock Service: A Cult Within the Church?* London: Mowbray.

Independent Inquiry into Child Sexual Abuse (2019) *The Anglican Church Case Studies: 1. The Diocese of Chichester 2. The Response to Allegations Against Peter Ball*. London: Independent Inquiry into Child Sexual Abuse.

Jenkinson, G. M. (2008) An investigation into cult pseudo-personality – what is it and how does it form? *Cultic Studies Review*, 7, 199–224.

Jenkinson, G. (2016) Freeing the authentic self: phases of recovery and growth from an abusive cult experience. PhD thesis, University of Nottingham.

Jenkinson, G. (2019) Out in the world: post-cult recovery. *BACP Therapy Today*, 30, 22–26.

Joseph, S. (2011) *What Doesn't Kill Us: The New Psychology of Posttraumatic Growth*. New York: Basic Books.

Katchen, M. (2018) Interrelated moral panics and counter-panics: the cult brainwashing panic and the false memory/ritual abuse moral panic. In R. Noblitt and P. P. Noblitt, eds., *Ritual Abuse in the Twenty-First Century: Psychological, Forensic, Social, and Political Considerations*. Bandon, OR: Robert D. Reed Publishers, pp. 193–236.

Kendall, L. (2006) A psychological exploration into the effects of former membership of 'extremist authoritarian sects'. PhD thesis, Buckinghamshire Chilterns University College.

Kernberg, O. (1986) Institutional problems of psychoanalytic education. *Journal of the American Psychoanalytic Association*, 34, 799–834.

Kurz, R. (2016) The cremation of care ritual: burning of effigies or human sacrifice murder? The importance of differentiating complex trauma from schizophrenia in extreme abuse settings. *European Psychiatry*, 33(Suppl.), S580.

Lacter, E. and Lehman, K. (2018) Guidelines to differential diagnosis between schizophrenia and ritual abuse/mind control traumatic stress. In R. Noblitt and P. P. Noblitt, eds., *Ritual Abuse in the Twenty-First Century: Psychological, Forensic, Social, and Political Considerations*. Bandon, OR: Robert D. Reed Publishers, pp. 85–154.

Lalich, J. (2004) *Bounded Choice: True Believers and Charismatic Cults*. Berkeley: University of California Press.

Lalich, J and McLaren, K. (2018) *Escaping Utopia: Growing Up in a Cult, Getting Out, and Starting Over*. New York: Routledge.

Lalich, J. and Tobias, M. (2006) *Take Back Your Life: Recovering from Cults and*

Abusive Relationships. Berkeley, CA: Baytree Publishing.

Langone, M. D., ed. (1993) *Recovery from Cults: Help for Victims of Psychological and Spiritual Abuse.* New York: W. W. Norton & Company.

Langone, M. D. (2007) Responding to Jihadism: a cultic studies perspective. *Cultic Studies Review*, 5, 268–306.

Lifton, R. J. (1989) Ideological totalism. In *Thought Reform and the Psychology of Totalism: A Study of 'Brainwashing' in China.* Chapel Hill: University of North Carolina Press, pp. 419–437.

Lifton, R. J. (1999) *Destroying the World to Save It: Aum Shinrikyo, Apocalyptic Violence, and the New Global Terrorism.* New York: Henry Holt and Company.

Lifton, R. J. (2019) *Losing Reality: On Cults, Cultism, and the Mindset of Political and Religious Zealotry.* New York: The New Press.

McKibben, J. A., Lynn, S. J. and Malinoski, P. (2000) Are cultic environments psychologically harmful? *Clinical Psychology Review*, 20, 91–111.

Martin, P. R. (1993) *Cult-Proofing Your Kids.* Grand Rapids, MI: Zondervan Publishing Company.

Martin, P. R., Langone, M. D., Dole, A. A. et al. (1992) Post-cult symptoms as measured by the MCMI before and after residential treatment. *Cultic Studies Journal*, 9, 219–240.

Masson, J. M. (1994) *Against Therapy.* Monroe, ME: Common Courage Press.

Matthews, C. and Salazar, C. F. (2014) Second-generation adult former cult group members' recovery experiences: implications for counseling. *International Journal for the Advancement of Counselling.* 36, 188–203.

Miller, A. (2018) Recognising and treating survivors of abuse by organised criminal groups. In R. Noblitt and P. P. Noblitt, eds., *Ritual Abuse in the Twenty-First Century: Psychological, Forensic, Social, and Political Considerations.* Bandon, OR: Robert D. Reed Publishers, pp. 443–478.

Moghadam, A. (2008) The Salafi-Jihad as a religious ideology. *CTC Sentinel*, 1, 14-16.

Murray, S. (2004) *Post-Christendom: Church and Mission in a Strange New World.* Milton Keynes: Paternoster Press.

Noblitt, J. R. and Noblitt, P. P., eds. (2018) *Ritual Abuse in the Twenty-First Century: Psychological, Forensic, Social, and Political Considerations.* Bandon, OR: Robert D. Reed Publishers.

Nogueira, F. (2019) The not so divine acts of medium 'John of God'. *Skeptical Inquirer.* 43, 11–13.

Noll, R. (2014) Speak, memory. *Psychiatric Times*, 19 March 2014. www.psychiatrictimes.com/view/speak-memory (accessed 15 December 2020).

Ofshe, R. J. (1992) Inadvertent hypnosis during interrogation: false confession due to dissociative state; mis-identified multiple personality and the Satanic cult hypothesis. *The International Journal of Clinical and Experimental Hypnosis*, 40, 125–156.

Ofshe, R. and Singer, M. R. (1986) Attacks on peripheral versus central elements of self and the impact of thought-reforming techniques. *Cultic Studies Journal*, 3, 3–24.

Pollan, M. (2019) *How to Change Your Mind: The New Science of Psychedelics.* London: Penguin Books.

Radcliffe, P. and Rix, K. (2019) DID in resurgence, not retreat. *BJPsych Advances*, 25, 296–298.

Raschke, C. (2018) The politics of the "false memory" controversy: the making of an academic urban legend. In R. Noblitt and P. P. Noblitt, eds., *Ritual Abuse in the Twenty-First Century: Psychological, Forensic, Social, and Political Considerations.* Bandon, OR: Robert D. Reed Publishers, pp. 177–192.

Raubolt, R., ed. (2006) *Power Games: Influence, Persuasion, and Indoctrination in Psychotherapy Training.* New York: Other Press.

Reber, A. S. and Reber, E. (2001) *The Penguin Dictionary of Psychology*, 3rd ed. London: Penguin.

Reinders, A. a. T. S. (2008) Cross-examining dissociative identity disorder: neuroimaging and etiology on trial. *Neurocase*, 14, 44–53.

Rodríguez-Carballeira, Á., Martín-Peña, J., Almendros, C. et al. (2010) A psychosocial analysis of the terrorist group as a cult. *International Journal of Cultic Studies*, 1, 49–60.

Schein, E. H. (1961) *Coercive Persuasion: A Socio-Psychological Analysis of 'Brainwashing' of American Civilian Prisoners by the Chinese Communists.* New York: W. W. Norton & Company.

Shaw, D. (2013) *Traumatic Narcissism: Relational Systems of Subjugation.* New York: Routledge.

Sinason, V. (1994) *Treating Survivors of Satanist Abuse.* London: Routledge.

Sinason, V., Galton, G. and Leevers, D. (2018) Where are we now? Ritual abuse, dissociation, police and the media. In R. Noblitt and P. P. Noblitt, eds., *Ritual Abuse in the Twenty-First Century: Psychological, Forensic, Social, and Political Considerations.* Bandon, OR: Robert D. Reed Publishers, pp. 363–380.

Singer, M. (2003) *Cults in Our Midst: The Continuing Fight Against Their Hidden Menace*, revised ed. Hoboken, NJ: Jossey-Bass.

Spring, C. (2016) *Recovery Is My Best Revenge: My Experience of Trauma, Abuse and Dissociative Identity Disorder.* Buxton: Carolyn Spring Publishing.

Stahelski, A. (2005) Terrorists are made, not born: creating terrorists using social psychological conditioning. *Cultic Studies Review* 4, 30–40.

Stein, A. (2017) *Terror, Love and Brainwashing.* New York: Routledge.

Storr, A. (1996) *Feet of Clay: A Study of Gurus.* New York: Free Press.

Tedeschi, R. G. and Calhoun, L. (2004) Posttraumatic growth: a new perspective on psychotraumatology. *Psychiatric Times*, 21, 58–60.

Temerlin, M. K. and Temerlin, J. W. (1982) Psychotherapy cults: an iatrogenic perversion. *Psychotherapy: Theory, Research & Practice*, 19, 131–141.

Temerlin, J. W. and Temerlin, M. K. (1986) Some hazards of the therapeutic relationship. *Cultic Studies Journal*, 3, 234–242.

Tylden, E. (1995) Psychological casualties. In J. Watt, ed., *The Church, Medicine and the New Age.* London: Churches' Council for Health and Healing, pp. 61–83.

Van der Hart, O., Nijenhuis, E. R. S. and Steele, K. (2006) *The Haunted Self: Structural Dissociation and the Treatment of Chronic Traumatization.* New York: W. W. Norton & Company.

Van Eck Duymaer Van Twist, A. (2015) *Perfect Children: Growing Up on the Religious Fringe.* New York: Oxford University Press.

Vergani, M., Iqbal, M., Ilbahar, E. and Barton, G. (2018) The three Ps of radicalization: push, pull and personal. A systematic scoping review of the scientific evidence about radicalization into violent extremism. *Studies in Conflict & Terrorism*, 43, 854.

Walsh, Y. and Bor, R. (1996) Psychological consequences of involvement in a new religious movement or cult. *Counselling Psychology Quarterly*, 9, 47–60.

West, L. J. and Martin, P. R. (1996) Pseudo-identity and the treatment of identity change in captives and cults. *Cultic Studies Journal*, 13, 125–152.

Winell, M. (2017) The challenge of leaving religion and becoming secular. In P. Zuckerman and J. R. Shook, eds., *The Oxford Handbook of Secularism.* New York: Oxford University Press, pp. 603–622.

World Health Organization (2020) *ICD-11: International Classification of Diseases 11th Revision.* Geneva: World Health Organization. Available at https://icd.who.int/en (accessed 11 December 2020).

Zeiders, C. and Devlin, P. (2020) *Malignant Narcissism and Power: A Psychodynamic Exploration of Madness and Leadership*. New York: Routledge.

Zimbardo, P. (1993) Understanding mind control: exotic and mundane mental manipulations. In M. D. Langone, ed., *Recovery from Cults: Help for Victims of Psychological and Spiritual Abuse*. New York: W. W. Norton & Company, pp. 104–125.

Ageing

18

Julia H. Head, Robert M. Lawrence and
Rachel J. Cullinan

Ageing brings with it the challenge of a personal journey into degrees of fragility and isolation that create fertile ground for increased vulnerability, and the generation of specific needs related to mental, emotional, physical and spiritual well-being. The relevance of a multidimensional and holistic approach therefore becomes paramount in the teaching, training and practice of any professionals dealing with older people.

In the assessment of older individuals, sufficient attention has to be paid to core aspects of being and personality which can convey important information about coping skills and how they influence responses to diagnoses, treatment and outcome. Deep among these core aspects lie the root constructs of a person's vision of life and personal meanings, and what some would describe as the presence of a spiritual/transcendent dimension.

This chapter will give a brief overview of the ageing process in relation to emerging psychopathologies of old age psychiatry, and especially the role of spirituality in ageing and the diverse ways in which individuals approach the transition to later life. We shall also consider an approach that goes beyond standard medical practice.

Physical, Psychosocial and Psychological Challenges of the Ageing Process

Levels of physical ageing vary between individuals. The mechanisms at play are both genetic and related to 'wear and tear' of body systems and organs. The expectation is that eyesight, hearing, skin, reproductive, neurological, metabolic and endocrinological functions, bone structure and mobility will become gradually less efficient, rendering individuals more prone to the development of disease (Bittles, 2002; Stuart-Hamilton, 2006; John et al., 2020).

Outward signs of ageing include greying of hair, skin and posture changes, and slowness and hesitancy in gait and coordination. Hearing and eyesight can also be affected. The reduction in bone density increases the risk of osteoporosis, and the urogenital system becomes less effective. There is an increased incidence of heart disease, hypertension and gastrointestinal pathologies. Respiratory function is reduced and atherosclerotic changes appear, bringing a risk of peripheral and cerebrovascular damage. In many individuals, cognitive functions slow down, with a reduction in the ability to learn new information (Persson et al., 2006; Townsend et al., 2006; MacKenzie, 2012) and difficulty in adapting to new situations.

All of this can challenge any individual's ability to hold on to a sense of personal integrity. The person is dealing with getting older and frailer, and may feel lonely, anxious, frightened or at best ambivalent about their future. Personal resources may be tested to the point of wavering under the strain, and may even collapse altogether when faced with the magnitude of the task at hand. Alongside these realities, there is the challenge of experiencing changes in one's role and position in society.

Social milestones in the transition to old age include retirement from employment, reduction in income and the ever-increasing likelihood of bereavement. Previous relationships and supportive networks shrink and may disappear altogether, and relationships with family members and friends may undergo significant changes. Health problems are likely to add to the burden of advancing years, contributing to the decision to move away from one's home and a familiar neighbourhood to retirement properties, sheltered housing or care homes. However, this challenge can also serve as a process that enables the individual to reaffirm his or her identity and self-esteem, and to adapt to the many changes that come with ageing.

There is no unitary personality theory that may be applied to ageing. However, it has been observed that introversion increases and neuroticism decreases with age, in principle promoting a quieter and more contented outlook (Eysenck and Eysenck, 1969). Erikson's theory of developmental stages throughout one's lifespan depends on the accomplishment or failure, partial or total, of successive life transitions. In this 'nested', multi-staged life history, chronological age is not as relevant as the outcome of transition from stage to stage (Erikson, 1963, 1982). Erickson posits a final stage from around the age of 65 years as 'integration v. despair,' which can be viewed as a basic conflict affecting many people who are seen in old age psychiatry services.

Within Western society, ageing may be stereotyped both by the young and by the old as a phase of decline, social and financial redundancy, and as the target of humour ranging from benevolence to outright disrespect. This phenomenon speaks of a 'financial, power-driven' morality present in modern society which may intrinsically disenfranchise the old. This 'morality' does not promote caring attitudes and intergenerational responsibility. However, a current of opinion is emerging today that considers it important to validate the role of older adults in society. Yet there is some way to go to shift the predominant trend, which is well rooted in our modern history (Department of Health, 2001; Age Concern and Mental Health Foundation, 2006; Department of Health and Care Services Improvement Partnership, 2006; Royal College of Psychiatrists, 2006; Lu et al., 2018).

Against the backdrop of multifactorial challenges posed by transitions in normal ageing also emerges the heightened vulnerability to both functional and organic psychiatric illness. The two most common pathologies encountered are depression and dementias, which often manifest together, whereas other psychopathologies are generally less represented.

Up to 15% of older people experience symptoms of depression and 3% have a depressive episode, but in association with physical illness and cognitive dysfunction the prevalence increases to about 20%, affecting about a third of those in residential and nursing homes (Baldwin, 2002; Åström et al., 2019). Depression in old age correlates with physical illness in general, and heightened vulnerability is seen in cerebrovascular disease and primary cortical neurodegeneration (Allen and Burns, 1995; Banerjee et al., 1996; Robert et al., 1997; Baldwin, 2007; Mewton et al., 2019). Depression is very common in the dementias, and is both a predisposing factor and integral to clinical presentation, as well as a reaction to awareness of the diagnosis and its implications (Amore et al., 2007; Chinello et al., 2007; Pfennig et al., 2007).

Depression strips individuals of positive feelings about themselves and the world. In older people this may find perverse validation in stereotypical self-degradation and lack of social support. They may begin to think that death or euthanasia are preferable, since there is nothing left in life to do or enjoy. There may be thoughts of 'altruistic suicide', where an individual, feeling a burden to others, may contemplate taking his or her life for their benefit. Depression is directly related to suicide, and older men are particularly vulnerable (Pearson et al., 1997; Pritchard and Baldwin, 2000). For men, the act of suicide is 'often planned and rational', indicating 'not an unwillingness to live or inability to live but a willingness to die' (Hassan, quoted in MacKinlay, 2001, p. 73).

Medication attempts to correct the biochemical imbalance, 'activities of daily living' training addresses rehabilitation, and psychology seeks to explain maintaining and precipitating factors. The care of older people steps into true human focus only when the person can be reached at more intimate emotional levels, starting with realistic acknowledgement of and respect for his or her singular and unique identity. This acknowledgement is based on a non-verbal disposition that allows respectful contact at a deep level, and in principle does not exclude those individuals for whom the gift of spoken language is irreparably lost or was never there.

Through a person-centred approach, the care of the older individual requires a holistic stance that reaches beyond the generic medical model. Clinicians working in old age psychiatry should be encouraged to develop skills in recognising and assessing a broader range of factors relevant to individual care patterns (Hummelvoll et al., 2015; Lucchetti et al., 2018; Royal College of Psychiatrists, 2018). These may include spiritual reawakening and validation, religious and spiritual coping, resurgence of faith, reactions to loss and death anxieties and their psychopathological manifestations.

It is not too difficult to see how the development of more compassionate and person-centred approaches can be vital to aspects of individual recovery for older people and uphold the importance of spiritual/transpersonal values (Lolak, 2013; Hummelvoll et al., 2015; Head, 2018; Royal College of Psychiatrists, 2018). All of these factors bring into focus the interface of spirituality/religion and physical, mental and emotional well-being in later life. They are also important in helping practitioners to understand how older people's perspectives on the meaning of life and suffering may influence the nature of therapeutic relationships and health outcomes. We shall discuss aspects of this interface next, before addressing the quest for meaning and integration in later life.

The Role of Spirituality/Religion in Ageing

Resurgence in Spiritual/Religious Interest in Older People

Older people often resume aspects of behaviour relating to formal religiousness (Idler et al., 2001, Wink and Dillon, 2002, 2003; Dalby, 2006), which suggests an internal shift towards seeking security and control when these become less accessible to the individual. Various studies and more recent findings in gerontology also suggest that people's spirituality increases across the lifespan, especially in the second half of life and during later adulthood. This makes the findings interesting in an age of increasing secularization, and important with regard to mental and emotional health benefits when facing challenges associated with ageing (Lavretsky, 2010; Moody, 2018).

Factors correlating with a return to spirituality in older people are religious upbringing, life events and personality traits. Personal meaning is in the affirmation of one's continuity despite changing appearance and a decline in physical strength and health (Ross, 1995; Isaia et al., 1999). The social meaning, especially in the context of religious networks and activities, also serves to counteract the feelings of isolation experienced through separation and bereavement (Lazarus and Folkman, 1984; Koenig et al., 1988a; Guignon, 2000; Zimmer et al., 2016).

Older people recognise the value of religion, the pursuit of specific interests, healthy lifestyles, will power and socialisation as coping mechanisms. They are also aware of the possible benefits of spiritual approaches in providing a framework of meaning for one's experience (Pieper, 1981). It seems that spirituality has an existential purpose, mediating a process of reconnection with oneself at the end of life (Sabat and Harre, 1992; Slater, 1995). In fact, spiritual conduct may be more relevant to outcome in terms of well-being than either social support or financial status (Koenig et al., 1988b; Fry, 2000; Koenig, 2006).

General Health Outcomes and Spirituality / Religion in Older People

Current evidence suggests that religion and spirituality have an important role in the health of older people (Lavretsky, 2010; Lolak et al., 2016). Spirituality has been linked with more positive perceptions of one's general health. Older people spontaneously refer to religious coping in health surveys (Bosworth et al., 2003), and to coping better with the pain and disability of a range of conditions, such as rheumatoid arthritis, cardiac surgery, hypertension, and mental and emotional health problems (Koenig et al., 1997, 1999; Bartlett, 2003; Koenig, 2012; Zimmer et al., 2016).

Spirituality has also been linked with higher self-esteem (Krause et al., 1999), more positive mood states and improved psychiatric treatment outcomes (Bosworth et al., 2003). A study in Hong Kong of 380 participants aged over 60 years showed a positive correlation between self-reported engagement in spiritual activity and improved cognitive function (Fung and Lam, 2013). Individuals with dementia may still clearly be concerned with spiritual themes. The qualitative analysis of interviews conducted with 23 individuals with early dementia (Katsuno, 2003) identified a primary separate category of 'faith in God', with six subcategories: belief, support from God, sense of meaning/purpose in life, private religious practice, public religious practice and changes due to dementia. Spiritual themes may also discretely nest in psychopathology. In a study of 'musical' hallucinations, older individuals with a diagnosis of dementia commonly described hearing religious tunes (Warner and Aziz, 2005). This phenomenon may relate to the uncovering of culture-bound unconscious mechanisms.

Religiousness also appears to be linked with better health outcomes through participation in more wholesome patterns of behaviour, such as not smoking, drinking in moderation, increased physical activity and socialisation (Koenig, 2012; Zimmer et al. 2016). In groups where social support networks are dedicated to mutual care, individuals become aware of problems in other members of the group, identification of problems may be easier and earlier, and compliance with treatment more likely than for those who are socially isolated (Koenig et al., 1999). Recent findings suggest that 'secure attachment to God' can be associated with improved optimism generally, but those who are more securely attached show higher levels of self-esteem and life satisfaction (Bradshaw and Kent, 2018).

Religious Practice and Health Outcomes

The importance of faith and formal religious practice in older people has been the subject of much psychosocial exploration in recent years. The evidence points to a positive correlation both with physical and mental health and with coping with disease (Koenig et al., 1988a; Koenig, 1994; Pargament, 1997; Krause et al., 1999; Fry, 2000; Post et al., 2000; Zimmer et al., 2016). In a project that focused on 2,676 individuals who were aged 17–65 years at baseline in 1965, and who were alive in 1994, those who worshipped regularly were found to be generally healthier, particularly women. The results suggested a reduction of around 23% in the risk of dying during the study period for those individuals who worshipped regularly (Strawbridge et al., 1997, 2001).

A Swiss longitudinal study of individuals over 80 years of age suggests that religious practice correlates with longevity (Spini et al., 2001), and in North Carolina a 6-year longitudinal study of individuals over 64 years of age (Koenig et al., 1999) reported generally healthier lifestyles and a survival rate as much as 46% higher among church attendees compared with non-attendees. Longer survival of older people has also been observed in religious compared with secular kibbutzim in Israel (Kark et al., 1996). Furthermore, religious beliefs have been associated with health and well-being in elderly men, to a greater extent than religious practice (Kroll and Sheehan, 1989). Conversely, in a study of elderly physically ill men, higher mortality during a 2-year follow-up was found to be associated with feelings of loss of faith, of being abandoned by God or of being the victim of evil forces (Pargament et al., 2001). One study suggests that further research is needed to identify (from a global health perspective) whether religion and spirituality result 'in longer healthy life rather than just longer life' (Zimmer et al., 2016).

Religious practice can protect against the more serious symptoms of depressive disorder (Koenig, 2012), although less has been reported about the actual correlation between depression and individual spiritual framework. However, the prevalence of depressive symptoms varies in populations drawn from different faith groups (Kennedy et al., 1996; Braam et al., 1997; Koenig et al., 1997; Butler and Orrell, 1998; Dein, 2006). Studies of older people suggest that rates of depressive illness are lower among some faith groups than others, which may reflect the extent of the support provided by a faith community, or may be more to do with differences in liturgy and/or ritual (Meador et al., 1992; Braam et al., 2001).

Religious practice can protect against depression when individuals are also physically ill (Wink et al., 2005), in hospital (Koenig, 2004) or in a nursing home (Milstein et al., 2003), and it can reduce anxiety symptoms linked to specific situations, such as fear of falling (Reyes-Ortiz et al., 2006). Studies have highlighted the complexity of the interactions between depression and the dimensions of organised, non-organised and intrinsic religiosity (Parker et al., 2003); here, individuals with less severe depression score higher on all three dimensions than do those with more severe depression. Conversely, depression and poor quality of life have been linked to lack of belief in external and/or divine agencies and a negative attitude towards faith communities and organised religion (Koenig et al., 1988b).

The potential for exploration in this area is endless, but researchers note that further research is needed into the relationship between 'religion and chronic mental disorders – schizophrenia, bipolar disorder, longstanding treatment-resistant depression and severe personality disorders' (Bonelli and Koenig, 2013, p. 670). In addition, researchers note the importance of clinicians being able to recognise the distinction between positive and more negative religious/spiritual coping and suffering and the impact on health outcomes and well-being in older people (Lolak et al., 2016).

Prayer and Ageing

Prayer can be an important coping mechanism, and is said to have both physical and mental health benefits (Mackenzie et al., 2000; Ai et al., 2002; Lavretsky, 2010). For example, prayer as therapy is a source of spirituality for the elderly with dementia (Abramowitz, 1993; Higgins, 2003; Shamy, 2003; Higgins et al., 2004).

Prayer is both personal and congregational. Fundamentally based on terms of relationship and hope, it can become an emotional bridge to 'optimism'. In the older individual, personal prayer reflects striving towards integrity of the mature self in the face of age-inherent weakness, in relation to a transcendent other believed to be watching, listening, understanding and holding the person in empathy and love. Personal prayer is more a function of individual 'connection', where the special relationship with the transcendent other affirms the self-worth of the older person (Krause, 2004).

In its congregational aspects, prayer acquires the symbolism of rituals performed as a group, where engagement enables adaptation and cohesion (Searle, 1992). Emotional validation, companionship and reconnection are therefore also promoted through a set of basic spiritual meanings represented in the performing together of specific acts derived from religious tradition and culture.

Spirituality, Meaning and Health Outcomes

We have noted the benefits of spirituality to mental and emotional health, yet research methods do not always reveal a unique, more complex inner process occurring within the individual. Malcolm Johnson notes how:

> The human spirit is capable of responding to the whole range of emotions and experiences that form the lifespan of an individual. . . . So reflecting on our past lives, as we all do, may be affirming and pleasurable. It may be harrowing, painful, full of guilt and anger. Or it may be a mixture of these two extremes. . . . As we get closer to the end of life this life review and self-evaluation becomes more frequent and more problematic. (Johnson, 2018, p. 198)

People have their own answers to existential questions, affording diverse degrees of appreciation, definition and expression of any individual's experience. Older people will have their own sense of why they are unwell, alongside what they are told by doctors, religious representatives or their own faith tradition. Some view suffering as just part of getting older, others regard it as a punishment from God, and yet others consider it to be confirmation that there is no God or higher power. Resentment or regret about one's life may develop, with individuals becoming passive in the face of what could be seen as life's final challenges. In an older person this private quest for meaning may be hijacked by higher levels of emotional disturbance and thrown into chaos by the experience of dementia.

Alternatively, a person's spiritual life may facilitate a sense of not feeling alone in the face of pain and distress. Ageing can be a period in which the individual brings real priorities into focus and achieves the contentment of having discovered the meaning and purpose of his or her life after all, and not least the resignation and freedom to accept his or her final fate. Spirituality enables connection with one's self at a deeper level. It can afford meaning even in the face of challenging life experiences, including death anxiety, which can apply to older people in a poignant way (Bamonti et al., 2016; Krause et al., 2018).

Why then should 'religion' and 'spirituality' help to give better outcomes? What is the nature of the relationship between these factors? Apart from rational and more superficial accounts of any individual's experience of illness, distress, pain and suffering, there is a deeper, symbolic level of meaning to the event. We suggest that this is what (consciously or unconsciously) influences the relationship with health outcomes, requiring the assuaging intervention of healing and coping methods. This is the level at which it is possible to discern and understand how spiritual and religious factors are embedded in health states; helping to make these more explicit is part of the caring and healing process. Ivan Illich illustrates this point well:

> When I suffer pain, I am aware that a question is being raised. . . . Pain is the sign for something not answered; it refers to something open, something that goes on the next moment to demand, 'What is wrong?', 'How much longer?' Observers who are blind to this referential aspect of pain are left with nothing but conditioned reflexes. They are studying a guinea pig, not a human being. A physician, were he able to erase this value-loaded question shining through a patient's complaints, might recognise pain as the symptom of a specific bodily disorder, but he would not come close to the suffering that drove the patient to seek help. (Illich, 1991, p. 149)

The symbolic level of meaning provides a strong argument for de-objectifying the experience of illness and distress in favour of a more anthropocentric and holistic approach. Creative use of pain and suffering by all individuals involved in the process means engaging more with the movement towards healing, recognising the 'mystery' of pain and suffering as part of the human condition, being creative with that experience and willing to explore the 'mystery'. An individual's ability to do this does not diminish with mental and emotional crises – it is often heightened by them – but doing so from a place of pain and distress can be a difficult and courageous journey (Head, 2004).

Individuals will have their own resources and will seek them out in order to counteract the loneliness, isolation and unsupported sense of self that often accompany the experience of disease and pain. For many, this includes their religious and spiritual resources as well as looking to their immediate carers as a major form of support. Studies relating to older people with mental health needs reveal powerfully the subjective nature of the experience that individuals go through at physical, psychological, social, emotional and spiritual levels. Psychological states that are involved in the process of ageing as it interfaces with mental and emotional disturbance and organic dysfunction include (Head, 2006):

loss	depression	grief	anxiety
despair	forgetfulness	terror	emptiness
isolation	alienation	deterioration	suspicion
paranoia	devaluation	denial	confusion
unpredictability	avoidance	fear	aggression
frustration	restlessness	anger	blaming
diminishment	sadness		

The practitioner who cannot hear questions associated with 'Why is this happening to me?' may miss a vital opportunity to improve outcomes and patient well-being. Not paying attention to these questions may also have the effect of causing or increasing spiritual distress (Scott, 2016).

Loss and Grief

Grief reactions form a natural and proper response to the losses that everyone – whether well or more frail – will experience one way or another through life, especially in its later stages (Oliver and Suleiman, 2004; Wattis and Curran, 2016).

Loss and bereavement can affect older people in mental health care and their caregivers to a disturbing degree (Head, 2006). How individuals cope with and integrate the multiple losses that mark later life may well depend on whether or not there is a 'lifelong narrative of successfully coping with change and loss' (Wattis and Curran, 2016). For an older person, the death of a partner or finding oneself to be increasingly the lone survivor of a long list of departed friends and relatives can easily tip the balance from coping with an already large number of adverse personal events to despair.

In addition to the demise of one's nearest and dearest, loss takes many other forms. The older person is leaving behind youth, physical fitness, looks, ambitions, unfulfilled dreams, employment, a more active role in society, public acknowledgement of his or her usefulness, autonomy and often a family home (Wattis and Curran, 2016). These realities can increase a sense of isolation and intensify feelings of loss, which need to be addressed with appropriate and effective care responses (Oliver and Suleiman, 2004). At such a difficult time, spiritual constructs, such as a belief in an afterlife or the contentment of having usefully achieved the completion of one's life cycle, can sustain the older person's emotional and psychological endurance (Fry, 2001).

Sadly, mental health changes can affect the successful negotiation and reframing of feelings of loss that reach into the very meaning of one's existence, compromising the journey to integrity. In some conditions, individuals lose the functional memory of their life journey, which can have a devastating and fearful effect.

The spiritual encounter here is dedicated to healing by patiently journeying with the individual, and sifting through themes that can still bring some clarity and comfort. This can include searching for traces of past conflict, guilt or lack of forgiveness for oneself or others, which are still nested in spiritual anguish and needing resolution. In dementia, one may need to go 'beyond words'. When the use of language is no longer accessible to the individual, touch, lights, colours and sounds from the past may still give a sense of connection and comfort (Lawrence, 2003, 2007; Kevern, 2019).

Caregivers and Spirituality

Myriads of devoted informal caregivers walk alongside older individuals who experience physical and/or mental distress. It is difficult enough to care for someone who is close to us, but additional problems arise when caring for older people. Diseases are more likely to be chronic and complex, accompanied by physical and emotional pain. The caregivers of the seriously and chronically ill are also vulnerable to stress and illness (Acton and Miller, 2003; Saffari et al., 2018), even more so because the individuals who care for an older person are likely to be either his or her partner and themselves elderly, or else his or her children. The old age psychiatrist is called to place caregivers, too, in a framework of holistic care and support and to understand their needs.

Reviews of available studies are inconclusive with regard to the real impact of spirituality or formal religious practice on caregivers' well-being (Acton and Miller, 2003). However, there are more than anecdotal indications of some positive effects, both on the caregivers and on those they care for. In relation to patients with terminal cancer, for example, the spiritual caregiver is described as being more willing to engage in carrying the burden of care and as deriving more satisfaction from the process (Hebert et al., 2006; Pearce et al., 2006). For those who lose a loved one to a terminal illness, the process of grief and vulnerability to depressive breakdown may be lessened by a foundation of faith in an afterlife and the support of a spiritual network (Walsh et al., 2002; Fenix et al., 2006). Caregivers of people with mental health needs may find support in spiritual means of coping (Saffari et al., 2018). Personal religiousness has been found to be more effective in this case than congregational activities (Murray-Swank et al., 2006).

There is evidence that caregivers of people with dementia not only pray frequently but also cope better with their role if they perceive it to be within a spiritual/religious context (Stolley et al., 1999; Acton and Miller, 2003; Hebert et al., 2007). Partners of individuals with dementia face a long journey during which their known relationship will erode from its original form and move to a completely different level. Intimacy is lost, communication levels change and responsibility is no longer shared, potentially resulting in partners becoming depressed and physically unwell (Meller, 2001). However, the more stable the relationship with the caregiver before dementia developed, and the more spiritual its foundation, the more successful the emotional itinerary of the caregiver appears to be (Dudley and Kosinski, 1990; Guberman et al., 1992; LobhoPrabhu et al., 2005).

The experience of caring for someone with dementia may thus produce a 'positive outcome' by providing the context for spiritual growth, counteracting in part the stress of the burden of care (Sanders, 2005). As the latter increases, so recourse to spiritual matters may grow (Skaff, 1995; Picot et al., 1997; Vernooij-Dassen et al., 1997; Chang et al., 1998). Church communities can also contribute to caregiver support by providing emotional and practical help (Ragno, 1995).

Negotiating End-of-Life Issues

End-of-life issues have both sociocultural and personal existential implications. From society's viewpoint, old age is linked to the expectation that individuals will make a final will and testament, assign lasting powers of attorney where appropriate and provide advance directives for their continued care and quality of life. End-of-life decisions reflect cultural and ethnic backgrounds. For example, qualitative analysis of a community of Chinese elders in Canada revealed that decisions concerning approaching death were intrinsically linked to concepts of hope and ending one's life cycle according to Buddhist, Taoist and Confucian perspectives (Bowman and Singer, 2001).

At an existential level, the ageing process is likely to mean facing the fear of one's own death. The negotiation of this process can be supported by faith constructs in an afterlife. Furthermore, a sense of personal esteem can be fed by the successful completion of one's life cycle, and by one's existence having contributed to future generations (Cicirelli, 2002). In being alongside individuals as they face this final challenge, the question is how clinicians can find encouragement to work with the full spectrum of Erikson's final stage of 'integration v. despair', mentioned earlier. This is not so much about prescribed modes of 'doing to' the patient as it is about modes of 'being with' those who are negotiating end-of-life issues as they interface with their mental and emotional health.

A starting point is for clinicians to be able to reflect on the meaning of suffering and the existential questions it raises – for the world of one's patients is never very far removed from one's own world. A fundamental aspect of the nature of suffering is that it changes one's sense of self, testing the way one approaches life and its exigencies (Head, 2006). Pain and suffering may impart a sense of meaninglessness, but it is more often about the way they disturb connections to others, as we struggle to remain connected to the world we know, which will never be quite the same again. It is important for practitioners to understand that people continue to be actors in events that threaten their personhood even when the effects may not be so visible to the outside world. It is virtually impossible to know when this movement towards personal development and spiritual integrity has ceased.

Our concern must be to uphold the dignity that belongs inherently to personhood in the midst of suffering, pain and decline. With people who are ageing, can we embrace the possibility that they may continue to be on their progressive journey towards 'spiritual maturity', even though there may be 'ways forward and ways backward ... directions which enhance our humanity, and ... directions which diminish and endanger it' (Macquarrie, 1982, p. 228)? Can we think that it is possible for us to journey with people in terms of their experiences being transforming and transcending, even when journeying together appears to come to nothing? When our own perspectives on the nature of suffering and pain do not allow for this, we might otherwise conclude that little can be done in terms of communication and interaction, and we are just waiting for death.

The suggestion here is that we still have the capacity in later years to transform and transcend old parts of ourselves. This can include examining our relationship to pain and suffering and recognising how the experience of these is an inevitable part of life – a perspective that can contribute to improved health outcomes and increased meaning and life satisfaction. McCarthy and Bockweg (2013) suggest that the notion of 'successful ageing' is often defined as the absence of disease development in old age, yet older adults consistently report ageing successfully even in the presence of chronic illness and functional decline. They argue that the concept of transcendence arising from the 'spiritual domain' should be considered 'a criterion for a holistic view of successful aging' (McCarthy and Bockweg, 2013, p. 91).

Elizabeth MacKinlay suggests that 'spiritual development and growth as a process towards achieving spiritual integrity has been identified as a developmental task of ageing' (MacKinlay, 2001, p. 220). Much of her language in discussing the interface between spirituality and ageing includes the notion of people transforming and transcending their difficulties. From her research, she identifies characteristics associated with growth and development that include:

> An openness to change and learning; an attitude of searching for the ultimate meaning in their lives; relationship with a confidante and/or membership of a long-term small group. It also included transcendence of disabilities and losses encountered in ageing; acceptance of their past life and a readiness to face the future, including the ability to live with uncertainty, and, finally, a sense of freedom and a move to a greater degree of interiority. (MacKinlay, 2001, p. 220)

The spiritual tasks of ageing include transcending disabilities and loss, finding final meaning and hope, and finding intimacy with God and/or others, all of which centre on responding to life's ultimate meaning (for further discussion of her model of spirituality and ageing, see MacKinley, 2018). Again the notion of interiority – of the individual's inner world – evokes the idea of a realm of thinking, feeling, desiring and imagining that is not always available to objective scrutiny yet holds vital energy in terms of the person's spiritual/transpersonal journey.

In our engagement with older people, it may be difficult for us to discern quite what is going on in their spiritual/religious life, particularly if communication through words is minimal. We may then have to be more creative in offering empathic responses that reach beyond the immediately obvious. John Killick's reflections on the experience of dementia remaining a fundamental mystery that is part of the broader mystery of life itself provides us with an example of such creative thinking:

> Looking at this woman before me I am led to speculate on her life – what events have shaped her, has she experienced the highs and lows of existence, or has she maintained an equilibrium, living largely uneventfully and untroubled? Has her frame been stirred with passion, and the only just supportable knowledge of its being returned? Or have her days been informed by a steady and constant affection, to lull her into the illusion of permanence? Does this love still sustain her in her present removed state? (Killick, 2002, p. 23)

Pain and suffering occur, and call for healing, at all levels – physical, psychological, social and spiritual. We are not dealing with suffering in later life as a static category, but with individuals from different contexts and cultures, with varying responses to life events all the way through their lives. We often deal with individuals who find it difficult to exercise autonomy over personal growth, who may desire to dwell in the past and who may be fearful of opening up to the future. On the other hand, we also encounter people who have been journeying with life's meanings and mysteries for many years.

It is important to recognise that in many cases we are not talking about major and one-off moments of transformation or transcendence. Neither are we talking about the linear progression of one's spiritual life such that it reaches its pinnacle with old age, although some kind of progression and maturity in this might be expected. In practice, we may be dealing with 'moments' of transformation/transcendence that may be quickly forgotten when working with some individuals who are cognitively impaired.

Spiritual Accompaniment and Care

Practitioners play a potentially important role in the spiritual care process. Suggestions abound for spiritual care interventions (e.g., Lavretsky, 2010; Lolak et al., 2016), but opinions vary on their effectiveness, how they are provided and what the role of spiritual advisors should be. Training and policies for providing spiritual care are often lacking and need further development (Lawrence et al., 2007; Goh et al., 2014; Scott, 2016).

Spiritual accompaniment and care is aimed at maintaining personhood and upholding the dignity and respect of individuals, which is particularly relevant for those whose mental powers are failing (Kitwood, 1997; Kevern, 2019). It is about being prepared to 'seek to understand and support each individual's own unique mindset, quest for meaning, purpose and connectedness' as well as appreciating background cultures and belief systems (Wattis and Curran, 2016), life philosophies and ultimate values and meanings. Key skills are empathic listening and providing a validating presence – concepts that hopefully are not unknown to practitioners.

Most people find themselves caught up in life's realities, which include pain and suffering. Sometimes the pain we face incapacitates our response to it. We need to try to stay with the tension of distress caused by people's suffering and frailty, and not aim for quick resolution or attempt to impose our own values on them (Wattis and Curran, 2016). This is the art of anyone who considers that there can be movements towards health even in the midst of pain and distress. Thus it is important for practitioners to revisit their personal philosophies on health and sickness. A factor which is often overlooked in the mental health context is that spiritual care depends first on being in a 'right relationship' with ourselves before we can be in an authentic relationship with others:

> Right relationships begin with ourselves. This exploration will inevitably transcend the very limited scientific view of what we are as human beings, and cause us to re-examine and incorporate spiritual values into our caring work. When this occurs, the healing potential expands. ... New relationships can come into existence which recognise the value of being with people as much as doing to them. Carers can let go of the intense effort required to give compassion, and relax into *being* compassionate, *being* healing, in short, *becoming* the sacred space in which healing occurs. (Wright and Sayer-Adams, 2000, p. 41)

People who have struggled with their own meaning can recognise the same spiritual endeavour in others. A person who is distressed needs another person who may be able to open up to them the experience of being genuinely understood. Those who are mentally distressed are very keenly aware of the chaos involved with the threat of loss of self. It is only when individuals can accept this within themselves, which they will do at many different levels, that the growth towards 'personhood' advances. What is important is that practitioners can commit themselves to 'be with' the person in distress. Sometimes giving a 'space' wherein the person may experience presence, but not necessarily have to act in it, is the only thing one can share with the other. The silence of encounter is more expressive and indicative of authentic solidarity than words could ever be.

To sit with someone who is not communicating is the real test of empathy in encounter – to listen to what the person might be trying to communicate in ways other than through language, and to think oneself into the experience of what life is like for him or her. This is the same for all forms of disturbance at any age, but the difference may show itself in how we attempt to enable a person's resources for communicating what he or she most needs. All of the elements of authentic relationship – presence, encounter, empathy and listening – will honour an individual's spiritual quest at any time of life, enabling the discernment and respecting of spiritual need and nurturing the dignity of personhood. In effect, we are working underneath individual stories, transcending the sight of the ageing process and reaching out to the ageless, spiritual/transpersonal core of the individual.

Ageing as Transformation in Beauty and Depth

Many contemporary writers posit an innate movement of human beings towards health and maintaining personhood, which often expresses itself precisely in the struggle to cope with adversity and decline. This struggle can lead to oscillation, an either/or position relating to Erikson's stage of integrity *v*. despair. Yet, given the right support, a different reality can emerge, that of adopting a more synthesised position of working with the 'given' (Head, 2006). The theologian John Macquarrie (1982) speaks of two possible reactions to pain and suffering–rebellion or resignation/passive acceptance. However, he effectively promotes a third way that synthesises these two positions and represents a more spiritual, transpersonal movement and journey:

> There is the possibility of realistically accepting that suffering is inevitable in the human condition, but at the same time of seeking to transform it and integrate it into human life in such a way that we come to see that life would be poorer without it. It may not be possible to integrate it without remainder. ... But at least we must see how far along this road we can go. (Macquarrie, 1982, p. 224)

If we can understand that life imposes its own wounding, leading us sometimes to lose sight of our selves/souls, then perhaps we can view life also as a journey to 'health', to reconnect to our selves/souls at any time in life. This stance is reflected in the suggestion by Hillman (1999, pp. xiii–xv) that 'ageing is no accident. It is necessary to the human condition, intended by the soul', and that old age is a '*structure* with its own essential nature'. Whereas one may think of ageing as being a process that leads to dying, Hillman desires to elevate thinking on this issue to suggest that 'the last years confirm and fulfil character'. In questioning whether the soul has to be 'aged' properly before it leaves, he suggests that we might then be able to 'imagine aging as a transformation in beauty as much as in biology'. He inquires:

> Can a person become an epiphany? Can we entertain the idea that all along our earthly life has been phenomenal, a showing, a presentation? Can we imagine that at the essence of human being is an insistence upon being witnessed – by others, by gods, by the cosmos itself – and that the inner force of character cannot be concealed from this display. The image will out, and the last years put a final finish to that. (Hillman, 1999, p. 201)

Thomas Moore, a contemporary spiritual writer, describes growing old as a 'matter of growing deep', growing into the earthiness of identity, becoming less interested in the 'surface glitter of culture' and living more from the soul than from the self. This is to understand oneself as being a part of nature and to conceive of the soul (the source of identity) as a piece of the world's soul. He suggests that our 'roots reach downward, not into the brain, but into the soil' (Moore, 2004, p. 294), and that all people can prepare through life for this opportunity of 'growing deep', although some people do so less readily than others. He tells us that we do not have to understand this deep level of our existence, but we do have to trust it:

> There can be no doubt that as you grow old, you must come to terms with the arc of your life, its rising and setting. You have to see its elephant ears as things of beauty and signals of a divine design. You have to move gracefully with that downturn and dimming so that you will benefit from its special powers. Then all your dark nights will begin to make sense and fold themselves into the ultimate passing of the light. You will enter the darkness knowing something about the territory. You will understand that it has its own luminosity and beauty. (Moore, 2004, p. 300)

Conclusion

Inevitably, the process of ageing draws the older person towards reappraising the meaning of life. Transition into old age involves the involution of physical strength and the need to readdress the continuum of one's own psychological identity. Here the human psyche bids for integrity in the light of less empirical yet increasingly transpersonal relationships. The feelings of hurt and joy posited in one's emotional memory, together with acquired and deeply held convictions and beliefs, now come to cushion the impact of the pain of growing older (Lawrence, 2003, 2007). Within a body that is weakening externally, the intimate core of one's constructs and personality comes to relatively outshine material parameters. This intimate core is one's whole unqualified 'I am', containing the zest of core experiences of childhood, the formative years of young adulthood, indeed all the hard and pleasant lessons learned along life's path.

References

Abramowitz, L. (1993) Prayer as therapy among the frail Jewish elderly. *Journal of Gerontological Social Work*, 19, 69–75.

Acton, G. and Miller, E. (2003) Spirituality in caregivers of family members with dementia. *Journal of Holistic Nursing*, 21, 117–130.

Age Concern and Mental Health Foundation (2006) *Promoting Health and Well-Being in Later Life: A First Report from the UK Inquiry*. London: Age Concern and Mental Health Foundation.

Ai, A. L., Peterson, C., Bolling, S. F. et al. (2002) Private prayer and optimism in middle-aged and older patients awaiting cardiac surgery. *Gerontologist*, 42, 70–81.

Allen, N. H. P. and Burns, A. (1995) The non-cognitive features of dementia. *Reviews in Clinical Gerontology*, 5, 57–75.

Amore, M., Tagariello, P., Laterza, C. et al. (2007) Subtypes of depression in dementia. *Archives of Gerontology and Geriatrics*, 44, 23–33.

Åström, E., Rönnlund, M., Adolfsson, R. and Carelli, M. G. (2019) Depressive symptoms and time perspective in older adults: associations beyond personality and negative life events. *Aging & Mental Health*, 23, 1674-1683.

Baldwin, R. (2002) Depressive disorders. In R. Jacoby and C. Oppenheimer, eds., *Psychiatry in the Elderly*. Oxford: Oxford University Press, pp. 627–676.

Baldwin, R. (2007) Recent understandings in geriatric affective disorder. *Current Opinion in Psychiatry*, 20, 539–543.

Bamonti, P., Lombardi, S., Duberstein, P. et al. (2016) Spirituality attenuates the association between depression symptom severity and meaning in life. *Aging & Mental Health*, 20, 494-499.

Banerjee, S., Shamash, K., Macdonald, A. et al. (1996) Randomised controlled trial of effect of intervention by psychogeriatric team on depression in frail elderly people at home. *British Medical Journal*, 313, 1058–1061.

Bartlett, S. J. (2003) Well-being and quality of life in people with rheumatoid arthritis. *Arthritis Care & Research*, 49, 778–783.

Bittles, A. H. (2002) Biological aspects of human ageing. In R. Jacoby and C. Oppenheimer, eds., *Psychiatry in the Elderly*. Oxford: Oxford University Press, pp. 3–24.

Bonelli, R. M. and Koenig, H. G. (2013) Mental disorders, religion and spirituality 1990 to 2010: a systematic evidence-based review. *Journal of Religion and Health*, 52, 657–673.

Bosworth, H. B., Park, K.-S., McQuoid, D. R. et al. (2003) The impact of religious practice and religious coping on geriatric depression. *International Journal of Geriatric Psychiatry*, 18, 905–914.

Bowman, K. W. and Singer, P. A. (2001) Chinese seniors' perspectives on end-of-life decisions. *Social Science and Medicine*, 53, 455–464.

Braam, A. W., Beekman, A. T., van Tilburg, T. G. et al. (1997) Religious involvement and depression in older Dutch citizens. *Social Psychiatry and Psychiatric Epidemiology*, 32, 284–291.

Braam, A. W., Van Den Eeden, P., Prince, M. J. et al. (2001) Religion as a cross-cultural determinant of depression in elderly Europeans: results from the EURODEP collaboration. *Psychological Medicine*, 31, 803–814.

Bradshaw, M. and Kent, B. V. (2018) Prayer, attachment to God, and changes in psychological well-being in later life. *Journal of Aging and Health*, 30, 667-691.

Butler, R. and Orrell, M. (1998) Late-life depression. *Current Opinion in Psychiatry*, 11, 435–439.

Chang, B., Noonan, A. E. and Tennstedt, S. L. (1998) The role of religion/spirituality in coping with caregiving for disabled elders. *Gerontologist*, 38, 463–470.

Chinello, A., Grumelli, B., Perrone, C. et al. (2007) Prevalence of major depressive disorder and dementia in psychogeriatric outpatients. *Archives of Gerontology and Geriatrics*, 44, 101–104.

Cicirelli, V. G. (2002) Fear of death in older adults: predictions from terror management theory. *Journals of Gerontology Series B: Psychological Sciences and Social Sciences*, 57B, 358–366.

Dalby, P. (2006) Is there a process of spiritual change or development associated with aging? A critical review of research. *Aging & Mental Health*, 10, 4–12.

Dein, S. (2006) Religion, spirituality and depression: implications for research and treatment. *Primary Care and Community Psychiatry*, 11, 67–72.

Department of Health (2001) *National Service Framework for Older People*. London: Department of Health.

Department of Health and Care Services Improvement Partnership (2006) *Everybody's Business: Integrated Mental Health Services for Older Adults: A Service Development Guide*. London: Department of Health and Care Services Improvement Partnership.

Dudley, M. G. and Kosinski, F. A. (1990) Religiosity and marital satisfaction: a research note. *Religious Research*, 32, 78–86.

Erikson, E. H. (1963) *Childhood and Society*. New York: W. W. Norton & Company.

Erikson, E. H. (1982) *The Life Cycle Completed: A Review*. New York: W. W. Norton & Company.

Eysenck, S. B. and Eysenck, H. J. (1969) Scores on three personality variables as a function of age, sex and social class. *British Journal of Social and Clinical Psychology*, 8, 69–76.

Fenix, J. B., Cherlin, E. J., Prigerson, H. G. et al. (2006) Religiousness and major depression among bereaved family caregivers: a 13-month follow-up study. *Journal of Palliative Care*, 22, 286–292.

Fry, P. S. (2000) Religious involvement, spirituality and personal meaning for life: existential predictors of psychological wellbeing in community-residing and institutional care elders. *Aging & Mental Health*, 4, 375–387.

Fry, P. S. (2001) The unique contribution of key existential factors to the prediction of psychological well-being of older adults following spousal loss. *The Gerontologist*, 41, 69–81.

Fung, A. W. T. and Lam, L. C. W. (2013) Spiritual activity is associated with better cognitive function in old age. *East Asian Archives of Psychiatry*, 23, 102-108.

Goh, A. M., Eagleton, T., Kelleher, R. et al. (2014) Pastoral care in old age psychiatry: addressing the spiritual needs of inpatients in an acute aged mental health unit. *Asia-Pacific Psychiatry*, 6, 127-134.

Guberman, N., Maheu, P. and Mailee, C. (1992) Women as family caregivers: why do they care? *The Gerontologist*, 32, 607–617.

Guignon, C. (2000) Authenticity and integrity: a Heideggerian perspective. In P. Young-Eisendrath and M. E. Miller, eds., *The Psychology of Mature Spirituality: Integrity, Wisdom, Transcendence.*. New York: Brunner-Routledge, pp. 62–74.

Head, J. (2004) 'Please pray for me': the significance of prayer for mental and emotional well-being. *Spirituality and Psychiatry Special Interest Group Newsletter*, 14 (April).

Head, J. (2006) A rich tapestry: emergent themes in spirituality in the care of older adults with mental health needs. *Spirituality and Psychiatry Special Interest Group Newsletter*, 21 (June).

Head, J. (2018) The spirituality of compassion. *Spirituality and Psychiatry Special Interest Group Newsletter*, 44 (February).

Hebert, R. S., Weinstein, E., Martire, L. M. et al. (2006) Religion, spirituality and the well-being of informal caregivers: a review, critique and research prospectus. *Aging & Mental Health*, 10, 497–520.

Hebert, R. S., Dang, Q. and Schulz, R. (2007) Religious beliefs and practices are associated with better mental health in family caregivers of patients with dementia: findings from the REACH study. *American Journal of Geriatric Psychiatry*, 15, 292–300.

Higgins, P. (2003) Holding a religious service for people with dementia. *Journal of Dementia Care*, 11, 10–11.

Higgins, P., Allen, R., Karamat, S. et al. (2004) Candlelight Group: a pilot project for people with dementia. *Spirituality and Psychiatry Special Interest Group Newsletter*, 14 (April).

Hillman, J. (1999) *The Force of Character: And the Lasting Life*. New York: Random House Publishing Group.

Hummelvoll, J. K., Karlsson, B. and Borg, M. (2015) Recovery and person-centredness in mental health services: roots of the concepts and implications for practice. *International Practice Development Journal*, 5 (Suppl.), Article 7.

Idler, E. L., Kasl, S. V. and Hays, J. C. (2001) Patterns of religious practice and belief in the last year of life. *Journals of Gerontology Series B: Psychological Sciences and Social Sciences*, 56, S326–S334.

Illich, I. (1991) *Limits to Medicine: Medical Nemesis – The Expropriation of Health*. London: Penguin.

Isaia, D., Parker, V. and Murrow, E. (1999) Spiritual well-being among older adults. *Journal of Gerontological Nursing*, 25, 15–21.

John, A., Desai, R., Richards, M. et al. (2020) Role of cardiometabolic risk in the association between accumulation of affective symptoms across adulthood and mid-life cognitive function: national cohort study. *British Journal of Psychiatry*, 218, 254–260.

Johnson, M. (2018) Spirituality, biographical review and biographical pain at the end of life in old age. In M. Johnson and J. Walker, eds., *Spiritual Dimensions of Ageing*. Cambridge: Cambridge University Press, pp. 198–294.

Kark, J. D., Carmel, S., Sinnreich, R. et al. (1996) Psychosocial factors among members of religious and secular kibbutzim. *Israel Journal of Medical Sciences*, 32, 185–194.

Katsuno, T. (2003) Personal spirituality of persons with early-stage dementia. *Dementia*, 2, 315–335.

Kennedy, G. J., Kelman, H. R., Thomas, C. et al. (1996) The relation of religious preference and practice to depressive symptoms among 1,855 older adults. *Journals of Gerontology Series B: Psychological Sciences and Social Sciences*, 51, 301–308.

Kevern, P. (2019) Spirituality and dementia. In L. Zsolnai and B. Flanagan, eds., *The Routledge International Handbook of Spirituality in Society and the Professions*. London: Routledge, pp. 223–230.

Killick, J. (2002) Approaching the mystery. *Journal of Dementia Care*, 10, 23.

Kitwood, T. (1997) *Dementia Reconsidered: The Person Comes First*. Buckingham: Open University Press.

Koenig, H. G. (1994) *Aging and God: Spiritual Pathways to Mental Health in Midlife and Later Years*. Binghamton, NY: Haworth Pastoral Press.

Koenig, H. G. (2004) Religion, spirituality, and medicine: research findings and implications for clinical practice. *Southern Medical Journal*, 97, 524–529.

Koenig, H. G. (2006) Religion, spirituality and aging. *Aging & Mental Health*, 10, 1–3.

Koenig, H. G. (2012) Religion, spirituality, and health: the research and clinical implications. *ISRN Psychiatry*, 2012, 278730.

Koenig, H. G., George, L. K. and Seigler, I. C. (1988a) The use of religion and other emotion-regulating coping strategies among older adults. *The Gerontologist*, 28, 303–310.

Koenig, H. G., Kvale, J. N. and Ferrel, C. (1988b) Religion and well-being in later life. *The Gerontologist*, 28, 18–28.

Koenig, H. G., Hays, J. C., George, L. K. et al. (1997) Modeling the cross-sectional relationship between religion, physical health, social support, and depressive symptoms. *American Journal of Geriatric Psychiatry*, 5, 131–144.

Koenig, H. G., Hays, J. C. and Larson, D. B. (1999) Does religious attendance prolong survival? A six-year follow-up study of 3,968 older adults. *Journals of Gerontology Series A: Biological Sciences and Medical Sciences*, 54, M370–M377.

Krause, N. (2004) Assessing the relationships among prayer expectancies, race, and self-esteem in late life. *Journal for the Scientific Study of Religion*, 43, 395–408.

Krause, N., Ingersoll-Dayton, B., Ellison, C. G. et al. (1999) Aging, religious doubt and psychological well-being. *The Gerontologist*, 39, 525–533.

Krause, N., Pargament, K. and Ironson, G. (2018) In the shadow of death: religious hope as a moderator of the effects of age on death anxiety. *The Journals of Gerontology Series B: Psychological Sciences and Social Sciences*, 73, 696–703.

Kroll, J. and Sheehan, W. (1989) Religious beliefs and practices among 52 psychiatric inpatients in Minnesota. *American Journal of Psychiatry*, 146, 67–72.

Lavretsky, H. (2010) Spirituality and aging. *Aging Health*, 6, 749–769.

Lawrence, R. M. (2003) Aspects of spirituality in dementia care: when clinicians tune into silence. *Dementia*, 2, 393–402.

Lawrence, R. M. (2007) Dementia: a personal legacy beyond words. *Mental Health, Religion and Culture*, 10, 553–562.

Lawrence, R. M., Head, J., Christodoulou, G. et al. (2007) Clinicians' attitudes to spirituality in old age psychiatry. *International Psychogeriatrics*, 19, 962–973.

Lazarus, R. S. and Folkman, S. (1984) *Stress, Appraisal, and Coping*. Berlin: Springer.

LobhoPrabhu, S., Molinari, V., Arlinghaus, K. et al. (2005) Spouses of patients with dementia: how do they stay together "till death do us part"? *Journal of Gerontological Social Work*, 44, 161–174.

Lolak, S. (2013) Compassion cultivation: a missing piece in medical education. *Academic Psychiatry*, 37, 285.

Lolak, S., Minor, D., Jafari, N. and Puchalski, C. (2016) Spiritual issues and interventions in mental health and aging. In H. Lavretsky, M. Sajatovic and C. F. Reynolds III, eds., *Complementary and Integrative Therapies for Mental Health and Ageing*. Oxford: Oxford University Press, pp. 257–272.

Lu, W., Pikhart, H. and Sacker, A. (2018) Socioeconomic determinants of healthy ageing: evidence from the English Longitudinal Study of Ageing. *The Lancet*, 392 (Special Issue), S54.

Lucchetti, A., Barcelos-Ferreira, R., Blazer, D. et al. (2018) Spirituality in geriatric psychiatry. *Current Opinion in Psychiatry*, 31, 373–377.

McCarthy, V. L. and Bockweg, A. (2013) The role of transcendence in a holistic view of successful aging: a concept analysis and model of transcendence in maturation and aging. *Journal of Holistic Nursing*, 31, 84–94.

Mackenzie, E. R., Rajagopal, D. E., Meibohm, M. et al. (2000) Spiritual support and psychological well-being: older adults' perceptions of the religion and health connection. *Alternative Therapies in Health and Medicine*, 6, 37–45.

MacKenzie, P. (2012) Normal changes of ageing. *InnovAiT: Education and Inspiration for General Practice*, 5, 605–613.

MacKinlay, E. (2001) *The Spiritual Dimension of Ageing*. New York: Jessica Kingsley Publishers.

MacKinlay, E. (2018) Ageing and spirituality across faiths and cultures. In M. Johnson and J. Walker, eds., *Spiritual Dimensions of Ageing*. Cambridge: Cambridge University Press, pp. 32–50.

Macquarrie, J. (1982) *In Search of Humanity: A Theological and Philosophical Approach*. London: SCM Press.

Meador, K. G., Koenig, H. G., Highes, D. C. et al. (1992) Religious affiliation and major depression. *Hospital and Community Psychiatry*, 43, 1204–1208.

Meller, S. (2001) A comparison of the well-being of family caregivers of elderly patients hospitalized with physical impairments versus the caregivers of patients hospitalized with dementia. *Journal of the American Medical Directors Association*, 2, 60–65.

Mewton, L., Reppermund, S., Crawford, J. et al. (2019) Cross-sectional and prospective inter-relationship between depressive symptoms, vascular disease and cognition in older adults. *Psychological Medicine*, 49, 2168–2176.

Milstein, G., Bruce, M. L., Gargon, N. et al. (2003) Religious practice and depression among geriatric home care patients. *International Journal of Psychiatry in Medicine*, 33, 71–83.

Moody, H. (2018) Stages of the soul and spirituality in later life. In M. Johnson and J. Walker, eds., *Spiritual Dimensions of Ageing*. Cambridge: Cambridge University Press, pp. 51–68.

Moore, T. (2004) *Dark Nights of the Soul: A Guide to Finding Your Way through Life's Ordeals*. New York: Avery.

Murray-Swank, A. N., Lucksted, A., Medoff, D. R. et al. (2006) Religiosity, psychosocial adjustment, and subjective burden of persons who care for those with mental illness. *Psychiatric Services*, 57, 361–365.

Oliver, R. and Suleiman, E. (2004) Bereavement. In S. Evans and J. Garner, eds., *Talking Over the Years: A Handbook of Dynamic Psychotherapy with Older Adults*. New York: Brunner-Routledge, pp. 265–280.

Pargament, K. I. (1997) *The Psychology of Religion and Coping: Theory, Research, Practice*. New York: Guilford Press.

Pargament, K. I., Koenig, H. G., Tarakeshwar, N. et al. (2001) Religious struggle as a predictor of mortality among medically ill elderly patients: a two-year longitudinal study. *Archives of Internal Medicine*, 161, 1881–1885.

Parker, M., Roff, L. L., Klemmack, D. L. et al. (2003) Religiosity and mental health in southern, community-dwelling older adults. *Aging & Mental Health*, 7, 390–397.

Pearce, M. J., Singer, J. L. and Prigerson, H. G. (2006) Religious coping among caregivers of terminally ill cancer patients: main effects and psychosocial mediators. *Journal of Health Psychology*, 11, 743–759.

Pearson, J. L., Conwell, Y., Lindesay, J. et al. (1997) Elderly suicide: a multi-national view. *Aging & Mental Health*, 1, 107–111.

Persson, J., Nyberg, L., Lind, J. et al. (2006) Structure–function correlates of cognitive decline in aging. *Cerebral Cortex*, 16, 907–915.

Pfennig, A., Littmann, E. and Bauer, M. (2007) Neurocognitive impairment and dementia in mood disorders. *Journal of Neuropsychiatry and Clinical Neurosciences*, 19, 373–382.

Picot, S. J., Debanne, S. M., Namazi, K. H. et al. (1997) Religiosity and perceived rewards of black and white caregivers. *The Gerontologist*, 37, 89–101.

Pieper, H. (1981) Church membership and participation in church activities among the elderly. *Activities, Adaptation & Aging*, 1, 23–30.

Post, S. G., Puchalski, C. M. and Larson, D. B. (2000) Physicians and patient spirituality: professional boundaries, competency and ethics. *Annals of Internal Medicine*, 132, 578–583.

Pritchard, C. and Baldwin, D. (2000) Effects of age and gender on elderly suicide rates in Catholic and Orthodox countries: an inadvertent neglect? *International Journal of Geriatric Psychiatry*, 15, 904–910.

Ragno, J. G. (1995) Volunteers of the spirit: quality of life programming with religious volunteers. *Activities, Adaptation & Aging*, 20, 35–39.

Reyes-Ortiz, C. A., Ayele, H., Mulligan, T. et al. (2006) Higher church attendance predicts lower fear of falling in older Mexican-Americans. *Aging & Mental Health*, 10, 13–18.

Robert, R., Kaplan, G. A., Shema, S. J. et al. (1997) Does growing old increase the risk for depression? *American Journal of Psychiatry*, 154, 1384–1390.

Ross, L. (1995) The spiritual dimension: its importance to patients' health, well-being and quality of life and its implications for nursing practice. *International Journal of Nursing Studies*, 32, 457–468.

Royal College of Psychiatrists (2006) *Raising the Standard: Specialist Services for Older People with Mental Illness. Report of the Faculty of Old Age Psychiatry*. London: Royal College of Psychiatrists.

Royal College of Psychiatrists (2018) *Person-Centred Care: Implications for Training in Psychiatry*. London: Royal College of Psychiatrists.

Sabat, S. and Harre, R. (1992) The construction and deconstruction of self in Alzheimer's disease. *Ageing and Society*, 12, 443–461.

Saffari, M., Koenig, H., O'Garo, K. and Pakpour, A. (2018) Mediating effect of spiritual coping strategies and family stigma stress on caregiving burden and mental health in caregivers of persons with dementia. *Dementia*, https://doi.org/10.1177/1471301218798082.

Sanders, S. (2005) Is the glass half empty or half full? Reflections on strain and gain in caregivers of individuals with Alzheimer's disease. *Social Work in Healthcare*, 40, 57–73.

Scott, H. (2016) The importance of spirituality for people living with dementia. *Nursing Standard*, 30, 41–50.

Searle, M. (1992) Ritual. In C. Jones, G. Wainwright, E. Yarnold and P. Bradshaw, eds., *The Study of Liturgy*. London: SPCK, pp. 51–58.

Shamy, E. (2003) *Worship for People with Alzheimer's Disease and Related Dementias: A Guide to the Spiritual Dimension of Care for People with Alzheimer's Disease and Related Dementias*. London: Jessica Kingsley Publishers.

Skaff, M. M. (1995) Religion in the stress process: coping with caregiving. Paper presented at the Annual Scientific Meeting of the Gerontological Society of America, Los Angeles, CA.

Slater, R. (1995) *The Psychology of Growing Old*. Buckingham: Open University Press.

Spini, D., d'Epinay, L. and Pin, S. (2001) Religious practice and survival in old age. *Médecine et Hygiène*, 59, 2258–2262.

Stolley, J. M., Buckwalter, K. C. and Koenig, H. G. (1999) Prayer and religious coping for caregivers of persons with Alzheimer's disease and related disorders. *American Journal of Alzheimer's Disease*, 14, 181–191.

Strawbridge, W. J., Cohen, R. D., Shema, S. J. et al. (1997) Frequent attendance at religious services and mortality over 28 years. *American Journal of Public Health*, 87, 957–961.

Strawbridge, W. J., Shema, S. J., Cohen, R. D. et al. (2001) Religious attendance increases survival by improving and maintaining good health behaviors, mental health and social relationships. *Annals of Behavioral Medicine*, 23, 68–74.

Stuart-Hamilton, I. (2006) *The Psychology of Ageing*. London: Jessica Kingsley Publishers.

Townsend, J., Adamo, M. and Haist, F. (2006) Changing channels: an fMRI study of aging and cross-modal attention shifts. *Neuroimage*, 31, 1682–1692.

Vernooij-Dassen, M., Felling, A. and Persoon, J. (1997) Predictors of change and continuity in home care for dementia patients. *International Journal of Geriatric Psychiatry*, 12, 671–677.

Walsh, K., King, M., Jones, L. et al. (2002) Spiritual beliefs may affect outcome of bereavement: prospective study. *British Medical Journal*, 324, 1551–1554.

Warner, N. and Aziz, V. (2005) Hymns and arias: musical hallucinations in older people in Wales. *International Journal of Geriatric Psychiatry*, 20, 658–660.

Wattis, J. and Curran, S. (2016) Stories of living with loss: spirituality and ageing. In C. Cook, A. Powell and A. Sims, eds., *Spirituality and Narrative in Psychiatric Practice: Stories of Mind and Soul*, pp. 160–172.

Wink, P. and Dillon, M. (2002) Spiritual development across the adult life course: findings from a longitudinal study. *Journal of Adult Development*, 9, 79–94.

Wink, P. and Dillon, M. (2003) Religiousness, spirituality and psychosocial functioning in late adulthood: findings from a longitudinal study. *Psychology and Aging*, 18, 916–924.

Wink, P., Dillon, M. and Larsen, B. (2005) Religion as moderator of the depression–health connection: findings from a longitudinal study. *Research on Aging*, 27, 197–220.

Wright, S. and Sayer-Adams, J. (2000) *Sacred Space: Right Relationship and Spirituality in Healthcare*. Edinburgh: Churchill Livingstone.

Zimmer, Z., Jagger, C., Chiu, C.-T. et al. (2016) Spirituality, religiosity, aging and health in global perspective: a review. *SSM - Population Health*, 2, 373–381.

Glossary

Christopher C. H. Cook

This glossary is offered as an aid to understanding the vocabulary of the interdisciplinary field of spirituality/religion and psychiatry. Terminology within this field can be confusing for a number of reasons:

1 Some of the words that are used are familiar in everyday usage, but also have a less obvious technical sense when used in spiritual or academic writing.
2 Some words are unfamiliar, or infrequently used, within the wider domain of psychiatry and mental health.
3 Quite a few terms – including the words 'spirituality' and 'religion' – are contested and controversial, some are differently defined within different academic disciplines, and others are differently interpreted within different cultures and faiths. Some of these terms, even though many people think they know exactly what they mean, are virtually undefinable.

In addition to the terminological confusion, there are a number of reasons for adding a glossary to the second edition of *Spirituality and Psychiatry*:

1 Some important topics are not covered within the main chapters of the book, and although they do not merit whole chapters to themselves, it seems appropriate that something should be said about them.
2 The glossary picks up on some of the key themes that run through the book. It draws attention to the varied perspectives taken on them by different professionals, patients and researchers, which in turn reflect different scientific, philosophical, spiritual and religious concerns.
3 The glossary offers pointers for further reading.

It is said by some that spirituality differs from religion in its emphasis on subjectivity and individuality. This can mean, when talking about spirituality, that the same words are used very differently by different writers, and often with important nuances and subtleties. (The same can be true, it must be said, in the field of religion.) Unlike Humpty Dumpty, in Lewis Carroll's *Through the Looking Glass*, I do not think that words can mean whatever I want them to mean. As a researcher I have to know what my colleagues and research subjects mean by them. As a clinician, I have to know what my patients mean by them. I also need to be able to explain, when asked, what I think I mean by them. This glossary is therefore both an attempt to explain what I mean by these terms, and an exercise in listening to how others use them in the wider literature.

A glossary such as this one inevitably represents the views and interests of its author, but I have also tried in each case to be inclusive of the diversity of usage of terms in the field, to draw attention to differences of understanding and to give examples from scholars with contrasting perspectives. The glossary was not made available to other contributors to the present volume before they wrote their chapters, and so has not influenced their contributions in any way. I have, however, drawn attention to where, and how, the terms have been used within this book.

Rather than including only short definitions for each term, as was the initial intention, during the course of writing this glossary has become rather more like a dictionary, with a number of longer entries. This reflects, to a large extent, the lack of agreement about what terms mean and the complexity of the debates surrounding them. I have, nonetheless, tried to avoid very long entries. I may therefore have oversimplified some of the arguments, and I hope that readers will consult the references cited for fuller accounts.

Terms have been selected for inclusion in this glossary with the following priorities in mind:

1 They are important to understanding the research base and/or debates around clinical practice and policy specifically in relation to the field of spirituality/religion and psychiatry.
2 They fill some of the gaps in relation to terms that have not been used or defined, and issues that have not been covered, within the rest of the book.
3 Some general terms from theology, religious studies and philosophy have been included, particularly where these might not be familiar to a psychiatric readership and/or where they have particular relevance to research and psychiatric practice.
4 Some terms have been included on the basis that it is helpful for the reader to be aware of practices, beliefs and theories that are controversial, are outside mainstream psychiatry or might be a cause for clinical concern.

Terms have not been included if they are not specific to the field of spirituality and psychiatry (e.g., wider psychiatric terminology) and are likely to be familiar to most readers. The lexicon that follows is far from exhaustive, and many more words could have been included, but I hope that it covers the major terms of interest. Inclusion of terms in this glossary in no way implies personal approval of or agreement with them by the author.

I am aware that there is a certain irony in creating a glossary for a book on spirituality. Words are often inadequate to communicate spiritual experience; metaphor, simile, poetry and visual images are more evocative than philosophical, theological or scientific definitions. Despite this, in most spiritual and mystical traditions, people have found the need to say all that they can before admitting that there is so much that cannot be said. In clinical practice, words remain the primary medium for communicating experiences, and the clinician needs to use them as effectively as possible. It is hoped that this glossary will be an aid to that end.

Where words are highlighted in **bold** type this indicates that they are included in the glossary under their own entry.

Agnosticism

Philosophically, agnosticism represents a belief that it is not possible, in principle, to know whether or not God exists, or what God might be like. In practice, and in many research surveys, it is often understood as 'not knowing' whether or not God exists, or not knowing what one believes. Along with atheists, agnostics are often included in research studies with others who have no religious affiliation – or **'nones'**.

Atheism

Literally and philosophically, atheism is the belief that there is no God. However, there are broader (negative) views of atheism as non-belief, and narrower (positive) views of atheism as itself a form of belief (i.e., that there is no God).

For further discussion, see Cliteur (2009), Speed and Fowler (2016) and Coleman et al. (2018). Atheism is arguably a **worldview** and, as such, may have similar benefits to **religion** in terms of health outcomes (Uzarevic and Coleman, 2020).

Cults

There is controversy about terms and definitions in relation to cults, sects and new religious movements. To some extent this is a matter of disciplinary perspective, with sociologists of religion seeing the differences primarily in terms of the extent to which new groups are schismatic or socially deviant. Thus, for example, sects may be understood as groups that have broken away from mainstream religious traditions, and cults as innovative and new religious groups (Stark and Bainbridge, 1979). On this basis, new religious movements are simply cults that have been around for longer and have become historically established. In psychiatry and the allied professions, much more emphasis is placed upon the psychological characteristics of the group, and in particular the psychological harm that it may cause to its members. Marc Galanter, for example, groups together cults, 'zealous self-help movements', and some new religious movements as 'charismatic groups' characterised by high social cohesiveness, intensely held beliefs and strong expectations of behavioural conformity (Galanter, 1990).

The definition and psychological characteristics of cults, with particular attention to the harm that they may cause, are considered in detail in Chapter 17.

Dark Night Experiences

The idea of a 'dark night' of spiritual experience originated with the Spanish mystic St John of the Cross (1542–1591), a significant reformer of the Carmelite order, a Christian community devoted to contemplative prayer. John's widely disseminated poem *En una noche oscura (On a Dark Night)*, later supplemented by a commentary, was written in the context of his experience of imprisonment and cruel treatment by rival Carmelites who disagreed with his approach to reform. The dark night, for John, is a spiritual experience of privation, absence, emptiness and abandonment, especially abandonment by God. It is, however, one within which he finds spiritual growth, faith and love. Often referred to now as the dark night 'of the soul', the concept has been appreciated by and found resonance within other faith traditions, in different biographical, historical and cultural contexts, in spirituality outside the context of religion, in psychotherapy, and in literature and the arts more widely. In these contexts it is diversely interpreted and applied. The relationship with depression, as a clinical disorder, is also diversely understood, but it is important to recognise (as discussed in Chapter 9) that the spiritual/religious significance of experiences of depression should be interpreted in context.

For further reading. see Culligan (2003), Foley (2018) and Chapter 9. For a book on the dark night written by a psychiatrist, see May (2003).

Disobsession

See **spirit release therapy**

Dualism

The understanding that there are two fundamental and opposing principles, energies or entities. Dualism can take many forms – for example, good and evil, mind and matter

(Cartesian dualism), body and soul, material and spiritual, yin and yang. Dualism is not currently popular in academia, and is equally out of favour among biological psychiatrists and psychologists (Bracken and Thomas, 2002; Searle, 2007; Maung, 2019; Glannon, 2020; Miller et al., 2020), but is widespread in popular religious belief. Indeed, it has even been suggested that human adults are natural dualists (Astuti, 2001). For an essay in defence of the compatibility of dualism with psychiatry, see Ng (2021).

Existentialism

In contrast to objective philosophies, existentialism is concerned with the individual in the context of his or her freedom and relationships. Having its origins in the work of the philosopher Soren Kierkegaard (1813–1855), it is now variously defined and understood. Although on the one hand it may be considered to be an atheistic **worldview**, finding no meaning and purpose in life, on the other hand it shares considerable overlap with the concept of spirituality, and sees it as the task of the individual to find his or her own meaning and purpose in life. The term transcends religious/secular divides, and many religious thinkers have been associated with existentialism, including the Christian Russian novelist Fyodor Dostoyevsky, as well as Kierkegaard himself.

Existential psychiatry recognises that existential concerns are relevant to the aetiology, phenomenology and outcome of mental disorders, and takes these concerns into account in evaluation and management (De Haan, 2017). It is perhaps an 'attitude' to other human beings, rather than a particular school of psychiatry (May, 1961). Existentialism has been influential in psychotherapy, as for example in the logotherapy of Viktor Frankl (Frankl, 1988) and the work of Irvin Yalom (Yalom, 1980).

According to May (1958, p. 11), 'Existentialism, in short, is the endeavour to understand man by cutting below the cleavage between subject and object which has bedeviled Western thought and science since shortly after the Renaissance'.

De Haan (2017, p. 528) defines it as follows: 'The existential dimension refers to our ability to relate to ourselves, our experiences, and our situation'.

For further reading in relation to spirituality, see Thompson (2007) and Webster (2004). A seminal text in existential psychiatry is that by May et al. (1958).

Exorcism

As a response to the plight of someone who is believed to be the subject of a **possession state**, exorcism usually takes the form of various prayers and/or rituals intended to release that person from an evil demonic/spiritual influence. Exorcism, in some form or another, is found in most religious traditions and generally aims to cast out, or expel, the malign entity. However, it may take very different forms. Disobsession (as it is known in Spiritism), or **spirit release therapy**, has a very different understanding of the nature of spiritual influences to that encountered in Christianity or Islam (for further discussion, see Chapter 16). 'Deliverance ministry' provides a somewhat broader, and less invasive, alternative response to perceived demonic influence within some Christian traditions.

Harmful Religion

Broadly speaking, harmful religion might be considered to refer to situations in which, for individuals or groups, religion becomes the cause of suffering. Sylvia Mohr and her colleagues have used the term in this way in their studies of spirituality/religion in people with schizophrenia (Mohr et al., 2011, 2012). It has been proposed (Walker, 1997) that there are two models of harmful religion: **religious addiction** and **religious abuse**. The former locates the problem within the individual (or victim), whereas the latter focuses more on the abuse of power (or the perpetrator). However, religion may be associated with suffering in other ways, as for example in negative forms of **religious coping**, or **religious/spiritual struggles**.

See also **pathological religion**

Higher Power

The idea of a Higher Power derives from Step 2 of the **Twelve-Step** programme of Alcoholics Anonymous (AA), founded in 1935. The 'steps' initially consisted of six steps that were written down by one of the founders, Bill Wilson, as an account of how his friend Ebby had found sobriety. Later, in 1939, expanded into 12 steps, they summarise the experiences of the early members of AA and are offered as a way for others to find recovery. The first three steps are as follows:

1 We admitted we were powerless over alcohol – that our lives had become unmanageable.
2 Came to believe that a Power greater than ourselves could restore us to sanity.
3 Made a decision to turn our will and our lives over to the care of God as we understood Him.
   (Alcoholics Anonymous World Services Inc., 1983, pp. 21–42)

The reference to a 'Power greater' – or a 'Higher Power' – seems to have been drawn from William James' book, *The Varieties of Religious Experience* (James, 1902). The phrase 'God as we understood him' may have come from Reverend Samuel Shoemaker, but is also very much in line with the psychological approach to religion taken by James. Wilson also acknowledged the debt that AA owed to the influence of Carl Jung, in particular the recognition of the importance of a spiritual or religious experience for recovery (Wilson and Jung, 1987). Members of AA are encouraged to find their own understanding of their Higher Power. For some this is AA as an organisation, or fellowship, and for others it may be God understood in traditional religious terms, but members have found diverse understandings of what a Higher Power might be (Dossett, 2013). In a recent study of members of Narcotics Anonymous, 98% of the participants were found to believe in a Higher Power, with slightly less than half of these individuals believing in God per se (Galanter et al., 2020). The term has since been taken up more widely, as for example in **transpersonal** psychology and among those who consider themselves **SBNR** (**spiritual but not religious**).

Immanence

Immanence is usually contrasted with **transcendence**. On the one hand, it can be employed as a reference to the tangible and objective immediate reality as studied by science. It is used in this sense, for example, by Charles Taylor, when he speaks of the 'immanent frame' of reference of our secular age being closed to transcendence (Taylor, 2007). On the other hand, the term is used within theistic religions to refer to the relationship between God and creation. In some religions, where immanence is emphasised, this relationship is conceived of as closer than in others. In pantheism the relationship is so close as to allow almost no distinction between God and the world. Many who identify as spiritual but not religious (**SBNR**) have a very immanent view of **spirituality** (Mercadante, 2014, p. 88). Most theistic religions maintain some kind of balance between the immanence and transcendence of God. In Christianity and Islam, for example, God is understood as both transcendent and immanent. Buddhism (a non-theistic religion) is generally more concerned with immanent experience, but even here some Buddhists would see nirvana (a state of release from attachment to immanent things) as a transcendent state.

For further discussion of immanence in relation to psychiatry, see Cook (2013).

Monism

Monism, not to be confused with monotheism, is the philosophical assertion that, despite the appearance of multiplicity, all things are interconnected and ultimately one. Some mystical experiences may be characterised as monistic (see Chapter 1), and many people who are spiritual but not religious (**SBNR**) hold monistic beliefs. Monism, as understood in a strictly theological/philosophical sense, is not compatible with the major theistic religions, which emphasise that God and the universe are distinct and separate, even though – at least according to the Abrahamic traditions – God is intimately and closely involved with creation. Non-duality, a closely related but subtly different concept deriving primarily from Eastern religious traditions, is variously defined but might be considered to be more concerned with experiences of non-dual awareness (Nash et al., 2013).

For further discussion of monism in relation to SBNR, see Mercadante (2014, pp. 116–125).

Moral Injury

Moral injury is essentially concerned with the impact of certain kinds of trauma upon the ethical and moral sensibilities of the survivor.

According to Jones (2020, p. 127), 'Moral injury is a term proposed to describe the distress that individuals feel when they perpetrate, witness or fail to prevent an act that transgresses their core ethical beliefs'.

Litz et al. (2009, p. 695) write that 'Potentially morally injurious events, such as perpetrating, failing to prevent, or bearing witness to acts that transgress deeply held moral beliefs and expectations may be deleterious in the long-term, emotionally, psychologically, behaviorally, spiritually, and socially (what we label as moral injury)'.

Although the concept behind the term is arguably very old, being concerned with the 'existential wounds of war', the term 'moral injury' appeared only very recently, in 2002 (Hodgson and Carey, 2017). There are numerous definitions, and the term is not universally accepted. Some emphasise elements of 'betrayal' (and thus the responsibility of those in military command), whereas others emphasise the acts perpetrated by the individual concerned. Some, taking a more holistic approach, emphasise the wider context, including the spiritual/religious dimension (Hodgson and Carey, 2017). Although the concept has its origins in discussion of combat-related trauma, its use has now broadened to other contexts, including traumatised refugees (Nickerson et al., 2015) and healthcare delivery in the context of the COVID-19 pandemic (Tracy et al., 2020).

The relationship to **spirituality** is debated, but arguably spirituality is central to an understanding of moral injury, and the spiritual consequences of moral injury can be significant (Hodgson and Carey, 2017). Among veterans suffering from moral injury, some experience significant **religious/spiritual struggles** (Currier et al., 2019; Sullivan and Starnino, 2019). Spiritual interventions are currently being evaluated and show promise (Pearce et al., 2018; Starnino et al., 2019).

Mysticism

Mystical theology has a long history, but the term 'mysticism' only appeared in the eighteenth century, at which time it was used mainly in a pejorative sense with reference to various expressions of religious enthusiasm, as for example among the Methodists and Quakers. In the nineteenth century, usage widened to refer to common elements within diverse groups and traditions (Tyler, 2011, pp. 6–7). Evelyn Underhill wrote, succinctly, that mysticism is 'the direct intuition or experience of God' (Underhill, 1925, p. 9). However, diverse definitions abound. With the mystical emphasis on direct experience of the divine, it is perhaps not surprising that mystics have often been controversial figures within their own faith traditions.

Christian mysticism has its roots in Judaism and the New Testament, and flourished in the Middle Ages. It has included such figures as Meister Eckhart (c.1260–c.1328), Julian of Norwich (c.1343–1416), St John of the Cross (1542–1591) and St Teresa of Avila (1515–1582), all of whom were controversial in their own time. Sufism (*tasawwuf*), the mystical tradition within Islam, has emphasised interior spiritual practice since the earliest days of Islam, and has included such noted adherents as Al-Ghazali (c.1058–1111) and the poet Rumi (1207–1273). Within Judaism, the Kabbalah represents a body of mystical teachings within which the *Zohar* ('Book of Splendour') occupies a central place. Although mysticism usually emphasises relationship with God, there are also non-theistic forms of mysticism, as in some strands of Buddhism, as well as some varieties of nature mysticism.

It has been suggested that a common 'core' of mystical experience can be identified in diverse religious traditions. For example, Tyler has suggested that mysticism is 'a universal form of religious experience that finds specific expression in distinctive movements: Buddhist mysticism, Indian mysticism, Spanish mysticism, German mysticism and so on' (Tyler, 2011, p. 7).

In an influential report on mysticism published in 1976, the Group for the Advancement of Psychiatry defined it as follows: 'mysticism involves a relationship with the supernatural which is not mediated by another person; the goal of mystical union is reached during the course of this relationship' (Committee on Psychiatry and Religion, 1976, p. 717).

Traditionally the domain of theology and religious studies, mystical experiences have in recent decades also been studied by the methods of neuroscientific research (see D'Aquili and Newberg, 1999; Cristofori et al., 2016).

For a review of psychiatry and mysticism, see Cook (2004).

Neurotheology

As defined by Andrew Newberg, neurotheology 'refers to the field of study linking the neurosciences with religion and theology' (Newberg, 2010, p. 45). Newberg sees this as requiring 'an openness to both the scientific as well as the spiritual perspectives' (Newberg, 2010, p. 1). It is thus in theory an interdisciplinary endeavour, and not aligned to any particular religious or theological tradition. However, in practice the interdisciplinary engagement appears to prioritise neuroscience, and neurotheology often seems to seek to 'explain religious experience and behaviour in neuroscientific terms' (Aaen-Stockdale, 2012, p. 520).

Nones

This is a term used to refer to people who profess no religious affiliation in response to surveys, questionnaires or interviews. Thus, typically, at the end of a list of other religious groups ('Christian, Muslim, Jewish, Hindu, Buddhist . . .') there may be a tick box labelled 'None'. This is clearly a very negative definition, and tells us only what these respondents are not. It does not tell us, in any positive sense, what they *are* (Vernon, 1968). The nones are a diverse group, and further research is needed to distinguish between its component groups in terms of health outcomes. They include, among others, atheists, agnostics and those who are **SBNR**. In one study in the USA, approximately one third of this group were identified as 'liminal nones', occupying a space somewhere on the margins of religious identity (Lim et al., 2010).

See also **atheism** and **agnosticism**.

Past Life Regression Therapy

This is a form of therapy in which an altered state of consciousness (a state of relaxation, often but not necessarily induced by hypnosis) is used to recover memories of 'past life' experiences. The premise is thus that a mental disorder may be caused by unresolved traumas that took place in a previous life. Although this would appear to assume a belief in **reincarnation** on the part of both therapist and patient, this is not considered essential by all practitioners.

Past life regression therapy is associated with significant ethical concerns (Andrade, 2017), and mainstream mental health professionals regard it as lacking an evidence base, such that it has been described by some researchers as 'discredited' (e.g. Norcross et al., 2006). The core controversy is around the generation of false memories (Spanos et al., 1994; Brainerd and Reyna, 2005). That false memories are generated in some cases is not widely disputed. The controversy seems to relate to whether or not past life memories, elicited according to good practice, are ever 'not false' – a question that is not readily amenable to empirical verification. There are various possible explanations for the experiences of patients in therapy, including cryptomnesia (a forgotten memory mistakenly misattributed to a past life), fantasy, confabulation or (according to a Jungian understanding; Read et al., 1959) emergence of material from the collective unconsciousness, as well as veridical memory of past lives. In response to criticisms of past life regression therapy, its advocates argue that (as with most psychotherapeutic interventions) much depends upon the skill and training of the therapist.

For some interesting clinical accounts by practitioners, see Woolger (1987), Modi (1997, pp. 105–189) and Powell (2018, pp. 29–31, 150–151).

Pathological Religion

The term 'pathological religion' seems to be used relatively infrequently in the professional/academic literature, and it overlaps with other terms and is not easily defined. In 1907, in *Obsessive Actions and Religious Practices*, Freud suggested that religion might be understood as a universal obsessional neurosis (Dickson, 1985, p. 40). On this basis, more or less all **religion** could be understood as pathological, a view with which the authors of this book have generally disagreed. Similarly, Jung took quite a different stance to Freud, identifying 'the existence of an authentic religious function in the unconscious mind', and seeing religious experience as potentially healing (Jung, 1938, p. 3, 114). However, he was not unaware of the possibility of a degenerate and corrupted form of religion that has 'lost the living mystery' (Jung, 1938, p. 37). Religion in general might thus be understood as normal and healthy, with terms such as **cult**, sect or **harmful religion** used to distinguish harmful (and usually more recent) deviations that are implicitly or explicitly 'pathological' (see Chapter 17). At the individual level, the concept of pathological religion might also be used to refer to **religious abuse**.

See also **harmful religion** and **pathological spirituality**.

Pathological Spirituality

If **spirituality** can be healthy, life giving and supportive of well-being, then the possibility also arises that aberrant forms of spirituality can be unhealthy, life denying, abusive or even contributory to mental disorder, including self-harm. Such aberrant forms of spirituality, within a medical vocabulary, might be termed 'pathological'. This pathology may originate within the psyche, and thus be a matter for psychotherapy (King, 2001), or it may be concerned with the adverse effects of recruitment into harmful groups of various kinds (whether referred to as **cults**, sects, religions or new religious movements). The pathology may be something that is harmful about the group itself or its teachings, or it may reside in the personality or mental disorder of a particular leader, guru or teacher within the group. Pathological spirituality may be religious or non-religious. It is explored further in Chapter 17.

See also **pathological religion**.

Possession State

The influence of discarnate spirits upon human well-being is recognised in most religious traditions worldwide, including all of the major monotheistic traditions, Hinduism and Spiritism. Details of beliefs vary from one tradition to another (and within traditions), but demonic possession may – in very general terms – be understood as concerned with the belief that a person's state of well-being has in some way been adversely affected by demonic entities.

'A possession state can be defined as the presence of a belief, delusional or otherwise, held by an individual (and sometimes others) that their symptoms, experiences and behaviour are under the influence or control of supernatural forces, often of diabolical origin' (Enoch and Ball, 2001, p. 224).

Roland Littlewood has suggested that possession may be the most common culture-bound psychiatric syndrome worldwide (Littlewood, 2004). Identification of possession as a psychiatric syndrome pathologises states that are culturally accepted as a normal part of life in large parts of the world. However, as Littlewood points out, possession beliefs may be employed culturally to explain a wide range of different psychiatric diagnoses.

Possession states may or may not be associated with an altered state of consciousness (trance). In some cultural/religious contexts, possession and/or trance is sought out (e.g., for the purpose of healing). In both DSM-5 Dissociative Trance (300.15) and ICD-11 Possession Trance Disorder (6B63), states that are a culturally accepted part of religious practice are excluded. The diagnosis of pathology therefore rests upon distress and upon the involuntary and/or unwanted nature of the possession/trance.

For further reading. see Littlewood (2004), Enoch and Ball (2001, pp. 224–244), Dein and Illaiee (2013) and Scrutton (2015).

See also **exorcism** and **spirit release therapy.**

Reincarnation

Also known as rebirth, transmigration of souls or metempsychosis, reincarnation is the belief that after death the eternal soul, or self, is reborn into a new body.

'Reincarnation may be defined as the belief that human beings do not, as most of us assume, live only once, but on the contrary live many, perhaps an infinite number of lives, acquiring a new body for each incarnation' (Edwards, 1996, p. 11).

Belief in reincarnation is widespread around the world, especially in Eastern religious traditions. Although such beliefs are less common in the Western world, they are not infrequent and are not confined to particular cultural or ethnic groups (Walker, 2000). Belief in reincarnation is closely related to (but should be distinguished from) a belief in karma – a law of cause and effect whereby actions have consequences that may carry over from past lives into the present (Sharma, 2000, pp. 344–345, 359–360).

Much evidence in support of reincarnation, including many case studies of children claiming to remember previous lives, was gathered by Ian Stevenson (1918–2007) (for a brief biography, see Tucker, 2008), a psychiatrist working at the University of Virginia, who wrote extensively on the subject (e.g., Stevenson, 1977, 2000). More recently, a collection of stories of children's memories of previous lives has been published by Jim Tucker, also at the University of Virginia (Tucker, 2021).

Beliefs in reincarnation should be treated sensitively and with respect in psychotherapy (Daie et al., 1992; Peres, 2012).

For a critical study of reincarnation, see Edwards (1996).

See also **past life regression therapy.**

Religion

The concept of religion, as discussed in Chapter 16, is amenable to diverse definitions, many of which reflect the disciplinary contexts within which they have arisen (Cox, 2010). Most scholars of theology and the study of religion would argue that the concept of religion defies definition. Just a small selection of definitions, relevant to the concerns of the present volume, will be offered here.

William James defined religion as 'The feelings, acts, and experiences of individual men in their solitude, so far as they apprehend themselves to stand in relation to whatever they may consider the divine' (James, 1902, p. 31).

According to Émile Durkheim, 'A religion is a unified system of beliefs and practices relative to sacred things, that is to say, things set apart and forbidden – beliefs and practices which unite into one single moral community called a Church, all those who adhere to them' (Durkheim, 1995, p. 44; originally published, in French, in 1912).

Clifford Geertz defines religion as follows: '(1) a system of symbols which acts to (2) establish powerful, pervasive, and long-lasting moods and motivations in men by (3) formulating conceptions of a general order of existence and (4) clothing these conceptions with such an aura of factuality that (5) the moods and motivations seem uniquely realistic' (Geertz, 1993, p. 90).

Finally, according to Harold Koenig and his colleagues, 'Religion involves beliefs, practices, and rituals related to the transcendent, where the transcendent is God, Allah, HaShem, or a Higher Power in Western religious traditions, or to Brahman, manifestations of Brahman, Buddha, Dao, or ultimate truth/reality in Eastern traditions' (Koenig et al., 2012, p. 45).

Religions

Whereas **religion** is difficult to define, it is relatively easy to define *a* religion.

A religion may be defined as 'a religious community of believers, followers, or adherents who hold there to be something distinctive in their beliefs, and who give their primary religious allegiance and loyalty to that religion' (Johnson et al., 2013, p. 139).

The focus is thus very much upon the individual believer, for whom a religion is often a significant part of their identity. There is much diversity within, as well as between, religions. It is therefore important in the clinical context to regard the patient as the expert from whom the clinician can learn, and not to make assumptions about beliefs or practices based upon textbook accounts. However, it is good to be well informed, and there are numerous books outlining the history, beliefs and practices of the world's major religions (e.g., Bowker, 2007).

For discussion of the issues that arise in psychiatry in relation to some of the major world religions, see Koenig (1998) and Moreira-Almeida et al. (2021). For a handbook that provides guidance on issues that arise in psychotherapy with patients who are followers of different religions, see Richards and Bergin (2000).

Religiosity

This refers to operationalised quantitative measures of individual differences in religiousness or religious commitment. It is thus concerned with such things as religious identity, feelings, experiences and practices.

For further discussion, see Chapter 16.

Religious Abuse

See **spiritual/religious abuse**

Religious Addiction

Religious addiction is closely related to the concept of **spiritual/religious abuse**. Like spiritual abuse, it features more in popular literature than in academic literature, and is not a recognised psychiatric diagnostic category. It may, however, be located within a wider body of literature that recognises various behaviours (e.g., gambling, exercise, shopping) that do not involve exogenous substances as having addictive potential (e.g., Johnson and Vanvonderen, 1991, pp. 189–191; Linn et al., 1995).

Religious Coping

In times of adversity, illness or stress, people draw on spiritual/religious resources in order to cope psychologically:

'We define [religious coping] as the use of religious beliefs or behaviours to facilitate problem-solving to prevent or alleviate the negative emotional consequences of stressful life circumstances' (Koenig et al., 1998, p. 513).

Spiritual/religious coping is often divided into positive and negative types. As originally proposed by Pargament et al. (1998, p. 712):

> positive religious coping methods [are] ... an expression of a sense of spirituality, a secure relationship with God, a belief that there is meaning to be found in life, and a sense of spiritual connectedness with others ...

> negative religious coping ... is an expression of a less secure relationship with God, a tenuous and ominous view of the world, and a religious struggle in the search for significance.

For further discussion of religious coping, see Chapter 16.

See also **religious/spiritual struggles**.

Religious or Spiritual Problem (V62.89)

This is a DSM category, first introduced in DSM-IV (Lukoff et al., 1998) under the heading of 'Other Conditions That May Be a Focus of Clinical Attention'. It is thus neither a diagnosis nor a mental disorder. Rather, it normalises spiritual/religious problems while also recognising their significance in terms of psychiatric assessment, diagnosis and treatment.

'This category can be used when the focus of clinical attention is a religious or spiritual problem. Examples include distressing experiences that involve loss or questioning of faith, problems associated with conversion to a new faith, or questioning of spiritual values that may not necessarily be related to an organized church or religious institution' (American Psychiatric Association, 2013, p. 725).

There is no explicitly equivalent category in ICD-10 (Abdul-Hamid, 2011), nor, despite proposals to this effect (Abdul-Hamid, 2011), has one been introduced in ICD-11. The most closely corresponding code in ICD-10 is Z65.8, 'Other Specified Problems Related to Psychosocial Circumstances'. Within ICD-11 the Z codes have been discontinued. 'Problems associated with social or cultural environment' are now located within 'Factors Influencing Health Status'. No detail is given about such problems, and spirituality/religion is not specifically mentioned in relation to this category at all.

For further discussion of religious and spiritual issues in DSM, see Peteet et al. (2011) and Chapter 12.

Religious/Spiritual Struggles

Spiritual/religious beliefs and practices are usually conducive to positive emotional states and well-being (Koenig et al., 2012, pp. 123–144). However, **spirituality** and **religion** may also be associated with psychological distress, as discussed in detail in Chapter 16.

'Religious/spiritual (r/s) struggles occur when some aspect of r/s belief, practice or experience becomes a focus of negative thoughts or emotions, concern or conflict' (Exline et al., 2014, p. 208).

Such experiences offer the possibility of spiritual and/or psychological growth, as for example in **dark night experiences**. However, in clinical practice and in research, 'struggles' provides an umbrella heading for a diverse group of experiences with correspondingly diverse outcomes. The term 'religious/spiritual struggles' is used more or less interchangeably with the term 'negative **religious coping**'.

For further reading that includes applications to psychotherapy, see Pargament and Exline (2022).

SBNR (Spiritual but Not Religious)

An important demographic in contemporary surveys of spirituality/religion, the category of SBNR provides a way of self-identifying as affirming the importance of a spiritual life but without identifying specifically with one or more religious traditions. In fact, people who identify as SBNR may draw on a variety of practices or beliefs from various religious traditions, and thus exemplify a form of **syncretism**, but nonetheless they do not personally identify as religious.

For further discussion, see Chapter 1.

Soul

Psychiatry, at least etymologically, is concerned with the treatment of the soul, the word being derived from the Greek words 'psyche', usually translated as 'soul' in English, and 'iatros', meaning physician. The soul, or psyche, may be equated with the mind, or may be understood as the essence of a person, or as the spiritual/immaterial part of a person (as also in the human **spirit**). With some variations in understanding, the concept of a soul is common to the Abrahamic religions (Judaism, Christianity and Islam) and also Hinduism (where Atman is the true self). In contrast, in Buddhism there is no enduring and immaterial human 'soul' – the individual self is ultimately illusory. The commonly understood Western concept of an immortal soul, which is widespread in Christianity, is actually Platonic in origin. In some religions, animals are also understood to have souls, and in animism even non-living things (e.g., rocks, rivers) are believed to have souls. With advances in the social and biological sciences, and in response to the critiques of Cartesian **dualism**, the idea of an immaterial soul has been largely replaced in scientific thinking with that of the self. However, academic disciplines have diverse conceptualisations of both soul and self, so there is now little agreement as to what constitutes either. Moreover, this does not resolve any of the difficult philosophical questions as to how a biological organ (the brain) relates to the non-material mind.

For a neurological approach to the generation of consciousness, see Damasio (2000). For a helpful review of the history of concepts of soul and self, see Martin and Barresi (2006). For a wide-ranging discussion of the place of the soul in psychiatric practice, see Powell (2017, 2018), and in relation to psychotherapy, see Chapter 6.

Spirit/spirit/spirits

Where used with an initial capital letter, the word 'Spirit' usually refers to the divine spirit, such as the Holy Spirit in Judaism and Christianity, or the Great Spirit of Native American religion. Where used with a lower-case initial letter, the word 'spirit' may refer to a life force in nature, an animating spirit in all living things (Steinhart, 2017) or the human spirit.

The human spirit is often understood to be more or less synonymous with 'mind', but usage of the term is variable. Conceptually, 'spirit' overlaps to a large extent with

soul, and for most purposes the two are probably best considered as synonymous. Where a distinction is made between soul and spirit, the distinction is often academically subtle and historically/theologically variable. For example, in Christianity, soul and spirit are not usually distinguished, but where they are the spirit is sometimes understood to be a higher part of the soul (intellect) and sometimes considered to be a lower part of the soul (imagination) (Boyd, 1995; Fokin, 2009). Similarly, soul and spirit are not usually distinguished in Islam, but it has been suggested that in Hadith literature there is a distinction on the basis of respective inclinations for the material and immaterial (Daftari, 2012), and in medieval Judaism there was debate as to whether the human spirit was more divine or material (Langermann, 2007). For a more clinical discussion in relation to psychotherapy, see Chapter 4.

Many religions also recognise various kinds of disembodied spirits, as for example in Spiritism and spiritualism,[1] in which communication with the spirits of the deceased is practised, or Christianity and Islam, where various discarnate spirits (angels and demons in Christianity, and angels and djinn in Islam) created by God are understood to have a role in human affairs. In certain circumstances, demons/djinn are said to 'possess' people. For more information about djinn in relation to psychiatry, see Dein and Illaiee (2013).

See also **possession state** and **spirit release therapy**.

Spirit Release Therapy

Spirit release therapy is a **transpersonal** approach to psychotherapy which seeks to release the patient from the influence of spiritual entities of various kinds, usually referred to as 'spirit attachment'. This is essentially a similar process to that described as disobsession within the religious context of Spiritism (see Chapter 16), and the two terms are used more or less interchangeably.

As with disobsession, spirit release differs from **exorcism** in that it has a much more positive understanding of the nature of the spirits concerned – they are 'attached' rather than possessing, they are not evil (they may, for example, be understood as the earthbound spirits of deceased people, or spirits of animals) and they are treated with compassion. They are 'released' rather than 'cast out', the aim being to allow them to continue on their journey to 'the light'.

Practitioners vary in their understanding of the ontological nature of the spirits concerned. Some would consider them to be psychological entities, aspects of the self (e.g., alter egos in dissociative identity disorder), whereas others would see them as 'real', but disembodied, forms of consciousness.

For further discussion, see Palmer (2014), Powell (2017, pp. 157–165), (Powell, 2018, pp. 2–11) and Chapter 6.

---

[1] Both of these religious movements are concerned with communication with spirits through mediums. Spiritism, which has a large number of adherents in Brazil, dates back to the nineteenth-century French writer Allan Kardec, but today is encountered as a syncretistic mix of various animistic traditions and Catholicism. Spiritualism has its origins in the USA, also in the nineteenth century, and has been more popular in the Anglophone world. Spiritism is arguably an offshoot of spiritualism, but the latter identifies as a religious movement and the former as a philosophical path. The beliefs of Spiritism, but not spiritualism, include **reincarnation**.

Spiritual Abuse

See **spiritual/religious abuse**.

Spiritual Awakening

Closely related to the concept of **spiritual emergency**, 'spiritual awakening' is a broader term, concerned with a dawning awareness or appreciation of a spiritual realm. It is in turn part of an even broader literature on 'awakening'. There is much diversity, confusion and overlap of terminology, with awakening belonging to a family of terms, such as enlightenment, cosmic consciousness and self-transcendence, all of which are concerned with identity and relationship (Kilrea, 2019).

There is no widely agreed definition, but according to Catherine Lucas, founder of the UK Spiritual Crisis Network, a spiritual awakening is 'a process of exploration and unfolding; a process of learning and growth, of healing and purification. It involves the whole of our beings and works on all levels, physical, emotional and psychological, as well as spiritual' (Lucas, 2011, p. 20).

Spiritual awakenings are not necessarily associated with any particular crisis or emergency, and may occur in a variety of different contexts. A spiritual awakening is referred to in step 12 of the **Twelve Steps** of Alcoholics Anonymous and its sister organisations, and is found by many members of these organisations to be very important in their recovery from addiction (Green et al., 1998). Spiritual awakening may occur in various religious contexts (e.g., Islam, Hinduism, Buddhism), as a part of non-religious spirituality (**SBNR**), or as part of a drug-induced experience. It may also occur in the course of **transpersonal** psychotherapy (Siegel, 2019).

Spiritual awakening comprises a diverse group of experiences, and critics have questioned whether or not it is a useful term (Hartelius, 2019). Spiritual awakenings may be sudden or gradual, and may be associated with experiences of ego dissolution or an energetic awakening (Taylor, 2018). In an interesting study of tourism, it was found that spiritual awakenings following transformative life events may generate a motivation to travel, and that travel, in turn, may be a deeply spiritual experience (Willson, 2017).

Spiritual Direction

Also known as spiritual accompaniment, or spiritual friendship, spiritual direction has been variously defined and understood. It is essentially a process in which one person meets with another in order to assist them in the growth of their spiritual life. The process is largely associated with the Christian tradition, but is becoming increasingly ecumenical and has its long-standing equivalents, albeit often known by other names (e.g., guru, spiritual master), in other faith traditions. It shares considerable common ground with some forms of psychotherapy and counselling, but meetings tend to be less frequent, and the focus is much more on growth in relationship with God through prayer and spiritual practices.

For a helpful exploration of spiritual direction in relation to psychotherapy, see Harborne (2012) and Saadeh et al. (2018). For a discussion by a psychiatrist, see May (1992). See also the discussion of spiritual direction in relation to affective disorder in Chapter 9.

Spiritual Emergency

This term was first introduced into the literature by Stanislav and Christina Grof (Grof and Grof, 1989). The word 'emergency' is intended to refer both to a crisis and also to an 'emergence' of a new level of spiritual awareness. The Grofs argue that some experiences and mental states traditionally diagnosed by psychiatrists as mental disorder actually have positive transformative potential. This idea has been taken up more widely by those who adopt a **transpersonal** approach (Lukoff, 2005), and by others (Clarke, 2010). Forms of spiritual emergency identified by the Grofs include various experiences drawn from traditional **religion** (e.g., shamanic crises, the Kundalini awakening of Indian religions, mystical experiences, **possession states**), channelling of spirits, encounters with UFOs, near death experiences, and past life experiences. Although their work has been controversial, the Grofs maintain a distinction between spiritual emergency and psychosis, recognising the importance of correct diagnosis.

Spiritual Healing

Spiritual healing can mean various things, including the use of spiritual practices to bring about physical or mental healing, healing of the spiritual aspect of the human being, or healing that is explained in terms of spiritual processes (Watts, 2011). All of these can be, and are, important in psychiatry (and in medicine more widely). Spiritual practices that may be important include, for example, prayer, various healing rituals and **exorcism/disobsession** (see Chapter 6 and Chapter 16). Because the human being is a spiritual and psychosomatic unity, the healing of the spiritual aspect is hardly separable from other aspects of healing, and is arguably the subject matter of all the chapters in this book. However, healing explained in terms of spiritual processes raises complex philosophical, theological and scientific problems. If understood in terms of divine intervention, as in most religious traditions, it raises the problem of the so-called 'causal joint', by way of which an immaterial God might be understood to intervene in a material world.

For further discussion of spiritual healing, see Watts (2011, pp. 6–8). For a meta-analysis of healing studies, see Roe et al. (2015).

Spiritual/Religious Abuse

There is a fairly large popular literature on spiritual/religious abuse, and it is therefore something that patients may well refer to in consultation with mental health professionals. However, it is not one of the ten types of abuse identified within the Care Act 2014 in the UK, nor is it one of the five types of abuse identified by the US Department of Justice. It is often associated with other forms of abuse. Thus, for example, it may be associated with child abuse (Kvarfordt, 2010), emotional abuse (Simonič et al., 2013) and domestic abuse (Dehan and Levi, 2009). It may also be directed at particular groups within a religious context, as in the case of LGBT+ people in conservative religious groups, for whom it may thus also lead to particular forms of **religious/spiritual struggles** (Super and Jacobson, 2011). Lisa Oakley, who in her earlier work proposed that spiritual abuse was a separate category of abuse, has more recently suggested that it should be seen as a sub-category of emotional and psychological abuse (Oakley et al., 2018). The distinctive features of spiritual abuse are concerned with the spiritual/religious context, recourse to scripture and/or divine authority to justify the abusive behaviour, and threats of spiritual/religious consequences for non-compliance.

There does not appear to be any widely accepted definition of either spiritual or religious abuse, and the two clearly overlap. By way of example, spiritual abuse has been defined in the following ways.

According to Johnson and Vanvonderen (1991, p. 20), it is 'the mistreatment of a person who is in need of help, support or greater spiritual empowerment, with the result of weakening, undermining or decreasing that person's spiritual empowerment'.

Ward (2011, p. 901) has defined it as 'A misuse of power in a spiritual context whereby spiritual authority is distorted to the detriment of those under its leadership'.

Finally, according to Oakley et al. (2018, p. 151), 'Spiritual abuse is a form of emotional and psychological abuse. It is characterised by a systematic pattern of coercive and controlling behaviour in a religious context. Spiritual abuse can have a deeply damaging impact on those who experience it'.

For a helpful discussion of spiritual abuse from a psychotherapeutic perspective, see Wehr (2000).

Spiritual Struggles

See **religious/spiritual struggles**.

Spirituality

There are numerous definitions of this word, none of which is universally accepted.

The following definition is employed in the Royal College of Psychiatrists' Position Statement, *Recommendations on Spirituality and Religion for Psychiatrists*:

> Spirituality is a distinctive, potentially creative and universal dimension of human experience arising both within the inner subjective awareness of individuals and within communities, social groups and traditions. It may be experienced as relationship with that which is intimately 'inner', immanent and personal, within the self and others, and/or as relationship with that which is wholly 'other', transcendent and beyond the self. It is experienced as being of fundamental or ultimate importance and is thus concerned with matters of meaning and purpose in life, truth and values. (Cook, 2004a, pp. 548–549)

For a discussion of the history of the term and conceptual issues, see Principe (1983) and Schneiders (2003). For a discussion of spirituality in different religious contexts, see Ferguson (2010). For a discussion of the history and use of the term in psychiatry, see Chapter 1, and for a patient perspective, see Chapter 15.

Spiritually Significant Voices

This term was introduced by Cook et al. (2020) to refer in a positive and non-judgemental way to voices that are 'distinctive by virtue of the spiritual interpretation that is placed upon them or – perhaps more correctly – is an integral part of the experienced voice'. Such voices may correctly be referred to as auditory verbal hallucinations, but the term avoids implications of pathology and is offered without judgement as to ontology or causation. People who hear such voices do not typically self-identify as 'voice hearers' (as they do, for example, within the Hearing Voices Movement), and the term avoids any judgement as to whether or not such voices are to be understood within the overall category of voice hearing experiences.

Syncretism

This term refers to drawing on beliefs and practices from a variety of sources. Religious syncretism is often a very individually selective process – as in the case of the **SBNR** – but may also be seen culturally and collectively (e.g., in the Caribbean). Some religions are essentially the product of a process of syncretism, as in the case of Spiritism, which comprises various mixtures of animism, Catholicism and mediumship. To a more limited extent, syncretism may be observed in many religious traditions, although there is some debate as to the difference between what counts as syncretism and what counts as inculturation, with the latter usually evaluated more positively than the former.

Theism

Theism is belief in a God or gods. It is sometimes taken to refer to belief in one God (monotheism), but more generally is also taken to include polytheism (belief in a number of gods). Theism tends to emphasise the **transcendence** of God, whereas pantheism (in which God and the universe are coterminous) emphasizes the **immanence** of God.

Transcendence

This term is used in a wide variety of ways, all of which allude to a spatial metaphor of going above or beyond. For example, various forms of 'self-transcendence' are concerned with the psychological transcendence of suffering, or the expansion of personal boundaries in some way (Cook, 2013, pp. 145–148). However, there are also theological forms of transcendence, which posit the existence of a transcendent reality. This is most often understood as God, but may or may not be conceived of as a personal being. The term 'transcendence' is usually compared or contrasted with the correlative term '**immanence**'. The transcendent order lies above/beyond the immanent order that we experience directly by means of sense perception.

For further discussion, see Cook (2013).

Transliminality

This is a concept arising from the work of Michael Thalbourne, according to which contents of the subconscious may emerge into consciousness in psychosis, as well as in mystical, paranormal or spiritual experiences.

Thalbourne and Delin (1994, p. 3) have defined it as 'the extent to which the contents of some preconscious (or "unconscious" or "subliminal") region of the mind are able to cross the threshold into consciousness (in its sense of "awareness"). There they may form the basis of paranormal belief, the experiencing of apparent psychic phenomena, some aspects of creativity, mystical experience, and psychotic-like symptoms'.

Although the term is an attempt to avoid pejorative alternatives, it is inevitably controversial.

For a helpful discussion, see Claridge (2010).

Transpersonal

The first use of this term appears to be attributable to William James (Vich, 1988). As an adjective, the term 'transpersonal' may be variously applied (e.g., transpersonal psychiatry, transpersonal psychology, transpersonal development, transpersonal philosophy, etc.). As with the term 'transcendence,' there is an implicit spatial metaphor of going above/beyond.

Walsh and Vaughan (1993, p. 203) define transpersonal experiences as 'experiences in which the sense of identity or self extends beyond (trans) the individual or personal to encompass wider aspects of humankind, life, psyche or cosmos'.

Bruce Scotton understands transpersonal as 'meaning beyond the personal, refers to development beyond conventional, personal, or individual levels' (Scotton, 1996, p. 3). Used in this way, the term is more or less synonymous with 'spiritual'. However, in practice, transpersonal psychiatry is not exactly the same as the field of **spirituality** and psychiatry, and has included some controversial concepts and practices, including the role of prenatal experience in the aetiology of psychiatric disorders, therapeutically induced non-ordinary states of consciousness, the concept of **spiritual emergency, past life regression therapy** and **spirit release therapy.**

For further discussion, see Read and Crowley (2009) and Scotton et al. (1996). See also Chapter 6 (p. 130; and case study on p. 132).

Twelve Steps

Alcoholics Anonymous (AA) was founded in 1935 by two men seeking recovery from their addiction to alcohol. Influenced by evangelical Christianity and the work of William James, the founders wrote down the principles for recovery that they had adopted as 12 'steps', starting with an admission of powerlessness over alcohol and concluding with a commitment to carry their message to others in need of similar help. The steps adopt a spiritual, but not religious, approach to recovery which involves accepting the need for help from a **Higher Power**. In time many other groups adopted similar principles, including Narcotics Anonymous (NA), Gamblers Anonymous (GA), Sex Addicts Anonymous, Overeaters Anonymous, Neurotics Anonymous and numerous others. Groups were also established to help families, such as AlAnon, for families of alcoholics, and Families Anonymous, for families of members of NA. These groups, or organisations, which adopt a non-professional, mutual-help approach, became collectively known as Twelve-Step groups. In time, institutional and professional treatment programmes were set up which drew on similar principles and sought to engage people in the non-professional approach to recovery encapsulated within the Twelve Steps (Cook, 1988a, 1988b). Twelve-Step Facilitation (TSF) is a professional approach to treatment which seeks to encourage patients in their engagement with Twelve-Step organisations (Humphreys, 1999).

For further discussion, see Chapter 8.

Worldviews

The concept of worldviews is proposed as a positive alternative to that of **religion** (or **spirituality**), and is inclusive of 'non-religions' such as **atheism** and **agnosticism**. **Existentialism** may, or may not, also be considered a worldview. Having its origins in the philosophy of Immanuel Kant, the concept of worldview (Weltanschauung) may be defined in terms of beliefs and assumptions about what does and does not exist, what can be known and goals that should be pursued in life (Koltko-Rivera, 2004). Alternatively, it may be defined in terms of the 'big questions' that human beings ask and reflect on, concerning what exists, and how we know what is true, what is good, what we should do, where we come from and where we are heading (Taves et al., 2018). The idea has been variously taken up by psychiatrists (Josephson and Peteet, 2004; Gray, 2011), but generally has not received the same attention within psychiatry as concepts such as religion or spirituality.

According to Gray (2011, p. 58), 'A worldview is a collection of attitudes, values, stories and expectations about the world around us, which inform our every thought and action'.

References

Aaen-Stockdale, C. (2012) Neuroscience for the soul. *The Psychologist*, 25, 520–523.

Abdul-Hamid, W. K. (2011) The need for a category of 'religious and spiritual problems' in ICD-11. *International Psychiatry*, 8, 60–61.

Alcoholics Anonymous World Services Inc. (1983) *Twelve Steps and Twelve Traditions*. New York: Alcoholics Anonymous World Services Inc.

American Psychiatric Association (2013) *Diagnostic and Statistical Manual of Mental Disorders. Fifth Edition. DSM-5.* Washington, DC, American Psychiatric Association.

Andrade, G. (2017) Is past life regression therapy ethical? *Journal of Medical Ethics and History of Medicine*, 10, 1–8.

Astuti, R. (2001) Are we all natural dualists? A cognitive developmental approach. *Journal of the Royal Anthropological Institute*, 7, 429–447.

Bowker, J. (2007) *Beliefs That Changed the World*. London: Quercus.

Boyd, J. H. (1995) The soul as seen through evangelical eyes, Part I: Mental health professionals and 'the soul'. *Journal of Psychology and Theology*, 23, 151–160.

Bracken, P. and Thomas, P. (2002) Time to move beyond the mind-body split. *British Medical Journal*, 325, 1433–1434.

Brainerd, C. J. and Reyna, V. F. (2005) *The Science of False Memory*. Oxford: Oxford University Press.

Carroll, L. (1872/2010) *Through the Looking Glass*. London: Collins.

Claridge, G. (2010) Spiritual experience: health psychoticism? In I. Clarke, ed., *Psychosis and Spirituality: Consolidating the New Paradigm*. Oxford: Wiley-Blackwell, pp. 75–87.

Clarke, I., ed. (2010) *Psychosis and Spirituality: Consolidating the New Paradigm*. Oxford: Wiley-Blackwell.

Cliteur, P. (2009) The definition of atheism. *Journal of Religion & Society*, 11, 1–23.

Coleman, T. J., Hood, R. W. and Streib, H. (2018) An introduction to atheism, agnosticism, and nonreligious worldviews. *Psychology of Religion and Spirituality*, 10, 203–206.

Committee on Psychiatry and Religion (1976) *Mysticism: Spiritual Quest or Psychic Disorder?* New York: Group for the Advancement of Psychiatry.

Cook, C. C. H. (1988a) The Minnesota Model in the management of drug and alcohol dependency: miracle, method or myth? Part I. The philosophy and the programme. *British Journal of Addiction*, 83, 625–634.

Cook, C. C. H. (1988b) The Minnesota Model in the management of drug and alcohol dependency: miracle, method or myth? Part II. Evidence and conclusions. *British Journal of Addiction*, 83, 735–748.

Cook, C. C. H. (2004) Psychiatry and mysticism. *Mental Health, Religion & Culture*, 7, 149–163.

Cook, C. C. H. (2013) Transcendence, immanence and mental health. In C. C. H. Cook, ed., *Spirituality, Theology & Mental Health*. London: SCM, pp. 141–159.

Cook, C. C. H., Powell, A., Alderson-Day, B. and Woods, A. (2020) Hearing spiritually significant voices: a phenomenological survey and taxonomy. *Medical Humanities*, https://doi.org/10.1136/medhum-2020-012021

Cox, J. L. (2010) *An Introduction to the Phenomenology of Religion*. London: Continuum.

Cristofori, I., Bulbulia, J., Shaver, J. H. et al. (2016) Neural correlates of mystical experience. *Neuropsychologia*, 80, 212–220.

Culligan, K. (2003) The Dark Night and depression. In K. J. Egan, ed., *Carmelite Prayer: A Tradition for the Twenty-first Century*. New York: Paulist Press, pp. 119–138.

Currier, J. M., Foster, J. D. and Isaak, S. L. (2019) Moral injury and spiritual struggles in military veterans: a latent profile analysis. *Journal of Traumatic Stress*, 32, 393–404.

D'Aquili, E. and Newberg, A. B. (1999) *The Mystical Mind: Probing the Biology of Religious Experience*. Minneapolis, MN: Fortress Press.

Daftari, A. (2012) The dichotomy of the soul and spirit in Shi'a Hadith. *Journal of Shi'a Islamic Studies*, 5, 117–129.

Daie, N., Wiztum, E., Mark, M. and Rabinowitz, S. (1992) The belief in the transmigration of souls: psychotherapy of a Druze patient with severe anxiety reaction. *British Journal of Medical Psychology*, 65, 119–130.

Damasio, A. (2000) *The Feeling of What Happens: Body, Emotion and the Making of Consciousness*. London: Heinemann.

De Haan, S. (2017) The existential dimension in psychiatry: an enactive framework. *Mental Health, Religion & Culture*, 20, 528–535.

Dehan, N. and Levi, Z. (2009) Spiritual abuse: an additional dimension of abuse experienced by abused Haredi (ultraorthodox) Jewish wives. *Violence Against Women*, 15, 1294–1310.

Dein, S. and Illaiee, A. S. (2013) Jinn and mental health: looking at jinn possession in modern psychiatric practice. *The Psychiatrist*, 37, 290–293.

Dickson, A., ed. (1985) *Sigmund Freud: 13. The Origins of Religion*. Harmondsworth: Penguin.

Dossett, W. (2013) Addiction, spirituality and 12-step programmes. *International Social Work*, 56, 369–383.

Durkheim, E. (1995) *The Elementary Forms of Religious Life*. New York: Free Press.

Edwards, P. (1996) *Reincarnation: A Critical Examination*. Amherst, NY: Prometheus Books.

Enoch, M. D. and Ball, H. N. (2001) *Uncommon Psychiatric Syndromes*, 4th ed. London: Hodder Arnold.

Exline, J. J., Pargament, K. I., Grubbs, J. B. and Yali, A. M. (2014) The Religious and Spiritual Struggles Scale: development and initial validation. *Psychology of Religion and Spirituality*, 6, 208–222.

Ferguson, D. S. (2010) *Exploring the Spirituality of the World Religions: The Quest for Personal, Spiritual and Social Transformation*. London: Continuum.

Fokin, A. R. (2009) The relationship between soul and spirit in Greek and Latin patristic thought. *Faith and Philosophy*, 26, 599–614.

Foley, M. (2018) *The Dark Night: Psychological Experience and Spiritual Reality*. Washington, DC: ICS Publications.

Frankl, V. E. (1988) *The Will to Meaning: Foundations and Applications of Logotherapy*. London: Meridian.

Galanter, M. (1990) Cults and zealous self-help movements: a psychiatric perspective. *American Journal of Psychiatry*, 147, 543–551.

Galanter, M., White, W. L., Ziegler, P. P. and Hunter, B. (2020) An empirical study on the construct of 'God' in the Twelve Step process. *American Journal of Drug and Alcohol Abuse*, 46, 731–738.

Geertz, C. (1993) Religion as a cultural system. In C. Geertz, ed., *The Interpretation of Cultures: Selected Essays*. New York: Fontana, pp. 87–125.

Glannon, W. (2020) Mind-brain dualism in psychiatry: ethical implications. *Frontiers in Psychiatry*, 11, 85.

Gray, A. J. (2011) Worldviews. *International Psychiatry*, 8, 58–60.

Green, L. L., Fullilove, M. T. and Fullilove, R. E. (1998) Stories of spiritual awakening. *Journal of Substance Abuse Treatment*, 15, 325–331.

Grof, S. and Grof, C., eds. (1989) *Spiritual Emergency: When Personal Transformation Becomes a Crisis*. New York: Jeremy P. Tarcher/Putnam.

Harborne, L. (2012) *Psychotherapy and Spiritual Direction: Two Languages, One Voice?* London: Karnac.

Hartelius, G. (2019) Does spiritual awakening exist? Critical considerations in the study of transformative postconventional development. *International Journal of Transpersonal Studies*, 37, iii–vi.

Hodgson, T. J. and Carey, L. B. (2017) Moral injury and definitional clarity: betrayal, spirituality and the role of chaplains. *Journal of Religion and Health*, 56, 1212–1228.

Humphreys, K. (1999) Professional interventions that facilitate 12-step self-help group involvement. *Alcohol Research & Health*, 23. 93–98.

James, W. (1902) *The Varieties of Religious Experience: A Study in Human Nature*. New York: Longmans, Green & Co.

Johnson, D. and Vanvonderen, J. (1991) *The Subtle Power of Spiritual Abuse: Recognizing and Escaping Spiritual Manipulation and False Spiritual Authority within the Church*. Bloomington, MN: Bethany House Publishers.

Johnson, T. M., Grim, B. J. and Bellofatto, G. A. (2013) *The World's Religions in Figures: An Introduction to International Religious Demography*. Chichester: John Wiley & Sons.

Jones, E. (2020) Moral injury in a context of trauma. *British Journal of Psychiatry*, 216, 127–128.

Josephson, A. M. and Peteet, J. R., eds. (2004) *Handbook of Spirituality and Worldview in Clinical Practice*. Washington, DC: American Psychiatric Publishing.

Jung, C. G. (1938) *Psychology and Religion*. New Haven, CT: Yale University Press.

Kilrea, K. (2019) Joy, not elsewhere classified: towards a contemporary psychological understanding of spiritual (and secular) awakening. *International Journal of Transpersonal Studies*, 37, 66–72.

King, S. (2001) Pathological spirituality: the story of false spiritual adult and bad child. *Self and Society*, 29, 12–18.

Koenig, H. G., ed. (1998) *Handbook of Religion and Mental Health*. London: Academic Press.

Koenig, H. G., Pargament, K. I. and Nielsen, J. (1998) Religious coping and health status in medically ill hospitalized older adults. *Journal of Nervous & Mental Disease*, 186, 513–521.

Koenig, H. G., King, D. E. and Carson, V. B., eds. (2012) *Handbook of Religion and Health*. New York: Oxford University Press.

Koltko-Rivera, M. E. (2004) The psychology of worldviews. *Review of General Psychology*, 8, 3–58.

Kvarfordt, C. L. (2010) Spiritual abuse and neglect of youth: reconceptualizing what is known through an investigation of practitioners' experiences. *Journal of Religion & Spirituality in Social Work: Social Thought*, 29, 143–164.

Langermann, Y. T. (2007) David Ibn Shoshan on spirit and soul. *European Journal of Jewish Studies*, 1, 63–86.

Lim, C., Macgregor, C. A. and Putnam, R. D. (2010) Secular and liminal: discovering heterogeneity among religious nones. *Journal for the Scientific Study of Religion*, 49, 596–618.

Linn, M., Linn, S. F. and Linn, D. (1995) *Healing Religious Addiction: Reclaiming Healthy Spirituality*. London: DLT.

Littlewood, R. (2004) Possession states. *Psychiatry*, 3, 8–10.

Litz, B. T., Stein, N., Delaney, E. et al. (2009) Moral injury and moral repair in war veterans: a preliminary model and intervention strategy. *Clinical Psychology Review*, 29, 695–706.

Lucas, C. G. (2011) *In Case of Spiritual Emergency: Moving Successfully Through Your Awakening*. Forres: Findhorn Press.

Lukoff, D. (2005) Spiritual and transpersonal approaches to psychotic disorders. In S. G. Mijares and G. S. Khalsa, eds., *The Psychospiritual Clinician's Handbook: Alternative Methods for Understanding and Treating Mental Disorders*. Binghamton, NY: The Haworth Reference Press™, pp. 233–257.

Lukoff, D., Lu, F. and Turner, R. (1998) From spiritual emergency to spiritual problem: the transpersonal roots of the new DSM-IV category. *Journal of Humanistic Psychology*, 38, 21–50.

Martin, R. and Barresi, J. (2006) *The Rise and Fall of Soul and Self*. New York: Columbia University Press.

Maung, H. H. (2019) Dualism and its place in a philosophical structure for psychiatry. *Medicine, Health Care, and Philosophy*, 22, 59–69.

May, G. G. (1992) *Care of Mind, Care of Spirit*. New York: HarperSanFrancisco.

May, G. G. (2003) *The Dark Night of the Soul*. New York: HarperSanFrancisco.

May, R. (1958) The origins and significance of the existential movement in psychology. In R. May, E. Angel and H. Ellenberger, eds., *Existence: A New Dimension in Psychiatry and Psychology*. New York: Basic Books, pp. 3–36.

May, R. (1961) Existential psychiatry: an evaluation. *Journal of Religion & Health*, 1, 31–40.

May, R., Angel, E. and Ellenberger, H. F., eds. (1958) *Existence: A New Dimension in Psychiatry and Psychology*. New York: Basic Books.

Mercadante, L. (2014) *Belief Without Borders: Inside the Minds of the Spiritual but Not Religious*. New York: Oxford University Press.

Miller, C. W. T., Ross, D. A. and Novick, A. M. (2020) "Not dead yet!": confronting the legacy of dualism in modern psychiatry. *Biological Psychiatry*, 87, e15–e17.

Modi, S. (1997) *Remarkable Healings: A Psychiatrist Discovers Unsuspected Roots of Mental and Physical Illness*.

Charlottesville, VA, Hampton Roads Publishing Company.

Mohr, S., Perroud, N., Gillieron, C. et al. (2011) Spirituality and religiousness as predictive factors of outcome in schizophrenia and schizo-affective disorders. *Psychiatry Research*, 186, 177–182.

Mohr, S., Borras, L., Nolan, J. et al. (2012) Spirituality and religion in outpatients with schizophrenia: a multi-site comparative study of Switzerland, Canada, and the United States. *International Journal of Psychiatry in Medicine*, 44, 29–52.

Moreira-Almeida, A., Mosqueiro, B. P. and Bhugra, D., eds. (2021) *Spirituality and Mental Health Across Cultures*. Oxford: Oxford University Press.

Nash, J. D., Newberg, A. and Awasthi, B. (2013) Toward a unifying taxonomy and definition for meditation. *Frontiers in Psychology*, 4, 806.

Newberg, A. B. (2010) *Principles of Neurotheology*. Farnham: Ashgate Publishing.

Ng, C. C.-W. (2021) Is mind–body dualism compatible with modern psychiatry? *BJPsych Advances*, 28, 132–134.

Nickerson, A., Schnyder, U., Bryant, R. A. et al. (2015) Moral injury in traumatized refugees. *Psychotherapy and Psychosomatics*, 84, 122–123.

Norcross, J. C., Koocher, G. P. and Garofalo, A. (2006) Discredited psychological treatments and tests: a Delphi poll. *Professional Psychology: Research and Practice*, 37, 515–522.

Oakley, L., Kinmond, K. and Humphreys, J. (2018) Spiritual abuse in Christian faith settings: definition, policy and practice guidance. *The Journal of Adult Protection*, 20, 144–154.

Palmer, T. (2014) *The Science of Spirit Possession*, 2nd ed. Newcastle upon Tyne: Cambridge Scholars Publishing.

Pargament, K. I. and Exline, J. J. (2022) *Working with Spiritual Struggles in Psychotherapy*. New York: Guilford Press.

Pargament, K. I., Smith, B. W., Koenig, H. G. and Perez, L. (1998) Patterns of positive and negative religious coping with major life stressors. *Journal for the Scientific Study of Religion*, 37, 710–724.

Pearce, M., Haynes, K., Rivera, N. R. and Koenig, H. G. (2018) Spiritually integrated cognitive processing therapy: a new treatment for post-traumatic stress disorder that targets moral injury. *Global Advances in Health and Medicine*, 7, 2164956118759939.

Peres, J. F. (2012) Should psychotherapy consider reincarnation? *The Journal of Nervous and Mental Disease*, 200, 174–179.

Peteet, J. R., Lu, F. G. and Narrow, W. E., eds. (2011) *Religious and Spiritual Issues in Psychiatric Diagnosis: A Research Agenda for DSM-V*. Arlington, VA: American Psychiatric Association.

Powell, A. (2017) *The Ways of the Soul: A Psychiatrist Reflects: Essays on Life, Death and Beyond*. London: Muswell Hill Press.

Powell, A. (2018) *Conversations with the Soul: A Psychiatrist Reflects: Essays on Life, Death and Beyond*. London: Muswell Hill Press.

Principe, W. (1983) Toward defining spirituality. *Studies in Religion*, 12, 127–141.

Read, H., Fordham, M., Adler, G. and McGuire, W., eds. (1959) *The Collected Works of C. G. Jung. Volume 9, Part I: The Archetypes and the Collective Unconscious*. Princeton, NJ, Princeton University Press.

Read, T. and Crowley, N. (2009) The transpersonal perspective. In C. Cook, A. Powell and A. Sims, eds., *Spirituality and Psychiatry*. London: RCPsych Publications, pp. 212–232.

Richards, P. S. and Bergin, A. E., eds. (2000) *Handbook of Psychotherapy and Religious Diversity*. Washington, DC: American Psychological Association.

Roe, C. A., Sonnex, C. and Roxburgh, E. C. (2015) Two meta-analyses of noncontact healing studies. *Explore (NY)*, 11, 11–23.

Saadeh, M. G., North, K., Hansen, K. L., Steele, P. and Peteet, J. R. (2018) Spiritual

direction and psychotherapy. *Spirituality in Clinical Practice*, 5, 273–282.

Schneiders, S. M. (2003) Religion vs. spirituality: a contemporary conundrum. *Spiritus*, 3, 163–185.

Scotton, B. W. (1996) Introduction and definition of transpersonal psychiatry. In B. W. Scotton, A. B. Chinen and J. R. Battista, eds., *Textbook of Transpersonal Psychiatry and Psychology*. New York: Basic Books, pp. 3–8.

Scotton, B. W., Chinen, A. B. and Battista, J. R., eds. (1996) *Textbook of Transpersonal Psychiatry and Psychology*. New York: Basic Books.

Scrutton, A. P. (2015) Schizophrenia or possession? A reply to Kemal Irmak and Nuray Karanci. *Journal of Religion and Health*, 54, 1963–1968.

Searle, J. R. (2007) Dualism revisited. *Journal of Physiology, Paris*, 101, 169–178.

Sharma, A. R. (2000) Psychotherapy with Hindus. In P. S. Richards and A. E. Bergin, eds., *Handbook of Psychotherapy and Religious Diversity*. Washington, DC: American Psychological Association, pp. 341–365.

Siegel, I. R. (2019) Spontaneous awakening in transpersonal psychotherapy. *The Journal of Transpersonal Psychology*, 51, 198–224.

Simonič, B., Mandelj, T. R. and Novsak, R. (2013) Religious-related abuse in the family. *Journal of Family Violence*, 28, 339–349.

Spanos, N. P., Burgess, C. A. and Burgess, M. F. (1994) Past-life identities, UFO abductions, and satanic ritual abuse: the social construction of memories. *The International Journal of Clinical and Experimental Hypnosis*, 42, 433–446.

Speed, D. and Fowler, K. (2016) What's God got to do with it? How religiosity predicts atheists' health. *Journal of Religion and Health*, 55, 296–308.

Stark, R. and Bainbridge, W. S. (1979) Of churches, sects, and cults: preliminary concepts for a theory of religious movements. *Journal for the Scientific Study of Religion*, 18, 117–131.

Starnino, V. R., Sullivan, W. P., Angel, C. T. and Davis, L. W. (2019) Moral injury, coherence, and spiritual repair. *Mental Health, Religion & Culture*, 22, 99–114.

Steinhart, E. (2017) Spirit. *Sophia*, 56, 557–571.

Stevenson, I. (1977) The explanatory value of the idea of reincarnation. *The Journal of Nervous and Mental Disease*, 164, 305–326.

Stevenson, I. (2000) The phenomenon of claimed memories of previous lives: possible interpretations and importance. *Medical Hypotheses*, 54, 652–659.

Sullivan, W. P. and Starnino, V. R. (2019) 'Staring into the abyss': veterans' accounts of moral injuries and spiritual challenges. *Mental Health, Religion & Culture*, 22, 25–40.

Super, J. T. and Jacobson, L. (2011) Religious abuse: implications for counseling lesbian, gay, bisexual, and transgender individuals. *Journal of LGBT Issues in Counseling*, 5, 180–196.

Taves, A., Asprem, E. and Ihm, E. (2018) Psychology, meaning making, and the study of worldviews: beyond religion and non-religion. *Psychology of Religion and Spirituality*, 10, 207–217.

Taylor, C. (2007) *A Secular Age*. Cambridge, MA: The Belknap Press of Harvard University Press.

Taylor, S. (2018) Two modes of sudden spiritual awakening? Ego-dissolution and explosive energetic awakening. *International Journal of Transpersonal Studies*, 37, 131–143.

Thalbourne, M. A. and Delin, P. S. (1994) A common thread underlying belief in the paranormal, creative personality, mystical experience and psychopathology. *Journal of Parapsychology*, 58, 3–38.

Thompson, N. (2007) Spirituality: an existentialist perspective. *Illness, Crisis & Loss*, 15, 125–136.

Tracy, D. K., Tarn, M., Eldridge, R. et al. (2020) What should be done to support the mental health of healthcare staff treating COVID-19 patients? *British Journal of Psychiatry*, 217, 537–539.

Tucker, J. B. (2008) Ian Stevenson and cases of the reincarnation type. *Journal of Scientific Exploration*, 22, 36–43.

Tucker, J. B. (2021) *Before: Children's Memories of Previous Lives*. New York: St Martin's Essentials.

Tyler, P. (2011) *The Return to the Mystical: Ludwig Wittgenstein, Teresa of Avila and the Christian Mystical Tradition*. London: Continuum.

Underhill, E. (1925) *Mystics of the Church*. Cambridge: James Clarke.

Uzarevic, F. and Coleman, T. J., 3rd (2020) The psychology of nonbelievers. *Current Opinion in Psychology*, 40, 131–138.

Vernon, G. M. (1968) The religious 'nones': a neglected category. *Journal for the Scientific Study of Religion*, 7, 219–229.

Vich, M. A. (1988) Some historical sources of the term 'transpersonal'. *The Journal of Transpersonal Psychology*, 20, 107–110.

Walker, A. (1997) Introduction: exploring harmful religion. In L. Osborn and A. Walker, eds., *Harmful Religion: An Exploration of Religious Abuse*. London: SPCK, pp. 1–11.

Walker, G. C. (2000) Secular eschatology: beliefs about afterlife. *OMEGA*, 41, 5–22.

Walsh, R. and Vaughan, F. (1993) On transpersonal definitions. *The Journal of Transpersonal Psychology*, 25, 199–207.

Ward, D. J. (2011) The lived experience of spiritual abuse. *Mental Health, Religion & Culture*, 14, 899–915.

Watts, F. (2011) Conceptual issues in spiritual healing. In F. Watts, ed., *Spiritual Healing: Scientific and Religious Perspectives*. Cambridge: Cambridge University Press, pp. 1–16.

Webster, R. S. (2004) An existential framework of spirituality. *International Journal of Children's Spirituality*, 9, 7–19.

Wehr, D. S. (2000) Spiritual abuse: when good people do bad things. In P. Young-Eisdendrath and M. E. Miller, eds., *The Psychology of Mature Spirituality: Integrity, Wisdom, Transcendence.* London: Routledge, pp. 47–61.

Willson, G. (2017) Spiritual awakening leading to a search for meaning through travel. *International Journal of Tourism and Spirituality*, 2, 10–23.

Wilson, W. and Jung, C. G. (1987) Spiritus contra Spiritum: the Bill Wilson/C. G. Jung letters. *Parabola*, 12, 68–71.

Woolger, R. J. (1987) *Other Lives, Other Selves: A Jungian Psychotherapist Discovers Past Lives.* London: Aquarian.

Yalom, I. D. (1980) *Existential Psychotherapy.* New York: Basic Books.

Index

Printed in the United States
by Baker & Taylor Publisher Services